EVIDENCE-BASED PSYCHOTHERAPIES FOR CHILDREN AND ADOLESCENTS

Evidence-Based Psychotherapies for Children and Adolescents

SECOND EDITION

Edited by
John R. Weisz
Alan E. Kazdin

THE GUILFORD PRESS
New York   London

© 2010 The Guilford Press
A Division of Guilford Publications, Inc.
72 Spring Street, New York, NY 10012
www.guilford.com

Printed in the United States of America

This book is printed on acid-free paper.

Last digit is print number: 9 8 7 6 5 4 3

Library of Congress Cataloging-in-Publication Data

Evidence-based psychotherapies for children and adolescents / edited by John R. Weisz
and Alan E. Kazdin. — 2nd ed.
    p. cm.
  Includes bibliographical references and index.
  ISBN 978-1-59385-974-9 (hardcover: alk. paper)
  1. Child psychotherapy. 2. Adolescent psychotherapy. 3. Evidence-based psychiatry.
I. Weisz, John R. II. Kazdin, Alan E.
  RJ504.E95 2010
  618.92′8914—dc22

                        2009049689

To Jenny, passionate advocate for children and families
—J. R. W.

To Fran, a model of courage, rationality, and caring
—A. E. K.

About the Editors

John R. Weisz, PhD, ABPP, is Professor of Psychology at Harvard University, Faculty of Arts and Sciences, and Professor at Harvard Medical School. He is also President and CEO of the Judge Baker Children's Center, an affiliate of Harvard Medical School specializing in child and adolescent mental health research, training, direct service, and media outreach. Dr. Weisz has previously held faculty positions at Cornell University, the University of North Carolina at Chapel Hill, and the University of California, Los Angeles. He has served as President of the Society of Clinical Child and Adolescent Psychology and of the International Society for Research in Child and Adolescent Psychopathology. Dr. Weisz is Director of the Research Network on Youth Mental Health, sponsored since 2001 by the MacArthur Foundation. His books and articles focus on youth problem behavior and psychotherapy for children and adolescents.

Alan E. Kazdin, PhD, ABPP, is the John M. Musser Professor of Psychology and Child Psychiatry at Yale University and Director of the Yale Parenting Center and Child Conduct Clinic, an outpatient treatment service for children and families. He has served as President of the American Psychological Association and received its Outstanding Lifetime Contribution to Psychology Award in 2009. At Yale, he has been Chairman of the Psychology Department, Director and Chair of the Yale Child Study Center at the School of Medicine, and Director of Child Psychiatric Services at Yale–New Haven Hospital. Dr. Kazdin's work focuses on child-rearing practices and the treatment of oppositional, aggressive, and antisocial behavior among children and adolescents. He has authored or edited more than 650 articles, chapters, and books. His 45 books focus on child and adolescent psychotherapy, parenting, aggressive and antisocial behavior, and methodology and research design.

Contributors

Alisha Alleyne, PhD, Judge Baker Children's Center, Boston, Massachusetts

Paula M. Barrett, PhD, Pathways Health and Research Centre, University of Queensland, School of Education, Queensland, Australia

Tammy D. Barry, PhD, Department of Psychology, University of Southern Mississippi, Hattiesburg, Mississippi

Sarah Kate Bearman, PhD, Judge Baker Children's Center, Boston, Massachusetts

Karen A. Blase, PhD, Frank Porter Graham Child Development Institute, University of North Carolina at Chapel Hill, Chapel Hill, North Carolina

Caroline L. Boxmeyer, PhD, Department of Psychology, University of Alabama, Tuscaloosa, Tuscaloosa, Alabama

David A. Brent, MD, Western Psychiatric Institute and Clinic, University of Pittsburgh School of Medicine, Pittsburgh, Pennsylvania

Janet L. Brody, PhD, Center for Family and Adolescent Research, Oregon Research Institute, Eugene, Oregon

Lauren I. Brookman-Frazee, PhD, Child and Adolescent Services Research Center, University of California, San Diego, San Diego, California

Elizabeth F. Bruno, PhD, Mary L. Johnson Developmental and Behavioral Unit, Lucile Packard Children's Hospital, Palo Alto, California

Lisa Burrows-MacLean, PhD, Center for Children and Families, University at Buffalo, The State University of New York, Buffalo, New York

Mary A. Cavaleri, PhD, New York State Psychiatric Institute, Columbia University, New York, New York

Patricia Chamberlain, PhD, Oregon Social Learning Center and the Center for Research to Practice, Eugene, Oregon

Bruce F. Chorpita, PhD, Department of Psychology, University of California, Los Angeles, Los Angeles, California

Gregory N. Clarke, PhD, Kaiser Permanente Center for Health Research, Portland, Oregon

Judith A. Cohen, MD, Center for Traumatic Stress in Children and Adolescents, Allegheny General Hospital, Pittsburgh, Pennsylvania

Eric L. Daleiden, PhD, Kismetrics, LLC, Satellite Beach, Florida

Lynn L. DeBar, PhD, Kaiser Permanente Center for Health Research, Portland, Oregon

Esther Deblinger, PhD, School of Osteopathic Medicine, University of Medicine and Dentistry of New Jersey, Stratford, New Jersey

Katie A. Devine, PhD, Department of Psychology, Loyola University Chicago, Chicago, Illinois

Michelle A. Duda, PhD, BCBA, Frank Porter Graham Child Development Institute, University of North Carolina at Chapel Hill, Chapel Hill, North Carolina

Sheila M. Eyberg, PhD, ABPP, Department of Clinical and Health Psychology, University of Florida, Gainesville, Gainesville, Florida

Gregory A. Fabiano, PhD, Center for Children and Families, University at Buffalo, The State University of New York, Buffalo, New York

Dean L. Fixsen, PhD, Frank Porter Graham Child Development Institute, University of North Carolina at Chapel Hill, Chapel Hill, North Carolina

Marion S. Forgatch, PhD, Implementation Sciences International, Inc., Oregon Social Learning Center, Eugene, Oregon

Martin E. Franklin, PhD, Department of Psychiatry, University of Pennsylvania School of Medicine, Philadelphia, Pennsylvania

Jennifer Freeman, PhD, Department of Psychiatry and Human Behavior, Brown University Medical School, Providence, Rhode Island

Jami M. Furr, MA, Child and Adolescent Anxiety Disorders Clinic, Temple University, Philadelphia, Pennsylvania

Elizabeth M. Gnagy, BS, Center for Children and Families, University at Buffalo, The State University of New York, Buffalo, New York

Andrew R. Greiner, BS, Center for Children and Families, University at Buffalo, The State University of New York, Buffalo, New York

Scott W. Henggeler, PhD, Department of Psychiatry and Behavioral Sciences, Medical University of South Carolina, Charleston, South Carolina

Kimberly Eaton Hoagwood, PhD, New York State Psychiatric Institute, Columbia University, New York, New York

Grayson N. Holmbeck, PhD, Department of Psychology, Loyola University Chicago, Chicago, Illinois

Viviana Horigian, MD, Department of Epidemiology and Public Health, University of Miami Miller School of Medicine, Miami, Florida

Arthur C. Houts, PhD, Department of Psychology, University of Memphis, Memphis, Tennessee

Stanley J. Huey, Jr., PhD, Department of Psychology, University of Southern California, Los Angeles, California

Colleen M. Jacobson, PhD, Department of Psychology, Iona College, New Rochelle, New York

Alan E. Kazdin, PhD, ABPP, Department of Psychiatry, Yale University, and Yale Parenting Center and Child Conduct Clinic, New Haven, Connecticut

Philip C. Kendall, PhD, Child and Adolescent Anxiety Disorders Clinic, Temple University, Philadelphia, Pennsylvania

Lynn Kern Koegel, PhD, Koegel Autism Center, Graduate School of Education, University of California, Santa Barbara, Santa Barbara, California

Robert L. Koegel, PhD, Departments of Clinical Psychology and Special Education, and Koegel Autism Center, University of California, Santa Barbara, Santa Barbara, California

Lauren S. Krumholz, MA, Department of Educational Psychology, University of Texas at Austin, Austin, Texas

Daniel le Grange, PhD, Department of Psychiatry, Section for Child and Adolescent Psychiatry, University of Chicago, Chicago, Illinois

Howard A. Liddle, EdD, ABPP, Departments of Epidemiology and Public Health and Psychology, and Center for Treatment Research on Adolescent Drug Abuse, University of Miami Miller School of Medicine, Miami, Florida

John E. Lochman, PhD, Department of Psychology, University of Alabama, Tuscaloosa, Tuscaloosa, Alabama

Robert G. Malgady, PhD, School of Education and Psychology, Touro College, New York, New York

Anthony P. Mannarino, PhD, Department of Psychiatry, Allegheny General Hospital, Pittsburgh, Pennsylvania

John S. March, MD, MPH, Department of Psychiatry and Behavioral Sciences, Duke University Medical School, Durham, North Carolina

Laura Mufson, PhD, Department of Psychiatry, College of Physicians and Surgeons of Columbia University, New York State Psychiatric Institute, New York, New York

Majella Murphy-Brennan, PhD, Parenting and Family Support Centre, University of Queensland, Woolloongabba, Queensland, Australia

Sandra F. Naoom, MSPH, Frank Porter Graham Child Development Institute, University of North Carolina at Chapel Hill, Chapel Hill, North Carolina

Kristine M. Pahl, PhD, Pathways Health and Research Centre, Woolloongabba, Queensland, Australia

Dustin A. Pardini, MA, Department of Psychiatry, University of Pittsburgh Medical Center, Pittsburgh, Pennsylvania

Puja Patel, MA, Department of Educational Psychology, University of Texas at Austin, Austin, Texas

Gerald R. Patterson, PhD, Implementation Sciences International, Inc., Oregon Social Learning Center, Eugene, Oregon

William E. Pelham, Jr., PhD, Center for Children and Families, University at Buffalo, The State University of New York, Buffalo, New York

Jennifer L. Podell, MA, Child and Adolescent Anxiety Disorders Clinic, Temple University, Philadelphia, Pennsylvania

Antonio J. Polo, PhD, Department of Psychology, DePaul University, Chicago, Illinois

Nicole P. Powell, PhD, Department of Psychology, University of Alabama, Tuscaloosa, Tuscaloosa, Alabama

M. Jamila Reid, PhD, School of Nursing Parenting Clinic, University of Washington, Seattle, Washington

Michael S. Robbins, PhD, Oregon Research Institute, Eugene, Oregon

Arthur L. Robin, PhD, Department of Child Psychiatry and Psychology, Children's Hospital of Michigan, Detroit, Michigan

Matthew R. Sanders, PhD, Parenting and Family Support Centre, University of Queensland, Woolloongabba, Queensland, Australia

Cindy Schaeffer, PhD, Department of Psychiatry and Behavioral Sciences, Medical University of South Carolina, Charleston, South Carolina

Sonja K. Schoenwald, PhD, Family Services Research Center, Medical University of South Carolina, Charleston, South Carolina

Stephen Scott, PhD, King's College London, Institute of Psychiatry, and National Academy for Parenting Practitioners, London, England

Dana K. Smith, PhD, Oregon Social Learning Center, Eugene, Oregon

Tristram Smith, PhD, Department of Pediatrics, University of Rochester Medical Center, Rochester, New York

Kevin D. Stark, PhD, Department of Educational Psychology, University of Texas at Austin, Austin, Texas

William Streusand, MD, Texas Child Study Center, University of Texas at Austin, Austin, Texas

José Szapocznik, PhD, Department of Epidemiology and Public Health, University of Miami Miller School of Medicine, Miami, Florida

Jessica Ucha, MEd, Department of Epidemiology and Public Health, University of Miami Miller School of Medicine, Miami, Florida

Ana Ugueto, PhD, Judge Baker Children's Center, Boston, Massachusetts

Melissa Van Dyke, LCSW, MSW, Frank Porter Graham Child Development Institute, University of North Carolina at Chapel Hill, Chapel Hill, North Carolina

Ty W. Vernon, PhD, Autism Research and Training Center, Graduate School of Education, University of California, Santa Barbara, Santa Barbara, California

Holly Barrett Waldron, PhD, Center for Family and Adolescent Research, Oregon Research Institute, Eugene, Oregon

Daniel A. Waschbusch, PhD, Center for Children and Families, University at Buffalo, The State University of New York, Buffalo, New York

Carolyn Webster-Stratton, PhD, School of Nursing Parenting Clinic, University of Washington, Seattle, Washington

V. Robin Weersing, PhD, Department of Psychology, San Diego State University, San Diego, California

John R. Weisz, PhD, ABPP, Department of Psychology, Harvard University, Faculty of Arts and Sciences, Cambridge, Massachusetts; Department of Psychiatry, Harvard Medical School, Boston, Massachusetts; and Judge Baker Children's Center, Boston, Massachusetts

Alison Zisser, MS, Department of Clinical and Health Psychology, University of Florida, Gainesville, Gainesville, Florida

Preface

It seems likely that behavioral, emotional, and social problems have always been a part of childhood, and that adults' efforts to help children with these problems are about as old as parenthood. Indeed, some of our most ancient documents include advice to parents on effective practices (e.g., "Train a child in the way he should go, and even when he is old he will not turn away from it," Proverbs 22:6). Given the long history of child problems and adult helping, it seems remarkable that formal systems of child and adolescent psychotherapy have taken shape only over the past century, and that the scientific study of psychotherapy is barely more than 50 years old. However, once research on child and adolescent psychotherapy began and built some momentum, it accelerated fast. One result has been a burgeoning collection of *evidence-based psychotherapies for children and adolescents*. The term refers to an array of psychological interventions that have been tested in studies and found to show evidence of beneficial effects. The studies have been designed in a number of different ways, and the criteria for establishing benefit have differed across the studies, but the commonalities are significant. There is general agreement, across variations in specific methods, that for a particular psychotherapy to be considered evidence based the intervention procedures must be well specified and documented (e.g., in the form of a treatment manual), treatment benefit must have been shown in well-controlled studies that rule out alternative explanations (e.g., showing that improvement could not reflect merely the natural time course of a problem), and beneficial effects must be robust across replication, ideally by investigators other than those who created the treatment program.

A substantial number of current psychotherapies satisfy these criteria, some more extensively than others. In addition, many programs of research now underway are developing psychotherapies; testing their effects; and investigating how, why, and for whom treatment works, what the necessary and sufficient components of intervention are, and how to create and implement treatments that will work well with understudied population groups and in new intervention settings. To understand the development, current status, and emerging future of the field, it is important to know about those venerable programs for which extensive support has already been compiled, others for which development and testing are well underway, and research pushing psychotherapies into new frontiers of implementation. This is the perspective that has guided our work shaping the present volume. We want to convey in this book the broad sweep of the field, capturing well-established treatments and illustrating the strategies being used by clinical scientists as they build treatments and enrich the evidence base in diverse ways.

There are pressing reasons to present the tapestry of evidence-based psychotherapies and the kinds of work needed to fill in that tapestry. At this writing, world economies are struggling, and nations around the world face the challenge of limited resources. Funds for health and mental health care are curtailed in many quarters. These conditions highlight the need for services that can be justified because they have been shown to work. The chapters in this book show that such services exist, and the number and array of such services are expanding rapidly. On the other hand, for most of the 200 disorders in the fourth edition of the *Diagnostic and Statistical Manual of Mental Disorders* that can be applied to children and adolescents, there are still no evidence-based psychotherapies designed specifically for use with young people. Moreover, most training programs in the major mental health professions—clinical psychology, child psychiatry, social work, counseling, and pediatrics—still provide relatively little training in the evidence-based psychotherapies. Each of these conditions is changing, but the changes may be best supported by efforts to identify, describe, and highlight the relevant evidence-based treatments, the evidence supporting them, and the most effective strategies used to build and implement them and disseminate information about them.

The book is designed to be useful to clinical scientists, including those early in their careers launching programs on effective intervention; to clinical practitioners, including those seeking to broaden their array of skills in the best tested practices and those willing to partner with clinical scientists in testing and improving psychotherapies; to policymakers and payers, who need hard data to inform hard decisions about support for new services; and to parents and other caring adults, who seek to navigate a landscape populated with claims and counterclaims about treatment options for their children. To make the book useful to such a diverse readership, we have worked with authors to generate concise, streamlined descriptions of the various psychotherapies, each one encompassing the conceptual basis for treatment, the intervention procedures used, evidence on the effects of treatment, challenges and directions that need to be pursued in the future, and resources available to those who want to learn more.

The discipline of concise chapters made it possible for us to broaden our coverage beyond that of our first edition in 2003. We have added chapters focusing on evidence-based psychotherapies for obsessive–compulsive disorder, substance use disorders, and posttraumatic stress disorder and other sequelae of trauma. We have provided an additional chapter on evidence-based psychotherapies in relation to minority youths. And we have now included a section focused entirely on implementation outside the boundaries of a typical study, including statewide, nationwide, and cross-national efforts, and efforts to navigate an array of policy contexts. Taken together, the chapters nicely capture the nature of the processes involved in creating evidence-based psychotherapies and making them available to young people and their families, a process that begins with conceptualizing clinical problems and conceiving of solutions, progresses into development and documentation of intervention procedures, moves directly to empirical testing—including, ideally, testing in contexts and with populations more and more like those for whom the intervention is ultimately intended and testing aimed at understanding the change processes through which intervention benefit comes about—and eventually may include implementation science, studying how to put a treatment into action in a new setting and make it effective there.

Although we have emphasized the content of the chapters, we should stress what might fairly be seen as the highlight of the book: the contributors. We were extremely fortunate to engage prominent investigators whose work is rigorous and highly thoughtful and whose contributions to the field are widely recognized. We are grateful to these accomplished authors for the time and care they have taken to convey their psychotherapy and research programs, as well as their valuable ideas about the field, in such clear and compelling ways. We also acknowledge with thanks several sources of support for our own research that we received during the period when this book was being prepared: the Annie E. Casey Foundation, Casey Family Programs, the John D. and Catherine T. MacArthur Foundation, the National Institute of Mental Health, the Norlien Foundation, the State of Connecticut Department of Social Services, and the William T. Grant Foundation. We both are especially indebted to our thoughtful colleagues, postdoctoral fellows, and graduate students, who are continuing sources of intellectual stimulation and sheer fun. We appreciate, very much, the care, commitment, and tireless good humor shown by Karen O'Connell, who worked with us on virtually every detail of book production to ensure a quality product. One of the editors, who shall go nameless, wishes to acknowledge what a pleasure it has been to work with the other editor, who will also go nameless. Finally, Seymour Weingarten, Editor-in-Chief of The Guilford Press, played a major role in conceptualizing the first edition of this book, and his support has been unflagging through the second. We are pleased to have the opportunity to work with him.

JOHN R. WEISZ
ALAN E. KAZDIN

Contents

III. IMPLEMENTATION AND DISSEMINATION: EXTENDING TREATMENTS TO NEW POPULATIONS AND NEW SETTINGS

IV. CONCLUSIONS AND FUTURE DIRECTIONS

I

FOUNDATIONS OF CHILD AND ADOLESCENT PSYCHOTHERAPY RESEARCH

1

Introduction

Context, Background, and Goals

ALAN E. KAZDIN and JOHN R. WEISZ

The focus of the book is on psychotherapy, which is defined broadly to include any intervention that is designed to reduce distress or maladaptive behavior or enhance adaptive functioning and that uses such means as counseling and structured and other planned psychosocial interventions (Weisz, Weiss, Han, Granger, & Morton, 1995). The goals of therapy consist of improving adjustment and functioning in both intrapersonal and interpersonal spheres and reducing maladaptive behaviors and various psychological and often physical complaints. The means by which the goals are achieved are primarily interpersonal contact; for most treatments this consists of verbal interaction. In child therapy, the means can include talking, playing, rewarding new behaviors, or rehearsing activities with the child. Also, the persons who carry out these actions can be therapists, parents, teachers, and peers. A variety of therapeutic aids such as puppets, games, stories, and videos may be used as the means through which treatment goals are pursued.

Psychotherapy has a remarkable history well beyond its formal delineation as a healing enterprise. A defensible place to begin would be with the work of Aristotle (384–322 B.C.E.), who emphasized the role of catharsis in tragic drama, comedy, and the arts more generally in arousing and alleviating emotional states (*Poetics*, 350 B.C.E.; *Politics* VIII, 350 B.C.E.).[1] The paths from Aristotle to psychotherapy could readily be charted by tracing medicine, religion, spiritualism, and less easily classified disciplines that have used practices such as suggestion, hypnosis, and assorted quasi-medical or expectancy-based interventions directed toward the alleviation of stress, maladjustment, and a broad scope of maladies (Shapiro & Shapiro, 1998). The formal delineation of psychotherapy as an area of study and clinical work can be traced to the past 100 years or so (Norcross, Vanden-Bos, & Freedheim, 2010). In this context, therapy grew directly from efforts to intervene to address impaired mental (psychiatric) function and problems of adjustment.

Empirical research on child therapy has a relatively brief history. The earliest reviews of the therapy literature identified a small number of studies that included children or adolescents (Levitt, 1957 [18 studies], 1963 [22 additional studies]). The reviews concluded that therapy did not seem to be more effective than the passage of time without formal intervention (i.e., no therapy). The rate of improvement among children (67–73%) was about the same whether or not treatment was provided. This conclusion was similar to the one reached by Eysenck (1952) in his pioneering and influential review of the effects of psychotherapy for adults. The conclusions reached in all three of these reviews were based on studies that, in most cases, were methodologically weak. For example, research included few randomized controlled trials, the samples were small, and the treatments were not well specified. Even so, the reviews had an important influence by showcasing an area and conveying the need for much more and better empirical research.

In the past 50 years, the quantity of studies on the effects of psychotherapy has greatly increased. There is no definitive count encompassing the world stage. However, as of 1999, a conservative count of studies within the English language alone estimated 1,500 controlled studies of psychotherapy with children and adolescents (Kazdin, 2000). The quality of research has improved over the years as well. The standards that need to be met for approval to begin a psychotherapy outcome study, to obtain funding to mount the study, and to publish the results have become increasingly demanding. For example, increasingly studies must meet special standards of reporting (e.g., Consolidated Standards of Reporting [CONSORT] *www.consort-statement.org/*), include clear statements about recruitment procedures and inclusion and exclusion criteria, provide treatment in manualized form, codify treatment fidelity, use multiple measures and multiple assessment methods, and assess therapeutic change using criteria beyond statistical significance (e.g., magnitude of effects, clinical significance). Also, more studies compare a proposed treatment against treatment as usual rather than no-treatment or wait-list control conditions. Comparison of two or more treatments makes demonstration of effects even more difficult than usual in light of the methodological demands (e.g., avoiding the diffusion of treatment; sustaining statistical power in light of smaller effect sizes from comparing two or more active treatments). The increases in quantity and quality of studies have coalesced to generate an impressive set of treatments with strong evidence in their behalf which serve as the basis for this book.

FOCUS ON EVIDENCE-BASED PSYCHOTHERAPIES

This book is about evidence-based psychotherapies for children and adolescents. "Evidence based" has many definitions and meanings in light of a large set of disciplines involved in their delineation, including clinical psychology, psychiatry, internal medicine, social work, public health, dentistry, law, and social policy. Evidence-based psychotherapies have been delineated by different professional organizations within and among countries (e.g., the Americas, European Union). Also, various private and public agencies are defining and delineating treatments that are considered to be evidence based. For example, one resource encompasses more than 30 federal, state, professional, and university sites that enumerate evidence-based interventions (*ucoll.fdu.edu/apa/lnksinter.html*). Perhaps the best known is the web-based resource provided by the Substance Abuse and Mental Health Services Administration (*www.nationalregistry.samhsa.gov*). With so many different parties involved, there is no single consensus definition of evidence-based psychotherapies.

For the most part, several criteria are commonly invoked to delineate an intervention as evidence based. These include at least two or more studies with the following:

1. Careful specification of the patient population.
2. Random assignment of participants to conditions.
3. Use of treatment manuals that document the procedures.
4. Multiple outcome measures (raters, if used, are naïve to conditions), including, of course, measurement of the problem or disorder targeted in treatment.
5. Statistically significant differences between treatment and a comparison group after treatment.
6. Replication of outcome effects, ideally by an independent investigator or research team.

There is little reason to make evidence based categorical. One might consider evidence based as a "spectrum," very much along the lines of the diagnosis of many psychiatric disorders (e.g., depression, conduct disorder, autism) in which a single cut point is difficult to defend. The spectrum is easily seen among treatments that have evidence. Some of the evidence-based psychotherapies have been replicated and supported in scores of trials, others in just a few. In this book, we are interested in presenting those treatments with strong empirical support in their behalf rather than drawing a line to classify them as evidence based or not. Also, we wish to eschew terms such as "promising" or "almost evidence based." We present evidence-based psychotherapies and feature exemplary research to illustrate the substantive advances and methodological quality of the research on which these advances are based. Given the definition provided at the beginning of the chapter, the focus is restricted to psychosocial interventions. Other treatments that might be used for childhood disorders (e.g., medication, diet) are omitted from the definition.

OVERVIEW OF ADVANCES FEATURED IN THIS VOLUME

Research on evidence-based psychotherapies has made remarkable progress. In the period since publication of the first edition, programs of research that were well in place have expanded, new programs have emerged, and our knowledge about specific techniques and their applicability has deepened. The rich literature now encompasses many findings on processes, outcomes, moderators, and new applications of existing techniques. Although this volume encompasses all these features, three characteristics of current research in child and adolescent therapy are particularly noteworthy in this volume.

First, treatment research has addressed a wide range of social, emotional, and behavioral problems of childhood and adolescence. These are delineated as problems insofar as they are associated with distress and impairment in daily functioning. The range of such problems children experience is vast. Considering psychiatric diagnoses alone, there are a variety of clinical disorders that emerge in infancy, childhood, and adolescence (e.g., pervasive developmental disorders, attention deficit and disruptive behavior disorders; American Psychiatric Association, 1994; World Health Organization, 1992). Many other disorders can emerge over the life span (e.g., anxiety, depression, eating disorders, adjustment disorder), although they may take different forms and have different features at different points in development.

As evidence-based psychotherapies have expanded, an increasing array of disorders and domains of child functioning have been addressed. In this volume, the expansion is illustrated nicely by coverage of multiple problems, including anxiety disorders, mood disorders, attention-deficit/hyperactivity disorder, anorexia nervosa, enuresis, autism, oppositional defiant disorder, conduct disorder, and substance abuse disorders. Interventions have been developed to evaluate different subtypes (e.g., obsessive–compulsive and posttraumatic stress among the anxiety disorders), different levels of severity for given problems (e.g., oppositional and aggressive behavior among disruptive behavior disorders), and at different points in development (e.g., conduct problems in young children and adolescents). These different foci also draw on different modes of intervention (e.g., with child, parent, family, school, and neighborhood resources) to accommodate the problems that children and adolescents experience.

Second, increased attention has been accorded developing and evaluating treatments with ethnically and culturally diverse children and families. Interventions are needed that are accessible and effective with diverse groups, not only for groups within our country or continent but as models that can address child and adolescent mental health needs worldwide. In North America (Canada, Mexico, United States), there are hundreds of ethnic and cultural groups; and there are thousands when one moves to the world stage (Marsella, 2008; *www.infoplease.com/ipa/A0855617.html*). Ethnicity and culture can influence symptom patterns and prevalence rates of clinical problems (Achenbach & Rescorla, 2007; Canino & Alegria, 2008). Many, but not all, treatments are effective across multiple ethnic groups (Miranda et al., 2005). Consequently, ethnicity and cultural issues need to be built into the development of evidence-based therapies (Bernal, 2006; Kazdin, 2008).

Advances in developing ethnically and culturally sensitive treatments are nicely illustrated in this volume. For example, programs of research for the treatment of Hispanic American children and adolescents convey the progress that has been made. Separate treatment techniques have been applied for youths of different ages and with different problems. Many of the applications have been tested with different subgroups of Hispanic American children. This is critical in light of the enormous heterogeneity, which usually is glossed over by such generic terms as Hispanic American, African American, Asian American, and European American. Evidence-based psychotherapies for diverse groups are critically important, and this volume highlights progress from programs of research.

Third, research has focused on implementing evidence-based psychotherapies in clinical practice settings. There are many research questions in developing therapies for children and more problems domains in need of attention. Even so, there are effective treatments available now that could make a difference in patient care and clinical outcomes if they could be extended to clinical training of mental health professionals and to those who are engaged in direct patient care. The challenges of implementation and dissemination are many and include those of diffusion of information and skills and increasing the scale of applications, each of which is daunting in its own right (Weisz & Gray, 2008; Weisz, Jensen-Doss, & Hawley, 2006).

New to this volume is a set of chapters on implementation and dissemination of treatment. The topics include critical issues and obstacles to dissemination of effective treatment, guidelines for how treatments can be disseminated, and essential components to sustain treatment quality. Dissemination of effective treatments requires integration of research findings with law, social policy, and local and federal or national legislation, all of which are addressed concretely in chapters in this volume.

Although the main features we have highlighted convey critical components of the book, the research is rich with other findings. For example, as evidence-based psycho-therapies were emerging, early concerns were voiced that perhaps the treatments could not be applied to children with multiple disorders (comorbidity), that they are not really effective with very severe cases, and that severely impaired families might not respond, among other concerns of this ilk. Advances in research have continued to address these concerns empirically. For example, our own work has shown that such factors as comor-bidity of disorders and complexity and stress in the families of clinically referred cases do not impede (or indeed necessarily moderate) treatment outcome with evidence-based treatments (Doss & Weisz, 2006; Kazdin & Whitley, 2006). The chapters that follow are rich in many such findings well beyond establishing the efficacy of treatment.

GOALS OF THIS BOOK

The book presents psychotherapies for children and adolescents that have evidence in their behalf and illustrates the type of research that is needed to place treatment on strong empirical footing. The chapters encompass many treatments that have been delineated as evidence based. However, as we mentioned, we did not invoke a rigid set of criteria to delineate what would and would not be covered in the book. Rather, we selected interventions and programs of research that we felt would be exemplary and where palpable progress has been made in controlled research. As the reader will note, some of the chapters cover treatments that have been very well established in controlled trials and with multiple replications. The book is designed to highlight advances among such evidence-based psychotherapies. In addition, we have presented treatments in vari-ous stages of development where programmatic studies are well underway. Although the book is intended to display the rich yield from years of research, the process of program-matic research also is nicely illustrated throughout the chapters. The purpose of this fea-ture of the book is to help researchers who are developing treatment and contemplating careers in intervention research by providing examples of ways to proceed in developing a research program.

The majority of chapters that follow are devoted to specific treatment techniques. For these chapters, contributors were asked to provide an overview of the clinical prob-lem they have been studying, the model or underlying assumptions of treatment, and the goals of treatment. Chapters include details of the intervention so the reader can discern the content of the treatment sessions, the sequence of material covered in the sessions, and the skills or tasks emphasized in treatment. Such details are not permitted in the usual publication outlets for research such as journal publication, so we as readers are often persuaded that a given intervention might work but do not really have an idea of what the intervention was in any detail. Contributors were encouraged to describe the intervention and to discuss how it is implemented, what treatment manuals are used and are available, who serves as therapists, how therapists are trained and supervised, and other details.

Contributors were also asked to describe the scope of the evidence for their treatment. The contributors are seasoned investigators with extensive programs of research. Consequently, asking them to present the outcome results in a brief space ranges somewhere between cruel and unfair. Even so, contributors met the challenge and provided us with a concise statement of the outcome evidence for the treatment they have covered and the questions that research has addressed in relation to that treatment. The chapters provide a concise statement of what the treatment is, to whom it is applied, the evidence bearing on outcomes of the treatment, and key questions that remain to be researched.

The chapters on implementation and dissemination of treatment represent at once a rich complement to research that has established treatment efficacy as well as the logical next step for programs of research. Programmatic research on implementation and dissemination has become a high priority, even as further work is needed on developing novel treatments for problems without evidence-based treatments. Challenges and successes at dissemination are covered and raise issues that may well influence considerations to be taken into account at the stage of developing new treatments.

We have attempted to weave the chapters together by placing treatments and dissemination in multiple contexts and in relation to broader issues. Our introductory and concluding chapters and those on development and ethical considerations convey critical issues in relation to research and practice. Our concluding chapter also points to next steps to help ensure that the trajectory of advances moves to new heights.

We are delighted to note that evidence-based psychotherapies, the range of disorders that can be treated, and the scope of dissemination efforts could not be comprehensively covered in the present volume. Our delight stems from the fact that scientific progress has been outstanding; separate volumes on evidence-based psychotherapies for internalizing or externalizing disorders, interventions with underrepresented groups, and models of and evidence for dissemination of treatment could easily be justified. This volume draws on extraordinary work from each of these areas and conveys continued progress to place therapies for children and adolescents on strong scientific footing.

NOTE

1. Tracing therapy back to Aristotle is not much of a stretch. Aristotle spoke about emotional states and how people suffering from emotional outbreaks can be cured by cathartic songs (*Politics* VIII 7.1342a4–16). Yet the connection is even more explicit in developing or charting a history of therapy. For example, Jacob Bernays (1824–1881), a relative of Freud by marriage, drew on Aristotle to note further that the cathartic benefits obtained via tragic drama are similar to a process of psychological healing (Bernays, 1857, 1880).

REFERENCES

Achenbach, T. M., & Rescorla, L. A. (2007). *Multicultural understanding of child and adolescent psychopathology: Implications for mental health assessment.* New York: Guilford Press.

American Psychiatric Association. (1994). *Diagnostic and statistical manual of mental disorders* (4th ed.). Washington, DC: Author.

Bernal, G. (2006). Intervention development and cultural adaptation research with diverse families. *Family Processes, 45,* 143–151.

Bernays, J. (1857). *Zwei Abhandlungen über die aristolische Theorie des Drama: I. Grundzüge der verlorenen Abhandlung des Aristoteles über Wirkung der Tragödie* [Two treaties about effective theory of drama: Part I. Fundamental part of the lost treatise of Aristotle about the effective tragedy]. Breslau, Germany.

Bernays, J. (1880). *Zwei Abhandlungen über die aristolische Theorie des Drama: II. Ergänzung zu Aristotle's Poetik* [Two treaties about effective theory of drama: Part II. Supplement to Aristotle's Poetic]. Breslau, Germany.

Canino, G., & Alegria, M. (2008). Psychiatric diagnosis—Is it universal or relative to culture? *Journal of Child Psychology and Psychiatry, 49,* 237–250.

Doss, A. J., & Weisz, J. R. (2006). Syndrome co-occurrence and treatment outcomes in youth mental health clinics. *Journal of Consulting and Clinical Psychology, 74,* 416–425.

Eysenck, H. J. (1952). The effects of psychotherapy: An evaluation. *Journal of Consulting Psychology, 16,* 319–324.

Kazdin, A. E. (2000). Developing a research agenda for child and adolescent psychotherapy research. *Archives of General Psychiatry, 57,* 829–835.

Kazdin, A. E. (2008). Evidence-based treatments and delivery of psychological services: Shifting our emphases to increase impact. *Psychological Services, 5,* 201–215.

Kazdin, A. E., & Whitley, M. K. (2006). Comorbidity, case complexity, and effects of evidence-based treatment for children referred for disruptive behavior. *Journal of Consulting and Clinical Psychology, 74,* 455–467.

Levitt, E. E. (1957). The results of psychotherapy with children: An evaluation. *Journal of Consulting Psychology, 21,* 189–196.

Levitt, E. E. (1963). Psychotherapy with children: A further evaluation. *Behaviour Research and Therapy, 60,* 326–329.

Marsella, A. J. (2008, September). *Psychology in a global era: Foundations, issues, directions.* Paper presented at the American Psychological Association Educational Leadership Conference, Washington, DC.

Miranda, J., Bernal, G., Lau, A. S., Kohn, L., Hwang, W. C., & LaFromboise, T. (2005). State of the science on psychosocial interventions for ethnic minorities. *Annual Review of Clinical Psychology, 1,* 113–143.

Norcross, J., VandenBos, G. R., & Freedheim, D. K. (Eds.). (2010). *History of psychotherapy: A century of change* (2nd ed.). Washington, DC: American Psychological Association.

Shapiro, A. K., & Shapiro, E. (1998). *Powerful placebo: From ancient priest to modern physician.* Baltimore: John Hopkins University Press.

Weisz, J. R., & Gray, J. S. (2008). Evidence-based psychotherapies for children and adolescents: Data from the present and a model for the future. *Child and Adolescent Mental Health, 13,* 54–65.

Weisz, J. R., Jensen-Doss, A., & Hawley, K. M. (2006). Evidence-based youth psychotherapies versus usual clinical care: A meta-analysis of direct comparisons. *American Psychologist, 61,* 671–689.

Weisz, J. R., Weiss, B., Han, S. S., Granger, D. A., & Morton, T. (1995). Effects of psychotherapy with children and adolescents revisited: A meta-analysis of treatment outcome studies. *Psychological Bulletin, 117,* 450–468.

World Health Organization. (1992). *International classification of diseases and health-related problems.* Geneva: Author.

2

Ethical Issues in Child and Adolescent Psychosocial Treatment Research

KIMBERLY EATON HOAGWOOD and MARY A. CAVALERI

E thical issues in research on mental health are occasionally treated as an after-thought—as an idea for a symposium topic, an academic seminar, or an after-dinner conversation—interesting but peripheral to scientific inquiry. Yet analysis of ethical issues in research cuts to the scientific core, revealing the *raison d'etre* for a study as well as the dialectical tensions between empirical inquiry and the study of human beings by human beings.

CENTRALITY OF ETHICAL ISSUES

Ethical dilemmas arise when harm to research participants—however small, unforeseen, or tenuous—enters into the design or implementation of a study or is experienced by a research participant during the course of a study. Such harm may occur inadvertently because of an unanticipated consequence from a procedure, measure, or process. Or it may be an explicitly stated risk about which a participant is informed in advance of entering into a protocol. In either case, however, the responsibility for estimating the potential for harm and building into the protocol safeguards to protect research participants falls directly upon the investigators and, consequently, such estimates have to be made before embarking on a study.

The key defense against vulnerability to harm through participation in research, as is described later, is the concept of informed consent. If participants knowingly enter into a study where the potential for harm to them is clearly listed, then the presumption exists that any untoward consequences were voluntarily entertained and that, therefore, the investigator has met his or her obligation. Yet, as will be seen, the clarity of this presumption is made much more complex in studies involving children and adolescents, especially those who also experience mental health problems.

The essential dialectic between scientific inquiry and social obligation is revealed perhaps most starkly in the field of child and adolescent mental health, where unevenness in the scientific knowledge base and urgent public health concerns about the status of children's mental health are in sharp relief. The lack of a strong scientific foundation on, for example, the effects of psychotropic drug treatments on children with mental illnesses creates an ethical problem. Prescriptions of such treatments and in particular the combination of such treatments are rapidly rising (Bhatara, Feil, Hoagwood, Vitiello, & Zima, 2002), but the knowledge base on the safety, efficacy, or long-term impact of the majority of the commonly prescribed medications does not yet exist (Jensen et al., 1999). Clearly, there is a need for strengthening knowledge about the effects of these medications, especially given the increase in their use. However, at the same time, constructing basic science studies into the safety and efficacy of psychotropic treatments, which may involve the use of these agents with normal controls, can introduce unforeseen harm to participants. A similar dilemma exists for psychosocial treatments, referred to in this book as psychotherapies, where a limited knowledge base, combined with widespread use of non-evidence-based treatments, creates a tension because of the need to accelerate study of the efficacy and effectiveness of treatments even as basic understanding of what constitutes risk to research participants is unavailable.

Added to this central ethical tension is the fact that the prevalence rates of unmet need for mental health services among children and adolescents with impairing forms of emotional, behavioral, or brain disorders are as high now as they were 20 years ago (National Advisory Mental Health Council's Workgroup, 2001). From a public health standpoint, the urgency of strengthening the science base on effective treatments has never been stronger. Yet equally urgent is the need to attend to a range of ethical issues that will inevitably arise when studying children and adolescents with mental health needs. Consequently, investigators embarking on studies of treatments for children's mental disorders have to shoulder an enormous responsibility to ensure that potential harm is considered, that such harm is minimized, and, simultaneously, that scientifically valuable and valid knowledge is created.

It is the purpose of this chapter to help investigators define and examine a range of ethical issues that may arise in studies of psychosocial treatments for youths. The chapter first describes the boundaries between ethical issues and legal regulations and the reasons why these categories are becoming increasingly indistinguishable. It then describes the primary federal regulations that guide approaches to studies of children and adolescents. This is followed by a description of some of the common research processes in which ethical dilemmas may arise. These include obtaining informed consent; weighing risks and benefits; engaging families or community stakeholders in studies; providing clinical feedback; offering incentives; and ensuring confidentiality.

Boundaries between Ethical Issues and Legal Issues

In research on child and adolescent mental health and illness, the boundaries between ethical issues—that is, the application of philosophically derived moral principles to questions of right and wrong—versus legal issues—that is, questions of what is or is not lawful—are often blurred. In fact, one can find articles about ethical issues in research that do little more than describe federal regulations (Vitiello, 2002).

It is easy to see why the boundaries between ethical and legal issues in research have become indistinguishable in many discussions about human subjects' protections. The historical starting point within the federal government that precipitated attention to ethical principles in research with human subjects was the Belmont Report, issued by the National Commission for the Protection of Human Subjects of Biomedical and Behavioral Research (1979) and from which the Code of Federal Regulations was later derived. In this report, the commission described three major principles that presumably dictate ethical practice in research with human beings.

1. *Respect for persons.* This principle prescribes that all individuals should be treated as autonomous and should be protected from risk. Protection is especially important for persons with diminished autonomy, including children and adolescents. Research issues related to informed consent, confidentiality, and voluntariness of participation are derived from this principle.

2. *Beneficence.* This principle reflects the perspective that not only must persons' decisions be respected and protected from harm, but that efforts to secure their well-being must also be made. Beneficence (i.e., to maximize good and minimize harm to individuals or to society) is thus an obligation.

3. *Justice.* This principle dictates that the benefits and burdens of research must be distributed fairly and equitably, and that research participants should be chosen for reasons related to scientific inquiry, not for reasons of accessibility or convenience. Additionally, persons with disabilities should not be asked to bear a disproportionate share of the burden.

All biomedical research must be guided by these three principles. Shortly after the Belmont Report was released in 1979, the first regulatory guidelines were issued (1983). Called the Code of Federal Regulations on the Protection of Human Subjects (CFR), this code was explicitly written to establish the basic beneficence-related requirements for research. The requirements are discussed later. However, the point here is that these guidelines essentially laid out the parameters of federal policy with respect to the ethical study of children and adolescents and thus from the outset combined regulatory language with issues of right and wrong.

An additional set of issues has led to the intermingling of ethical and legal perspectives on mental health research. This involves the nature of psychological and psychiatric research itself. Because the focus of study often involves individuals with emotional or mental impairments, legal issues often by necessity arise. For example, laws governing consent, custody, or involuntary commitment may enter into the implementation of a study protocol even if such issues are not a primary or even a secondary focus of the project. Legal considerations can dictate parameters of studies that may not have been previously anticipated.

Finally, there are anecdotal reports that ethical and legal concerns may increasingly be vying for ascendancy within university-based institutional review boards (IRBs). The current increase in lawsuits directed against universities involved in human subject research (Icenogle, 2003) has led to a climate wherein concerns about human subjects' protections are weighed against concerns about potential litigation within the review deliberations that occur in IRBs. This is an inevitable result of the mixed purposes that academic institutions have, in which attracting large research grants leads to institutional accreditation, credibility, and stature; however, large-scale scientific projects, especially in new or untested areas of science, such as genetic therapies, therapeutic development of new agents, or therapies with high-risk patients (e.g., those who are suicidal), also entail increased potential for harm to research subjects and increased likelihood of litigation against the university if harm occurs.

Guidelines and Federal Regulations

Although the foundational principles underpinning protection of human subjects in research have remained unchanged since the 1970s, the application of these principles to subpopulations and their interpretation is dynamic and changeable (Hoagwood, Jensen, & Fisher, 1996). Research ethics involving children and adolescents with mental health needs has been the subject of recent federal attention (Charney, 2000). In 1998, the National Bioethics Advisory Commission issued its report, "Research Involving Persons with Mental Disorders that May Affect Decision-making Capacity." In 1999 the National Institute of Mental Health (NIMH) created a work group of the National Advisory Mental Health Council to provide additional safeguards and reviews of human subject concerns for grant applications involving challenging designs, methods, or techniques. In 2000 the National Human Research Protections Advisory Committee, which was replaced in 2002 by the Office for Human Research Protections, met to review ethical issues inherent in research involving children and formed a work group to examine the adequacy of the existing regulations in subpart D (described later).

In 2000 the National Institutes of Health (NIH) issued new requirements governing the education of clinical investigators in the protection of research subjects. The NIMH also issued program announcements specifically targeting studies of research ethics (NIH, 2009) and in 2008 instituted a series of conferences to provide an educational forum by which mental health researchers can convene to discuss pressing ethical issues and form a panel to provide guidance and offer recommendations for best practices concerning ethical issues in research via publications in peer-reviewed periodicals (NIMH, 2009). All of these activities reflect the heightened awareness at the federal level of the need to attend carefully to issues of human subject protection while ensuring the growth and solidity of the scientific foundation on issues of public health significance.

From a public health scientific standpoint, in addition to the three principles defined in the Belmont Report (National Commission, 1979), there are several fundamental requirements without which the ethical grounding of a scientific study can be questioned. The first is that the potential yield of the study must be significant in its promise of improving public health. Investigators have been cautioned to focus on scientific issues of genuine significance rather than questions that may be interesting but trivial or unrelated to general societal benefit (Hyman, 1999). Second, the experimental design must be sound, and alternative designs should be considered carefully with respect to both ethical and practical concerns (Vitiello, Jensen, & Hoagwood, 1999). In addition, the balance between risk and potential benefit should be weighed favorably toward the study participants. Finally, research participants must be fully informed of the risks, benefits, implications, and alternatives to participation.

Federal Regulations

The specific policy that sets the standards for federally funded research was first issued in 1983 as the CFR on the Protection of Human Subjects. Within this code were requirements for the establishment of IRBs, criteria for IRB approval, criteria for determining the hierarchy of risks, circumstances under which parental permission was needed or waivers obtainable, and special protections for children involved as subjects in research. A revision of this code in 1991 included more specific discussion on protection of children and adolescents as research subjects (U.S. Department of Human Services [DHHS], 1991a, 1991b; see especially subpart D). The main requirements of the policy included the necessity of obtaining permission or consent, which is fully informed, by the parent or other legal guardian for a child's participation in research; obtaining assent, when possible, from the child; and ensuring that the risk–benefit ratio is favorable to the child.

In evaluating the concept of risk, several variants are described in the federal code. Minimal risk is defined as risk that is not greater than that ordinarily encountered in daily life or during routine physical or psychological assessments (section 46:102(i) in DHHS 1991a). Minimal risk is not equivalent to no risk, and the ways in which it is calibrated and defined differ considerably from one investigation to another and from one IRB to another. Research that involves greater than minimal risk but also includes the prospect of direct benefit is justified if the potential benefit outweighs the potential harm (section 46.405 in DHHS 1991b). According to 45CFR46, a benefit must be reasonably expected if a study is to be considered to have the prospect of direct benefit. Risks, however, must be presented if they are foreseeable. This is much broader and could include possible but unlikely problems. Treatment studies tend to fall into this category. Deliberation of the risks and benefits involves careful consideration of the severity of the child's illness, the availability of alternative treatments, and the estimates of the safety and efficacy of the experimental treatment, which the child may receive if enrolled in the study. Table 2.1 lists the kinds of research by level of risk and the decisional elements to weigh when considering involvement of children.

Research that does not contain direct benefit to the participant is among the most controversial. Examples of these kinds of studies include invasive medical procedures, exposure to situations that may provoke anxious or upsetting responses, and administration of agents that are potentially toxic. Federal regulations stipulate that this kind of research may be conducted only if, in addition to the other requirements, the following conditions are also met:

1. The study involves only a minor increase over minimal risk;
2. The procedure involves "experiences to the subjects that are commensurate with those inherent in their actual or expected medical, dental, psychological, social or educational situations";
3. The study has the potential to provide knowledge that is of "vital importance" to understanding or treating the pediatric illness; and
4. Parental permission and child assent are obtained. (DHHS, 1991b, section 46.406)

The final category of risk involves projects that present greater than a minor increase over minimal risk. These studies are rarely proposed and are considered only if they have the potential to increase scientific knowledge about a serious public health problem affecting children. They require special review and approval by the DHHS.

TABLE 2.1. Elements to Consider in Evaluating the Ethics of Research in Children

Type of research	Critical elements
1. Research that has potential benefit to research participants	Risk–benefit must be favorable to the research participants.
2. Research that has no potential benefit to the research participants	No greater than minimal risk is allowed.
	Research is likely to generate important knowledge to justify the minimal risk involved.
3. Research that has no potential benefit but relevant knowledge can be gained	No more than a minor increase over minimal risk is allowed.
	Participants are exposed to experiences reasonably commensurate with those inherent in their lives.
	Research is likely to yield knowledge that is of vital importance for amelioration of the condition.
4. Research that is not otherwise approvable under the prior criteria	Secretary of DHHS can determine that proposed research presents a reasonable opportunity to further understanding, prevention, or alleviation of a serious problem affecting health/ welfare of children.

Note. DHHS, U.S. Department of Health and Human Services.

Obtaining Informed Consent

Informed consent is, in some sense, the ethical cornerstone on which human subject protections rest. It requires that individuals understand and are free to choose whether to participate. Ethical dilemmas on consent may arise in any type of treatment or intervention study, including pharmacological, psychosocial, preventive, and service trials. As a rule, the consent process should include specific elements: an invitation to participate; a statement of the purpose of the study; the basis of participant selection; and explanation of procedures, risks, and discomforts; how untoward consequences will be handled; benefits of participation; alternatives to participation; financial consideration; confidentiality; opportunities for continuing disclosure; and measures for ensuring that a person's decision to participate is voluntary (Fisher, 2004).

Informed consent goes beyond merely providing information, but should advance potential subjects' comprehension and voluntary decision making relating to their participation (Brody, McCullough, & Sharp, 2005) and is the first step toward a process by which potential participants integrate and personalize the information in order to make a decision that is concordant with their values (Lidz, Appelbaum, Grisso, & Renaud, 2004).

Bruzzese and Fisher (2003) suggest that assessing the adequacy of a study's informed consent procedures entails answering several key questions such as, do the participants understand what the purpose of the research is, their rights (i.e., participation is voluntary, they may discontinue participation), and aspects related to confidentiality)? If their rights are violated, do they know they can take measures to protect themselves. Similarly, Appelbaum (2007) identified four central criteria to consider when assessing the adequacy of informed consent procedures: capacity, understanding, reasoning, and ability to express a choice. Capacity involves the ability of the individuals to provide consent. Although it is not the same as competence, which is a legal term, it refers to a basic capacity for understanding language, linguistic convention, and the meaning attached to words.

Understanding refers to the ability of individuals to comprehend the terms of the agreement involved in consent. Understanding is sometimes believed to have occurred if individuals can repeat back what has been heard, but new methods of ensuring understanding are being developed for consent involving adult patients with potential limitations (e.g., patients with schizophrenia; see Dunn, Candilis, & Roberts, 2006, for a review) as well as children and adolescents (Bruzzese & Fisher, 2003), such as educational tools (e.g., videos and computer-based slide shows as well as measures that provide information about the key elements of informed consent). Reasoning refers to the ability of individuals to balance risks and benefits and to foresee or anticipate both. Finally, the ability of individuals to express a choice is essential to the concept of informed consent. It is separate from understanding in a receptive sense, because it entails the active ability to weigh options and select according to one's preferences. It is probably a key aspect of the consent process and yet has rarely been studied.

Informed Consent with Children and Adolescents

Certain complexities arise when obtaining consent for research with children and adolescents. Adolescents' consent to participate generally must involve both the adolescents and their parents or guardians. Children, by virtue of their limited legal status and because they cannot legally consent to research participation, are often considered to be a vulnerable population. In research involving minimal risk, it has sometimes been sufficient to obtain informed consent of one parent. In research with greater than minimal risk, obtaining permission of both parents (if available) is generally advisable. However, even if one or both parents authorize their child to participate, the child's decision trumps the parent's consent in most situations (Bruzzese & Fisher, 2003), although there have been cases in which the youth's dissent is overruled (Collogan & Fleischman, 2005).

Children with psychiatric disorders may, but do not necessarily, have limitations with respect to understanding the conditions by which their participation is being solicited (Yan & Munir, 2004). Therefore, special efforts must be made to ensure that children's assent to participate is voluntary and that they understand fully the risks and benefits of participation. It is often prudent to ask whether a particular study's aims could be directed toward a less vulnerable population first. A clear rationale should be provided as to why children with psychiatric disorders, as opposed to children or adolescents without these conditions, are the population of interest for a particular study.

States vary in their laws authorizing minors to consent to either treatment or participation in research. In all but three states (in which the age is 19), adolescents who are 18 or older are legally adults (Hoagwood, Jensen, & Leshner, 1997). There are circumstances under which children can give their own consent, based upon their status (e.g., mature minors, who are not legally emancipated but are considered able to understand the risks and benefits of participating in a given treatment or research), specific services sought (e.g., treatment for mental health difficulties and substance abuse), or type of study (e.g., high-risk populations; Collogan & Fleischman, 2005; English, 1991; Fisher, 2004).

Some states allow minors who are living apart from their parents (e.g., homeless, emancipated minors, married minors) to consent to receive health or mental health care (English, 1991). Laws relating to consent for minors are changing in many states and thus subject to variation. As a consequence, it is advisable for researchers to become well acquainted with the laws governing minor status and consent in the state in which the research is to be conducted.

Impairments in decisional capacity, as may occur with children whose cognitive capacities are developing or among psychiatrically impaired individuals, have implications for informed consent procedures. These impairments may be transient, intermittent, or permanent (Roberts, 1998). Clinical syndromes may create distortions of thought, impaired attention or memory, ambivalence, emotional lability, lack of motivation, distractibility, or impulsivity (Expert Panel Report to the National Institutes of Health, 1998; Roberts, 1998). In studies involving persons with mental illnesses that may impair their judgment, investigators should strongly consider using independent qualified professionals to assess potential participants' capacity to provide informed consent. Children, whose cognitive, affective, and physiological development is emerging, do not possess full decisional capacity and thus are usually dependent on others—generally the parents—for providing such (Munir & Earls, 1992). However, among adolescents, there are cases in which independent professionals have been engaged in research projects, and paid as independent consultants, to assess adolescents' understanding of the informed consent protocol and to ensure that participation is entirely voluntary (Fisher, 1996).

A variety of features may be included in protocols to improve the process of obtaining informed consent. These include repeated exposure to the information in the protocol; multiple avenues of communication (e.g., verbal, written); language use that is simple, in small units, and comprehensible; use of patient educators, who review relevant information with the potential subject, explain the study's purpose and process, and answer any questions; and specific attention to particular aspects of consent, including motivation, culture, or personal history of involvement in research projects (Fisher, 2004; Roberts, 1998).

Weighing Risks and Benefits

The risks and benefits of participation in research are analyzed by the investigators, and the appropriateness of the balance is ascertained by the IRB. The purpose of the study must include demonstration of the potential benefits of the study as well as an explicit discussion as to how the investigators intend to minimize risk. In assessing risks, investigators occasionally overlook some of the distinct advantages to participation in research. For example, in addition to the increased access to treatment that is available from participation in treatment trials, participation in research can also provide youths with information about the effectiveness of treatments, the availability of community services, and the perceptions of their peers (Hoagwood et al., 1996).

However, the weighing of risks and benefits in research on child and adolescent mental health can be among the most complex to address. The primary premise is that risks and benefits should be viewed from the standpoint of the research participant, not the investigator or institution. No risk is considered acceptable if the research does not have the potential to benefit the participant or if it will not strengthen knowledge about the condition or treatment for that condition.

The scientific validity of the design is one factor that is important for evaluating the potential benefit of a study. The design should reduce risks to the maximum extent possible while preserving the scientific integrity of the design. For example, active treatment comparison arms are desirable, as opposed to wait-list controls or placebo conditions. Whenever feasible, the design should also maximize benefits to increase the likelihood that advantages to individual participants or to other populations will be accrued. For example, a study of the comparative effectiveness of two empirically validated treatments might confer benefit and reduce risk for all subjects enrolled in the study. Finally, a careful assessment of the range of potential positive outcomes, both direct and indirect, should be taken into account when determining the likely impact of a treatment (Fisher, 1996).

Just as there are both direct and indirect benefits that must be considered, there are also direct and indirect risks. The notion of what constitutes a risk needs to be assessed broadly to encompass physical risks, psychological risks, and social dimensions of risk (Roberts, 1998). The latter include risks such as stigma, labeling, and community distrust. For example, some studies of service interventions have been viewed as "hit-and-runs," with services put into place temporarily for the purposes of studying them but no provision being made from the outset to try to ensure continuation of services, if they are found to be effective, after the study is completed (Hoagwood et al., 1996). In some ways, risks from medication trials may be easier to identify than risks from psychosocial treatments or service interventions. For example, the risks from medication treatment trials may include dizziness, sleeplessness, tics, and heart palpitations, whereas most often the risks from participation in psychosocial treatment trials are harder to quantify or predict. Nevertheless, they must be considered and included in the informed consent protocol. Such possibilities as memory flashbacks, transient discomforts, and increased restlessness or anxiety through exposure to memories or events may be among the risks associated with participation in psychosocial treatment trials.

The other side of the risk coin, however, is that the lack of a scientifically valid and useful knowledge base about effective psychosocial treatments for children and adolescents has created a situation wherein millions of children are exposed to treatments or interventions everyday in schools, mental health clinics, or other service venues for which there is no evidence whatsoever of their impact. In fact, most estimates of the percentage of programs for youths who receive public mental health services through either the mental health, welfare, education, or justice systems indicate that upward of 90% of such programs have no evidence to support their impact, and some, in fact, are known to be harmful (Bickman, 2008; Burns & Hoagwood, 2004, 2005; U.S. DHHS, 1999). The ethics of a public mental health system that delivers untested clinical services and treatments should certainly be called into question.

Placebos

Concerns about the use of placebos have been voiced for decades. Foremost among these is the argument that the ethical duty of clinical investigators is to avoid harm and that placebo arms, by definition, promote risk by providing no treatment at all for a period of time. This argument is at the core of the World Medical Association's (WMA; 2000) revision of the Declaration of Helsinki, which argues that clinical research involves an ethical obligation of investigators to conduct research based on the therapeutic value for the participants.

The WMA first developed the Declaration of Helsinki in 1964 as a statement to guide physicians and others in medical research involving human subjects. The declaration contains a series of statements about what ought and ought not to occur in medical research (WMA, 2000). In 2000, the WMA issued a revision tightening its stance against the use of placebos by stating that in any medical trial all patients, including those in control conditions, must be assured of receiving an active treatment. In essence, this statement precluded the use of placebos in research. However, the statement aroused considerable controversy and discussion, including a major conference by the NIH in November 2000. In fall 2001, the WMA stated that, under certain circumstances, placebo-controlled trials could be ethically acceptable if sound methodological reasons were provided. The interpretation of this has yet to achieve any consensus internationally, and some countries (e.g., Brazil) continue to ban all placebo-controlled studies, while international groups such as the Canadian Institutes of Health Research and national organizations such as the American Academy of Child and Adolescent Psychiatry have held conferences to address the myriad ethical and clinical issues involved in using placebos in research.

Although questions about the ethical appropriateness of placebos arise more often in pharmacological treatment trials than in studies of psychosocial treatments, the principles are the same: Withholding treatments for children who have clear treatment needs and for whom an effective treatment exists creates an ethical problematic. However, use of placebo treatment arms is also one of the strongest scientific strategies for demonstrating treatment impact vis-à-vis nonspecific factors (e.g., attention). The issues investigators must weigh in deciding in favor of or against inclusion of a placebo arm include the appropriateness of comparison treatments for the population to be studied (e.g., has it only been used with adults?), the status of the scientific evidence supporting alternative treatments (e.g., is the support for alternative treatments reasonably commensurate with one another?), and the nature of the research questions being examined. Improvements in designs can also provide additional protections, as described by Charney (2000) and Baldwin et al. (2003).

It is also important to note that high-risk protocols that involve placebo arms may require special preparation to incorporate into consent forms or other research materials the perspectives of families or other stakeholders. Further discussion of the models for establishing formal means of enlisting community stakeholder perspectives is provided later.

Deception

The use of deception is another ethically laden issue that has several historical precedents, including the Public Health Service Syphilis Study, in which treatment was purposely withheld from participants in order to study the natural progression of syphilis, and Milgram's Obedience Study, in which subjects thought they were administering sometimes lethal shocks to actors posing as students when they answered incorrectly in order to understand deference to authority. The use of deception, particularly with research involving children, is controversial because these studies involve a falsification of information on which potential subjects base their decision to participate, and runs counter to children's expectations and beliefs that they are assenting to a particular study and associated procedures. Further, debriefing, which is a standard safeguard in deception research, can actually increase harm to the children greater than the deception itself, because telling children they were mislead can lead to mistrust of adults, or the children may refuse to believe that they were deceived or may be forced to confront aspects of themselves in the research trial (e.g., participating in cheating or becoming angry or upset) that they otherwise would not be confronted with (Fisher, 2005).

When using deception in research involving children, Fisher (2005) recommends asking children whether they would still participate if they were put in situations that reflected poorly on their behavior and that adults would know about or warning them that deception might be used in the study, although disclosing this information compromises methodological aspects of the study (e.g., the validity of data that is collected) because the children know that they may be deceived and thus may act differently than they would if they were unaware.

Engaging Families, Youth, and Community Stakeholders

Because the issues about the weighing of relative risks and benefits depend in large measure on community norms, and because federally funded studies must demonstrate adequate representation of the population diversity that exists within the communities being examined, a growing number of studies are establishing formal means of incorporating community perspectives into the research protocol. In fact, some researchers have called such inclusion the only means of ensuring that an ethical compact exists (Jensen, Hoagwood, & Trickett, 1999). There are a variety of ways in which community or stakeholder perspectives can be incorporated into research studies, from advising to collaborating in the design and implementation of the study (Brody et al., 2005), and many of the more robust models have arisen from work within the HIV/AIDS community. For example, McKay and colleagues have adapted an advisory board model from an HIV prevention program to their work with families of youths with mental illnesses (McKay & Paikoff, 2007). In mental health care, collaborative models for involving community leaders or other relevant stakeholders, such as parents of youths with mental health issues, are being used increasingly to gain traction and improve the sustainability of effective practices (Hoagwood & Horwitz, 2009; Hoagwood, Jensen, McKay, & Olin, in press). These approaches often involve the establishment of a community advisory board composed of parents or caretakers of youths with mental illnesses and community stakeholders, case managers, or policymakers. These boards are actively engaged in every phase of the research project, from its inception (including design, selection of measures, recruitment, implementation) to the final dissemination of the results.

Another model for enlisting community collaboration in research studies entails the involvement of special consultants with knowledge of the values, attitudes, or perspectives of the community in which the project will be carried out. These expert consultants may be involved at any phase of the project to provide advice and guidance about the suitability or acceptability of designs, measures, or recruitment of vulnerable populations. Often they are included on a scientific advisory board and meet once or twice a year to provide input into these issues as the study is designed and conducted. This model is less intense and elicits far less substantive guidance about the perspectives of stakeholders, but it is a more common model selected by investigators, in part because it seems to be less time consuming and intrusive to the overall objectives of the scientific enterprise. However, those perceptions may well be false. A number of recently launched large clinical trials have encountered serious obstacles to recruitment and acceptance of the study in a range of communities because the investigators failed to include in a substantive way community input into the design and conduct of the study from the beginning. In addition, there is no evidence to suggest that the involvement of community perspectives will undermine the scientific validity of the study; to the contrary, some have argued that this is the only way to create an ethically valid and grounded science base (Hoagwood & Horwitz, 2009; Jensen, Hoagwood, & Trickett, 1999).

One question that often arises in either of these models, however, is the extent to which any individual person or group of persons can realistically "speak" for a "community." In fact, the notion of what constitutes a community is itself controversial (Fisher et al., 2002). However, it behooves the would-be investigator to attempt to understand the context in which the study is to occur, and often this will entail special attention to the perspectives of those who will be the ultimate beneficiaries of the outcomes of the study (i.e., the families, caseworkers, providers, administrators, or policymakers in the community where the treatment will or can be provided).

Beyond consideration of community perspectives in the design and conduct of treatment studies, there are those who have argued that research subjects themselves are best seen as active collaborators in the research process (Attkisson, Rosenblatt, & Hoagwood, 1996; Conroy & Harcourt, 2009; Hoagwood & Horwitz, 2009). The relationship between investigators and research participants is most respectful when it is structured as a collaborative partnership. This stance requires that participants be fully informed about the risks and benefits of the study, that they understand that the partnership is voluntary, and that they can discontinue participation at any time. This role of the research participants as actively engaged in the study, as collaborators, contrasts to the passive stance that has typically described much medical research in the past.

Models of research–participant collaboration between researchers and children and adolescents have also been proposed as a means to maximize investment in the research, facilitate informed consent, and gain insight into palatable studies for these populations (Conroy & Harcourt, 2009; Fisher, 1996). As Attkisson et al. (1996) point out, the role of research participants as collaborators is an ideal that is never fully realized in any study; there are numerous obstacles to it. The principles of collaboration, whether directed at community stakeholders or at research participants themselves, are especially important in studies involving psychosocial treatments for children and adolescents in part because profound misunderstandings of what constitutes mental illnesses and misperceptions about the need for and consequences of treatments have created a climate wherein distrust and suspicion about research and researchers abound. These are compounded by widespread ignorance about the goals of science, what evidence-based practice is, and the reasons why application of research findings to practice is needed. Direct and open communication among stakeholders and researchers will not be a panacea, but it is probably an essential element for creating an ethical and valid science base on psychosocial treatments for youths.

Providing Clinical Feedback: The Therapeutic Dilemma

The Blueprint Report of the NIMH (National Advisory Mental Health Council's Workgroup, 2001) called for an increase in the number of studies of treatment efficacy, effectiveness, and process for children and adolescents with mental disorders. In the past 5 years, the number of pediatric trials of treatments—both pharmacological and psychological—has quadrupled. Expansion of child and adolescent treatment trials is expected to continue, in large part because of the urgency of the public health need for scientific knowledge about effective interventions. In addition, however, there is an increasing interest in studies that attend to issues of treatment process, not only outcome. Such studies are essential if the active ingredients that lead to therapeutic change are to be discovered.

For psychosocial treatment researchers, especially those involved in long-term treatment studies, issues about the extent of investigators' responsibility to inform subjects about their progress or about comorbid conditions can arise. The appropriateness of providing feedback is generally thought to depend on the research goal and the definition of clinical services. For example, one IRB ruled that because information about a participant was obtained by nonclinicians (i.e., graduate students), it was not clinical and thus no obligation existed to inform the participant about treatment needs or to refer the participant for treatment. However, some standards of clinical responsibility suggest that any investigator undertaking a treatment research project is simultaneously agreeing to either provide appropriate intervention when needed or refer the participant to another resource (Fisher, 1996).

Using Incentives

Recruitment for participation involves consideration of several questions in advance. How significant are the study's aims? Why are particular populations, especially if they are vulnerable populations, needed for answering the questions of interest? Can the study be conducted on less vulnerable populations first? For studies supported by public health funds, there is a public health responsibility to ensure that the highest quality of science is supported and that only issues of genuine importance are targeted for such studies (Hyman, 1999).

Incentives for research participation need to be considered with respect to two issues: respect for the participants' time and compensation for such and lack of coercion (Roberts, 1998). Investigators working with populations that are socioeconomically disadvantaged have special responsibilities to ensure that access to both research benefits and risks are not unfairly distributed. Once again, the establishment of community advisory boards can be helpful in ascertaining the community's perceptions of risks associated with recruitment and the types of recruitment strategies that may be viewed as coercive. Perceptions of risk and coercion vary enormously according to cultural norms, previous experiences that members of a community may have had with research, and attitudes toward different kinds of treatments or services (e.g., concerns about medications and risk; concerns about custody and how disclosure about a child's behavior might affect one's rights as a parent).

Monetary incentives provided to research participants, may be viewed as inducements that are deemed to be fair compensation for one's time. On the other hand, such compensation can also be viewed as coercive in some communities, because it may be seen as offering inducements that are outside the bounds of convention and that will be used to manipulate rather than compensate. The perceptions of the ways in which monetary inducements may be viewed within particular community contexts need to be carefully considered by investigators before designing a study. Community advisory boards can be helpful in reflecting back to investigators the community values, expectations, and beliefs about incentives.

Ensuring Confidentiality

Research on psychosocial treatments for children and adolescents may involve divulging sensitive information about a child or family that may not have been previously revealed to others or that could be harmful if discovered. Ethical considerations about recruitment and consent can provide important safeguards against the revelation of confidential information, but additional protections are needed to ensure that information remain confidential. Investigators are obligated to ensure that information collected during a research protocol is not divulged to others in a manner inconsistent with the participant's understanding. Procedures for protecting confidentiality must ensure that a participant retains control over what is shared and to whom (Fisher, 1996).

Routine procedures for maintaining confidentiality of data include the use of subject codes rather than identifiers, secure storage, limited access to data, disposal of unnecessary identifying information, and appropriate supervision of research personnel. With newer technologies available for protecting electronic information, but with the additional risks that electronic transmission poses, investigators must be especially cautious to ensure that identifiable information collected during research projects is safeguarded.

The Certificate of Confidentiality is a federally sponsored document that provides immunity to investigators from any governmental or civil order to disclose identifying information from research records. The certificate is granted under §301(d) of the Public Health Service Act. The certificate provides additional protection against disclosure of confidential information to outside parties. When a Certificate of Confidentiality is granted, both its protections and its limitations should be explained to the child and caregiver. The application for the certificate can be obtained by most federal research institutions.

Other Special Considerations and Strategies

Roberts (1998) has developed a process for helping investigators develop protocols to ensure that ethically important research elements—design, informed consent, and assurances of confidentiality, for example—explicitly deal with human subject protections. The Research Protocol Ethics Assessment Tool is an evaluative checklist for use with participants who may have mental health problems. Although not designed to be used with child and adolescent populations, it can be useful for investigators who wish to ensure that key aspects of the research project are adhering to the highest ethical standards (Roberts & Dyer, 2004).

Other resources exist for investigators seeking guidance about obtaining informed consent. In 1998 the NIH convened a conference to provide practical advice to IRBs on issues related to involving individuals with questionable capacity to consent. A summary of the conference is available from the NIH (Expert Panel Report, 1998). Finally, the NIH now requires all investigators and key personnel seeking funding for research to obtain and document evidence of continuing education in the protection of human subjects, although discretion is left to each institution to provide a sufficient training program. The requirement for such is described in the NIH (2000) guide.

SUMMARY AND CONCLUSIONS

It is as unethical to conduct studies that have not ensured adequate human subject protections as it is to withhold examination of treatments from children who need them. Creating an ethically grounded science base requires more than attending to the jots and tittles within legally grounded regulations or guidelines. It requires principled commitment to the intrinsic value of science and to the belief that no harm must ensue from participation in research. It requires attention to the values, histories, and beliefs of the culture or the community into which the researchers enter. These are principles that need thoughtful consideration at the beginning of investigations, not at the end.

As noted in the Surgeon General's Report on Mental Health (U.S. Department of Health and Human Services, 1999), research on the efficacy and effectiveness of treatments and other mental health services for children and adolescents lags far behind the adult field and remains one of the most significant public health arenas in which to advance the health of the nation's children. However, the task of constructing designs that will provide adequate safeguards against potential harm is complex and requires deliberate attention to a range of issues. As has been described in this chapter, these include ensuring that truly informed consent has been obtained from the participants. What constitutes understanding of a study has yet to be fully examined scientifically, but the elements involved in consent include capacity, understanding, reasoning, and ability to express choices. If children or adolescents with limited cognitive abilities are part of a research population, then procedures must be in place to ensure that a guardian, caretaker, or independent professional with the best interests of the child in mind can make that decision.

Striking a balance between the benefits that can accrue to individuals or to society as a whole through research versus the potential harm from participating in a particular study requires that investigators carefully consider the varieties of harm, both direct and indirect, that may ensue as well as the varieties of potential benefit. The primary standpoint from which such decisions are made is that of research participants, not the investigators or institutions. Designs can often be constructed that will maximize benefit and minimize harm, such as the use of active treatment comparisons.

Consideration of issues such as the use of monetary incentives often rests on the values implicit within the particular community, neighborhood, or setting in which the study is to be carried out. Such consideration can often benefit from guidance provided by community leaders, families of children with mental health problems, or stakeholders. Models of ways to establish formal means of enlisting such guidance are being used in a variety of studies on HIV/AIDS, chronic physical illnesses, and, more recently, childhood mental illnesses. Beyond obtaining consultation from community stakeholders, however, the active participation of persons who represent the perspectives of the ultimate beneficiaries of science augments the validity and generalizability of the findings and, most importantly, provides an ethical grounding by which to determine whether the findings are intrinsically important and meaningful or can be relegated to dusty academic shelves.

Although the challenges to conducting research on psychosocial treatments for youth may appear daunting, the alternative, which is the status quo for the majority of children in the public mental health system—namely to provide untested or even harmful treatments or services—is simply untenable. From a public health standpoint, scientific knowledge about the impact of treatments and their delivery, especially in real-world service settings, are urgently needed, and the pace of implementation must be accelerated. The ethical principles that undergird this urgency extend beyond those described in the Belmont Report. In addition to ensuring that research participants experience no harm (beneficence) and are treated respectfully (respect) and equitably (justice), one can add a higher order principle: namely that the rational generation and transformation of the knowledge base must be ceaseless. It is through constant examination, reexamination, analysis, and reanalysis that the self-correcting process of science, as a method for generating both knowledge as well as uncertainty, can be sustained.

REFERENCES

Appelbaum, P. S. (2007). Assessment of patients' competence to consent to treatment. *New Eng land Journal of Medicine, 357*, 1834–1840.

Attkisson, C. C., Rosenblatt, A., & Hoagwood, K. (1996). Research ethics and human subjects protection in child mental health services research and community studies. In K. Hoagwood, P. S. Jensen, & C. B. Fisher (Eds.), *Ethical issues in mental health research with children and adolescents* (pp. 43–58). Mahwah, NJ: Erlbaum.

Baldwin, D., Broich, K., Fritze, J., Kasper, S., Westernberg, H., & Moller, H. J. (2003). Placebo controlled studies in depression: Necessary, ethical and feasible. *European Archives of Psychiatry and Clinical Neuroscience, 253*, 22–28.

Bhatara, V., Feil, M., Hoagwood, K., Vitiello, B., & Zima, B. (2002). Trends in combined pharmacotherapy with stimulants for children. *Psychiatric Services, 53*, 244–245.

Bickman, L. (2008). Why don't we have effective mental health services? *Administration in Policy in Mental Health and Mental Health Services Research, 35*, 437–439.

Brody, B. A., McCullough, L. B., & Sharp, R. R. (2005). Consensus and controversy in clinical research. *Journal of the American Medical Association, 294*, 1411–1414.

Bruzzese, J. M., & Fisher, C. B. (2003). Assessing and enhancing the research consent capacity of children and youth. *Applied Developmental Science, 7*, 13–26.

Burns, B. J., & Hoagwood, K. (2004). Evidence-based practices: Part I. A research update. *Child and Adolescent Psychiatric Clinics of North America, 13*, xi–xiii.

Burns, B. J., & Hoagwood, K. (2005). Evidence-based practices: Part II. Effecting change. *Child and Adolescent Psychiatric Clinics of North America, 14*, 241–254.

Charney, D. S. (2000). The use of placebos in randomized clinical trials of mood disorders: Well justified, but improvements in design are indicated. *Biological Psychiatry, 47*, 687–688.

Collogan, L. K., & Fleischman, A. R. (2005). Adolescent research and parental permission. In E. Kodish (Ed.), *Ethics and research with children: A case-based approach* (pp. 77–99). New York: Oxford University Press.

Conroy, H., & Harcourt, D. (2009). Informed agreement to participants: Beginning the partnership with children in research. *Early Child Development and Care, 179*, 157–165.

Department of Health and Human Services. (1991a). *Protection of human subjects. Basic HHS policy for protection of human research subjects. Code of Federal Regulations, Title 45, Public Welfare: Part 46, Subpart A: 46.101-46.124.* Washington, DC: Office of the Federal Register, National Archives and Records Administration.

Department of Health and Human Services. (1991b). *Protection of human subjects, Subpart D: Additional protections for children involved as subjects in research, Code of Federal Regulations, Title 45,*

Public Welfare: Part 46, Subpart D: 46.401-46.409. Washington, DC: Office of the Federal Register, National Archives and Records Administration.

Dunn, L. B., Candilis, P. J., & Roberts, L. W. (2006). Emerging empirical evidence on the ethics of schizophrenia research. *Schizophrenia Bulletin, 32,* 47–68.

English, A. (1991). Runaway and street youth at risk for HIV infections: Legal and ethical issues in access to care: Homeless youth [Special issue]. *Journal of Adolescent Health, 12,* 504–510.

Expert Panel Report to the National Institutes of Health. (1998). *Research involving individuals with questionable capacity to consent: Ethical issues and practical considerations for institutional review boards (IRBs).* Washington, DC: National Institutes of Health.

Fisher, C. B. (1996). Casebook on ethical issues in research on child and adolescent mental disorders. In K. Hoagwood, P. Jensen, & C. B. Fisher (Eds.), *Ethical issues in child and adolescent mental health research* (pp. 135–166). Mahwah, NJ: Erlbaum.

Fisher, C. B. (2004). Informed consent and clinical research involving children and adolescents: Implications of the revised APA Ethics Code and HIPAA. *Journal of Clinical Child and Adolescent Psychology, 33,* 832–839.

Fisher, C. B. (2005). Deception research involving children: Ethical practices and paradoxes. *Ethics and Behaviors, 15,* 271–287.

Fisher, C. B., Hoagwood, K., Duster, R., Frank, D. A., Grisso, T., Levine, R. J., et al. (2002). Research ethics for mental health science involving ethnic minority children and youth. *American Psychologist, 57,* 1024–1040.

Hoagwood, K. E., & Horwitz, S. M. (2009). Balancing science and services: The challenges and rewards of research. In A. R. Stiffman (Ed.), *The field research survival guide* (pp. 3–22). New York: Oxford University Press.

Hoagwood, K., Jensen, P. S., & Fisher, C. (Eds.). (1996). *Ethical issues in child and adolescent mental health research.* Mahwah, NJ: Erlbaum.

Hoagwood, K., Jensen, P. S., & Leshner, A. I. (1997). Ethical issues in research on child and adolescent mental disorders: Implications for a science of scientific ethics. In S. W. Henggeler & A. B. Santos (Eds.), *Innovative approaches for difficult-to-treat populations* (pp. 459–476). Washington, DC: American Psychiatric Press.

Hoagwood, K., Jensen, P. S., McKay, M., & Olin, S. (in press). *Children's mental health research: The power of partnerships.* New York: Oxford University Press.

Hyman, S. E. (1999). Protecting patients, preserving progress: Ethics in mental health research. *Academic Medicine, 74,* 258–259.

Icenogle, D. L. (2003). IRBs, conflict and liability: Will we see IRBs in court and when? *Clinical Medicine and Research, 1,* 63–68.

Jensen, P. S., Bhatara, V., Vitiello, B., Hoagwood, K., Feil, M., & Burke, L. B. (1999). Psychoactive medication prescribing practices for U.S. children: Gaps between research and clinical practice. *Journal of the American Academy of Child and Adolescent Psychiatry, 38,* 557–565.

Jensen, P. S., Hoagwood, K., & Trickett, E. (1999). Ivory tower or earthen trenches?: Community collaborations to foster real-world research. *Journal of Applied Developmental Science, 3,* 206–212.

Lidz, C. W., Appelbaum, P. S., Grisso, T., & Renaud, M. (2004). Therapeutic misconception and the appreciation of risks in clinical trials. *Social Science and Medicine, 58,* 1689–1697.

McKay, M., & Paikoff, R. (Eds.). (2007). *Community collaborative partnerships: The foundation for HIV prevention research efforts in the United States and internationally.* West Hazleton, PA: Haworth Press.

Munir, K., & Earls, F. (1992). Ethical principles governing research in child and adolescent psychiatry. *Journal of the American Academy of Child and Adolescent Psychiatry, 31,* 408–414.

National Advisory Mental Health Council's Workgroup Report on Child and Adolescent Mental Health Intervention Development and Deployment. (2001). *Blueprint for change: Research on child and adolescent mental health.* Bethesda, MD: National Institute of Mental Health.

National Bioethics Advisory Commission. (1998). *Research involving persons with mental disorders that may affect decisionmaking capacity.* Retrieved January 1, 2000, from *www.bioethics.gov.*

National Commission for the Protection of Human Subjects of Biomedical and Behavioral Research. (1979). *The Belmont Report: Ethical principles and guidelines for the protection of human subjects of research.* Washington, DC: U.S. Government Printing Office.

National Institute of Mental Health. (2009). *Ethics in mental health research.* Retrieved May 1, 2009, from *www.emhr.net.*

National Institutes of Health. (2000). *Required education in the protection of human research participants* (NIH guide OD-00-039). Retrieved April 27, 2009, from *grants.nih.gov/grants/guide/notice-files/NOT-OD-00-039.html.*

National Institutes of Health. (2009). *Research on ethical issues in human subjects research* (NIH guide PA-07-277). Retrieved April 27, 2009, from *grants.nih.gov/grants/guide/pa-files/PA-07-277.html.*

Roberts, L. W. (1998). Ethics of psychiatric research: Conceptual issues and empirical findings. *Comprehensive Psychiatry, 39,* 99–110.

Roberts, L. W., & Dyer, A. D. (2004). *Concise guide to ethics in mental health care.* Arlington, VA: American Psychiatric Publishing.

U.S. Department of Health and Human Services. (1999). *Mental health: A report of the surgeon general.* Rockville, MD: U.S. Department of Health and Human Services, Substance Abuse and Mental Health Services Administration.

Vitiello, B. (2002). Ethical issues in pediatric psychopharmacology research. In D. R. Rosenberg, P. A. Davanzo, & S. Gershon (Eds.), *Pharmacotherapy for Child and Adolescent Psychiatric Disorders* (2nd ed., pp. 7–22). New York: Marcel Dekker.

Vitiello, B., Jensen, P. S., & Hoagwood, K. (1999). Integrating science and ethics in child and adolescent psychiatry research. *Biological Psychiatry, 46,* 1044–1049.

World Medical Association. (2000). *Declaration of Helsinki: Ethical principles for medical research involving human subjects.* Retrieved August 12, 2009, from *www.wma.net/e/policy/pdf/17c.pdf.*

Yan, E. G., & Munir, K. M. (2004). Regulatory and ethical principles in research involving children and individuals with developmental disabilities. *Ethics and Behavior, 14,* 31–49.

3

Developmental Issues and Considerations in Research and Practice

GRAYSON N. HOLMBECK, KATIE A. DEVINE, and ELIZABETH F. BRUNO

Suppose that a 6-year-old and a 16-year-old are referred for problematic levels of aggressive behavior. Although the presenting symptoms for the two children may be similar, it is unlikely that identical treatments could be provided with equivalent effectiveness to both children. Multiple developmental differences between children of different ages would likely necessitate the use of different assessment and treatment strategies. Even the degree to which such behaviors are viewed as problematic would vary as a function of age. Unfortunately, we know little about how or when a given treatment should be modified for use with children functioning at different developmental levels. That is, the proposition that treatment outcomes for children and adolescents will be enhanced if clinicians attend to developmental issues is largely an untested assumption. On the other hand, it is our contention that the effectiveness of child and adolescent treatments will be improved if treatment is tailored to the developmental level of the target child, although we acknowledge that more research is needed on this issue (Holmbeck, O'Mahar, Abad, Colder, & Updegrove, 2006; Kingery et al., 2006; Shirk, 2001; Silverman & Ollendick, 1999; Weisz & Hawley, 2002).

The goal of this chapter is to discuss ways that developmental issues can be incorporated into the treatment of children and adolescents. First, we examine the degree to which developmental issues have been considered in the design and implementation of child psychotherapy. Evidence that treatment effects vary as a function of age and developmental level is reviewed. Second, we discuss how developmental level can serve as a moderator or a mediator of treatment effects on outcome. Third, we argue that knowledge of certain developmental issues will likely improve the quality of treatment manuals and the effectiveness of child psychotherapy. Finally, we provide recommendations for therapists and researchers who wish to incorporate development into their work.

PAST WORK ON DEVELOPMENTAL ISSUES AND PSYCHOLOGICAL TREATMENTS

Developmental Level and Treatment Outcome: Studies of Adolescents

In this section, we target literature reviews on the developmental sensitivity of treatments for adolescents, given that comprehensive reviews from a developmental perspective have not yet been conducted for other age groups. Holmbeck, O'Mahar, and colleagues (2006) conducted a review of recent treatment outcome studies employing cognitive-behavioral treatments (CBT) with adolescents. It was encouraging that approximately 70% of the empirical articles reviewed mentioned developmental issues when designing and evaluating the treatments. This percentage contrasts sharply with our earlier review of the literature from 1990–1998 (Holmbeck et al., 2000), where the percentage of empirical articles that focused on developmental issues was 26%. Specifically, two of nine (22%) empirical articles in our 2000 review considered issues relevant to parent involvement, but by 2006 this number grew to 10 of 20 (50%) articles. Although none of the studies in the 2000 review included treatments that focused on the contexts in which adolescents interact (i.e., family, peer, school), three of the 20 studies in the 2006 review focused on contexts.

Although these findings are encouraging, less than half of the studies in the 2006 review that included a discussion of development interpreted research findings in relation to developmental issues (33% in the 2000 review; 25% in the 2006 review). Also, very few studies in either review used a developmental variable as a moderator of treatment effects (one of nine in the 2000 review; two of nine in the 2006 review). In the 2006 review, age was the moderator in both instances. The failure to use developmental markers as moderators of treatment effectiveness was also noted in Weisz and Hawley's (2002) review of the larger literature on interventions with adolescents (i.e., only 6% of the studies they reviewed used age as a moderator even though all of the studies included information on participants' ages). There was also an apparent drop in the percentage of studies in which the treatment was developed via consideration of developmental issues (56% in the 2000 review; 35% in the 2006 review). Although many authors suggest possible adaptations of treatment manuals to make them more developmentally sensitive, few provide methods for doing so (Weisz & Hawley, 2002; for an exception, see Kingery et al., 2006). Several authors recommend that therapists assess adolescents' cognitive developmental level; again, however, little advice has been forthcoming for how to do this. Clearly, the integration of the developmental psychology and treatment literatures remains a challenge.

In their comprehensive review of the literature on the treatment of adolescents, Weisz and Hawley (2002) examined 25 empirically supported psychotherapies that have been used with children and adolescents. According to these authors, 14 of the 25 therapies have been shown to be effective with adolescents. Interestingly, seven are downward adaptations of treatments originally designed for adults and six are upward adaptations of treatments originally designed for children, leaving only one that was developed specifically for adolescents. In other words, few of the 14 empirically supported treatments that have been used with adolescents were designed with a focus on the primary developmental tasks of adolescence.

Developmental Level and Treatment Outcome: Meta-Analyses

Although recognition of the importance of developmental factors has increased, few researchers who evaluate treatment outcomes actually include specific measures of cognitive developmental level in their research protocols (see Owens et al., 2003, who used child IQ as a moderator). Therefore, meta-analysts have not had access to data from measures of developmental level and have chosen to rely on age as a proxy for cognitive or overall developmental level (e.g., Weisz, McCarty, & Valeri, 2006). However, there are disadvantages to using age as a proxy for cognitive developmental level, because cognitive development is heterogeneous even within the same age group.

Meta-analyses focused on age (as a proxy for cognitive developmental level) have generally shown greater effect sizes for psychotherapy with preadolescents and adolescents compared with children (but see Weisz, McCarty, & Valeri, 2006). These results fit well with the idea that the main components of CBT and other cognitive therapies require more complex, symbolic, abstract, metacognitive (i.e., the ability to think about one's own thinking), consequential (i.e., the ability to reflect on the outcomes of a particular pattern of thinking), and hypothetical thinking consistent with the greater cognitive sophistication of adolescents (Grave & Blissett, 2004; Holmbeck, O'Mahar, et al., 2006).

DEVELOPMENTAL LEVEL AS A MEDIATOR AND MODERATOR OF TREATMENT EFFECTIVENESS

In this section, we explain differences between mediator and moderator effects (see Baron & Kenny, 1986; Holmbeck, 1997; Kraemer, Kiernan, Essex, & Kupfer, 2008). A moderator is a variable that specifies conditions under which a given predictor is or is not related to an outcome (see Figure 3.1, top). For example, it may be that the impact of a given intervention on a given outcome varies as a function of some moderator (e.g., developmental level, age, gender, social class). In this way, the treatment may be more effective at one level of the moderator than at another. A significant mediator is a variable that specifies a mechanism by which a predictor has an impact on an outcome (see Figure 3.1, bottom). With mediation, the predictor (e.g., treatment condition) is associated with the mediator (e.g., change in developmental level), which is, in turn, associated with the outcome (e.g., adjustment). The mediator accounts for a significant portion of the relationship between predictor and outcome.

Developmental Level as a Moderator

By examining moderators of treatment effectiveness, we are interested in isolating conditions that determine when a treatment is particularly effective or ineffective (see Figure 3.1; e.g., Owens et al., 2003). One relevant moderator that is expected to have an impact on effectiveness is cognitive-developmental level (Bierman, Nix, Greenberg, Blair, & Domitrovich, 2008).

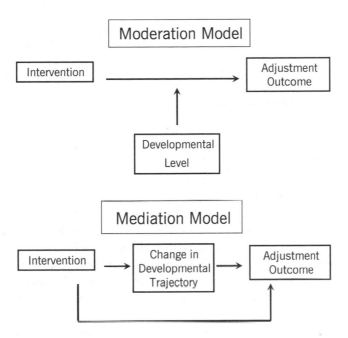

FIGURE 3.1. Moderation (top) and mediation (bottom) models of treatment outcome: The potential role of developmental level.

Although there is general agreement that a shift in thinking occurs during the transition from childhood to adolescence, theorists have described these changes in different ways, which may influence which factors are attended to in any given treatment. Piaget (1972) identified adolescence as the period in which formal operational thinking typically emerges. Adolescents who have achieved such abilities are able to think more complexly, abstractly, and hypothetically as well as take the perspective of others and use future-oriented thinking. Critics of the Piagetian approach have suggested alternatives. Proponents of the information-processing perspective, for example, suggest that specific changes in processing capacity or efficiency, knowledge base, and cognitive self-regulation account for advances in thinking (Keating, 1990). Alternatively, Vygotsky (1978) suggested that psychological processes have a social basis, focusing on children's socially relevant cognitions. This social-contextual perspective aligns closely with Erikson's belief that developmental processes are driven by the interaction between a child and the social and cultural world (Erikson, 1950). Specifically, the development of social-emotional competencies such as role taking and empathy skills, the understanding of moral issues, the role of affect in understanding people, attributional processes in social situations, the establishment of a personal identity, and prosocial behavior are a few of the social-cognitive-developmental tasks that may influence progress with interventions.

Given this list of cognitive changes during childhood and adolescence, it seems reasonable to propose that the degree to which a child has developed these skills will enhance or limit the potential effectiveness of a given psychotherapeutic intervention (Bierman et al., 2008; Ingram, Nelson, Steidtmann, & Bistrickly, 2007). It is even possible that more advanced cognitive abilities may exacerbate some types of psychopathology (e.g., depressogenic cognitions). Although a thorough review is beyond the scope of this chapter, several measures of cognitive development have been developed that may be relevant to therapy and treatment–outcome research.

Change in Developmental Level as a Mediator

Examining developmental level as a mediator addresses a different set of questions (see Figure 3.1). Once it is established that a given treatment affects a given outcome, researchers are likely to examine possible mechanisms by which the treatment affects the outcome of interest (Kazdin, 1997; Kendall & Treadwell, 2007). From this perspective, a mediator is assumed to account for at least a portion of the treatment effect. A mediator is viewed as causally antecedent to the outcome, such that change in the mediator is expected to be associated with subsequent changes in the outcome (Kraemer et al., 2008). In some cases, the mediator (rather than the adjustment outcome) may be the preferred target of treatment because of some known causal connection between the mediator and the outcome or a belief that the mediator is a necessary catalyst for change (e.g., negative self-statements could be a mediator of treatment effects; Kendall & Treadwell, 2007).

An important corollary of this discussion is that specific developmental constructs or processes (e.g., perspective taking, cognitive-developmental level, emotion regulation, and self-control) could be the focus of treatment (see Figure 3.1; Eyberg, Schuhmann, & Rey, 1998; Shirk, 1999). That is, if research suggests that children who have failed to master a certain developmental task or successfully navigate a specific developmental milestone are more likely to exhibit certain symptoms, such tasks and milestones could be the target of the intervention. For example, adolescents may benefit from treatment that initially focuses on changing or accelerating cognitive-developmental processes, particularly if lack of development in this domain has been linked with subsequent increases in symptoms.

Moderated mediation is also possible. For example, it may be that increased perspective taking is a significant mediator of treatment effectiveness for aggression, but only for adolescent participants. In this way, the mediational model is moderated by age. If one found such an effect, it might be that a different treatment is needed for younger children or that this treatment works for younger children but the mechanism by which it works differs across age. Alternately, both may be true; different treatments may be needed at different ages because the mediational mechanisms vary with age. Despite the plausibility of these speculations, it is important to note that time-limited child treatments may not have dramatic affects on development. One must also consider the possibility of multiple moderating factors in addition to developmental level influencing treatment outcomes. Further research is required to examine these hypotheses.

CONSIDERATION OF DEVELOPMENTAL FACTORS WHEN CONDUCTING THERAPY

Developmental Level and Milestones

In Table 3.1, we review important developmental stages and milestones that are relevant at different ages and developmental periods. One implication of this list of milestones is that therapists who work with children and adolescents may need to address not only

TABLE 3.1. Developmental Milestones and Stages across Childhood, Adolescence, and Emerging Adulthood

Age	Corresponding stage of cognitive development	Characteristics
Infancy: birth–2 years	Piaget's sensorimotor stage	• Infants explore world via direct sensory/motor contact • Emergence of emotions • Object permanence and separation anxiety develop • Critical attachment period: Secure parent–infant bond promotes trust and healthy growth of infant; insecure bond creates distrust and distress for infant • Initial use of sounds and words to communicate • Emerging comprehension of cause and effect
Toddler/ preschool: 2–6 years	Piaget's preoperational stage	• Use of multiple words, gestures, and symbols to communicate • Learns self-care skills, including toileting, feeding, cleaning • Mainly characterized by egocentricity, but preschoolers appreciate differences in perspectives of others • Use of imagination, engagement in symbolic play • Increasing sense of autonomy and control of environment • Moral reasoning is imposed from environment rather than internal intentions • Development of school readiness skills
School age: 6–10 years	Piaget's concrete operational stage	• Development of social, physical, and academic skills • Logical thinking and reasoning develops • Understanding of multiple perspectives • Increased interaction with peers • Increasing self-control and emotion regulation
Adolescence: 10–18 years	Piaget's formal operations stage	• Pubertal development; sexual development • Development of metacognition (i.e., thinking about one's own thinking) • Higher cognitive skills develop, including abstraction, consequential thinking, hypothetical reasoning, and perspective taking • Transformations in parent–child relations; increase in family conflicts • Peer relationships increasingly important and intimate • Making transition from childhood to young adulthood • Developing sense of identity and autonomous functioning, can lead to identity crisis
Emerging adulthood: 18–26 years	Continuation of Piaget's formal operations stage	• Establishment of meaningful and enduring interpersonal relationships • Identity explorations in areas of intimacy, work, and worldviews • Peak of certain risk behaviors • Obtaining education and training for long-term adult occupation

clients' presenting symptoms (e.g., attention-deficit/hyperactivity disorder [ADHD] and aggressiveness) but also the normative skills (e.g., self-control, emotion regulation) that may have failed to develop as a result of severe behavior problems. It is also clear that the context and targets of treatment are likely to change dramatically as one moves across the first two decades of life. For example, whereas cognitive factors and peer relationships are less relevant when applying parent training in families of preschool children, such factors become highly salient in the treatment of youths in middle childhood and adolescence (Forehand & Wierson, 1993). It is also important that therapists distinguish between recent traumatic events versus events that occurred during childhood that are now being revisited anew during adolescence. Indeed, treatment for a given trauma (e.g., early child abuse) may need to be administered intermittently at different critical periods as the original trauma is reexperienced at new developmental stages. Finally, another implication of the developmental milestones noted in Table 3.1 is that there is considerable interindividual and intraindividual variability with respect to each of these milestones and processes. That is, different children develop at different rates with respect to each of these milestones, and they will make developmental advances in each of these domains at different rates (e.g., perspective taking vs. emotion regulation). Thus, therapists should not assume that advances in one developmental domain are indicative of advances in others.

With respect to developmental level, Weisz and Weersing (1999) detailed ways in which cognitive-developmental level affects the process of therapy and the types of treatments selected. Children's cognitive-developmental level may limit (or enhance) their understanding of the purpose and process of therapy. Similarly, the degree to which children are able to use abstract reasoning or perspective-taking skills may determine, in part, whether certain cognitive or insight-oriented techniques as well as strategies that require hypothetical thinking (e.g., role-playing exercises) can be implemented.

Developmental Psychopathology

Developmental psychopathology is an extension of developmental psychology insofar as the former is concerned with variations in the course of normal development (Cicchetti & Rogosch, 2002; Holmbeck, Friedman, Abad, & Jandasek, 2006). Research based on a developmental psychopathology perspective has informed us about the developmental precursors and future outcomes of child and adolescent psychopathology. Moreover, the field of developmental psychopathology has provided us with a vocabulary with which to explain phenomena that are relevant to therapists and that researchers seek to explain empirically (e.g., risk and protective processes, cumulative risk factors, resilience, developmental trajectories; Cicchetti & Rogosch, 2002). Developmental psychopathologists have also informed us about boundaries between normal and abnormal and how such distinctions are often blurred at certain stages of development for certain symptoms (e.g., substance abuse vs. normative experimentation with substances during adolescence).

Research indicates that the frequency and nature of most disorders vary as a function of age. Scholars have documented important differences between those with early-onset problem behaviors versus those with later-onset problem behaviors. Interestingly, roughly half of all adolescent disorders are continuations of those seen in childhood (Rutter, 1980). Those that emerge anew during adolescence (e.g., anorexia) tend to be quite different than those that began during childhood (e.g., ADHD), with the symptomatology of most adolescent disorders being manifestations of problems a child has had navigating particular stages of development.

The terms equifinality, multifinality, and heterotypic continuity are also likely to be useful to clinicians who work with children and adolescents. Interestingly, it appears that equifinality and multifinality are more the rule than the exception (Cicchetti & Rogosch, 2002). Specifically, equifinality is the process by which a single disorder is produced via different developmental pathways. Multifinality involves the notion that the same developmental event may lead to different adjustment outcomes across different individuals (some adaptive, some maladaptive). Given past research support for the concepts of equifinality and multifinality (Cicchetti & Rogosch, 2002), it appears that therapists are best served by gathering as much developmental and historical information as possible about a given child. Put another way, if equifinality proves to be an adequate explanatory model for most child psychopathologies, then treatments that are based on single causal/mediational models will likely not be effective for sizable proportions of affected children (Cicchetti & Rogosch, 2002). Finally, heterotypic continuity involves the notion that a given pathological process will be exhibited differently with continued development. For example, behavioral expression of an underlying conduct disorder may change over time even though the underlying disorder and meaning of the behaviors remain relatively unchanged (Cicchetti & Rogosch, 2002). Thus, an understanding of developmental factors is important for assessing and conceptualizing the history of a presenting problem.

DIRECTIONS FOR PRACTICE AND FOR RESEARCH

In this section, we provide recommendations for therapists and researchers who seek to incorporate developmental principles into their work.

Recommendations for Therapists

1. *Stay current with the developmental literature.* It is recommended that therapists subscribe to journals such as *Development and Psychopathology, Child Development, Developmental Psychology, Developmental Neuropsychology, Journal of Consulting and Clinical Psychology,* and the *Journal of Research on Adolescence.* Interestingly, all of these journals regularly publish articles that examine clinical issues within a developmental context. Further, students would benefit from training programs that integrate their clinical–child programming with offerings from a developmental program. Continuing education workshops that focus on evidence-based developmentally sensitive interventions is another important way for clinicians to remain current.

2. *Consider cultural factors.* Cultural factors likely have an impact on how and when children and their families are referred for treatment as well as their attributions about the cause and meaning of problematic behaviors. Research on this topic is limited at this time, but there is increased recognition of the importance of cultural factors for diagnostic assessment and treatment (Barrett, 2000). Therefore, it is important to assess how children and parents view the children's behavior within the context of their culture and background, because these beliefs may influence their engagement in treatment and other factors related to treatment outcome.

3. *Use developmentally sensitive techniques.* Researchers who conduct interventions with young children (ages 4–8) often have success using techniques that incorporate videotape modeling strategies, play, or life-sized puppets rather than strict cognitive approaches. Many young children have difficulty distinguishing between different types of emotions; thus, drawings and pictures from media publications may be useful.

4. *Focus on developmental tasks and milestones that the child is attempting to master.* Although Weisz and Hawley (2002) argued that group trends that emerge in developmental research may not apply to a specific case, they provide useful suggestions for incorporating knowledge of developmental tasks into one's clinical work. First, they suggest using knowledge of developmental findings to identify specific domains of functioning that are likely salient at a given age. Second, therapists may prioritize certain presenting complaints over others depending on which are most developmentally atypical or pathological. Finally, therapists can use their knowledge to select treatment strategies or modules from a more comprehensive set of treatments that are developmentally appropriate for a given individual.

5. *When working with older children and adolescents, think multisystemically and consider the children's context.* Working with adolescents, Henggeler, Schoenwald, Borduin, Rowland, and Cunningham (1998) have documented the importance of attending to the multiple systems (family, peer, school) in which children interact. Incorporating peers or teachers as "therapists" in addition to parents may be a particularly useful strategy.

6. *Help parents (and other relevant adults such as teachers) to become developmentally sensitive.* Parents are likely to manage their children differently if they know, for example, that increases in parent–child conflict over certain issues is normative during the transition to adolescence than if they did not have this knowledge.

7. *To prevent exacerbation of symptomatology and maintain gains from successful therapy, anticipate future developmental tasks and milestones.* For example, therapists can discuss the normative tasks of adolescence with a family seeking treatment for a preadolescent. Discussing how such future tasks may affect a particular child with certain vulnerabilities can be helpful.

8. *Consider the concept of equifinality when conducting treatment.* As noted earlier, different developmental pathways may lead to the same psychopathological outcome. In keeping with this perspective, Shirk, Talmi, and Olds (2000) have suggested that treatment should not be guided exclusively by diagnostic status. Indeed, treatments may be unsuccessful for some children because the developmental precursors for their symptoms differ from those of symptoms for children exhibiting successful treatment outcomes.

9. *Consider alternative models of treatment delivery.* Kazdin (1997) provided a useful discussion of how different types of psychopathology may require different types of treatment delivery. Indeed, it is likely that most children will not derive maximum benefit from traditional time-limited treatment. Kazdin (1997) describes six such models of treatment delivery, which vary with respect to dosage, number of systems targeted, and degree to which the treatment is continuous or intermittent. He draws parallels between treatment for psychological symptoms and treatments for various medical conditions. For example, some psychopathologies may require continued care, much like ongoing treatment for diabetes, which is modified over time but never discontinued. Other psychopathologies may be best treated with a "dental model," where the child is monitored at regular intervals (particularly during important developmental transition points).

Recommendations for Researchers

1. *Know your disorder.* Before developing or evaluating a treatment, it is critical that investigators generate a thorough developmentally oriented conceptualization of the disorder in question. In this way, the investigators come to understand developmental antecedents in relation to the onset, maintenance, and escalation of the disorder, the developmental course of the symptoms, and any subtypes (Kazdin, 1997).

2. *Include measures of developmental level in treatment–outcome studies and use them to evaluate moderation effects.* If evaluations of age differences in treatment–outcome studies were to become the norm, this would be progress for the field. However, it would be even better if researchers began to include specific measures of developmental level. Examples of such variables would be cognitive-developmental level, pubertal development, social skills and friendship quality, emotion regulation and self-control, autonomy development, and change in parent–child relationships (see Table 3.1 for examples of characteristics that typically correspond to different ages). Researchers can document the developmentally sensitive modifications they make to their treatments so that these modifications can be evaluated and replicated (e.g., see Diamond et al., 2002). User-friendly measures of various cognitive-developmental constructs are sorely needed. Clinician-friendly measures of social perspective taking, empathy skills, self-control, future-oriented thinking, and decision making would have considerable utility, although paper-and-pencil measures may provide somewhat limited and less ecologically valid assessments of cognitive skills than would observations of real-life encounters.

3. *Examine mediators of treatment effects.* Knowledge of mediational processes inform us about mechanisms through which treatments have their effects (Bierman et al., 2008; Hinshaw, 2007). Developmentally oriented variables, such as those noted previously, could be examined as intervening causal mechanisms.

4. *Begin to examine the efficacy and effectiveness of alternative modes of treatment.* As noted by Kazdin (1997), most treatment–outcome studies examine time-limited interventions. As reviewed earlier, there are other ways that we can conduct our treatments (e.g., continued care, intervention followed by regular monitoring). The effectiveness of these strategies could be compared with traditional treatments.

5. *Build development into treatment strategies.* When discussing mediational effects, it was noted that developmental outcomes could be the target of treatment efforts. Change in these developmental mediators may then impact the primary treatment outcomes (Kraemer et al., 2008).

SUMMARY AND CONCLUSIONS

Although it appears that most treatments for children and adolescents are not developmentally oriented (because many of them are downward or upward extensions of treatments for individuals of ages other than the target population), there is great potential for the integration of developmental research with clinical practice. Ways in which developmental variables could serve as mediators or moderators of treatment effects were highlighted. We also reviewed various types of developmental research that could be informative for therapists who work with children and adolescents and for researchers who develop new treatments or evaluate existing ones. Knowledge of normative development can aid therapists in formulating appropriate treatment goals, provide a basis for designing alternate versions of the same treatment, and guide the stages of treatment.

We have also provided a number of recommendations for clinicians and researchers who wish to integrate developmental principles into their work. Despite increased attention to and understanding of developmental issues in treatment, the impact of adding developmentally sensitive strategies to treatment remains mostly untested at this point. Although developmentally adapted treatments exist, we lack a body of evidence demonstrating the improvements these treatments provide relative to treatment approaches that do not consider developmental level. One next step for treatment–outcome studies is to evaluate the impact of developmentally sensitive techniques as well as the potential moderating and mediating role of different aspects of development. We hope that this chapter will prompt greater attention to developmental factors from both researchers and clinicians.

ACKNOWLEDGMENTS

Completion of this chapter was supported in part by a research grant from the National Institute of Child Health and Human Development (No. R01-HD048629).

REFERENCES

Baron, R. M., & Kenny, D. A. (1986). The moderator–mediator variable distinction in social psychological research: Conceptual, strategic, and statistical considerations. *Journal of Personality and Social Psychology, 51,* 1173–1182.

Barrett, P. M. (2000). Treatment of childhood anxiety: Developmental aspects. *Clinical Psychology Review, 20,* 479–494.

Bierman, K. L., Nix, R. L., Greenberg, M. T., Blair, C., & Domitrovich, C. E. (2008). Executive functions and school readiness intervention: Impact, moderation, and mediation in the Head Start REDI program. *Development and Psychopathology, 20,* 821–843.

Cicchetti, D., & Rogosch, F. A. (2002). A developmental psychopathology perspective on adolescence. *Journal of Consulting and Clinical Psychology, 70,* 6–20.

Diamond, G., Godley, S. H., Liddle, H. A., Sampl, S., Webb, C., Tims, F. M., et al. (2002). Five outpatient treatment models for adolescent marijuana use: A description of the Cannabis Youth Treatment Interventions. *Addiction, 97,* 70–83.

Erikson, E. H. (1950). *Childhood and society.* New York: Norton.

Eyberg, S., Schuhmann, E., & Rey, J. (1998). Psychosocial treatment research with children and adolescents: Developmental issues. *Journal of Abnormal Child Psychology, 26,* 71–81.

Forehand, R., & Wierson, M. (1993). The role of developmental factors in planning behavioral interventions for children: Disruptive behavior as an example. *Behavior Therapy, 24,* 117–141.

Grave, J., & Blissett, J. (2004). Is cognitive behavior therapy developmentally appropriate for young children?: A critical review of the evidence. *Clinical Psychology Review, 24,* 399–420.

Henggeler, S. W., Schoenwald, S. K., Borduin, C. M., Rowland, M. D., & Cunningham, P. B. (1998). *Multisystemic treatment of antisocial behavior in children and adolescents.* New York: Guilford Press.

Hinshaw, S. P. (2007). Moderators and mediators of treatment outcome for youth with ADHD: Understanding for whom and how interventions work. *Journal of Pediatric Psychology, 32,* 664–675.

Holmbeck, G. N. (1997). Toward terminological, conceptual, and statistical clarity in the study of mediators and moderators: Examples from the child–clinical and pediatric psychology literatures. *Journal of Consulting and Clinical Psychology, 65,* 599–610.

Holmbeck, G. N., Colder, C., Shapera, W., Westhoven, V., Kenealy, L., & Updegrove, A. (2000). Working with adolescents: Guides from developmental psychology. In P. C. Kendall (Ed.), *Child and adolescent therapy: Cognitive-behavioral procedures* (pp. 334–385). New York: Guilford Press.

Holmbeck, G. N., Friedman, D., Abad, M., & Jandasek, B. (2006). Development and psychopathology in adolescence. In D. A. Wolfe & E. J. Mash (Eds.), *Behavioral and emotional disorders in adolescents: Nature, assessment, and treatment* (pp. 21–55). New York: Guilford Press.

Holmbeck, G. N., O'Mahar, K., Abad, M., Colder, C., & Updegrove, A. (2006). Cognitive-behavioral therapy with adolescents: Guides from developmental psychology. In P. C. Kendall (Ed.), *Child and adolescent therapy: Cognitive-behavioral procedures* (3rd ed., pp. 419–464). New York: Guilford Press.

Ingram, R. E., Nelson, T., Steidtmann, D. K., & Bistrickly, S. L. (2007). Comparative data on child and adolescent cognitive measures associated with depression. *Journal of Consulting and Clinical Psychology, 75,* 390–403.

Kazdin, A. E. (1997). A model for developing effective treatments: Progression and interplay of theory, research, and practice. *Journal of Clinical Child Psychology, 26,* 114–129.

Keating, D. P. (1990). Adolescent thinking. In S. S. Feldman & G. R. Elliott (Eds.), *At the threshold: The developing adolescent* (pp. 54–89). Cambridge, MA: Harvard University Press.

Kendall, P. C., & Treadwell, K. R. H. (2007). The role of self-statements as a mediator in treatment of youth with anxiety disorders. *Journal of Consulting and Clinical Psychology, 75,* 380–389.

Kingery, J. N., Roblek, T. L., Suveg, C., Grover, R. L., Sherrill, J. T., & Bergman, R. L. (2006). They're not just "little adults": Developmental considerations for implementing cognitive-behavioral therapy with anxious youth. *Journal of Cognitive Psychotherapy: An International Quarterly, 20,* 263–273.

Kraemer, H. C., Kiernan, M., Essex, M., & Kupfer, D. J. (2008). How and why criteria defining moderators and mediators differ between the Baron & Kenny and MacArthur approaches. *Health Psychology, 27(2,* Suppl.), S101–S108.

Owens, E. B., Hinshaw, S. P., Kraemer, H. C., Arnold, L. E., Abikoff, H. B., Cantwell, D. P., et al. (2003). Which treatment for whom for ADHD?: Moderators of treatment response in the MTA. *Journal of Consulting and Clinical Psychology, 71,* 540–552.

Piaget, J. (1972). Intellectual evolution from adolescence to adulthood. *Human Development, 15,* 1–12.

Rutter, M. (1980). *Changing youth in a changing society: Patterns of adolescent development and disorder.* Cambridge, MA: Harvard University Press.

Shirk, S. R. (1999). Developmental therapy. In W. K. Silverman & T. H. Ollendick (Eds.), *Developmental issues in the clinical treatment of children* (pp. 60–73). Boston: Allyn & Bacon.

Shirk, S. R. (2001). Development and cognitive therapy. *Journal of Cognitive Psychotherapy, 15,* 155–163.

Shirk, S., Talmi, A., & Olds, D. (2000). A developmental psychopathology perspective on child and adolescent treatment policy. *Development and Psychopathology, 12,* 835–855.

Silverman, W. K., & Ollendick, T. H. (Eds.). (1999). *Developmental issues in the clinical treatment of children.* Boston: Allyn & Bacon.

Vygotsky, L. (1978). *Mind in society: The development of higher psychological processes.* Cambridge, MA: Harvard University Press.

Weisz, J. R., & Hawley, K. M. (2002). Developmental factors in the treatment of adolescents. *Journal of Consulting and Clinical Psychology, 70,* 21–43.

Weisz, J. R., McCarty, C. A., & Valeri, S. M. (2006). Effects of psychotherapy for depression in children and adolescents: A meta-analysis. *Psychological Bulletin, 132,* 132–149.

Weisz, J. R., & Weersing, V. R. (1999). Developmental outcome research. In W. K. Silverman & T. H. Ollendick (Eds.), *Developmental issues in the clinical treatment of children* (pp. 457–469). Boston: Allyn & Bacon.

II

TREATMENTS AND PROBLEMS

A

Internalizing Disorders and Problems

4

Child-Focused Treatment of Anxiety

PHILIP C. KENDALL, JAMI M. FURR, and JENNIFER L. PODELL

OVERVIEW OF THE TREATMENT MODEL

Anxiety disorders are common in youths, with prevalence rates of 10–20% in the general population and primary care settings. These disorders are associated with difficulties in academic achievement, social and peer relations, and future emotional health. Anxiety places children at increased risk for comorbidity and psychopathology in adulthood. Given the prevalence of and interference caused by anxiety disorders, effective treatments must be developed and evaluated.

The treatment program, *Coping Cat* (Kendall, 1990; Kendall & Hedtke, 2006a, 2006b),[1] was developed at the Child and Adolescent Anxiety Disorders Clinic (CAADC) at Temple University and is targeted for anxiety-disordered children ages 7–13 years. A teen program, the *C.A.T. Project*, is also available (Kendall, Choudhury, Hudson, & Webb, 2002).[2] Representative of cognitive-behavioral therapy (CBT), the program consists of a treatment manual to guide the therapist and a workbook for use by each child client. Both are tailored for children with a principal diagnosis of separation anxiety disorder (SAD), generalized anxiety disorder (GAD), or social phobia (SP). Although the strategies outlined in the treatment manual could also benefit children with other anxiety disorders (specific phobias, obsessive–compulsive problems, posttraumatic stress), the program addresses the basic similarities within SAD, GAD, and SP.

Many youths with anxiety disorders also have other comorbid conditions, such as attention-deficit/hyperactivity disorder and depression. The CAADC accepts comorbid conditions (we exclude psychosis and IQ less than 80 but have included children with pervasive development disorders) provided that an anxiety disorder is the principal diagnosis. For example, the program is appropriate for children with GAD and comorbid depressive symptomatology. When depression is more severe and impairing than anxiety, then treatment for depression would be recommended instead of anxiety treatment. Our assessment process determines whether anxiety is the primary problem.

45

First, an initial phone screen reduces the probability of inappropriate cases. Once the families present for evaluation, parents and children participate in structured interviews conducted separately. We rely on clinician severity ratings of interference and distress to determine which diagnoses are principal/primary, and based on these we proceed with treatment. During treatment, the focus is on the anxiety diagnoses, not the comorbid diagnoses. Interestingly, the treatment has been found to have beneficial effects on some comorbid conditions in addition to the targeted principal diagnoses (Kendall, Brady, & Verduin, 2001).

Guiding Theory and Main Treatment Themes

Anxiety can be conceptualized as a tripartite construct involving physiological, cognitive, and behavioral components. From an evolutionary perspective, anxiety is a normal and expected emotional response that serves an adaptive and protective function. If we did not have any anxiety, we might not be cautious when caution is warranted. Anxiety can even enhance performance at times. Being a little nervous about a test motivates test takers to study harder, and being nervous before a game may help athletes to perform better. It is important to note that youths experience fear and anxiety as part of normal development. It is not uncommon for a young child to be afraid of the dark or to feel mild distress when separating from a parent. As children get older, anxiety regarding appearances and peer relationships is normal. Too much anxiety, however, can cause a great deal of distress. It gets in the way of school and work as well as relationships with friends and family. Youths who suffer from anxiety tend to perceive the world as a dangerous place. They live in a constant state of worry, which often is accompanied by physical symptoms such as headaches and stomachaches. They tend to avoid situations that make them anxious, and this, in turn, serves to reinforce their anxiety.

CBT for anxious youths targets the somatic, cognitive, and behavioral aspects of anxiety. The majority of CBTs include several main treatment components: psychoeducation, somatic management skills, cognitive restructuring, gradual exposure to feared situations, and relapse prevention plans. During the early stages of treatment, affective awareness is increased and corrective information about anxiety provided; explanations often include normalizing the experience of anxiety. Youths are then assisted in identifying different somatic reactions to anxiety (e.g., fast heartbeat, sweaty palms, upset stomach), and somatic management techniques (e.g., relaxation procedures) are introduced. Cognitive restructuring techniques focus on identifying and challenging maladaptive thoughts (self-talk) and shifting toward coping-focused thinking. Following the skill-building portion of treatment, graduated and controlled behavioral exposure to feared situations and stimuli is conducted. Finally, relapse prevention plans are discussed, with a focus on consolidating and generalizing treatment gains over time.

Characteristics of the Treatment Program

The Coping Cat is cognitive-behavioral intervention to help children with anxiety problems. The overall goal is to teach children to recognize signs of anxious arousal and to implement strategies to better cope with the challenges in their lives. The program is divided into two segments. The first focuses on skills training and the second on skills practice. For a summary of the sequence and content of specific sessions, see Table 4.1.

TABLE 4.1. Overview of the Sequence and Content of the Coping Cat Program for Anxious Children (and C.A.T. Project for Anxious Teens/Adolescents)

Session	Purpose of session
1	Build rapport; provide orientation and overview of the program; encourage the child's participation and verbalizations during sessions; Introduce STIC tasks and rewards; play a "Personal Facts" game; have some fun!
2	Talk about treatment goals; introduce **F** step: **F**eeling frightened? Identify different feelings and somatic responses to anxiety; normalize fear/anxiety; develop hierarchy of anxiety-provoking situations; play "Feelings Charades"; create a "Feelings Dictionary."
3	Review distinguishing anxious feelings from other feelings; learn more about somatic responses to anxiety; identify individual somatic responses to anxiety.
4 (parent session)	Provide information about treatment to the parents; give parents opportunity to discuss concerns and situations in which the child becomes anxious; provide ways in which parents may be involved.
5	Introduce relaxation training; review recognition of somatic cues; make version for child to practice at home; let child show skills to a parent.
6	Review relaxation training. Introduce **E** step: **E**xpecting bad things to happen? Use cartoons to identify self-talk; help child recognize anxious self-talk; help child generate less anxiety-provoking self-talk.
7	Review anxious self-talk and reinforce changing anxious self-talk into coping self-talk. Introduce **A** step: **A**ttitudes and **A**ctions that might help. Introduce cognitive strategies to manage anxiety; review relaxation training.
8	Introduce **R** step: **R**esults and **R**ewards. Introduce self-evaluation; review skills by putting steps together into the FEAR plan. Make a FEAR plan poster and a wallet-sized card with the FEAR mnemonic.
9 (parent session)	Explain second half of treatment; acknowledge that this portion of treatment may provoke greater anxiety; encourage parents to discuss concerns.
10	Practice the four-step coping (FEAR) plan under low anxiety provoking conditions, both imaginal and *in vivo*.
11	Continue practicing skills for coping with anxiety in low-level imaginal and *in vivo* situations.
12	Practice skills for coping with anxiety in imaginal and *in vivo* scenarios that provoke moderate anxiety.
13	Practice skills for coping with anxiety in *in vivo* situations that produce moderate levels of anxiety.
14	Practice skills for coping with anxiety in imaginal and *in vivo* situations that produce high anxiety; begin planning "commercial."
15	Practice skills for coping with anxiety in situations that produce high anxiety; continue planning "commercial."
16	Final practice of skills for coping with anxiety in *in vivo* situations that produce high levels of anxiety; review and summarize the program; make plans with parents to help the child maintain and generalize newly acquired skills; bring closure to the therapeutic relationship; tape the "commercial"; award the certificate.

In individual treatment (Kendall, 1994; Kendall & Hedtke, 2006a), the therapist works primarily with the anxious child (e.g., once a week typically for 16 weeks) and meets with the parents on two occasions (i.e., to address issues regarding parents' response to the child's anxiety and to inform parents of upcoming features of the treatment). Meeting with the child individually provides an opportunity for the child to trust and build a relationship with the therapist. Throughout the program, the therapist serves as a collaborative and supportive coach.

Children learn a four-step "FEAR plan" to organize the steps used to cope with anxiety. They then apply the FEAR plan to the real situations that they associate with anxiety (e.g., taking tests, being away from a parent, talking to a peer). A key component of Coping Cat is practicing the application of anxiety management strategies in real, anxiety-provoking situations. Children start by applying the FEAR plan in low-anxiety situations and then move to practicing it in higher anxiety situations in a gradual progression that suits their needs.

The First Half: Building the FEAR Plan

The first half (educational phase) of treatment introduces several basic concepts to the child, concepts that are later integrated and summarized into the mnemonic FEAR (**F**eeling frightened? **E**xpecting bad things to happen? **A**ttitudes and **A**ctions that might help; **R**esults and **R**ewards), plan to help the child remember the concepts. To facilitate the child's involvement in and ownership of the program, provide some fun activities, and ensure effective communication and learning of the various concepts, chapters in the *Coping Cat Workbook* parallel the treatment sessions provided by the therapist. The child and therapist work with the session content and homework assignments (Show That I Can tasks); the plan manual privately guides the therapist, while both the child and therapist use the workbook in sessions.

Feeling Frightened?

First, the child is asked, "Are you **F**eeling frightened?" An awareness of physical symptoms related to anxiety cues the child to do something to address the arousal (e.g., taking a deep breath; using relaxation techniques). Relaxation training helps the child recognize that he or she does have control over physical reactions. In relaxation training, the body's major muscle groups are sequentially relaxed through tension-releasing exercises designed to inform the child of states of tension and to use perceived muscle tension as a cue to initiate relaxation procedures. The particular muscle groups and somatic sensations that accompany anxiety are specific to each child, so greater awareness of the child's unique responses permits targeting specific muscle groups when anxious. Pictures in the workbook, with guidance from the therapist, assist the child in learning about symptoms of **F**eeling frightened.

Relaxation techniques are practiced via coping modeling and role plays. The therapist describes anxiety-provoking scenarios and models recognition of anxious feelings and accompanying tension and somatic responses. The therapist demonstrates coping by taking deep breaths and relaxing specific muscle groups, describing what is being done step by step. The child tags along with the therapist during a similar sequence. Once the child has learned some relaxation skills, parents are invited into the session and the child teaches the parents.

Expecting Bad Things to Happen?

Next, the child is asked whether he or she is Expecting bad things to happen. The child's faulty expectations are first identified and later challenged. After this identification, the child can then test out and eventually reduce these faulty beliefs. To modify maladaptive expectations (anxious self-talk), the therapist helps to identify unfairly negatively biased self-statements for the child. Together, the child and therapist try out new ways of viewing situations, using different expectations and coping self-talk as a framework to replace the anxiety-producing misinterpretations.

Children are not known for their willingness to tell adults what they are thinking. Any experienced therapist will confirm that when a child is asked, "What are you thinking?," the likely answer is "Nothing" or "I dunno." Using the *Coping Cat Workbook*, the therapist introduces the idea of self-talk using cartoons with empty thought bubbles. The therapist describes nonstressful situations and asks the child to provide examples of thoughts that might accompany the events. The child is then asked to develop different sets of possible thoughts for more ambiguous situations. The child and therapist fill in the possible thoughts for the different cartoon situations before the child is asked about his or her own thoughts and before the thoughts are targeted for change. The concept of self-talk is expanded to anxiety-provoking situations, progressing from low to high degrees of anxiety.

Modeling and role plays are used to help the child practice the skill of identifying and challenging negative self-talk. Accurate assessment and understanding of the child's characteristic dysfunctional thoughts are crucial to effective building of a coping template. It is worth noting that the goal is not to completely eradicate perceptions of stress but rather to teach the child to recognize and change unfounded perceptions of stress to more realistic perceptions, which are then used as cues to initiate coping strategies. The emphasis is not on teaching positive self-talk but on identifying and reducing negative self-talk.

Attitudes and Actions That Might Help

The third step in the FEAR plan—Attitudes and actions that might help—is taught as problem solving. The goal is to develop the child's confidence in his or her ability to meet daily challenges. The therapist points out that it might be helpful to take some action that will help change the anxious situation or the reaction to it. Problem solving begins with the therapist helping the child to understand that problems are a part of everyday life and encouraging the child not to rely on initial reactions that might be maladaptive. The child is asked to reconsider a problem in clearly defined ways and with clearly defined goals. Next, the child and therapist generate alternative solutions for the problem, and each solution is evaluated for possible outcomes. The therapist and child discuss the suggested alternatives, determine which may be the most feasible alternative, and make a plan to put the solution into action. Throughout this step, the therapist models problem solving and asks the child to tag along. Skills are practiced in session under conditions involving gradually increasing degrees of anxiety, and the therapist has the child try out and record (in the workbook) problem solving in situations outside of session.

Results and Rewards

The last step of the FEAR plan—Results and Rewards—is based on self-monitoring and contingent reinforcement. Approach behavior is strengthened and anxious behavior reduced through shaping, appropriate rewards, and positive reinforcement. Some children diagnosed with anxiety disorders have self-doubting thoughts, low self-confidence, or exceptionally high standards of achievement and are unforgiving if they fail to meet these standards. The therapist addresses these maladaptive expectations by rewarding the child for minor achievements and partial successes as well as for all forward-moving effort. Perfection is not an option and never expected.

For the young child, the therapist may introduce the concept of self-rating and reward by describing a reward as something that is given when someone is pleased with work that was done (e.g., parental evaluation and rewards). For the older child, the therapist gradually introduces the idea of self-rating by describing how a child can decide whether he or she is satisfied with his or her own work. Once the child understands self-monitoring/self-rating, the therapist provides opportunities for the child to practice making self-ratings and rewarding him- or herself for effort. The therapist uses coping modeling and role-play techniques to demonstrate self-rating and self-reward.

The Second Half: Exposure and Practice

The second segment of the program is largely devoted to the application and practice of the newly acquired FEAR plan within exposure to increasingly anxiety-provoking situations. The main strategy used is exposure, both imaginal and *in vivo*. Exposure tasks involve placing the child in situations that are fear evoking, having the child experience distress, and having the child become accustomed to the situation and practicing using coping strategies. The program follows a graduated-exposure model, in which the child moves up a hierarchy of anxiety-provoking situations, as determined by the child's anxiety level. When the child experiences anxiety during exposure tasks, it is important that his or her anxiety level not be so high as to result in the child's perception of the need for even greater avoidance. For all exposure tasks, the therapist collaborates with the child to make sure that the child understands the situation, ways to handle the situation, and the intended goal of the experience.

The therapist uses the following strategies when guiding the training and practice of the new skills. The process begins with an imaginal, in-office exposure to a nonstressful situation. Situations presented to each child are individually designed based on the child's particular fears and worries (as assessed during the initial evaluation, the ongoing sessions, and the collaborative development of the hierarchy). Future sessions also involve imaginal, in-office exposure, but the situations are designed to produce low levels of anxiety and are followed by actual *in vivo* experiences in low-stress situations. Subsequent sessions involve exposure to situations that cause gradually increasing levels of stress in the child, again first in imaginal settings and, once these are mastered, in *in vivo* situations. For example, a child may initially have to ask a secretary for a key to a room, whereas a later task may require that the child purchase a chosen snack from a streetside food vendor. Exposure tasks need not be of long duration and several can be arranged for one session; but it is important for the child to endure the exposure until the anxiety decreases (e.g., approximately 50%).

Part of the practice segment of the program includes giving the child the chance to practice telling others about how to manage anxiety. When nearing the completion of the program, the child with the therapist's help, creates a product or "commercial" (e.g., video, booklet) summarizing his or her experiences that can help inform other children about how to manage anxiety. This gives the child a chance to be the expert, gives the therapist a chance to see what the child has learned, and provides an opportunity for the child and therapist to share what has been accomplished with others to help reinforce treatment-produced gains.

Although the treatment manual offers a structured session-by-session approach, an important emphasis within the manual-based treatment is therapist flexibility (Chu & Kendall, 2004). The therapist, mindful of the goals of each session and features of the child, adapts the protocol to the individual needs of the child, tailoring the program to an optimal fit, which increases the child's engagement in the treatment process and predicts greater improvement. Although the manual provides solid guidelines from which to work, the therapist is nevertheless required to be flexible and creative in applying the manual in treatment (Kendall, Gosch, Furr, & Sood, 2008).

Parental Involvement in Treatment

Parental involvement in treatment is integral to help children overcome clinically meaningful anxiety. Consistent with this, the Coping Cat program now has a parent companion book (Kendall, Podell, & Gosch, 2010) that provides an overall description as well a session-by-session guide for parents and caregivers. Although the program focuses on helping the individual child to learn to think and behave differently, parents nevertheless play a role. Parental involvement in treatment can vary. Parents can be consultants (e.g., provide information), collaborators (e.g., assist with the child's acquisition of coping skills), or co-clients (e.g., learn skills to manage their own anxiety). In the individual treatment, parents are involved as consultants and collaborators. Parents are important in determining accurate child diagnoses and in ensuring the child's participation. Therapists also meet individually with the parents during two sessions (i.e., one during the skill-building phase and one just before beginning exposures) to collaborate with them on treatment plans and to maintain their cooperation. Parents discuss their concerns and provide further information that might be helpful. Unstructured conversations often include parents discussing their concerns and impressions of their child's anxiety and the therapist's offering specific ways that the parents might help in fostering positive outcomes.

Parents may play a role in the development and maintenance of childhood anxiety, and programs have been developed to increase parental involvement in treatment. Increasing parental involvement may provide an opportunity to directly address parenting behaviors that are maintaining the child's anxiety or, conversely, may impede the child from developing independence. The benefits of increased involvement vary (see Barmish & Kendall, 2005, for a review).

Even outside a family-oriented treatment, therapists need be aware of the problems that families of anxious children experience. For example, some parents may experience increased anxiety and particular problems in parenting styles (e.g., overprotectiveness, intolerance of negative emotions). Parents of anxious youths are often more encouraging of avoidant behavior, more intrusive, and less encouraging of autonomy than parents of nonanxious youths. When parents are controlling or overly involved, children may experience decreased self-efficacy and increased anxiety.

A family-based Coping Cat program (Howard, Chu, Krain, Marrs-Garcia, & Kendall, 2000) was developed at the CAADC to examine the efficacy of increased parental involvement. The same strategies as the child-focused treatment are used, but all of the sessions include the parents. A randomized controlled trial (RCT) examined the efficacy of the child-focused Coping Cat treatment (individual CBT [ICBT]), the family-based Coping Cat treatment (family CBT [FCBT]), and a family-based education/support/attention (FESA) condition. The results, in general, indicated that the ICBT and FCBT conditions outperformed the FESA condition. ICBT outperformed both family treatments on teacher reports of child anxiety, whereas FCBT outperformed ICBT on child reports of anxiety when both parents had an anxiety disorder (Kendall, Hudson, Gosch, Flannery-Schroeder, & Suveg, 2008).

Flexibility within Fidelity

Critics of manual-based treatment offer potentially reasonable objections, many of which rest on the assumption that manuals involve a prearranged and rigid approach to treatment. Critics often assume that manuals are designed to implement specific procedures using a steadfast, linear approach, precluding any therapist individuality. Clearly, such assumptions are unwarranted, and there is a rational middle ground between the complete freedom of an unstructured treatment and the rigid adherence to a manual. This middle ground consists of using the manual as a guide and with integrity, yet allowing it to become vibrant and alive when put into practice. Practitioners are best prepared to achieve flexible applications of manual-based treatments when there is an understanding of the treatment on multiple levels, including the model on which the treatment is based and the elements involved in the process of treatment.

The Coping Cat program can be used both with necessary fidelity and desired flexibility. The model/strategy (cognitive change and behavioral exposure tasks) drives the treatment, not specific sentences or exact techniques. However, affective and educational factors affect the therapeutic relationship, and the child's involvement in treatment (a variable that is influenced by a lively, flexible manual and an engaging therapist) is associated with overall progress (Chu & Kendall, 2004). We assign a key role to child involvement, a factor that is facilitated by a living, breathing therapist manual. For example, in each session and across sessions, the therapist can adapt the treatment goals to the needs and interests of the child. There are many opportunities for such flexibility within fidelity (see Kendall, Gosch, et al., 2008, for descriptions of flexible applications of the program). A child may modify the acronym FEAR to his or her own liking. One child completing the program transformed the FEAR plan into a military-inspired "scouting, intelligence, battle, and recon" plan. Flexibility can also include schedule adjustments, other adaptations, and tailoring of the treatment. However, some children may not require all 16 sessions of treatment to obtain success, suggesting that fewer skill-building or exposure sessions may be necessary for successful outcome. Our group is currently working to adapt the 16-session treatment into a shorter, focused eight-session treatment with fewer skill-building and exposure sessions, with more, we hope, to report in the future!

EVIDENCE ON THE EFFECTS OF TREATMENT

In this section, we summarize the results of outcome research using applications of the Coping Cat program with anxious children. Drawing on the foundations provided by the American Psychological Association Task Force on Psychological Intervention guidelines, a scheme was created for determining when a psychological treatment for a specific problem or disorder may be considered to be efficacious or possibly efficacious (American Psychological Association, 2006). According to their system, a treatment may be considered efficacious (i.e., established) or possibly efficacious (i.e., promising but in need of replication) if it has been shown to be more effective than no treatment, a placebo, or an alternate treatment across multiple trials conducted by different investigative teams. Treatments that meet these criteria, except for replication or independent replication, are designated as probably efficacious. According to recent reviews, the Coping Cat program for childhood anxiety is probably efficacious.

Randomized Clinical Trials

Building on a promising initial evaluation of the Coping Cat program using a multiple baseline design (Kane & Kendall, 1989), several RCTs have been conducted (Kendall, 1994; Kendall et al., 1997; Kendall, Hudson, et al., 2008). The first RCT (Kendall, 1994) evaluating the Coping Cat program included 47 children, ages 9–13 years, who were referred from multiple community sources. Participants received a principal anxiety disorder diagnosis of overanxious disorder (OAD), avoidant disorder (AD; Kendall & Warman [1996]) found that children meeting *Diagnostic and Statistical Manual of Mental Disorders* (third edition [DSM-III], American Psychiatric Association [APA], 1980) criteria for OAD/AD were not dissimilar to those diagnosed by DSM-IV (American Psychiatric Association, 1994) criteria as GAD/SP, or SAD. The results indicated that, compared with wait-list control children, children who received the treatment evidenced a significant positive change from pre- to posttreatment on self-report, parent report, and behavioral observation measures. Based on the independent diagnostic evaluation, both children's and parents' diagnostic interview data indicated that 64% of the treated children no longer met diagnostic criteria for their principal diagnosis at posttreatment, whereas only 5% of the wait-list control children no longer met diagnostic criteria at posttreatment. Treatment-produced gains were maintained at 1-year follow-up. In a longer follow-up study, Kendall and Southam-Gerow (1996) reassessed 36 of the 47 children treated in the 1994 clinical trial. The length of time from completion of the treatment program to long-term assessment ranged from 2–5 years ($M = 3.35$ years). On both self-report and parent report measures and in terms of diagnostic status, treatment-produced gains were maintained at 3.35-year follow-up.

A second RCT (Kendall et al., 1997) involved 94 children, ages 9–13 years. Participants received a principal diagnosis of one of the target anxiety disorders. The outcomes of the study supported the efficacy of the treatment for childhood anxiety, with 50% of treated patients being free from their principal anxiety disorder at posttreatment. For those patients in whom the principal anxiety diagnosis remained at posttreatment, analyses showed significant reductions on severity scores. Children who received the Coping Cat treatment demonstrated significant positive change on self-report, parent report, and some behavioral observation measures. The average scores of the treated children returned to within the normative range on these measures, indicating clinically significant gains. The gains were maintained at 1-year follow-up. It is also worth noting that a 7.4-year follow-up of 90% of the cases treated in the 1997 study revealed evidence of the long-term maintenance of gains and some positive impacts on.the sequelae of anxiety (e.g., substance abuse; Kendall, Safford, Flannery-Schroeder, & Webb, 2004).

A third RCT (Kendall, Hudson, et al., 2008), mentioned briefly earlier, compared ICBT, FCBT, and FESA. Participants included 161 anxiety-disordered youths ages 7–13 years and their parents. As in previous trials, all child participants had a principal diagnosis of SAD, GAD, or SP or a combination. Children evidenced treatment gains across conditions, although FCBT and ICBT were superior to FESA in reducing the presence and principality of the principal anxiety disorder. In some instances, ICBT outperformed FCBT and FESA (i.e., on teacher reports of child anxiety) and FCBT outperformed ICBT (i.e., when both parents had an anxiety disorder). Treatment gains, when found, were maintained at 1-year follow-up.

To examine the efficacy of the Coping Cat program in a group format, Flannery-Schroeder and Kendall (2000) compared group treatment, individual treatment, and a wait-list control condition providing services for 37 children, ages 8–14 years. All of the children were diagnosed with principal anxiety disorders (i.e., GAD, SAD, SP). When diagnostic status was considered at posttreatment, significantly more of the treated youths (73% individual, 50% group) than the wait-list youths (8%) were free of the principal anxiety diagnosis they had received at pretreatment. Only children receiving individual treatment showed significant improvements on self-report measures of anxious distress; and the three conditions did not differ with regard to measures of social functioning. At a 3-month follow-up assessment, treatment gains were maintained.

A recent emotion-focused modification of the Coping Cat program (emotion-focused CBT; Suveg, Kendall, Comer, & Robin, 2006) integrates into all treatment sessions the component of emotion recognition, understanding, and regulation regarding anxiety and other emotions. A pilot study examined six children ages 7–13 years with principal anxiety disorders (i.e., GAD, SAD, or SP). At posttreatment, all children showed a decrease in the severity of their principal anxiety disorder, and 67% did not meet criteria for their pretreatment principal anxiety disorder. In addition, 83% evidenced an increase in their awareness of emotional experiences, use of emotion-related language, and understanding of hiding and changing emotions, and all demonstrated a decrease in their emotional inflexibility and dysregulated negative affect.

Variables that Potentially Affect Treatment Outcome

Demographic and Diagnostic Variables

Researchers have considered potential moderating factors such as gender, ethnicity, comorbidity, symptom severity, and cognition. Very few of these factors have been found to significantly predict differential treatment outcome. Children diagnosed with a childhood anxiety disorder have been found to have similar prevalence or intensity of fears as a function of gender or ethnicity based on child, parent, teacher, and diagnostic ratings of the anxious youths. Moreover, reductions in anxious symptomatology and the absence of anxiety disorder diagnoses as a result of treatment have also been found to be comparable across gender and ethnicity. A review of ICBT and FCBT for anxious youths supports similar findings with gender or age and treatment outcome.

Although very few variables identify differential treatment response, one study found differences between treatment completers and noncompleters. Kendall and Sugarman (1997) examined treatment completers ($n = 146$, who completed 16–20 sessions of treatment), noncompleters ($n = 44$, including 23 dropouts, who started treatment but terminated before the end of treatment), and refusers ($n = 21$, who were evaluated and offered treatment but never received it), and found that noncompleters were more likely to live in a single-parent household, be ethnic minorities, and have child-reported less anxious symptomatology than treatment completers. No differences were found between completers and noncompleters on mother and teacher reports of child internalizing and externalizing behavior. Follow-up interviews suggest that these factors influenced decisions to discontinue treatment. Socioeconomic status and level of parental education, however, were not predictors of early treatment termination.

Southam-Gerow, Kendall, and Weersing (2001) investigated the correlates of good versus poor treatment response in 135 children and adolescents (ages 7–15) who received CBT. Although participants had generally improved, analyses of the combined data identified several correlates of a less favorable response, including higher levels of maternal- and teacher-reported child internalizing psychopathology at pretreatment, higher levels of maternal self-reported depressive symptoms, and older child age. However, ethnicity, gender, family income, family composition (i.e., dual- vs. single-parent household), child-reported symptomatology, and maternal-reported level of child externalizing problems were not correlated with treatment response.

Kendall and colleagues (2001) examined comorbidity as a potential moderator of treatment outcome for 173 children (ages 9–13) who had been treated for a DSM-III-Revised (APA, 1987)/DSM-IV primary anxiety disorder diagnosis. Comorbidity was high: 79% of the participants received at least one comorbid diagnosis at pretreatment. At posttreatment, 68% of noncomorbid children were free of their principal diagnosis compared with 71% of the comorbid children. Both groups showed significant reductions in pretreatment diagnosis and on parent and child self-report measures. These results suggest that treatment was comparably effective with comorbid and noncomorbid anxious children.

In-Session Variables

Within the treatment of anxiety in youths, subjective units of distress scale (SUDS) ratings are frequently used (e.g., Kendall & Hedtke, 2006a). Benjamin, Crawley, Beidas, Martin, and Kendall (2009) examined SUDS ratings as a process variable and potential predictor of treatment outcome. The magnitude of change in SUDS ratings, as reported by anxiety-disordered youths during the exposure task portion of CBT, was associated with treatment outcome. The SUDS scores, on average, were halved over the course of the exposure. Specifically, SUDS change scores for easy exposure sessions were associated with teacher-reported improvement, for medium exposure sessions were correlated with both teacher- and child-reported improvement at posttreatment, and for difficult exposure sessions were not correlated with teacher- or child-report measures, suggesting that change in SUDS on easy- and medium-exposure sessions plays a significant role in the learning process. During exposures, youths with the highest level of anxiety and those who had the greatest level of change in SUDS scores showed the most child- and teacher-reported improvement in outcome.

Exposure tasks increase the distress the child may experience in session, but do they negatively impact the therapeutic relationship? Kendall et al. (2009) compared the pattern of alliance ratings before in-session exposure tasks and after engagement in exposure tasks (i.e., within-subjects examination). For treatments with and without exposure tasks, therapist, child, mother, and father ratings indicated significant growth in alliance regardless of the use of exposure tasks. In short, the data did not indicate a rupture in therapeutic alliance following the introduction of in-session exposures.

To examine a mediator of treatment response, Kendall and Treadwell (2007) conducted a second investigation on features of self-statements as predictors of anxiety in 145 children (ages 9–13) with and without an anxiety disorder and the impact of treatment on anxiety disorders. Treadwell and Kendall (1996) found that children's negative self-statements and states-of-mind (SOM)[3] ratios (but not positive self-statements) significantly predicted anxiety, and changes in self-statements predicted improvement in anxiety after treatment and mediated treatment gains. Similar results were found in the 2007 study: Children's anxious, but not positive or depressed, self-statements predicted improvement in anxiety in children with and without anxiety disorders. Importantly, changes in anxious self-statements again mediated treatment gains. The treatment-produced gains were mediated by reductions in the children's negative self-talk, underscoring the power of nonnegative thinking!

When medications are considered in combination with CBT for the treatment of child anxiety disorders, one study compared the Coping Cat (CBT) condition, medication (sertraline) condition, and their combination with a pill placebo condition (Walkup et al., 2008). This large multisite (Temple University, Duke University, Johns Hopkins University, Columbia University, University of California, Los Angeles, and Western Psychiatric Institute and Clinic) RCT included 488 children (ages 7–17) with principal anxiety disorders (i.e., GAD, SAD, SP). Results indicate that the combination of CBT and sertraline produced the best positive response. A significant percentage of children were found to be much or very much improved at posttreatment in the combination therapy (80.7%), which was greater than found in either monotherapy (59.7% CBT; 54.9% sertraline); and all therapies demonstrated greater improvement than placebo (23.7%). It is possible that the synergistic effects of the combination of the two treatments could account for the increased efficacy, but the authors report that there was also greater contact time in the combination therapy, which cannot be ruled out as a possibility for greater response.

Transporting Treatment from a Research Clinic to the Practice Clinic

Although evidence from research supports the efficacy of the Coping Cat treatment program for childhood anxiety, there remains a disjunction between empirically supported therapies (ESTs) and treatments used in practice settings. There are calls to broaden the range of treatment delivery models to help bridge the gap and growing efforts to transport ESTs to the community.

Despite the difficulties, promising and innovative models have been developed to increase the transportability of treatments to the community. One approach is computer-based or computer-assisted treatment. Computer-assisted CBT may be an efficient, cost-effective, and community-friendly method of service delivery (Khanna & Kendall, 2007). One computer-based CBT program for anxiety in youths, developed by a team of researchers, child psychologists, programmers, and graphic designers, is Camp Cope-A-Lot: The Coping Cat DVD (CCAL; Kendall & Khanna, 2008a, 2008b). CCAL combines the empirically supported CBT protocol with state-of-the-art computer flash animation and interactive computer-based training with audio, two-dimensional animations, photographs, video, schematics, and a built-in reward system. As in the Coping Cat treatment, CCAL includes affective education, relaxation training, identification and labeling of anxiety-related cognition, problem solving, social reward and shaping, exposure tasks, role plays, and homework. The entire 12-level program is designed to be completed over 12 weeks, with the participant completing one level per week. The first six levels, which the user completes independently, are skill building; the remaining six levels, completed with the assistance of a coach, consist of exposure tasks and rehearsal in specific anxiety-provoking situations. Two parent sessions are conducted by the therapist/coach while child participants are working on Levels 3 and 7. CCAL is geared for a variety of mental health professionals who work in a range of community settings (i.e., schools, training programs, community clinics). Preliminary results from an RCT comparing the CCAL with traditional CBT (i.e., Coping Cat) and an education/support/attention (ESA) control indicate that children receiving either version of the Coping Cat (individual sessions; computer-assisted program) outperformed the ESA controls.

DIRECTIONS FOR RESEARCH

The development and evaluation of the treatment reported herein began in 1984. Much has been accomplished over the past two decades, but we still have far to go. The CAADC and colleagues are continuing research to examine the transportability of the Coping Cat into the community, the efficacy and effectiveness of computer-assisted adaptations (i.e., Camp Cope-A-Lot) and brief versions of the Coping Cat, the specific components associated with positive treatment outcome, the optimal role of parents, and the role of medications in the overall treatment of anxiety disorders in youths.

In general, the literature supports the belief that including parents in the treatment of child psychopathology can have a beneficial effect on outcomes. For anxious youths, some data suggest that including parents as co-clients in treatment sessions is not essential for positive child gains. However, for those whose parents have an anxiety disorder, increased parental involvement was beneficial (Kendall, Hudson, et al., 2008). Parents of anxious youths may be overinvolved in their children's lives, and the preferred intervention may be to have them less involved (and not in sessions). With the parents out of the session, the children can develop a relationship with the therapist and begin to have favorable experiences with new ways of thinking and behaving. In contrast, parents may be needed in sessions when the therapist directly addresses granting more autonomy to the children, demonstrating greater tolerance of negative emotions, and encouraging the children to have learning experiences (as opposed to avoiding experience to be safe).

Once an intervention has been found to have efficacy with regard to outcomes (see also Silverman, Pina, & Viswesvaran, 2008), it is fruitful to examine the processes and therapeutic mechanisms that contribute to psychological change. Some data suggest that reduction in negative thinking mediates positive outcomes. Process variables within our manual-based treatment, such as therapeutic alliance, therapist flexibility, and child involvement, are currently being examined.

However, despite the significant percentage of children who have a positive outcome, approximately 25–30% do not have optimal outcomes posttreatment. Advances are likely to be found in (1) the addition of booster sessions and further contacts for those patients not reaching preferred level of improvement at the end of the time-limited treatment, (2) investigations of developmental factors (cognitive, social, emotional, or physical) that may help to individually tailor treatments and increase the percentage of improved patients, and (3) getting to know more about how nonanxious youths manage their unwanted distress. Some of the processes involved in normal adjustment to anxious arousal may contribute meaningfully to the further refining of our current program.

CONCLUSIONS

Anxiety disorders in youths are significant and prevalent forms of psychological distress. Using appropriate methodologies for evaluations, CBT has a favorable record of success in treating anxious youths who have a high incidence of comorbid conditions. As noted, the treatment integrates an understanding of cognition, behavior, and emotional functioning within a larger social context.

The Coping Cat program and its adaptations work to build positive therapeutic alliance and educate children and their parents about the normality of anxiety, the signs of anxiety, anxious and coping self-talk, relaxation skills to reduce anxious arousal, and problem-solving skills. The second half of this treatment relies on the hierarchical use of exposure tasks to address anxious distress. The main features of the educational phase are summarized with a four-step FEAR plan, and the plan is implemented and practiced in the second half of the program. The therapist is active and serves as a coping model who appropriately self-discloses and arranges the challenging *in vivo* exposure tasks for the child patients. Roughly two-thirds of those children treated, including children of both genders, various ethnicities, and several principal anxiety disorders, have been found to benefit meaningfully. Initial evidence suggests that older children with more severe co-occurring psychopathology may do less well after treatment.

Additional scientific investigations are needed to improve the treatment for those who, to date, have not been positive treatment responders. Also there is a need for a greater understanding of the role of developmental factors in the nature and treatment of anxiety disorders in children and youths.

NOTES

1. Contact the publisher for these references at *www.WorkbookPublishing.com*.
2. Contact the publisher for this references at *www.WorkbookPublishing.com*.
3. The SOM model proposes categories of self-talk, including positive dialogue (considered

optimal for adaptation), negative dialogue (associated with moderate anxiety or depression), internal dialogues of conflict (associated with self-doubt, worry, and mild anxiety/depression), positive monologue (positive self-statements possibly indicating grandiosity), and negative monologue (low positive self-statements associated with severe depression).

ACKNOWLEDGMENTS

The research reported in this chapter was supported by grants from the National Institutes of Health (e.g., MH63747, MH59087, MH64484, MH067481).

REFERENCES

American Psychiatric Association. (1980). *Diagnostic and statistical manual of mental disorders* (3rd ed.). Washington, DC: Author.

American Psychiatric Association. (1987). *Diagnostic and statistical manual of mental disorders* (3rd ed., rev.). Washington, DC: Author.

American Psychiatric Association. (1994). *Diagnostic and statistical manual of mental disorders* (4th ed.). Washington, DC: Author.

American Psychological Association. (2006). Evidence based practice in psychology. *American Psychologist, 61,* 271–285.

Barmish, A. J., & Kendall, P. C. (2005). Should parents be co-clients in cognitive-behavioral therapy for anxious youth? *Journal of Clinical Child and Adolescent Psychology, 34,* 569–581.

Benjamin, C., Crawley, S., Beidas, R. S., Martin, E., & Kendall, P. C. (2009). *Distress during exposure tasks: A treatment process predicting anxiety outcomes in youth using subjective units of distress.* Manuscript submitted for publication, Temple University.

Chu, B. C., & Kendall, P. C. (2004). Positive association of child involvement and treatment outcome within a manual-based cognitive-behavioral treatment for children with anxiety. *Journal of Consulting and Clinical Psychology, 72,* 821–829.

Flannery-Schroeder, E. C., & Kendall, P. C. (2000). Group and individual cognitive-behavioral treatments for youth with anxiety disorders: A randomized clinical trial. *Cognitive Therapy and Research, 24,* 251–278.

Howard, B. L., Chu, B., Krain, A., Marrs-Garcia, A., & Kendall, P. C. (2000). *Cognitive-behavioral family therapy for anxious children: Therapist manual* (2nd ed.). Ardmore, PA: Workbook.

Kane, M., & Kendall, P. C. (1989). Anxiety disorders in children: A multiple-baseline evaluation of a cognitive-behavioral therapy. *Behavior Therapy, 20,* 499–508.

Kendall, P. C. (1990). *Coping Cat workbook.* Ardmore, PA: Workbook.

Kendall, P. C. (1994). Treating anxiety disorders in children: Results of a randomized clinical trial. *Journal of Consulting and Clinical Psychology, 62,* 100–110.

Kendall, P. C., Brady, E., & Verduin, T. (2001). Comorbidity in childhood anxiety disorders and treatment outcome. *Journal of the American Academy of Child and Adolescent Psychiatry, 40,* 787–794.

Kendall, P. C., Choudhury, M. S., Hudson, J. L., & Webb, A. (2002). *The C.A.T. Project.* Ardmore, PA: Workbook.

Kendall, P. C., Comer, J. S., Marker, C., Creed, T., Puliafico, A., Hughes, J., et al. (2009). In-session exposure tasks and therapeutic alliance across the treatment of childhood anxiety disorders. *Journal of Consulting and Clinical Psychology, 77,* 517–525.

Kendall, P. C., Flannery-Schroeder, E., Panichelli-Mindel, S., Southam-Gerow, M., Henin, A., & Warman, M. (1997). Therapy for youth with anxiety disorders: A second randomized clinical trial. *Journal of Consulting and Clinical Psychology, 65,* 366–380.

Kendall, P. C., Gosch, E., Furr, J. M., & Sood, E. (2008). Flexibility within fidelity. *Journal of the American Academy of Child and Adolescent Psychiatry, 47,* 987–993.

Kendall, P. C., & Hedtke, K. A. (2006a). *Cognitive-behavioral therapy for anxious children: Therapist manual* (3rd ed.). Ardmore, PA: Workbook.

Kendall, P. C., & Hedtke, K. A. (2006b). *Coping Cat Workbook* (2nd ed.). Ardmore, PA: Workbook.

Kendall, P. C., Hudson, J., Gosch, E., Flannery-Schroeder, E., & Suveg, C. (2008). Cognitive-behavioral therapy for anxiety disordered youth: A randomized clinical trial evaluating child and family modalities. *Journal of Consulting and Clinical Psychology, 76,* 282–297.

Kendall, P. C., & Khanna, M. (2008a). *Camp Cope-A-Lot: The Coping Cat CD-ROM.* Ardmore, PA: Workbook.

Kendall, P. C., & Khanna, M. (2008b). *Coach's Manual for Camp Cope-A-Lot: The Coping Cat CD-ROM.* Ardmore, PA: Workbook.

Kendall, P. C., Podell, J. L., & Gosch, E. A. (2010). *The Coping Cat: Parent companion.* Ardmore, PA: Workbook.

Kendall, P. C., Safford, S., Flannery-Schroeder, E., & Webb, A. (2004). Child anxiety treatment: Outcomes in adolescence and impact on substance use and depression at 7.4-year follow-up. *Journal of Consulting and Clinical Psychology, 72,* 276–287.

Kendall, P. C., & Southam-Gerow, M. (1996). Long-term follow-up of a cognitive-behavioral therapy for anxiety-disordered youth. *Journal of Consulting and Clinical Psychology, 64,* 724–730.

Kendall, P. C., & Sugarman, A. (1997). Attrition in the treatment of childhood anxiety disorders. *Journal of Consulting and Clinical Psychology, 65,* 883–888.

Kendall, P. C., & Treadwell, K. (2007). The role of self-statements as a mediator in treatment for anxiety-disordered youth. *Journal of Consulting and Clinical Psychology, 75,* 380–389.

Kendall, P. C., & Warman, M. J. (1996). Anxiety disorders in youth: Diagnostic consistency across DSM-III-R and DSM-IV. *Journal of Anxiety Disorders, 10,* 452–463.

Khanna, M., & Kendall, P. C. (2007). New frontiers: Computer technology in the treatment of anxious youth. *The Behavior Therapist, 30,* 22–25.

Silverman, W., Pina, A., & Viswesvaran, C. (2008). Evidence-based psychosocial treatments for phobic and anxiety disorders in children and adolescents. *Journal of Clinical Child and Adolescent Anxiety, 37,* 105–130.

Southam-Gerow, M. A., Kendall, P. C., & Weersing, V. R. (2001). Examining outcome variability: Correlates of treatment response in a child and adolescent anxiety clinic. *Journal of Clinical Child Psychology, 30,* 422–436.

Suveg, C., Kendall, P. C., Comer, J. S., & Robin, J. (2006). Emotion-focused cognitive behavioral therapy for anxious youth: A multiple baseline evaluation. *Journal of Contemporary Psychotherapy, 36,* 77–85.

Treadwell, K. R. H., & Kendall, P. C. (1996). Self-talk in youth with anxiety disorders: States of mind, content specificity, and treatment outcome. *Journal of Consulting and Clinical Psychology, 64,* 941–950.

Walkup, J. T., Albano, A. M., Piacentini, J., Birmaher, B., Compton, S. N., Sherrill, J. T., et al. (2008). Cognitive behavioral therapy, sertraline, or a combination in childhood anxiety. *New England Journal of Medicine, 359,* 2753–2766.

5

Interventions for Anxiety Disorders in Children Using Group Cognitive-Behavioral Therapy with Family Involvement

KRISTINE M. PAHL and PAULA M. BARRETT

OVERVIEW OF THE TREATMENT MODEL

The Clinical Problem

Anxiety disorders are among the most prevalent psychiatric disorders affecting children and adolescents, with prevalence rates ranging from 3–24% (Cartwright-Hatton, McNicol, & Doubleday, 2006). Once present, childhood anxiety disorders tend to be chronic and recurrent. They rarely remit without treatment and can subsequently affect several areas of life, including academic performance, social interaction, self-confidence, and the ability to enjoy everyday life experiences. Fortunately, researchers have demonstrated that anxiety disorders in childhood can be successfully treated with brief psychosocial interventions. Cognitive-behavioural therapy (CBT) has been classified as a "probably efficacious" individual treatment (Ollendick & King, 1998; Silverman, Pina, & Viswesvaran, 2008) and group treatment for childhood anxiety (Silverman et al., 2008). For a treatment to be classified as probably efficacious, at least two good experiments must demonstrate that the treatment is superior to a wait-list control group (see Ollendick & King, 1998; Silverman et al., 2008). CBT treatment modalities for childhood anxiety often involve parents and families in the treatment process to increase generalizability and sustainability of the skills learned. This chapter focuses on family-based group CBT interventions for childhood anxiety with a particular focus on the FRIENDS programs (Barrett, 2004, 2005, 2007a, 2007b). Although several anxiety disorders exist, the most common anxiety disorders treated in the FRIENDS programs include social phobia, specific phobia, separation anxiety, and generalized anxiety disorder.

Conceptual Model Underlying Treatment

As in individual CBT (ICBT), family-based cognitive-behavioral treatment (FCBT) focuses on dysfunctional cognitions and how these affect and interact with the child's emotions and behavior. Cognitive distortions play an important role in the maintenance of anxiety symptoms; however, the family—parents and siblings—is seen as the optimal environment for effecting change in the child's dysfunctional cognition. Parents are in a unique position to facilitate new experiences in which the child can test dysfunctional beliefs, and parents living with the child can assist in the processing of new experiences on a daily basis. Also, parents are influential role models in their child's life: A parent modeling adaptive beliefs and cognitive processing of day-to-day events and rewarding a child for approaching situations in an optimistic manner can be especially helpful for anxiety reduction. Our family-based approach focuses on the reciprocal interactions in the family. All family members learn skills to become more brave, confident, and happy. Our model follows a strength-based approach to treatment where attention is paid to an individual's strengths and his or her ability to cope in a given situation.

This chapter focuses on family-based group treatment for anxiety disorders in children, with a central focus on treatment–outcome research conducted by our research team and international colleagues. The majority of this chapter describes three developmentally tailored, FCBT intervention programs for anxious children: the Fun FRIENDS program (Barrett, 2007), the FRIENDS for Life for Children program (Barrett, 2004), and the FRIENDS for Life for Youth program (Barrett, 2005). The program name FRIENDS is an acronym for the strategies taught in the programs. Throughout the chapter, the term FRIENDS groups applies to all three developmental versions unless otherwise stated. The term children is used to represent both children and adolescents.

FRIENDS for Life for Children and Youth

Feelings
Remember to relax. Have quiet time.
I can do it! I can try my best!
Explore solutions and coping step plans.
Now reward yourself! You've done
    your best!
Don't forget to practice.
Smile! Stay calm for life!

Fun FRIENDS:

Feelings
Relax
I can try!
Encourage
Nurture
Don't forget to be brave
Stay happy

Main Themes of the Treatment Program

The FRIENDS programs follow a cognitive-behavioral model for child anxiety that addresses cognitive, physiological, and learning processes that are thought to interact in the development, maintenance, and experience of anxiety. Cognitive processes are addressed by teaching children positive thinking strategies and encouraging flexibility in thinking through challenging negative thoughts/self-talk. Physiological processes are addressed by teaching children to become aware of their internal, physiological body cues (termed "body clues" in the programs) by teaching skills that enable them to self-regulate emotional distress and physiological arousal. Finally, learning processes are addressed through the acquisition of new skills that help children cope with and manage anxiety and anxiety-provoking situations.

The underlying philosophy of the FRIENDS programs is strength based; it empowers families to make positive change in their lives and values the unique knowledge and experiences that parents, siblings, and children bring to the group. A collaborative team approach is emphasized in which the therapist, parents, siblings, and child work together with a shared goal of increasing both the child's and family's confidence and coping skills.

CHARACTERISTICS OF THE TREATMENT PROGRAM

Participants and Program Format

The child component of the FRIENDS for Life program (Barrett, 2004, 2005) originated with the development of the Coping Koala program (i.e., Barrett, Dadds, & Rapee, 1996), an Australian adaptation of Kendall's Coping Cat program (Kendall, 1990). The program later became FRIENDS when it was adapted for group treatment delivery (i.e., Barrett, 1998; Shortt, Barrett, & Fox, 2001). The FRIENDS for Life program (4th edition; Barrett, 2004, 2005) includes two developmentally tailored workbooks for use with either children, 7–11 years (Barrett, 2004), or youths, 12–16 years (Barrett, 2005). Most recently, Paula Barrett created a downward extension of the FRIENDS for Life program for children ages 4–6 years – called the Fun FRIENDS program (Barrett, 2007a, 2007b). Each program caters to the developmental differences in children's abilities, which are reflected in the session content and activities.

All of the FRIENDS programs can be run in both group and individual settings, although the group treatment is the more preferred mode of delivery. Clinical experience indicates that individual motivation to overcome fears appears to increase within a group setting, and children can acquire and practice the new skills learned in a safe and interactive environment, which fosters supportive peer learning through experiential group exercises. Group therapy also enhances cost-effectiveness because it allows more efficient use of the therapist's time.

Content of Treatment

The FRIENDS programs consist of 10 weekly sessions and two booster sessions held 1 and 3 months after the completion of treatment. Each session is designed to run for approximately 1 to 1½ hours. The typical size of an effective group would be between six and 10 children, which allows adequate time for everyone in the group to share ideas. The use of cofacilitators in group therapy is very helpful both to manage the group process by offering reinforcement to children who are trying their best and to assist children with any reading or writing difficulties. An overview of the program content for the Fun FRIENDS program is displayed in Table 5.1, Table 5.2 displays content for the FRIENDS for Life for Children program, and Table 5.3 displays content for the FRIENDS for Life for Youth program. These illustrate how each strategy is represented by each letter of the FRIENDS acronym.

TABLE 5.1. Outline of Fun FRIENDS Session Content

Session no.	Content of session—major learning objectives
1	Developing a sense of identity. Introduction of "being brave" concept. Acceptance of differences and similarities among people.
2	Feelings Awareness of feelings, understanding of feelings in others. Normalization of feelings, expressing feelings.
3	Feelings Problem solving with feelings, coping strategies.
4	Relax Identifying physiological symptoms of worry ("body clues"). "Milkshake breathing," progressive muscle relaxation, visualization.
5	I can try! Identifying self-talk, introducing helpful green thoughts and unhelpful red thoughts.
6	I try! Challenging unhelpful red thoughts.
7	Encourage Coping step plans. Friendship skills: helping, sharing, listening, smiling.
8	Nurture Discussing our role models.
9	Don't forget to be brave (practicing the FRIENDS skills). Support teams.
10	Stay happy! Review of all skills and party.
Boosters 1 and 2	Review of Fun FRIENDS strategies and preparing for future challenges.
Additional social-emotional learning content	Developing a sense of self and positive self-identity. Social skills. Responsibility for self and others, self-direction, and independence. Prosocial behavior.

Family Skills

In the current edition of FRIENDS for Life for Children (Barrett, 2004) and Youth (Barrett, 2005), two structured parent sessions are outlined in the leader's manuals for flexible use within multiple settings such as community clinics and schools. In the clinic setting, these sessions are generally held outside of the allotted group time (e.g., in the evening) and typically last 2 hours each. During these sessions, program content is explained in detail and behavior management strategies are discussed (e.g., planned ignoring, quiet time, time-out).

Parents and siblings are also invited to attend the last 20–30 minutes of every session to discuss the session content. During this time, parents and siblings may be asked

TABLE 5.2. Outline of FRIENDS for Life for Children Session Content

Session no.	Content of session—major learning objectives
1	Rapport building and introduction of group participants. Establishing group guidelines. Normalization of anxiety and individual differences in anxiety.
2	Affective education and identification of various emotions. Introduce the relationship between thoughts and feelings.
3	Feelings. Identifying physiological symptoms of worry. Remember to relax. Have quiet time. Relaxation activities.
4	I can do it! I can try my best! Identifying self-talk, introducing helpful green thoughts and unhelpful red thoughts.
5	Attention training—looking for positive aspects in all situations. Challenging unhelpful red thoughts. Explore solutions and coping step plans. Coping step plans and setting goals.
6	Problem-solving skills (six-stage problem-solving plan). Coping role models. Social support plans.
7	Now reward yourself. You've done your best!
8	Don't forget to practice. Smile. Stay calm for life! Reflect on ways to cope in difficult situations.
9	Generalizing skills of FRIENDS to various difficult situations. Coaching others in how to use the FRIENDS coping skills.
10	Skills for maintenance of the FRIENDS strategies. Preparing for minor setbacks that may occur.
Boosters 1 and 2	Review of FRIENDS strategies and preparing for future challenges.

to engage in an activity related to the program skills (e.g., playing a "red" and "green" thoughts game) to reinforce the learning component. With younger children, parents are assigned homework activities, which involve the entire family in skill acquisition. The process of these parent sessions may vary to meet the needs and preferences of the groups. For example, during this time, younger children (Fun FRIENDS and FRIENDS for Life for Children) are often taken to another area of the clinic with one or two of the cofacilitators, leaving one facilitator to discuss the concepts and strategies with the parents and siblings. For older children and adolescents, group participants tend to stay in the room (if room size allows), with the parents and siblings with cofacilitators dispersed throughout the room to assist in managing the process.

TABLE 5.3. Outline of FRIENDS for Life for Youth Session Content

Session no.	Content of session—major learning objectives
1	Rapport building and introduction of group participants. Establishing group guidelines. Normalization of anxiety and individual differences.
2	Enhancing self-esteem in self and others. Recognition of individual's strengths.
3	Affective education, friendship skills. Introduction to relationship between thoughts and feelings.
4	**F**eelings. Identifying physiological symptoms of worry. **R**emember to relax. Have quiet time. Relaxation activities.
5	**I** can do it! I can try my best! Identifying self-talk, challenging unhelpful thoughts. Attention training (environmental, intrapersonal, and interpersonal).
6	**E**xplore solutions and coping step plans. Introducing coping step plans and setting goals.
7	Coping role models. Social support plans. Conflict and communication styles: assertive, aggressive, passive. CALM: conflict resolution plan.
8	Six-stage problem-solving plan. **N**ow reward yourself. You've done your best! Thinking like a winner, focusing on positive aspects in every situation.
9	**D**on't forget to practice. **S**mile. Stay calm for life! Generalizing skills of FRIENDS to various difficult situations. Coaching others in how to use the FRIENDS coping skills.
10	Skills for maintenance of the FRIENDS strategies. Preparing for minor setbacks that may occur.
Boosters 1 and 2	Review of FRIENDS strategies and preparing for future challenges.

Skills Emphasized in Treatment

Most of the general anxiety management concepts are consistent among all three programs. However; method of delivery varies to match the developmental needs of each age group. The program skills are discussed to coincide with the FRIENDS acronym.

- **Feelings.** This skill involves affective education, focused on understanding feelings in one's self and in others. The focus is on empathy building, awareness of one's own emotional responses, and emotional regulation. Children are taught to specifically identify physiological indicators (or body clues, e.g., butterflies in the stomach, racing heart) and behavioral indicators (e.g., avoiding anxiety-provoking situations) of anxiety.

Fun FRIENDS variation: The feelings concept is introduced through play and activity and uses colorful pictures to demonstrate feelings. Children are introduced to the concept of being brave. Brave behaviors (i.e., social skills) can include looking people in the eye, using a brave voice, smiling, standing up tall, and giving something a try. To assist in the promotion of a positive self-identity, children are also taught to accept similarities and differences among people.

Family skills: Parents and siblings are encouraged to focus on their physiological responses to fear and anxiety. Families are encouraged to accept individual differences, particularly in response to feelings, and to normalize and validate each other's personal emotional responses. Family members are asked to discuss feelings openly with each other.

• **R**emember to relax. Have quiet time/**R**elax. Children are taught that they can feel more calm and brave if they repair their body clues (physiological arousal) by practicing relaxation exercises. Children are encouraged to think of relaxation as a skill like riding a bike that needs to be practiced regularly before they can really enjoy it and notice its benefits. Relaxation strategies include diaphragmatic breathing, progressive muscle relaxation, and visualization.

Fun FRIENDS variation: When discussing body clues, numerous examples must be provided by the facilitator, because it is often difficult for young children to make the connection between the physical symptoms of anxiety and the situations that make them feel worried. This can be demonstrated by providing pictures of other people's body clues (provided in the Fun FRIENDS manual; Barrett, 2007a, 2007b). When working with young children, it is helpful to establish relaxation rules before beginning relaxation. Such rules may include keeping hands to one's self, keeping the eyes closed, listening to the facilitator, and staying quiet.

Family skills: Families are encouraged to learn relaxation strategies and to practice these strategies regularly as a family by creating family relaxation plans, in which all members of the family practice relaxation on scheduled days. The importance of quiet time is emphasized as a preventive measure for stress and anxiety. Parents are encouraged to ensure the family has regular periods of quiet time, whereby everyone in the family can regulate their stress and achieve relaxation. Examples of quiet time include lying on the grass under a tree, listening to quiet music at home, going for a walk along the beach or on a nature trail, reading stories, and drawing pictures.

• **I** can do it! I can try my best!/**I** can try! This step introduces the cognitive strategies of the program. Children are taught to become aware of and pay attention to their inner thoughts or self-talk. Self-talk is described in terms of two different kinds: green helpful thoughts and red unhelpful thoughts. Children are taught that green thoughts are helpful because they make us feel good, happy, and brave, whereas red, unhelpful thoughts make us feel sad, worried, or scared. They are encouraged to identify their unhappy red thoughts and to challenge those thoughts and come up with alternate helpful green thoughts. Children are also taught attention-training strategies and are encouraged to always look for and pay attention to the positive aspects in every situation.

• Fun FRIENDS variation: The concept of red and green thoughts is introduced to the children using the analogy of a traffic light: Green means go, red means stop. When we have happy green thoughts, we want to go! When we have unhappy red thoughts, we want to stop! Red and green *Fun FRIENDS* puppets are used to practice identifying red and green thoughts along with other play-based activities that involve dancing, "driving cars," art, and role play.

Family skills: Parents are encouraged to become aware of their own cognitive style and how they model optimism or pessimism to their children through their individual responses to stress and challenges. Families are encouraged to use positive green thoughts to help them cope in difficult situations and to notice and reward each other for trying to think in helpful ways. Families are encouraged to challenge one another's thoughts using questions such as, "Is that really true?" or "Are you 100% sure that will happen?"

• **Explore solutions and coping step plans/Encourage.** This step aims to teach children ways to solve problems in difficult or worrying situations through a number of proactive plans. First, the Six-Block Problem-Solving Plan (used in the children and youth versions) involves thinking through a number of steps to solve a problem, including (1) What is the problem—Define it!, (2) Brainstorm—List all possible solutions, (3) List what might happen for each solution, (4) Select the best solution based on the consequences, (5) Make a plan for putting this solution into practice and do it!, and (6) Evaluate the outcome in terms of strengths and weaknesses, and if it did not work return to step 2 and try again.

The second plan for dealing with anxiety-provoking situations is the coping step plan (used in all three versions). In the coping step plan, children construct a graded-exposure hierarchy that they will implement during the remainder of the program; it involves exposure and response prevention to feared situations. In implementing the step plan, children are encouraged to use the strategies covered in previous sessions to assist them as they climb each step.

Third is the CALM model, used only in the youth version. CALM is a conflict resolution plan that teaches teenagers conflict resolutions using the following steps: (C) **C**alm down when in a conflict situation, (A) **A**ctively listen to the other person and what he or she wants, (L) **L**ist their own needs in the situation, and (M) **M**ake a solution that is based on a compromise between both person's needs.

Fun FRIENDS variation: With this young age group, the coping plans work best when created with the parents because they are often more aware of which fears/difficult situations their children ought to conquer. Although the coping step plans are a primary focus of the parenting session, children are taught friendship skills—sharing, helping, listening, and smiling—using game-based activities. Parents are encouraged to praise and reward their children when they demonstrate friendship behaviors.

Family skills: All family members are taught how to use the problem-solving plan and create coping step plans. Everyone in the family is encouraged to create their own coping step plan so that they can practice setting goals, focusing on solutions and working toward outcomes. Parents are encouraged to be positive role models for their children (e.g., approaching difficult situations rather than avoiding them and encouraging their child to do the same).

• **Now reward yourself! You've done your best!/Nurture.** This step teaches children to evaluate their performance in terms of partial success and to set reasonable, achievable goals. Children are encouraged to reward themselves whenever they try their best.

The importance of support networks (called support teams) and role models within the home, school, and wider community are discussed.

Family skills: Parents are encouraged to attend to the positive, desirable behaviors of their anxious children by providing praise or reward. Attending to positive behavior acts to reinforce the behavior and increases the likelihood that the positive behavior will be repeated in the future. Children and parents are encouraged to extend and strengthen their support networks.

- **D**on't forget to practice/**D**on't forget to be brave and **S**mile! Stay calm for life!/ **S**tay happy. Step **D** reminds children that the skills and strategies learned in the FRIENDS programs need to be practiced on a regular basis. Step **S** reminds children that they can stay calm because they have effective strategies for coping. Children are encouraged to plan ahead for challenging situations and to identify how they can use their *FRIENDS* plan to help them cope.

Family skills for **D** and **S**: Families are encouraged to always discuss and review challenging situations. Because children with anxiety tend to focus on situations in the future, it is important for parents to always talk about upcoming challenges with children. Families are taught to focus on the positive aspects of the upcoming situation and to discuss how they can use the FRIENDS skills to help them cope.

Fun FRIENDS variation: In addition to the cognitive-behavioral skills already mentioned, the Fun FRIENDS program also focuses on resilience promotion through the development of social and emotional learning. The following skills are incorporated: developing a self-identify, emotion regulation and feelings management, becoming responsible for oneself and others, and increasing prosocial behaviors by promoting social skills and friendships skills. All of these skills are administered in a play-based manner with multiple activities per session lasting approximately 5–10 minutes each.

Facilitator Manuals and Workbooks

One of the goals in creating the FRIENDS programs was to ensure that they were user friendly and could be implemented in research and community settings. To this end, all three programs are manualized and consist of two parts:

1. A group leader's manual that clearly describes the activities the facilitator needs to implement in each session and detailed content for the parenting sessions.
2. A workbook for each child or youth to complete while working through the program. In Fun FRIENDS, a family activity workbook (called Family Adventure Workbook) is available.

The FRIENDS for Life children and youth manuals are published by Australian Academic Press and can be ordered from the FRIENDS website *www.friendsinfo.net/*. Fun FRIENDS manuals can be ordered from the Fun FRIENDS website *www.ourfunfriends. com.au*. Facilitators must attend an accredited training workshop before implementing the programs (see recommendations regarding implementation in practice). Other supporting materials, including relaxation eye pillows and red and green thoughts koala puppets, are available through the Pathways Health and Research Centre website: *www. pathwayshrc.com.au/resources*.

EVIDENCE ON THE EFFECTS OF TREATMENT

How Treatment Is Evaluated

A multiple-informant, multimethod approach to the assessment of anxiety is recommended. Clinical interviews with the child (if age appropriate) and his or her parents, self-report measures, and parent and teacher behavior ratings should be included as matter of course at the beginning, middle, and end of treatment. Follow-up assessments at 6 and 12 months posttreatment should be included when possible.

When evaluating family-based treatments, there is a clear need to include measures of family functioning, parental psychopathology, and observations of parent–child interaction. It is important to obtain data from both parents, particularly fathers. We believe it is important to assess children's level of positive coping, strength, resilience, and happiness to obtain more data on individual strengths and positive changes over time. These measures are now becoming increasingly available in the literature for all age groups. In addition, recent evidence has highlighted the need to examine the contribution of emotional regulation skills training in CBT treatment programs (Hannesdottir & Ollendick, 2007) for childhood anxiety disorders.

Status of the Evidence

Since Kendall's (1994) study, researchers have espoused the importance of *parental involvement* in helping anxious children and have extended the role of parents in treatment from the typically more passive role of consultants and collaborators to engaging them (and family members) as co-clients in therapy. Barrett et al. (1996) conducted the first randomized controlled trial of CBT plus family anxiety management (FAM) training. In this study (Barrett et al., 1996), FAM involved (1) training parents in contingency management, (2) giving parents skills to better manage their own anxiety, and (3) training parents in problem-solving and communication skills. Barrett et al. (1996) randomly assigned 79 children (ages 7–14 years) to either ICBT, CBT + FAM, or a wait-list condition. At posttreatment, 61% of children in the ICBT group were diagnosis free compared with 88% of children in the combined treatment and less than 30% in the wait-list condition. At 12-month follow-up, the relative superiority of CBT + FAM was maintained.

Interestingly, age and gender appeared to moderate the effectiveness of the additional parent component. Specifically, younger children (ages 7–10 years) and girls who completed the CBT + FAM condition were more likely to be diagnosis free than their peers in the ICBT condition. For boys and children ages 11–14 years, the ICBT was as effective as CBT + FAM at posttreatment and at follow-up. Barrett et al. (1996) suggested that enhancing parenting skills and involvement in child anxiety management may be important for younger children, but for older children individual work may be sufficient to reduce anxiety, possibly because of growing need for autonomy that occurs during adolescence. In a long-term follow-up study, Barrett, Duffy, Dadds, and Rapee (2001) assessed 52 of the 79 original participants. Of these 52 participants, 31 had received ICBT and 21 had received CBT + FAM. The follow-up results continued to support the efficacy of ICBT and CBT + FAM across all measures, but no significant differences were found between the two conditions on any measure at the follow-up.

In the first controlled trial of group FCBT intervention for childhood anxiety disorders, Barrett (1998) randomly assigned 60 children (ages 7–14 years) to three treatment conditions: group CBT (GCBT), group CBT plus family management (GCBT + FAM), and wait-list control. At posttreatment, 56% of children in the GCBT condition, 71% in the GCBT + FAM condition, and 25% in the wait-list condition no longer met criteria for any anxiety disorder diagnosis. At 12-month follow-up, 65% in the GCBT and 85% in the GCBT + FAM conditions were diagnosis free. At posttreatment and 12-month follow-up, comparison of the GCBT and GCBT + FAM conditions revealed that children in the latter showed significant improvements on measures of diagnostic status, parent perception of their ability to deal with the child's behavior, and change in family disruption by child's behavior. These results suggest that FCBT interventions for childhood anxiety disorders can be effectively administered in a group format. In support of the findings from Barrett et al.'s (1996) earlier study, the addition of a family management component led to more favorable outcomes.

Following her 1998 study, Barrett developed the FRIENDS program, a family-based group CBT (FGCBT). Shortt et al. (2001) conducted the first randomized clinical trial evaluating the efficacy of the FRIENDS program for children. Seventy-one children ranging in age from 6–10 years who met diagnostic criteria for an anxiety disorder were randomly assigned to the FRIENDS group or wait-list control. Children in the treatment group participated in 10 weekly sessions in addition to two booster sessions that occurred 1 and 3 months after treatment. Results indicated that children who completed the program showed greater improvement than the wait-list condition. Sixty-eight percent of the children who completed the FGCBT were diagnosis free compared with 6% of those in the wait-list condition. At 12-month follow-up, treatment gains were maintained, with 76% of the children in the treatment group being diagnosis free. These results are positive and demonstrate the efficacy of the FRIENDS program with familial involvement in decreasing anxiety immediately after program implementation and over time.

More recently, Liber et al. (2008) examined individual CBT (ICBT) versus GCBT in the delivery of the Dutch translation of the FRIENDS for LIFE for Children program (Utens, de Nijs, & Ferdinand, 2001) with a group of referred anxious children (N = 133). Children were randomly assigned into the ICBT or GCBT conditions and received the FRIENDS program. All of the parents received four sessions of CBT parent training. Liber et al. (2008) found no significant difference in treatment outcome between ICBT and GCBT. Similar decreases were found at posttreatment for participants who no longer met criteria for any anxiety disorder (ICBT, 48%; GCBT, 41%) and for those who no longer met the criteria for their primary disorder (ICBT, 62%; GCBT, 54%). These results suggest that anxious children benefited equally from the FRIENDS program delivered in both individual and group formats with parental involvement, as evidenced by decreased anxiety at posttreatment. No control group was used in this study.

In summary, research by our team provides positive support for the utilization of GCBT with parent/familial involvement. In recent years, our research interests have expanded. We have adopted a joint focus on both treatment and prevention and early intervention to intervene before the development of significant anxiety symptomatology. The decision to adopt a joint focus is based on our belief that treating children who are already experiencing significant anxiety problems may not be the most effective or efficient means of reducing the incidence of childhood anxiety in the general population. The FRIENDS program has accumulated an evidence base as a universal prevention program, with significant decreases in anxiety found immediately after program implementation (Barrett & Turner, 2001; Lowry-Webster, Barrett, & Dadds, 2001; Stallard et al., 2005; Stallard, Simpson, Anderson, Hibbert, & Osborn, 2007) and effects maintained at 12-month (Lock & Barrett, 2003; Lowry-Webster, Barrett, & Lock, 2003; Stallard, Simpson, Anderson, & Goddard, 2008) and a 3-year (Barrett, Farrell, Ollendick, & Dadds, 2006) follow-up.

To date, one universal, school-based controlled trial has been conducted ($N = 263$) examining the Fun FRIENDS program (Pahl & Barrett, 2009a). Results have indicated nearly significant decreases in anxiety, significant decreases in behavioral inhibition (BI) and increases in social-emotional strength for children following the intervention program for children in the intervention group and wait-list control group. Interestingly, girls improved more than boys on BI and social-emotional strength. Teacher report indicated that children in the intervention group improved significantly more than children in the wait-list group on BI and social-emotional strength immediately following the program. At 12-month follow-up, significant improvements in anxiety were found from preintervention measures, and significant decreases in BI were evident at all time points for girls but not for boys. Improvements on social-emotional strength were found from preintervention to 12-month follow-up, with girls scoring significantly higher than boys at all time points, although boys' scores did increase over time (Pahl & Barrett, 2009a). As a result of ethical restrictions, there was no comparison group at 12-month follow-up; therefore, we lacked the evidence to suggest that the intervention was solely responsible for the long-term positive changes that occurred in the children who received the intervention. Nevertheless, these results are promising and highlight the possible long-term positive impact of the program. Social validity data collected throughout the trial demonstrated that teachers and parents enjoyed the program. The results from this trial demonstrate that intervention programs can be successfully adapted for use with young children ages 4–6 years. Our research team is currently undertaking a large treatment trial of the Fun FRIENDS program setting. See Table 5.4 for a summary of research findings.

Overall Evaluation of the Treatment

The programs encompass a family approach to empower everyone in the family to recognize their skills and strengths and to use these skills to help each other become more brave and confident. This family approach helps to maintain long-term sustainability of the skills through continual reinforcement and modeling among all family members. The approach differs from isolated CBT interventions, which focus solely on treating the child or on treating the parents (i.e., parenting management training only). The FRIENDS programs are child centered and maintain a focus on developing reciprocal interactions in the family as all members learn positive coping skills. In metaphorical terms, this approach can be compared with learning a language. Attempting to learn a language by oneself or in isolation from others will prove to be difficult and may lead to limited success. In contrast, learning a language as a family unit, where all family members practice the language several nights per week, will increase the chance of success and the likelihood that the language will be learned and maintained.

The programs also encourage the inclusion of extended family networks, including grandparents. Grandparents are seen as important participants in the promotion of mental health. They can represent positive, supportive role models to many young children and can provide children with invaluable knowledge regarding familial history and the continuity of culture and identity. In the FRIENDS programs, grandparents are welcomed and encouraged to attend sessions and to be actively involved in their grand-children's lives whenever possible.

A limitation to our research is the lack of available data assessing positive, strength-based traits such as happiness, resilience, and coping and the subsequent effect the FRIENDS programs have on such traits. It is important to obtain these data to examine the positive changes (i.e., increased happiness) that occur following the FRIENDS programs and over time. Currently research evaluating the Fun FRIENDS program has incorporated assessment measures examining resilience and social-emotional strength. Assessment is also warranted to examine the unique contribution of the emotional regulation skills taught in the program (see Hannesdottir & Ollendick, 2007) and to potentially make this a larger component of the program in future revisions.

RECOMMENDATIONS REGARDING IMPLEMENTATION IN PRACTICE

Family Involvement

Emerging evidence supports the inclusion of fathers in treatment for various types of developmental psychopathology; such inclusion has led to better long-term mental health outcomes (Bögels & Phares, 2008). However, fathers have been neglected in research on the cause, prevention, and treatment of childhood anxiety even though research has highlighted the important role of fathers in the socialization of children and in the protection against severe anxiety and their potentially important role in the treatment of child anxiety (Bögels & Phares, 2008). In their review, Bögels and Phares (2008) recommended that every effort be made to involve *all* fathers in anxiety research. A recent modeling study by Pahl and Barrett (2009b) demonstrated the important role of fathers in the etiology of early childhood anxiety. The study examined risk factors of early childhood anxiety in a sample of 4- to 6-year-olds ($N = 236$). Results indicated that mother's parenting stress and negative affect (anxiety and depression) significantly predicted early childhood anxiety. Mediational analyses revealed that father's parenting stress may affect child anxiety via mother's parenting stress, indicating a reciprocal family interaction of stress and anxiety. These direct and mediational effects demonstrate the contributing role of both parents in the development and maintenance of anxiety and reinforce the need to involve both parents in the treatment and intervention process.

Frequently, family involvement overlooks siblings; however, our research has demonstrated the negative effects that anxiety disorders have on siblings and the potential significance and benefits of involving siblings in therapy (i.e., Fox, Barrett, & Shortt, 2002). Family involvement in therapy, including parents and siblings, increases the social support for the child with anxiety, enhances consistency in contingency management, and encourages greater practice of skills and generalization of skills by having everyone use the same strategies and approaches in managing stress and anxiety. Practicalities for clinicians in increasing the likelihood of family attendance is to offer after-hour appointments for families, including weekend sessions, to ensure they are aware of the expectations for all to attend in advance, to strongly reinforce fathers and siblings who attend sessions, and to provide specific homework tasks for all family members so that they feel their presence is valued and worthwhile.

TABLE 5.4. Treatment and Prevention Studies Examining the FRIENDS Programs

Author(s)	N	Format	Comparison group	Postintervention effects	Maintenance effects
Barrett et al. (1996)	79 (ages 7–14 years)	ICBT CBT + FAM	WL	ICBT, 61% diagnosis free CBT + FAM, 88% diagnosis free WL, 30% diagnosis free	At 12-month FU, CBT + FAM superior to ICBT
Barrett et al. (2001)	52 6-year FU for Barrett et al. (1996)	ICBT CBT + FAM	WL		Efficacy of ICBT and CBT + FAM supported. No significant differences between groups.
Barrett (1998)	60 (ages 7–14 years)	GCBT GCBT + FAM	WL	GCBT, 56% diagnosis free GCBT + FAM, 71% diagnosis free WL, 25% diagnosis free	12-month FU: GCBT, 65% diagnosis free GCBT + FAM, 85% diagnosis free
Shortt et al. (2001)	91 (ages 6–14 years)	FGCBT	WL	FGCBT, 68% diagnosis free WL, 6% diagnosis free	12-month FU: FGCBT, 76% diagnosis free
Liber et al. (2008)	133 (ages 8–12 years)	ICBT + parent involvement GCBT + parent involvement	No	No longer met criteria for anxiety disorder: ICBT, 48% GCBT, 41% No longer met criteria for primary disorder: ICBT, 62% GCBT, 54%	
Barrett & Turner (2001)	489 (ages 9–10 years)	Universal, school-based intervention	Psychologist- versus teacher-led conditions MT	Significant reductions in anxiety in psychologist- and teacher-led conditions compared with MT	
Lowry-Webster et al. (2001)	594 (ages 10–13 years)	Universal, train-the-trainer model, preventive intervention	MT	Significant reductions in anxiety in the IG and MT group. Significant reduction in self-reported symptoms of depression for IG only. High-risk status: IG, 75.3% no longer at risk MT, 54.8% no longer at risk	
Lowry-Webster et al. (2003)	594 Long-term FU of Lowry-				Prevention effects maintained at 12-month FU with lower anxiety scores for IG versus MT.

Study	Sample	Type	Comparison	Results	Follow-up
Webster et al. (2001)					85% at high risk in IG were diagnosis free at FU compared with 31.2% in MT.
Lock & Barrett (2003)	737 $N = 336$ (ages 9–10 years) $N = 401$ (ages 14–16 years)	Universal school-based preventive intervention	MT	Significant reductions in anxiety in both IG and MT. Reductions larger for IG. Significant decreases in grade 6 compared with grade 9.	At 12-month FU, significant reductions in anxiety in both IG and MT. Reductions larger for IG. Significant reductions in depressive symptoms for IG.
Barrett et al. (2006)	669 Long-term FU (12, 24, 36 months) for Lock & Barrett (2003)	Universal school-based preventive intervention	MT		Significantly lower anxiety in IG. No significant group differences for grade 9 students at FU points. Females in IG reported significantly lower anxiety than MT at 12- and 24-month FU but not 36-month FU. Fewer at high risk in IG at 36-month FU.
Stallard et al. (2005)	213 (ages 9–10 years)	Universal school-based preventive intervention	No	Significant improvement in anxiety and self-esteem. Significant improvement in more than half of children with severe emotional problems.	
Stallard et al. (2007)	106 (ages 9–10 years)	Universal school-based preventive intervention	No	Postassessment conducted at 3-month FU. Significant improvements in anxiety and self-esteem	
Stallard et al. (2008)	63 Long-term FU of Stallard et al. (2007)	Universal school-based preventive intervention	No		Significant effects maintained at 12-month FU. 67% of high-risk children at baseline were low risk at 12-month FU.
Pahl & Barrett (200x)	263 (ages 4–6 years)	Universal, school-based preventive intervention	WG at postintervention only	Parent report: nearly significant decreases in anxiety, significant decreases in BI, and significant improvements in social-emotional strength for both conditions. Teacher report: significant improvements in BI and social-emotional strength for children in the intervention group.	Significant improvements in anxiety, BI (girls only), and social-emotional strength. There was no comparison group at 12-month follow-up.

Note. BI, behavioral inhibition; CBT, cognitive-behavioral therapy; FAM, family; FGCBT, family group cognitive-behavioral therapy; FU, follow-up; GCBT, group cognitive-behavioral therapy; ICBT, individual cognitive-behavioral therapy; IG, intervention group; MT, monitoring group; WL, wait-list control group.

Program Delivery and Process

The FRIENDS programs can be successfully run in clinic and school settings following the required training (see Program Training section later). When conducting the *FRIENDS* groups within each setting, it is crucial to consider process issues important to successful program delivery. These can be broken down into several main areas, applicable to all settings:

1. *Family.* It is important to involve parents, siblings, and extended family when possible. In the school setting, parents can be invited to cofacilitate sessions to act as mentors and role models but should be separated from their own children when doing activities. Mentors may be recruited from higher grades to act as positive mentors and role models.

2. *Setting up the group for an optimal learning experience.* It is often helpful to break the larger group into smaller groups for activities to optimize the learning experience and allow greater opportunity for all children to have a turn and share ideas. Ideas should then be shared with the larger group. After sharing ideas, all group members should applaud each child and the facilitator can use positive feedback such as "good idea" or "thanks for being so brave and sharing with us" to reinforce their effort. Children should be seated strategically, with a cofacilitator beside any disruptive children to impose behavior management strategies. If siblings are in a group together, we recommend seating them apart whenever possible to foster individual independence. As a facilitator, it is important to allow all children in the group a turn to speak to the group, to reinforce the shy, introverted children, and to always follow up their efforts with praise.

3. *Behavior management.* Behavior management strategies ought to be considered before the program commences. Facilitators should have a clear idea of what behavior management skills will be implemented if disruptive behavior occurs. These may include planned ignoring for mild to moderate misbehavior and time-out for severe misbehavior. For young children, reward charts may be used to reinforce positive behaviors.

Booster Sessions and Follow-Up

The FRIENDS programs incorporate two booster sessions to be held 1 month and 3 months after treatment. The booster sessions focus on a review of all skills learned in the programs and focus on preparing children for future challenges. We recommend offering longer term follow-up sessions (e.g., at 6 months and 12 months) to assist in skill maintenance.

Program Training

A requirement for implementing the FRIENDS programs is to attend an accredited training workshop to learn successful delivery of the program skills. Training workshops are frequently held across Australia and worldwide. Training is available internationally through a license agreement with Pathways Health and Research Centre. The license agreement grants access to specialized training protocols and systems for dissemination of the program by schools, clinics, governmental and nongovernment organizations, universities, and private companies. For more information, please visit the Pathways website: *www.pathwayshrc.com.au.*

DIRECTIONS FOR RESEARCH

Issues for future research in child anxiety treatment include extended evaluations of family-based treatments focused on outcomes addressing the role of the family in maintaining anxiety as well as in improving outcomes for child anxiety disorders. Although parental psychopathology and family interaction variables may play a role in the maintenance of anxiety, little is known about how these issues can be addressed in treatment and how family members and family characteristics (such as interactions) may actually improve outcomes in therapy. Controlled trials evaluating FCBT, which include the entire family in therapy, versus child-focused therapy alone and child plus parent therapy (without siblings) are warranted to determine the genuine effectiveness of family involvement in CBT for child anxiety disorders. Further investigation is also required in the specific role of fathers in the etiology and treatment of childhood anxiety.

There is an increasing need to improve available measurement devices. Rating scales used to compare variants of CBT generally show nonstatistically significant differences between treatment conditions (with or without parental involvement). This lack of significant difference may be due in part to insensitivity of the existing measures in detecting the specific skills that are being targeted in treatment programs. For example, the specific parenting skills targeted in parenting programs may be inadequately assessed with the available measures (Silverman et al., 2008). In addition to efficient assessment of anxiety disorders, we believe strength-based measures should be incorporated into standard assessment procedures, including those examining positive coping, resilience, happiness, self-esteem, and social-emotional competence. Such assessments would allow for the examination of alternate outcomes from CBT and shift the focus from psychopathology to strength-based assessment. Further research is needed to examine the contributing role of emotional regulation skills in CBT programs for child anxiety.

There is a need to conduct randomized treatment trials of the Fun FRIENDS program to assess its effectiveness in treating young anxious children. Research indicates that approximately 10–15% of young children experience internalizing problems (Egger & Angold, 2006), yet research and available treatment programs remain scarce for this age group. This may be due to the difficulties posed by assessing this young age group. There is uncertainty as to whether current diagnostic categories for anxiety are reliable or valid for this young age group because fears during the preschool years are common, normal part of development. Furthermore, diagnostic assessment tools for preschool children are scarce and still under development. Additional research examining FCBT with young children is required along with the development of appropriate assessment measures.

CONCLUSIONS

Research investigating anxiety disorders in children has revealed that successful treatment outcome can be achieved through group-based interventions (e.g., the FRIENDS program) involving parents and families. The FRIENDS programs are offered in three developmentally tailored versions and deliver cognitive-behavioral skills. The programs aim to empower families to develop positive coping skills and to work as a team in increasing brave and confident behaviors. Research to date by our team has highlighted the usefulness of the child and youth versions of the FRIENDS program in decreasing anxiety immediately after completion of the group program and at long-term follow-up. The results have also suggested that parents play a positive role in the maintenance and sustainability of program skills.

Additional research is required to examine the influence of family-based treatment with the inclusion of siblings and parents. We believe that involving all family members is extremely important for skill acquisition, reinforcement, generalization, and long-term maintenance. We foresee a shift in treatment paradigms over the next 10 years to involve all family members in treatment, including extended family members (e.g., grandparents), as normative, standard practice, with multiple benefits being observed in child mental health.

We also foresee a shift in the focus of assessment from psychopathology-based to strength-based assessment (positive coping, happiness, resilience) and the implementation of treatment and intervention programs earlier in the developmental trajectory (e.g., the preschool years). In our opinion, these advances (involving entire families in treatment and early initiation of treatment/interventions in the developmental trajectory) would significantly benefit the mental health of many children and families.

REFERENCES

Barrett, P. M. (1998). Evaluation of cognitive-behavioral group treatments for childhood anxiety disorders. *Journal of Clinical Child Psychology, 27,* 459–468.

Barrett, P. M. (2004). *FRIENDS for Life program—Group leader's workbook for children* (4th ed.). Brisbane, Queensland: Australian Academic Press.

Barrett, P. M. (2005). *FRIENDS for Life Program—Group leader's workbook for youth* (4th ed.). Brisbane, Queensland: Australian Academic Press.

Barrett, P. M. (2007a). *Fun FRIENDS. Family learning adventure: Resilience building activities for 4, 5, & 6-year-old children.* Brisbane, Australia: Fun FRIENDS.

Barrett, P. M. (2007b). *Fun FRIENDS. The teaching and training manual for group leaders.* Brisbane, Australia: Fun FRIENDS.

Barrett, P. M., Dadds, M. R., & Rapee, R. (1996). Family treatment of childhood anxiety: A controlled trial. *Journal of Consulting and Clinical Psychology, 64,* 333–342.

Barrett, P. M., Duffy, A., Dadds, M., & Rapee, R. (2001). Cognitive-behavioral treatment of anxiety disorders in children: Long term (6 year) follow up. *Journal of Consulting and Clinical Psychology, 69,* 135–141.

Barrett, P. M., Farrell, L. J., Ollendick, T. H., & Dadds, M. (2006). Long-term outcomes of an Australian universal prevention trial of anxiety and depression symptoms in children and youth: An evaluation of the FRIENDS program. *Journal of Clinical Child and Adolescent Psychology, 35,* 403–411.

Barrett, P. M., & Turner, C. M. (2001). Prevention of anxiety symptoms in primary school children: Preliminary results from a universal school-based trial. *British Journal of Clinical Psychology, 40,* 399–410.

Bögels, S., & Phares, V. (2008). Fathers' role in the etiology, prevention and treatment of child anxiety: A review and new model. *Clinical Psychology Review, 28,* 539–558.

Cartwright-Hattton, S., McNicol, K., & Doubleday, E. (2006). Anxiety in a neglected population: Prevalence of anxiety disorders in pre-adolescent children. *Clinical Psychology Review, 26,* 817–833.

Egger, H. L., & Angold, A. (2006). Common emotional and behavioral disorders in preschool children: Presentation, nosology, and epidemiology. *Journal of Child Psychology and Psychiatry, 47,* 313–337.

Fox, T., Barrett, P. M., & Shortt, A. (2002). Sibling relationships of anxious children: A preliminary investigation. *Journal of Clinical Child and Adolescent Psychiatry, 31*, 375–383.

Hannesdottir, D. K., & Ollendick, T. H. (2007). The role of emotion regulation in the treatment of child anxiety disorders. *Clinical Child and Family Psychology Review, 10*, 275–239.

Kendall, P. C. (1990). *Coping Cat workbook*. Ardmore, PA: Workbook.

Kendall, P. C. (1994). Treating anxiety disorders in youth: Results of a randomised clinical trial. *Journal of Consulting and Clinical Psychology, 62*, 100–110.

Liber, J. M., Van Widenfelt, B. M., Utens, E. M., Ferdinand, R. F., Van der Leeden, A. J., Van Gastel, W., et al. (2008). No differences between group versus individual treatment of childhood anxiety disorders in a randomised clinical trial. *Journal of Child Psychology and Psychiatry, 49*, 886–893.

Lock, S., & Barrett, P. M. (2003). A longitudinal study of developmental differences in universal preventive intervention for child anxiety. *Behavior Change, 20*, 183–199.

Lowry-Webster, H. M., Barrett, P. M., & Dadds, M. R. (2001). A universal prevention trial of anxiety and depressive symptomatology in childhood: Preliminary data from an Australian study. *Behavior Change, 18*, 36–50.

Lowry-Webster, H. M., Barrett, P. M., & Lock, S. (2003). A universal prevention trial of anxiety symptomatology during childhood: Results at 1-year follow-up. *Behavior Change, 20*, 25–43.

Ollendick, T. H., & King, N. J. (1998). Empirically supported treatments for children with phobic and anxiety disorders: Current status. *Journal of Clinical Child Psychology, 27*, 156–167.

Pahl, K. M., & Barrett, P. M. (2009a). *Preventing anxiety and promoting social and emotional strength in preschool children: A universal evaluation of the Fun FRIENDS program*. Manuscript submitted for publication.

Pahl, K. M., & Barrett, P. M. (2009b). *Examining potential risk factors for anxiety and behavioral inhibition in preschool aged children*. Manuscript submitted for publication.

Shortt, A., Barrett, P. M., & Fox, T. (2001). Evaluating the FRIENDS program: A cognitive-behavioral group treatment of childhood anxiety disorders. *Journal of Clinical Child Psychology, 30*, 525–535.

Silverman, W. K., Pina, A. A., & Viswesvaran, C. (2008). Evidence-based psychosocial treatments for phobic and anxiety disorders in children and adolescents. *Journal of Clinical Child and Adolescent Psychology, 37*, 105–130.

Stallard, P., Simpson, N., Anderson, S., Carter, T., Osborn, C., & Bush, S. (2005). An evaluation of the FRIENDS programme—A cognitive behavior therapy intervention to promote emotional resilience. *Archives of Disease in Childhood, 90*(10), 1016–1019.

Stallard, P., Simpson, N., Anderson, S., & Goddard, M. (2008). The FRIENDS emotional health prevention programme: 12 month follow-up of a universal UK school based trial. *European Journal of Child and Adolescent Psychiatry, 17*, 283–289.

Stallard, P., Simpson, N., Anderson, S., Hibbert, S., & Osborn, C. (2007). The FRIENDS Emotional Health Programme: Initial findings from a school-based project. *Child and Adolescent Mental Health, 12*, 32–37.

Utens, E. M. W. J., de Nijs, P., & Ferdinand, R. F. (2001). *FRIENDS for children—Manual for group leaders [Dutch translation]*. Rotterdam, the Netherlands: Department of Child and Adolescent Psychiatry Erasmus Medical Centre/Sophia Children's Hospital Rotterdam.

6

Treating Pediatric Obsessive–Compulsive Disorder Using Exposure-Based Cognitive-Behavioral Therapy

MARTIN E. FRANKLIN, JENNIFER FREEMAN, and JOHN S. MARCH

OVERVIEW

At any given time, up to 1 in 100 children and adolescents suffers from clinically significant obsessive–compulsive disorder (OCD; e.g., Flament et al., 1988), and up to one half of adults with OCD developed the disorder during childhood or adolescence (Rasmussen & Eisen, 1990). Thus, besides reducing morbidity and functional impairment associated with pediatric OCD, improvements in treatment and in making empirically supported treatments more readily available have the potential to reduce OCD symptoms and related dysfunction into adulthood. Fortunately, significant advances have been made over the past decade and, as is the case with adult OCD, cognitive-behavioral therapy (CBT) has emerged as the initial treatment of choice for pediatric OCD (Abramowitz, Whiteside, & Deacon, 2005; March, Frances, Kahn, & Carpenter, 1997). The evidence on which these expert opinions are based has strengthened considerably in the last decade, lending further credence to experts' recommendation that families be vigorously encouraged to seek CBT for children and adolescents suffering from this often disabling condition.

Our review begins with a discussion of the fundamental principles on which the treatment is based, and we then provide a brief review of our CBT protocol for use in both clinical and research settings (March & Mulle, 1998). Next, we briefly summarize empirical studies supporting the use of CBT with children and adolescents, including discussion of multisite comparative treatment trials involving CBT as an initial treatment for pediatric OCD (Franklin, Foa, & March, 2003; Pediatric OCD Treatment Study Team, 2004), as an adjunctive treatment for children and adolescents who have experienced a partial response to serotonergic medication for OCD (Freeman et al., 2009), and as a treatment for very young children with OCD (Freeman et al., 2007, 2008). We then provide some recommendations for future research.

THE TREATMENT MODEL AND THE ROLE OF ASSESSMENT

Treatment of OCD in children and adolescents should always begin with proper assessment and psychoeducation. In our view, an adequate assessment of pediatric OCD should include (1) a comprehensive evaluation of current and past OCD symptoms; (2) current OCD symptom severity and associated functional impairment; and (3) comorbid psychopathology. The strengths of the child and family, as well as their knowledge of OCD and its treatment, should also be considered.

In documenting past and current OCD symptoms and current symptom severity, it is important to determine whether the child should be interviewed with or without the parents present. The decision can be informed by discussing the alternatives with the parents in advance and observing the child and family's behavior in the waiting area and even during the interview itself, if necessary. For example, if it becomes clear that a patient is reluctant to discuss certain symptoms with parents present (e.g., sexual or extremely violent obsessions), the clinician can save some time at the end of the interview to revisit these potentially sensitive issues alone with the patient.

Before initiating the formal assessment, the evaluator should define obsessions and compulsions, using specific examples if the child or parents have difficulty grasping the key concepts. We also let families know about the prevalence, nature, and treatment of OCD, which may increase their willingness to disclose specific symptoms once the semistructured interview begins. Children may be particularly vulnerable to feeling as though they are the only ones suffering from certain obsessive fears, such as intrusive images of hurting a loved one, so prefacing examples with "I once met a kid who ... " to allay this concern immediately may improve the quality of the assessment.

THE APPLICATION OF CBT FOR PEDIATRIC OCD

Exposure and Ritual Prevention

As applied to OCD, the exposure principle relies on the fact that anxiety usually attenuates after sufficient duration of contact with a feared stimulus that is not inherently dangerous. Thus, a child with fear of germs must confront fear-relevant but objectively low-risk situations and allow his or her anxiety to decrease naturally over time. Repeated exposure is associated with decreased anxiety across exposure trials (between-session habituation), with anxiety reduction largely specific to the domain of exposure, until the child no longer fears contact with specifically targeted phobic stimuli. Adequate exposure depends on blocking the negative reinforcement effect of rituals or other avoidance behavior, a process termed response or ritual prevention. For example, a child with germ worries must not only touch "germy things" but must refrain from ritualized washing until his or her anxiety diminishes substantially. Exposure and ritual prevention (EX/RP) is typically implemented in a gradual fashion (sometimes termed graded exposure), with exposure targets developed in an interactive process between patients and therapists. Intensive approaches may be especially useful for treatment-resistant OCD or for patients who desire a very rapid response (Franklin et al., 1998; Storch, Geffken, Merlo, Mann, et al., 2007).

Cognitive Techniques

A wide variety of cognitive interventions have been used to provide the child with a "tool kit" to facilitate compliance with EX/RP. The goals of such interventions, which may be more or less useful or necessary depending on the child and the nature of his or her specific OCD symptoms, typically include increasing a sense of personal efficacy, predictability, controllability, and self-attributed likelihood of a positive outcome within EX/RP tasks. Specific interventions include (1) constructive self-talk and "bossing-back OCD" and (2) cultivating nonattachment or, stated differently, learning to simply notice obsessions and then allowing them to come and go of their own accord instead of engaging in inherently futile thought suppression attempts. Each of these discussions must be individualized to match the specific OCD symptoms that afflict the child and must mesh with the child's cognitive abilities, developmental stage, and preference among the two techniques. Such methods are routinely incorporated into EX/RP programs, wherein cognitive procedures are used to support and complement EX/RP rather than to replace it (Franklin & Foa, 2008).

Of critical importance is emphasizing the futility of thought suppression efforts of any kind, including distraction, because these efforts provide negative reinforcement and thus are likely to provide only temporary relief while simultaneously strengthening the connection between obsession and compulsion. In trying to underscore this point in a developmentally sensitive manner, we tell our pediatric patients that we want them to change their approach to their obsessions, learning how to "let them go away instead of trying to make them go away." We have an expectation based on outcome studies and experimental data that by eliminating efforts to make bad thoughts and anxiety go away, a reduction in the frequency and intensity of these obsessions will likely follow eventually. However, we take care to de-emphasize in treatment the goal of living obsession free, and instead emphasize the importance of refraining from rituals and avoidance behaviors when obsessions do arise.

Ritual Prevention

Because blocking rituals or avoidance behaviors removes the negative reinforcement effect of the rituals or avoidance, ritual prevention technically is an extinction procedure. By convention, however, extinction is usually defined as the elimination of OCD-related behaviors through removal of parental positive reinforcement for rituals. For example, for a child with reassurance-seeking rituals, the therapist may ask parents to refrain from providing the child with reassurance in response to an OCD-specific question. Extinction frequently produces rapid effects but can be difficult to implement when the child's behavior is bizarre (e.g., screaming out "God forgive me!" in response to obsessional thoughts about the devil regardless of the social context) or very frequent (e.g., asking "Am I OK?" over and over again). In addition, nonconsensual extinction procedures often produce unmanageable distress on the part of the child, disrupt the therapeutic alliance, miss important EX/RP targets that are not amenable to extinction procedures, and, most importantly, fail to help the child internalize a strategy for resisting OCD.

Thus, as with the rest of the EX/RP plan, placing the extinction of reassurance under the child's control leads to increased compliance and improved outcomes, and we provide ample coaching and role-playing examples in session to teach parents and children how to weaken OCD by depriving it of this important source of fuel.

Operant Procedures

Clinically, positive reinforcement seems not to directly alter OCD symptoms but rather helps to encourage compliance with EX/RP procedures and thereby produces a noticeable, if indirect, clinical benefit. In contrast, punishment (defined as imposition of an aversive event) and response–cost (defined as removal of a positive event) procedures have proven to be unhelpful in the treatment of OCD. Most CBT programs use liberal positive reinforcement for compliance with EX/RP tasks and proscribe aversive contingency management procedures unless targeting disruptive behavior outside the domain of OCD. Because OCD itself is a powerful aversive stimulus, successful EX/RP promotes willingness to engage in further EX/RP via negative reinforcement (e.g., reduction of OCD symptoms boosts compliance with EX/RP) as manifested by unscheduled generalization to new EX/RP targets as treatment proceeds.

Involvement of the Family in OCD and in Treatment

Family psychopathology is neither necessary nor sufficient for the onset of OCD; nonetheless, families affect and are affected by the disorder. More specifically, it appears that family accommodation to the child's OCD symptoms is the norm (Peris et al., 2008; Storch, Geffken, Merlo, Jacob, et al., 2007), and that family conflict and comorbid externalizing symptoms are worse when families attempt to refrain from accommodation (Peris et al., 2008). Hence, although dismantling studies in pediatric OCD have yet to indicate clearly the optimal amount of family involvement necessary for robust and durable symptom reduction, clinical observations suggest that some combination of individual and family sessions is best for most patients age 9 and older. In our protocol, we include several whole-family sessions and typically involve the family at the end of each session to ensure that both the parents and the children understand the EX/RP homework assignment and their respective roles in implementing them. Some investigators have emphasized family work even more in the development of their CBT protocols (e.g., Piacentini, Bergman, Jacobs, McCracken, & Kretchman, 2002), and family-based group (FGCBT) CBT has been found to be as effective as individual CBT at reducing OCD symptoms (Barrett, Healy-Farrell, & March, 2004). With younger patients, the role of the family in the OCD process and treatment is larger; our work with very young children with OCD includes parents as part of every session and essentially teaches parents to conduct EX/RP with their children (Freeman et al., 2007).

Our CBT Protocol

Our pediatric OCD treatment protocol (Franklin et al., 2003; Freeman et al., 2009; Pediatric OCD Treatment Study Team, 2004), which is fairly typical of a gradual-exposure regimen (March & Mulle, 1998), consists of 14 visits over 12 weeks across five phases: (1) psychoeducation, (2), cognitive training, (3) mapping OCD, (4), EX/RP, and (5) relapse prevention and generalization training. With the exception of the first 2 weeks, in which patients visit twice weekly, all visits are administered on a once/weekly basis, last 1 hour, and include one between-visit 10-minute telephone contact scheduled during weeks 3–12. Psychoeducation, defining OCD as the identified problem, cognitive training, and development of a stimulus hierarchy (mapping OCD) take place during visits 1–4; EX/RP occurs during visits 5–12, with the last two sessions incorporating generalization training and relapse prevention. Each session includes a statement of goals, review of the previous week, provision of new information, therapist-assisted practice, homework for the coming week, and monitoring procedures.

Parents are centrally involved at sessions 1, 7, and 11, with the latter two sessions devoted to guide the parents about their central role in assisting their child to accomplish the homework assignments. Sessions 13 and 14, which are devoted to relapse prevention and celebration of accomplishments in treatment, also require significant parental input. Parents check in with the therapist at each of the other sessions, and the therapist provides feedback describing the goals of each session and the child's progress in treatment. The therapist works with parents to assist them in refraining from suggesting inappropriate EX/RP tasks. It is not uncommon for parents (and sometimes children as well) to have expectations of moving up the hierarchy too quickly and expecting behavioral change that is much too difficult for a given point in treatment. This sometimes comes from frustration with lack of progress but can also come from excitement from initial success (e.g., parents see that a child has one symptom under control and expect that the child should be able to face all symptoms). In some cases, extensive family involvement in rituals and the developmental level of the child require that family members play a more central role in treatment, as is the case with younger children (Freeman et al., 2007) and children with developmental disabilities. It is important to note that the CBT protocol provides sufficient flexibility to accommodate variations in family involvement dictated by the OCD symptom picture and the developmental level of the child.

Critical to the success of any CBT protocol for children and adolescents is the delivery of treatment in a developmentally appropriate fashion. We promote developmental appropriateness by allowing flexibility in CBT within the constraints of fixed session goals, which Kendall, Gosch, Furr, and Sood (2008) termed "flexibility within fidelity." More specifically, the therapist adjusts the level of discourse to the cognitive functioning, social maturity, and capacity for sustained attention of each patient. Younger patients require more redirection and activities to sustain attention and motivation. Adolescents are generally more sensitive to the effects of OCD on peer interactions, which, in turn, require more discussion. Cognitive interventions in particular require adjustment to the developmental level of the patient, so, for example, adolescents are less likely to appreciate giving OCD a "nasty nickname" than younger children. Developmentally appropriate metaphors relevant to the child's areas of interest and knowledge are also used to promote active involvement in the treatment process.

EVIDENCE ON THE EFFECTS OF CBT

As has typically been the case with pediatric anxiety and mood disorders, the building of the CBT outcome literature in pediatric OCD began with age-downward extension of protocols found efficacious with adults, then publication of single-case studies, case series, and open clinical trials involving these protocols. Collectively, the published uncontrolled evaluations (e.g., Franklin et al., 1998; March, Mulle, & Herbel, 1994; Piacentini et al., 2002) yielded remarkably similar and encouraging findings across settings and cultures: At posttreatment, the vast majority of patients were responders, with significant symptom reductions. This pilot work set the stage for randomized studies evaluating the efficacy of CBT, one of which was published in the late 1990s (de Haan, Hoogduin, Buitelaar, & Keijsers, 1998), four that have been published more recently (Barrett et al., 2004; Bolton & Perrin, 2008; Pediatric OCD Treatment Study Team, 2004; Storch, Geffken, Merlo, Mann, et al., 2007), and one that has recently been completed (J. Piacentini, personal communication, December 4, 2008). Next, we review some of the key findings from this literature. Notably, these six randomized controlled trials (RCTs) have differed considerably with regard to the specific nature of the intervention (individual, family, group), intensity of the treatment, and type of comparison condition, making it difficult to draw definitive comparisons across trials.

Study Design and Treatment Outcome

In the first RCT to compare CBT and medication treatments, de Haan and colleagues (1998) randomly assigned 22 children ages 8–17 to 12 weeks of clomipramine (mean dose, 2.5 mg/kg) or twice-weekly EX/RP. Both treatments led to significant improvement; however, the mean level of symptom reduction following exposure treatment was significantly greater than that for the clomipramine group (59.9% vs. 33.4% decrease in OCD symptoms). The response rate was also higher for the exposure group compared with the clomipramine group (66.7% vs. 50%). No control condition was used in this study, however. Thus, the effects of the passage of time, therapist contact, and repeated assessment on symptom reduction cannot be parsed out. The comparative treatment trial conducted by our group (Pediatric OCD Treatment Study Team, 2004) and discussed later replicated the results of de Haan et al. by repeating the comparison of CBT and a pharmacotherapy of established efficacy and extended their findings by greatly increasing the sample size and including a pill placebo condition as well as a combined treatment arm.

Barrett and colleagues (2004) compared individual family-based CBT (FCBT), (FGCBFT), and wait-list control (WL) in 77 youngsters with OCD ages 7–17 years. Both active treatments consisted of a 14-week manualized protocol that included both parent and sibling components. Participants in the WL group were assessed at baseline and 4–6 weeks later. Both active treatments were associated with significant improvement compared with the truncated WL group. At posttreatment, 88% of FCBT, 76% of FGCBT, and 0% of WL youngsters no longer met criteria for OCD according to parent report on structured interviews. FCBT was associated with a 65% reduction in OCD symptoms according to child-only reports compared with 61% for FGCBT and no change for WL. Observed gains were largely maintained over a 6-month follow-up. Of interest, there were no treatment-related gains on any of the family measures.

Bolton and Perrin (2008) were interested in examining the effects of a more behaviorally oriented protocol that clearly emphasized a habituation model of change, and compared 5 weeks of intensive exposure with response prevention treatment with a WL control in 20 OCD children and adolescents ages 8–17. The exposure protocol was strictly behavioral and did not involve cognitive elements or psychoeducation, as found in many pediatric OCD treatment programs. The program was also delivered intensively, with up to 10 sessions over 7 weeks, and none of the participants were taking medication for their OCD. The authors report a statistically and clinically significant reduction in OCD symptoms for the exposure group at the end of treatment and at 14-week follow-up.

To examine the advantage of intensive versus less intensive CBT, Storch, Geffken, Merlo, Mann, et al. (2007) compared 14 sessions of CBT delivered in a standard weekly protocol with 14 sessions of daily (or intensive) CBT in 40 participants with OCD ages 7–17 years. The authors found no significant overall differences in symptom reduction between the two groups. When global measures of functioning were considered, there appeared to be a slight advantage for daily treatment immediately posttreatment, but there were no group differences at 3-month follow-up. These results suggested that the more easily transported weekly protocol is sufficient to treat OCD in patients with mild to moderately severe OCD.

Both of the studies just reviewed that used comparison conditions (Barrett et al., 2004; Bolton & Perrin, 2008) failed to control for nonspecific effects of therapist contact time, thus leaving unresolved the question of whether the specific techniques of CBT are responsible for the observed symptom reductions. In a recent RCT at University of California, Los Angeles, Piacentini and colleagues compared individual CBT (EX/RP plus cognitive therapy) supplemented with a weekly manualized family intervention (F/ERP) with a psychosocial comparison condition, relaxation training/psychoeducation, in 71 participants ranging in age from 8–17 years (Piacentini, March, & Franklin, 2006). The family intervention was designed to (1) reduce the level of conflict and feelings of anger, blame, and guilt; (2) facilitate disengagement from the child's OCD symptoms, (3) rebuild normal (OCD free) family interaction patterns; and (4) foster an environment conducive to maintaining treatment gains. Both treatments consisted of 14 manualized sessions delivered over 12 weeks. Initial results from this study indicate that F/ERP was superior to relaxation training in terms of clinician-rated response rate (clinical global improvement score of much or very much improved), but differences on primary continuous outcome measures of OCD symptoms, although favoring F/ERP, did not reach statistical significance. The lack of significant differences on the continuous outcomes is somewhat surprising given that relaxation training has not been shown effective for adult OCD. However, these findings are consistent with RCTs of other pediatric anxiety disorders in that CBT and a psychosocial comparison condition (psychoeducation/support) failed to separate from one another, and that both were associated with significant symptom reductions for non-OCD child anxiety disorders (e.g., Silverman et al., 1999).

Dose and Time Response

Most of the studies of CBT outcome in pediatric OCD have used a weekly therapy regimen. Franklin et al. (1998) found no differences between 14 weekly sessions over 12 weeks or 18 sessions over 4 weeks, but interpretation of this finding is hampered by the lack of random assignment. As noted previously, the Storch, Geffken, Merlo, Mann, et al. (2007) study suggests that patients respond well to CBT delivered either weekly or intensively. Both of these studies were too small to provide sufficient power to examine predictors of response to one regimen or the other; thus, at this point, clinical judgment must be used to determine whether a patient might need more than the standard weekly treatment.

Durability

Epidemiological studies suggest that OCD is a chronic condition. The three pediatric OCD pilot studies (Franklin et al., 1998; March et al., 1994; Wever & Rey, 1997) and one recently published randomized trial (Bolton & Perrin, 2008) support the durability of EX/RP, with therapeutic gains maintained up to 9 months post-treatment. Moreover, because relapse commonly follows medication discontinuation, the finding of March et al. (1994) that improvement persisted in six of nine responders after the withdrawal of medication provides limited support for the hypothesis that CBT inhibits relapse when medications are discontinued. Follow-up data from Barrett et al.'s (2004) study further indicate the durability of gains made in CBT for pediatric OCD (Barrett, Farrell, Dadds, & Boulter, 2005).

Availability, Acceptability, and Tolerability

Experts have recommended CBT as a first-line treatment for OCD in children and adolescents (March et al., 1997), yet several barriers may limit its widespread use. First, few therapists have extensive experience with CBT for pediatric OCD; thus, CBT may be only accessible near major medical centers associated with its development and empirical evaluation. Second, even when CBT is available, some patients and families reject the treatment as "too difficult." Once involved in CBT, some patients find the initial distress when confronting feared thoughts and situations while simultaneously refraining from rituals so aversive that they drop out of treatment. In our protocol, we use hierarchy-driven EX/RP, actively involve the patient in choosing exposure exercises, and include anxiety management techniques for the few who need them. As a result, the dropout rates in our pilot studies and clinical trials have been quite low, suggesting that the vast majority of children and adolescents can tolerate, and will benefit from, CBT when it is delivered in a clinically informed and developmentally sensitive fashion.

CBT for pediatric OCD is, unfortunately, often difficult to find outside of academic medical settings associated with the development and empirical evaluation of these protocols, most of which share the common elements of EX/RP. Hence, it is not feasible in many settings to actually follow the Expert Consensus Guidelines (March et al., 1997) to begin treatment with CBT or with combined treatment (CBT plus a serotonin reuptake inhibitor) for pediatric OCD. A recently completed open trial that examined the efficacy of CBT in community clinics as delivered by master's-level clinicians who were not OCD experts provides encouragement for the transportability of this treatment. Valderhaug, Larsson, Götestam, and Piacentini (2007) tested a supervision of supervisors model in providing the psychologists who were supervising these clinicians in rural Norway with access to expert supervision. Findings indicated both statistically significant and clinically meaningful reductions in OCD and related symptoms at posttreatment that were maintained at follow-up (11 months). Benchmarking these outcomes against findings from pilot studies conducted in our respective clinics (Franklin et al., 1998; March et al., 1994) demonstrates comparability of outcomes at both acute and follow-up assessments and indicates that CBT can indeed be disseminated well beyond the academic context and hence transported to the kinds of clinical settings that most families who have a child with OCD are able to access. Larger randomized studies with comparison conditions are needed to extend these findings and to continue building this important bridge to improved access to CBT for families in need.

Moderators of CBT Response

Although many have suggested that the presence of comorbidity, especially with the tic disorders, lack of motivation or insight, and the presence of family psychopathology might predict a poor outcome in children undergoing CBT, there is as yet little empirical basis on which to predict treatment outcome in children undergoing psychosocial treatment. In the Pediatric OCD Treatment Study I (POTS I) we found that comorbid tic diagnosis predicted response to medication but not to CBT (March et al., 2007); Storch, Geffken, Merlo, Mann, et al. (2007) found that externalizing conditions such as oppositional defiant disorder predicted poorer response to CBT. We are currently examining other moderators and mediators of response in the context of our National Institute of Mental Health collaborative studies, although we recognize that limited statistical power will likely render their exploration an exercise in hypothesis generation rather than a definitive evaluation of the influence of these variables on treatment outcome.

COMPARATIVE TREATMENT TRIALS: CBT AND MEDICATION

Pediatric OCD Treatment Study I

The POTS I was the first randomized trial in pediatric OCD to directly compare the efficacy of an established medication (sertraline), OCD-specific CBT, and their combination with a pill placebo control condition in the acute treatment of pediatric OCD.

A volunteer sample of 112 individuals between the ages of 7–17 inclusive with a primary *Diagnostic and Statistical Manual of Mental Disorders* (fourth edition; American Psychiatric Association, 1994) diagnosis of OCD entered the study; the sample was evenly split between boys and girls and included approximately equal numbers of adolescents, ages 12–17, and younger children, ages 7–11. Consistent with an intention-to-treat (ITT) analytic model, all patients, regardless of responder status, returned for all scheduled assessments, and the main dependent variables were assessed by an independent evaluator. Specifically, in stage I (12 weeks), patients were assessed at baseline and weeks 4, 8, and 12; in stage II, patients were evaluated at weeks 16, 20, 24, and 28.

Results of our ITT analyses indicated a significant advantage for all three active treatments—combined treatment, CBT, and sertraline—compared with placebo (Pediatric OCD Treatment Study Team, 2004). With respect to comparisons of active treatments, overall combined treatment was particularly effective; it proved superior to both CBT and sertraline, which did not differ from one another. Approximately 54% of the patients who received combined treatment and 39% of those who received CBT alone achieved OCD symptom remission compared with approximately 21% of those who received sertraline and 3% who received placebo. We also detected site x treatment effects such that CBT alone at the University of Pennsylvania was superior to CBT at Duke University, whereas the reverse was true for sertraline alone. Notably, no site x treatment effects were found for combined treatment or for the pill placebo condition, suggesting that the effects of combined treatment are relatively less vulnerable to site effects.

On the basis of these results, we recommended that children and adolescents with OCD begin treatment with either the combination of CBT plus a selective serotonin reuptake inhibitor (SSRI) or CBT alone. The addition of medication to CBT alone may be particularly important when CBT is attenuated for some reason or if the child has a comorbid tic disorder (March et al., 2007).

Pediatric OCD Treatment Study II

Despite the growing evidence base for CBT, for most pediatric patients with OCD treated in the community, the first-line treatment remains monotherapy with an SSRI. Unfortunately, recommended doses of these medications leave the great majority of patients with clinically significant residual symptoms (Freeman et al., 2009), and the chances for excellent response (as defined previously) are lower with medication alone. For example, POTS I indicated that the rate of excellent response in children treated with sertraline only was just 21%. Accordingly, our next phase of research was designed to address the issue of treatment augmentation (adding an additional treatment to a current treatment) as well as treatment transportability (developing a treatment in a research setting specifically for use in community clinical settings). In the POTS II study, we compare the relative efficacy of augmentation of (1) medication management (MM) provided by a study psychiatrist (MM only), (2) MM plus OCD-specific CBT as delivered by a study psychologist (MM + CBT), and (3) MM plus instructions in CBT (MM + I-CBT) delivered by the study psychiatrist assigned to provide MM. The primary questions of interest to be addressed are as follows: (1) Can CBT augment medication management? (2) Is a more transportable treatment, in the form of MM + I-CBT, as effective as full CBT by a psychologist (MM + CBT)? We have just recently completed recruitment of more than 120 children and adolescents ages 7–17 who were already taking an SSRI for OCD and yet still experiencing clinically significant OCD symptoms.

Family-Based Treatment of Early Childhood OCD

Recent work also supports the success of family-based CBT for young children (5–8 years) with OCD compared with family-based relaxation training (Freeman et al., 2008). Inclusion and exclusion criteria were identical to the other POTS trials described previously except that at least one parent was required to participate in every session. Both treatment protocols (CBT and relaxation training) consisted of 12 sessions delivered over the course of 14 weeks. Our FCBT program draws on extant approaches for older children but contains novel elements that have been tailored to young children with OCD. These elements include (1) attention to developmental stage and concomitant levels of cognitive and socioemotional skills, (2) awareness of a child's involvement in and dependence on a family system, and (3) the incorporation of parent training and behavior management techniques.

Using the ITT sample, 11 of 22 (50%) participants randomized to CBT were classified as achieving clinical remission after 12 weeks of treatment compared with 4 of 20 (20%) participants in the relaxation training group; this difference in response rates was statistically and clinically significant. Using the completer sample, 11 of 16 (69%) participants randomized to CBT were classified as achieving clinical remission compared with only three of 15 (20%) participants in the relaxation training group, which was again statistically and clinically significant. Given the small sample size, the results are very encouraging and indicate that CBT is associated with a moderate and clinically relevant treatment effect (ITT effect size, 0.53). This is especially promising given that the control condition was also an active treatment and not a WL control, as is common in treatment development studies. We have now begun recruitment on a new multisite replication and extension of that study, with Brown University, University of Pennsylvania, and Duke University, which will also allow us to examine predictors of response with a much larger sample.

DIRECTIONS FOR RESEARCH

Using the POTS collaborations as a stepping stone, current research efforts in the field of pediatric OCD are now (or shortly will be) focusing on the following key areas: (1) more controlled trials comparing medications, CBT, and combination treatment to determine whether medications and CBT are synergistic or additive in their effects on symptom reduction; (2) comparisons of individual- and family-based treatments to determine which is more effective in which children; (3) development of innovative treatment for OCD subtypes, such as obsessional slowness or hoarding, that may not respond well to EX/RP; (4) development of treatment innovations to target specific factors, such as family dysfunction and externalizing comorbidity, that constrain the application of CBT to patients with OCD; (5) once past initial treatment, the management of partial response, treatment resistance, treatment maintenance, and discontinuation; and (6) exporting research treatments to divergent clinical settings and patient populations in order to judge the acceptability and effectiveness of CBT as a treatment for child and adolescent OCD in real-world settings. We are truly excited by the new possibilities that these and other initiatives will yield and look forward to another decade's worth of progress in identifying and treating OCD in young people before the illness disrupts developmental trajectories that are difficult to get back on track.

CONCLUSIONS

CBT for pediatric OCD has blossomed in the last decade into an empirically supported treatment for this often disabling condition, with randomized studies from around the world attesting to its efficacy relative to various comparison conditions and to active medication. As is the case in treatment studies for adults suffering from OCD, the effects of CBT for children and adolescents appear to be both robust and durable, with the available follow-up studies indicating that the effects of treatment last for up to 1 year after treatment has ended. Weekly treatment for approximately 12–14 weeks appears to be sufficient, although future studies should examine whether symptom severity, comorbidity, readiness for change, and case complexity (e.g., family problems) necessitate more intensive approaches. Both alone and in combination with SSRIs, CBT provides a viable treatment alternative to SSRIs alone, although the paucity of therapists trained in its use makes it difficult in some regions to heed the Expert Consensus Guidelines to begin treatment with CBT alone or in combination. Dissemination of CBT for pediatric OCD thus remains a pressing challenge for the field, although encouraging data currently available suggest that a supervision of supervisors model can yield impressive results comparable to those achieved in academic medical settings that have developed the CBT protocol use with children and adolescents. A modified CBT protocol that centrally involves parents in the treatment of young children ages 5–8 with OCD has now been developed and its efficacy evaluated in a small initial study. Findings from that randomized trial indicate that the treatment can be delivered effectively to this population as well, which might encourage earlier intervention for those whose symptoms are already evident in young childhood.

REFERENCES

Abramowitz, J. S., Whiteside, S. P., & Deacon, B. J. (2005). The effectiveness of treatment for pediatric obsessive–compulsive disorder: A meta-analysis. *Behavior Therapy, 36*, 55–63.

American Psychiatric Association. (1994). *Diagnostic and statistical manual of mental disorders* (4th ed.). Washington, DC: Author.

Barrett, P., Farrell, L., Dadds, M., & Boulter, N. (2005). Cognitive-behavioral family treatment of childhood obsessive–compulsive disorder: Long-term follow-up and predictors of outcome. *Journal of the American Academy of Child and Adolescent Psychiatry, 44*, 1005–1014.

Barrett, P., Healy-Farrell, L., & March, J. S. (2004). Cognitive-behavioral family treatment of childhood obsessive–compulsive disorder: A controlled trial. *Journal of the American Academy of Child and Adolescent Psychiatry, 43*, 46–62.

Bolton, D., & Perrin, S. (2008). Evaluation of exposure with response-prevention for obsessive compulsive disorder in childhood and adolescence. *Journal of Behavior Therapy and Experimental Psychiatry, 39*, 11–22.

de Haan, E., Hoogduin, K. A., Buitelaar, J. K., & Keijsers, G. P. (1998). Behavior therapy versus clomipramine for the treatment of obsessive–compulsive disorder in children and adolescents. *Journal of the American Academy of Child and Adolescent Psychiatry, 37*, 1022–1029.

Flament, M. F., Whitaker, A., Rapoport, J. L., Davies, M., Berg, C. Z., Kalikow, K., et al. (1988). Obsessive compulsive disorder in adolescence: An epidemiological study. *Journal of the American Academy of Child and Adolescent Psychiatry, 27*, 764–771.

Franklin, M. E., & Foa, E. B. (2008). Obsessive–compulsive disorder. In D. H. Barlow (Ed.), *Clinical handbook of psychological disorders* (4th ed., pp. 164–215). New York: Guilford Press.

Franklin, M. E., Foa, E. B., & March, J. S. (2003). The Pediatric OCD Treatment Study (POTS): Rationale, design and methods. *Journal of Child and Adolescent Psychopharmacology, 13*(Suppl. 1), 39–52.

Franklin, M. E., Kozak, M. J., Cashman, L. A., Coles, M. E., Rheingold, A. A., & Foa, E. B. (1998). Cognitive-behavioral treatment of pediatric obsessive–compulsive disorder: An open clinical trial. *Journal of the American Academy of Child and Adolescent Psychiatry, 37*, 412–419.

Freeman, J. B., Choate-Summers, M. L., Garcia, A. M., Moore, P. S., Sapyta, J., Khanna, M., et al. (2009). The Pediatric Obsessive-Compulsive Disorder Treatment Study II: Rationale, design and methods. *Child and Adolescent Psychiatry and Mental Health, 3*, 4.

Freeman, J. B., Choate-Summers, M. L., Moore, P. S., Garcia, A. M., Sapyta, J. J., Leonard, H. L., & et al. (2007). Cognitive behavioral treatment of young children with obsessive compulsive disorder. *Biological Psychiatry, 61*, 337–343.

Freeman, J. B., Garcia, A. M., Coyne, L., Ale, C., Przeworski, A., Himle, M., et al. (2008). Early childhood OCD: Preliminary findings from a family-based cognitive-behavioral approach. *Journal of the American Academy of Child and Adolescent Psychiatry, 47*, 593–602.

Kendall, P. C., Gosch, E., Furr, J. M., & Sood, E. (2008). Flexibility within fidelity. *Journal of the American Academy of Child and Adolescent Psychiatry, 47*, 987–993.

March, J., Frances, A., Kahn, D., & Carpenter, D. (1997). Expert Consensus Guidelines: Treatment of obsessive–compulsive disorder. *Journal of Clinical Psychiatry, 58*(Suppl. 4), 1–72.

March, J. S., Franklin, M. E., Leonard, H., Garcia, A., Moore, P., Freeman, J., et al. (2007). Tics moderate the outcome of treatment with medication but not CBT in pediatric OCD. *Biological Psychiatry, 61,* 344–347.

March, J. S., & Mulle, K. (1998). *OCD in children and adolescents: A cognitive-behavioral treatment manual.* New York: Guilford Press.

March, J. S., Mulle, K., & Herbel, B. (1994). Behavioral psychotherapy for children and adolescents with obsessive–compulsive disorder: An open trial of a new protocol-driven treatment package. *Journal of the American Academy of Child and Adolescent Psychiatry, 33,* 333–341.

Pediatric OCD Treatment Study Team. (2004). Cognitive-behavioral therapy, sertraline, and their combination for children and adolescents with obsessive–compulsive disorder: The Pediatric OCD Treatment Study (POTS) randomized controlled trial. *Journal of the American Medical Association, 292,* 1969–1976.

Peris, T. S., Bergman, R. L., Langley, A., Chang, S., McCracken, J. T., & Piacentini, J. (2008). Correlates of accommodation of pediatric obsessive–compulsive disorder: Parent, child, and family characteristics. *Journal of the American Academy of Child and Adolescent Psychiatry, 47,* 1173–1181.

Piacentini, J., Bergman, R. L., Jacobs, C., McCracken, J. T., & Kretchman, J. (2002). Open trial of cognitive behavior therapy for childhood obsessive–compulsive disorder. *Journal of Anxiety Disorders, 16,* 207–219.

Piacentini, J. C., March, J. S., & Franklin, M. E. (2006). Cognitive-behavioral therapy for youth with obsessive–compulsive disorder. In P. C. Kendall (Ed.), *Child and adolescent therapy: Cognitive-behavioral procedures* (pp. 297–321). New York: Guilford Press.

Rasmussen, S. A., & Eisen, J. L. (1990). Epidemiology of obsessive compulsive disorder. *Journal of Clinical Psychiatry, 53*(Suppl.), 10–13; discussion, 14.

Silverman, W. K., Kurtines, W. M., Ginsburg, G. S., Weems, C. F., Rabian, B., & Serafini, L. T. (1999). Contingency management, self-control, and education support in the treatment of childhood phobic disorders: A randomized clinical trial. *Journal of Consulting and Clinical Psychology, 67,* 675–687.

Storch, E. A., Geffken, G. R., Merlo, L. J., Jacob, M. L., Murphy, T. K., Goodman, W. K., et al. (2007). Family accommodation in pediatric obsessive–compulsive disorder. *Journal of Clinical Child and Adolescent Psychology, 36,* 207–216.

Storch, E. A., Geffken, G. R., Merlo, L. J., Mann, G., Duke, D., Munson, M., et al. (2007). Family-based cognitive-behavioral therapy for pediatric obsessive–compulsive disorder: Comparison of intensive and weekly approaches. *Journal of the American Academy of Child and Adolescent Psychiatry, 46,* 469–478.

Valderhaug, R., Larsson, B., Götestam, K. G., & Piacentini, J. (2007). An open clinical trial of cognitive-behaviour therapy in children and adolescents with obsessive–compulsive disorder administered in regular outpatient clinics. *Behaviour Research and Therapy, 45,* 577–589.

Wever, C., & Rey, J. M. (1997). Juvenile obsessive compulsive disorder. *Australian and New Zealand Journal of Psychiatry, 31,* 105–113.

7

Cognitive-Behavioral Therapy for Depression
The ACTION Treatment Program for Girls

KEVIN D. STARK, WILLIAM STREUSAND, LAUREN S. KRUMHOLZ, and PUJA PATEL

The ACTION treatment program was developed over years of outcome research and clinical experience. Originally (Stark, Reynolds, & Kaslow, 1987), the intervention program was a downward extension of Rehm's (Fuchs & Rehm, 1977) self-control treatment for depressed adults. Subsequently, it was modified to include more of a cognitive intervention (Stark, 1990). In both of these early investigations, the intervention was designed to be used when treating both males and females. In its latest form, the intervention has been designed specifically for treating girls. However, with modifications to the procedures used for teaching participants the core therapeutic skills, it could be made appropriate for boys. The core therapeutic components and the order in which they are delivered would be the same for boys who are experiencing depression. In this chapter, we describe the latest version of the ACTION program that is specific to the treatment of depressed girls.

OVERVIEW OF THE CLINICAL PROBLEM

Adolescence is a critical time of susceptibility to depression, because the rate of depressive disorders dramatically increases during this period (Costello, Erkanli, & Angold, 2006). This is especially true for girls, whose rates are twice as high as those of boys during adolescence (Angold, Erkanli, Silberg, Eaves, & Costello, 2002). One of the potential causal factors for this gender difference may be an increased cognitive vulnerability among females. Girls' responses to negative events often appear to be characterized by rumination and a negative inferential style (Hankin & Abramson, 2001). In other words, girls relative to boys tend to worry about problems rather than actively try to solve them and tend to choose more passive and less effective strategies for solving problems. In addition, girls possess a more negative orientation in general to problems relative to boys (Maydeu-Olivares, Rodriguez-Fornells, Gomez-Benito, & D'Zurilla, 2000). Furthermore, girls compared with boys make more negative inferences about the self when facing problems or undesirable outcomes (Hankin & Abramson, 2002). This difference in inferential style appears to mediate gender differences in depressive symptoms (Hankin & Abramson, 2002).

Depressive disorders produce serious long-term impairment in major domains of life, including academic, social, and mental health functioning. Youth depression is also a strong predictor of recurrent depression in adulthood as well as of long-term functional impairment (Geller, Zimerman, Williams, Bolhofner, & Craney, 2001). Most concerning, depressed youths are at increased risk for suicide, which is the third leading cause of death during adolescence.

ASSUMPTIONS UNDERLYING TREATMENT

There are multiple pathways to the development of a depressive disorder. Each child will have her own unique pathway. The pathways consist of a diathesis or an accumulation of diatheses, that, when combined with stress, produces a depressive disorder. The diathesis may originate in a disturbance in cognitive, neurochemical, behavioral, or family functioning as well as deficits in emotion regulation skills. Furthermore, a reciprocal relationship exists between these disturbances, and the disturbances reciprocally interact with a deficit in emotion regulation. Thus, a disturbance in one area would affect, and be affected by, each of the other domains. For a more complete discussion of the theoretical tenets that underlie the ACTION treatment program, see Stark, Hargrave, Hersh, Greenberg, Herren, and Fisher (2008).

GOALS AND MAIN THEMES OF THE TREATMENT PROGRAM

Child Program

Perhaps the main goals and themes of the ACTION treatment program are captured in one of the cards from the girls' Coping Kit, which reads:

1. If you feel bad and you don't know why, use coping skills.
2. If you feel bad and you can change the situation, use problem solving.
3. If you feel bad and it is due to negative thoughts, change the thoughts.

Although these three statements are purposely simplistic and written for 9- to 13-year-old girls, they capture the central goals of treatment: (1) The girls will learn and effectively apply coping skills to manage their emotions and stress; (2) the girls will learn to recognize problems that they can impact and effectively apply problem solving to manage them; (3) the girls will recognize and restructure maladaptive cognitions to build core beliefs that they are lovable, worthy, and efficacious.

To accomplish each of the aforementioned overarching goals, a number of subgoals must be attained. Some of these subgoals are designed to build a therapeutic context that will maximize change, whereas others are related to learning and applying the three core therapeutic skills. A critical subgoal is that depressed girls will become behaviorally activated. All three of the core therapeutic strategies are designed to accomplish this. However, coping skills training and pleasant events scheduling through the use of the Catch the Positive Diary (CPD) most directly help the girls achieve this subgoal. Depressed children experience more problems than their nondepressed peers. Furthermore, they believe that they are helpless in the face of these problems, and they tend to use more passive and less effective problem-solving strategies. Thus, a primary subgoal of treatment is that the girls will be able to recognize when a problem exists and use problem solving to manage the impact of or eliminate the problem. If the problem is outside of their control, then coping skills are the preferred strategies because they help the patients to manage the emotional impact of the problem. Another primary subgoal is to produce lasting and meaningful change, which is most likely to occur when depressive core beliefs are restructured. The girls learn to recognize negative thoughts and beliefs and then evaluate their validity and either let them go or combat them through use of the cognitive restructuring. Another core goal or theme to the ACTION treatment program is that the girls will apply the skills and new ways of thinking.

Parent Training

There are a few overarching goals to the parent training program. One of the primary goals is to help parents model the use of therapeutic skills and healthier ways of thinking and reinforce their daughters' use of the therapeutic strategies. To change the affective tone of the family and the communication that occurs within the family, the parents are taught empathic listening and conflict resolution skills. Another goal is to create a supportive environment that sends positive messages to the girls. Parents are taught to increase their use of reinforcement to manage their daughters' behavior and to act in ways that help their daughters perceive themselves as important, valued, and loved.

CHARACTERISTICS OF TREATMENT PROGRAM

Who Is Seen and in What Format

The ACTION program is designed for girls ages 9–13 with a primary diagnosis of depression and their caregivers (referred to as parents). The intervention has proven equally effective with relatively large samples of Hispanic and European American girls. It also has been equally effective with girls of African American descent and for girls of diverse socioeconomic status. During the ACTION program, girls receive cognitive-behavioral therapy (CBT) in their schools in small groups ($n = 2$–5). The group format offers several advantages, such as providing some degree of normalization of the problem; facilitating friendships, which engenders opportunities to enhance social skills and build confidence about engaging in interpersonal relationships; and providing a window to observe and assess the girls' interpersonal behaviors.

Treatment consists of 20 group meetings and two individual meetings over 11 weeks. Additional individual meetings are scheduled on an as-needed basis. The length of each meeting ranges from 45–75 minutes depending on the time prescribed by school principals. Ideally, we recommend tailoring the duration of the meetings to the developmental level of the girls.

The parent training component also involves a small-group format. Parents of the girls meet with the same therapist as their daughters once per week for 10 weeks. The girls attend the meetings with their parents every other week. These meetings last approximately 90 minutes. Both parents are encouraged to attend if they can act in a constructive way toward each other and their daughter. Similarly, stepparents are encouraged to attend meetings as long as everyone behaves in a constructive fashion.

Content of the Treatment and Sequence of Therapy Sessions

ACTION is a manualized, gender-specific, developmentally appropriate treatment program for depressed girls and includes six core therapeutic components: (1) affective education, (2) goal setting, (3) coping skills training, (4) problem solving, (5) cognitive restructuring, and (6) building a positive sense of self. The sequence of the child sessions and objectives for each session are presented in Table 7.1. As a general overview, the first nine sessions focus on affective education and the acquisition of coping and problem-solving skills. Sessions 10–19 emphasize the continued application of coping and problem-solving strategies, learning and applying cognitive restructuring, and enhancing girls' core beliefs about the self.

The parent training component includes positive behavior management, family problem solving, communication skills, conflict resolution, and changing behaviors that support depressive core beliefs. Positive behavior management strategies are taught to parents first to try to change the affective tone in the home so that it supports the effort to improve their daughters' mood through coping skills training and increasing engagement in pleasant events. Parents are taught family problem solving so that they can model the procedure for their daughters, help them acquire the skill, and support them as they adopt a general problem-solving attitude. Parents are then taught effective communication skills (e.g., empathic listening) followed by conflict resolution skills, because these can contribute to a more positive family environment. To support the desired cognitive change that the girls are working toward, it is necessary to decrease conflict in the family and enhance positive interpersonal interactions between family members. Finally, with the children and families functioning more adaptively, the parents can collaboratively assess their own behaviors that support their daughters' negative core beliefs. Subsequently, they work at changing these behaviors so that instead they communicate positive messages to their daughters. Once again, this supports the cognitive restructuring that their daughters are simultaneously learning and applying.

Skills and Accomplishments Emphasized in Treatment

As mentioned, the core therapeutic components of the ACTION program are affective education, goal setting, coping skills training, problem solving, cognitive restructuring strategies, and building a positive self-schema. Specific skills are used to teach the components of treatment in a developmentally sensitive fashion.

Affective Education

Affective education is the component in which girls learn about the experience of depression and the CBT model of depression, including its causes and how they are

TABLE 7.1. Descriptions of Primary Child Treatment Components and Objectives for Meetings

Meeting no.	Primary child treatment component	Objective by meeting
1	Introductions and discussion of pragmatics	Discuss parameters of meetings. Introduce counselors and participants. Establish rationale for treatment. Discuss confidentiality. Establish group rules. Build group cohesion. Establish within group incentive system.
2	Affective education and introduction to coping	Introduce participants to chat time and agenda setting. Establish pragmatics of completing homework. Introduce mood meter and Take ACTION List. Complete within-session coping activity.
Individual meeting 1		Review therapeutic concepts. Develop treatment goals.
3	Affective education and coping skills	Discuss importance of thinking about meetings and doing practice. Introduce clients to various therapeutic components, including focusing on the positive, affective education, and coping strategies.
4	Extend group cohesion; review participant goals, application of coping skills	Extend group cohesion. Review participant goals and strategies. Discuss application of coping strategics. Complete coping skills activity within session.
5	Extend coping skills, introduction to problem solving	Experience impact of coping skills activity within session. Introduction, extension, and application of problem solving. Introduction to brainstorming step of problem solving.
6	Cognition and emotion, introduction to cognitive restructuring	Demonstrate the role of cognition in emotion and behavior. Introduce connection of thoughts to feelings. Enactment of coping skills activity within session.
7	Apply problem solving	Apply problem solving to real-life situations. Practice brainstorming activity. Experience coping skills activity within session.
8	Apply problem solving	Apply problem solving to teasing. Experience coping skills activity within session.
9	Apply problem solving	Apply problem solving to interpersonal problems. Experience coping skills activity within session.
Individual meeting 2		Review therapeutic concepts. Identify common negative thoughts. Individualize Catch the Positive Diaries. Introduce cognitive restructuring.
10	Prepare for cognitive restructuring and introduction to cognitive restructuring	Prepare for cognitive restructuring. Experience coping skills activity within session. Practice cognitive restructuring.
11	Cognitive restructuring	Introduce how perceptions are constructed. Illustrate how depression distorts thinking. Provide rationale for changing negative thoughts.

(cont.)

TABLE 7.1. *(cont.)*

Meeting no.	Primary child treatment component	Objective by meeting
12	Cognitive restructuring and self-maps	Practice identifying negative thoughts of group members. Introduce client strengths through a self-map. Practice cognitive restructuring.
13	Cognitive restructuring and self-maps	Practice identifying negative thoughts. Continue identifying strengths for the self-maps. Practice cognitive restructuring with questions using alternative interpretations.
14	Cognitive restructuring and self-maps	Continue identifying negative thoughts, adding strengths to the self-maps, and practicing cognitive restructuring.
15	Cognitive restructuring and self-maps	Continue identifying negative thoughts and adding strengths to the self-maps. Introduce examining evidence as a tool for cognitive restructuring.
16	Cognitive restructuring and self-maps	Continue identifying negative thoughts and adding strengths to the self-maps. Practice cognitive restructuring. Prepare for termination.
17	Cognitive restructuring and self-maps	Continue adding strengths to the self-maps. Integrate and apply cognitive restructuring. Continue preparing for termination.
18	Cognitive restructuring and self-maps	Continue adding strengths to the self-maps. Integrate and apply all of the learned skills. Continue preparing for termination.
19	Cognitive restructuring and self-maps	Draw conclusions from self-maps. Empowerment activity for clients to continue using skills on their own. Prepare for group termination.
20	Bring it all together and termination activity	Say goodbye to the group. Say goodbye to negative thoughts and feelings. Terminate.

going to learn to manage it. The affective education component helps girls become more self-aware, particularly of therapeutically relevant experiences such as their depressive thoughts, unpleasant emotions, and other depressive symptoms. Girls are then taught to use these experiences as cues to engage in the therapeutic strategies.

Girls are taught to identify their emotions by acting like "emotion detectives," who investigate their own experience of the "three Bs": **B**ody (how their body is reacting), **B**rain (what they are thinking), and **B**ehavior (how they are behaving). This process increases awareness of emotional experiences. For example, during the meetings, when a girl states that she is feeling a particular emotion, the therapist asks her to describe what is happening in her body, what she is thinking, and how she is behaving. Simultaneously, the therapist may use a simple cookie cutout drawing of a girl to illustrate what is happening in her body, brain, and behavior. The girls also complete therapeutic homework assignments in which they identify their emotional experiences and assess their experience of the three Bs.

Goal Setting

The therapist meets with each girl individually to collaboratively identify her first three goals. The therapist then describes how each of the core treatment procedures will be used to achieve each goal. Before the end of the goals meeting, the therapist asks permission to share the girl's goals with the group. During the next group meeting, with each girl's permission, the goals are shared with the other group members, and then the group brainstorms how they can help each other reach their goals. At the beginning of every other meeting, there is a "goals check-in" time to report progress toward goal attainment and to celebrate progress. The therapist plots the rating of each goal on a poster. If there is no progress, problem solving is used. As goals are achieved, additional goals are collaboratively established.

Coping Skills Training

In the ACTION program, coping skills are taught both as a general strategy for enhancing mood and as a specific strategy when a girl is experiencing an undesirable or stressful situation that she cannot change. Children must experience the benefits of coping skills before they will try to use them; therefore, only discussing the skills is not sufficient.

Mood Monitoring

When a coping strategy is taught, the therapist asks the girls to recall a stressful event and rate their mood at that moment on a scale from 1–10 using a mood meter, with 1 being the worst and 10 being the best that one can feel. Then the girls participate in a coping activity and rerate their mood following completion of the activity. The mood meter provides the girls with direct evidence of the benefit of coping. As the girls apply coping skills outside of meetings, they are asked to self-monitor and describe their use and impact in their workbooks.

Five ACTION Coping Skills

Five broad categories of coping skills are taught: (1) Do something fun and distracting, (2) do something soothing and relaxing, (3) seek social support, (4) do something that expends lots of energy, and (5) change your thinking. The girls are taught and experience the benefits of examples of coping skills from each of five broad categories within treatment sessions. The therapist chooses coping skills to be taught and applied during each meeting based on what he or she believes is most needed by the group. For example, group members may be exhibiting flat affect. The therapist would then do something fun and energizing as a means of enlivening the group. In addition to teaching coping strategies, the therapist helps the girls identify situations where it is most advantageous to use specific coping skills. The improvement in mood resulting from utilizing coping strategies sets the stage for problem solving and cognitive restructuring, which are taught later.

Catch the Positive Diary

As the name suggests, the CPD is designed to help girls catch (attend to) positive events by helping them self-monitor and record the occurrence of a variety of therapeutically important positive events. When treating depressed youths, the CPD is used to (1) behaviorally activate the girls through monitoring and encouraging engagement in fun activities, (2) redirect the girls' attention from negative to positive events, (3) increase the girls' completion of therapeutically relevant activities, and (4) help the girls find evidence that supports new, more adaptive beliefs and counters negative beliefs.

Self-monitoring of enjoyable activities leads to an increase in the frequency of engagement in these activities. Participation in fun, distracting activities as a means of enhancing mood and coping with stress is the first coping strategy taught. To further increase involvement in these activities, the therapist educates the girls about the mood-enhancing quality of engaging in recreational activities and gives the girls therapeutic homework to do as many of the enjoyable activities on their list as they can each day. An overarching goal of the treatment program and of the CPD is to improve mood by increasing the frequency and types of coping skills used by the girls.

Problem Solving

As the girls acquire a better understanding of their emotions, accurately identify them, recognize their impact on behavior and thinking, and understand that they can take action to moderate the intensity and impact of their emotions, they learn that some of the undesirable situations that lead to unpleasant emotions can be changed. Problem solving is the strategy used to develop a plan for changing undesirable situations using a five-step problem-solving sequence. Before the problem-solving strategy can be applied, the group learns to identify what constitutes a problem. The next step is to determine whether or not the problem can be changed. Problem solving is applied to situations that are within the girls' control.

Five Ps

Girls are taught to break problem solving down into five steps through education, modeling, coaching, rehearsal, and feedback. To simplify the process and to help the girls remember the steps, the therapist refers to the steps as the "five Ps": (1) problem definition (**P**roblem), (2) goal definition (**P**urpose), (3) solution generation (**P**lans), (4) consequential thinking (**P**redict and pick), and (5) self-evaluation (**P**at on the back). The steps are defined in a developmentally sensitive manner, and activities are used to illustrate the meaning and purpose of each step.

Cognitive Restructuring

To effectively restructure youngsters' distorted thoughts and beliefs, it is necessary to first establish a relationship among negative thoughts, unpleasant mood, and other depressive symptoms. The activities are designed to extend the girls' understanding of the nature of cognition and its relationship to emotional adjustment. When establishing the rationale for cognitive restructuring with the girls, another important concept to teach is that often their thoughts are not true. "Just because you think it, it doesn't mean that it is true" (Beck, 2005). This is a surprising revelation for children. They are under the assumption that if they think something, then it has to be true. Another important message to relay is that we are continually confronted with multiple ways of thinking about situations and that we are making choices about what we want to think and believe. In many situations, we can choose what we want to believe because there is no clear-cut, definitive way of thinking that is correct. The girls should be taught that sometimes we have to look at the practical outcome of believing a negative thought and then weigh the advantages of choosing to believe a viable and possibly true, alternative thought. Real-life situations and a number of activities completed during the meetings are used to illustrate these points.

Catch Negative Thoughts

To independently restructure negative thoughts and the beliefs that underlie them, the girls must become aware of their own thoughts. The extent to which girls need direct training in the metacognitive process of recognizing their own thoughts is a function of developmental level. Adolescents can do this much more readily than younger girls. Regardless of age, it is easier to recognize when someone else expresses negative thoughts; therefore, we begin by asking the girls to identify others' negative thoughts as a bridge to recognizing and identifying their own. Within-session activities and experiences are used to help the girls learn to identify negative thoughts.

Thought Detective

Once a negative thought has been identified, a girl asks one of the two Thought Detective questions to evaluate the thought's validity and to develop adaptive thoughts to replace negative thoughts: (1) What is another way to think about it? (2) What is the evidence? (Beck, Rush, Shaw, & Emery, 1979). The girls learn to differentiate which question is best suited for specific negative thoughts. "What is another way to think about it?" is the easiest cognitive restructuring question for early adolescent girls to learn. They use this question to generate alternative, plausible, and positive thoughts. This is a good question to use when the girls draw a negative conclusion from a situation that has many other viable conclusions. "What is the evidence?" is used when the objective facts do not support negative thoughts.

Muck Monster

The standard cognitive restructuring procedure is difficult to teach 9- to 13-year-old girls. One powerful tool to enhance the accessibility of cognitive restructuring is an activity that the girls refer to as "Talking Back to the Muck Monster." When girls are having difficulty changing or letting go of negative thinking, we refer to this as being "stuck in the negative muck." When they are stuck in the negative muck, it is the Muck Monster that is filling them with negative thoughts and keeping them from extricating themselves from the muck.

Establishing the Muck Monster as the source of depressive thoughts is useful in a number of ways. It depersonalizes the negative thinking; it creates emotional distance between the girl and her depressive thinking; and it becomes a common opponent to defeat. The term Muck Monster is not used with adolescents, rather, we ask them to either give the source of their depression a name or just refer to it as "that is your depression talking to you."

When completing the Muck Monster activity, an extra chair is brought to group meetings. The chair is for the Muck Monster. The therapist moves to the empty chair and acts like the Muck Monster, stating the target child's negative thoughts. The girl forcefully uses the two Thought Detective questions to guide her talking back to the Muck Monster. Group members help her do this by providing additional evidence or alternative interpretations. The girls may be encouraged to forcefully talk back to the Muck Monster by yelling at it. Other group members assist and cheer the girl on as she evaluates negative thoughts and then replaces them with more realistic positive thoughts. The workbook guides the process of catching, evaluating, and replacing negative thoughts outside of treatment.

Building a Positive Sense of Self

One of the tools used to help girls develop more positive beliefs about themselves is the self-map. Overall, the self-map helps girls broaden their self-definition and recognize more personal strengths than they previously acknowledged. Girls are asked to complete each bubble within the self-map with relevant strengths. In addition, parents and teachers are interviewed by the therapist to identify their perceptions of their daughters' strengths in each of the domains. This information is provided to the girls by the therapist. We have found that this information has a powerful impact. The girls are often quite surprised that these adults think positively about them. In addition to adult input, group members provide each other with positive feedback for each bubble. Once again, receiving this information from peers appears to be poignant and believable to the girls.

DURATION AND HOW TO DETERMINE WHEN TREATMENT IS "FINISHED"

Based on the results of our research, it is clear that the girls varied greatly in the number of sessions it took until they no longer reported experiencing a depressive episode. Some of the girls were rapid responders, who reported significant improvements within the first three sessions. Others did not report significant improvement until the last few meetings. Girls who participated in an interview after completion of treatment and the posttreatment assessment reported that they experienced significant improvement after the acquisition of specific skills. Some improved following acquisition and application of coping skills, others stated that problem solving was the skill that helped them the most, whereas still others reported that they benefitted most from changing their thinking. Thus, there is no simple answer to how long is long enough for participation in treatment.

We have used the Beck Depression Inventory for Youth (BDI-Y; Beck, Beck, & Jolly, 2001) to monitor participants' progress during treatment. Children can complete the measure in 5–10 minutes, and it provides information about depressive thoughts as well as depressive symptoms. Thus, it can help guide cognitive restructuring. We rely on a clinical interview, the present episode version of the Schedule for Affective Disorders and

Schizophrenia for School-Aged Children (K-SADS-IV-R; Ambrosini & Dixon, 2000), as a means of determining when treatment is complete. The K-SADS-IV-R yields a measure of the presence and severity of depressive symptoms. Its semistructured nature allows the interviewer the freedom to ask questions to determine the duration of various symptoms and whether a symptom is still being experienced or has improved and no longer impacts the child's life. In the clinical setting, when a child reports minimal symptoms on the BDI-Y (mood disturbance no longer exists and other symptoms are below the clinical level) for at least two consecutive administrations (4 weeks in a row), the K-SADS-IV-R is administered to determine whether the depressive episode has been successfully treated. Treatment is considered to be complete when the child no longer reports experiencing a disturbance in mood and all of the other symptoms have improved to subclinical levels. It is important to continue treatment until the child's mood, self-concept, helplessness, vegetative symptoms, and suicidal ideation have normalized and the child is at decreased risk for relapse.

MANUALS AND OTHER SUPPORTING MATERIALS

Structured therapist manuals and workbooks are available for the child (Stark, Simpson, Schnoebelen, Hargrave, Glenn, & Molnar, 2006; Stark, Schnoebelen, Simpson, Hargrave, Glenn, & Molnar, 2006) and parent (Stark, Yancy, Simpson, & Molnar, 2006; Stark, Simpson, Yancy, & Molnar, 2006) portions of treatment.

EVIDENCE ON THE EFFECTS OF TREATMENT

How Is Treatment Evaluated?

Treatment is evaluated in a number of ways depending on the question being asked. At the most basic level, the question is, "Has participation in treatment produced a significant improvement in the depressive disorder (i.e., child is no longer experiencing a depressive disorder)? This question is answered using multiple raters and multiple methods, including self-report, semistructured interviews of the child and her primary caregiver, and completion of behavior rating scales before and after treatment. Progress in treatment is evaluated by asking the child to regularly complete the BDI-Y, and effectiveness of the treatment program is evaluated based on the child's and the primary caregiver's completed K-SADS-P-IV-R. Another question could be, "Has the child acquired the therapeutic skills?" This question is evaluated by asking the child to complete a number of skills quizzes and by monitoring her completion of therapeutic homework. It is also desirable to determine whether the girl's core beliefs have changed to become more positive and realistic. This can be accomplished through completion of the Cognitive Triad Inventory for Children (CTI-C: Kaslow, Stark, Printz, Livingston, & Tsai, 1992).

Status of the Evidence

The current ACTION treatment is the culmination of a programmatic line of research that has been designed to evaluate and guide the development of a treatment for depressed youths. In the first of the outcome studies (Stark et al., 1987), a downward extension of a self-control treatment for depressed adults (Fuchs & Rehm, 1977) was found to be more effective than a wait-list condition for 8- to 12-year-old boys and girls who reported elevated depressive symptoms. Thus, it was apparent that a relatively simple intervention that included psychoeducation, pleasant events scheduling and monitoring, and self-evaluation training directed at reducing children's excessive standards and negative evaluations, along with training in self-reinforcement for working toward personal improvement, was effective for those who reported elevated depressive symptoms. In the next study (Stark, 1990), an expanded version of the original treatment was evaluated relative to a traditional supportive counseling intervention to determine whether the treatment was more effective than the standard of care in the schools. In addition, the participants included boys and girls in grades 4–7 who reported a depressive disorder on a semistructured diagnostic interview. The self-control treatment components (Stark et al., 1987) were expanded to include a broader array of positive events that were self-monitored, a problem-solving component, and a fairly circumscribed and simplistic cognitive restructuring component. Results indicated that this intervention was more effective than the supportive counseling program for the treatment of moderately depressed (based on a semistructured diagnostic interview) boys and girls. Thus, the intervention demonstrated promise as a treatment for depressed boys and girls. The intervention was further expanded and in some ways simplified over the ensuing years. The expansion included teaching the children to use emotion regulation skills. Problem solving was expanded to include identification of goals for problem solving. A goal-setting component that included self-monitoring of goal attainment was added as a means of further building the therapeutic alliance and client motivation for change. The greatest change was the addition of a more sophisticated cognitive restructuring component. This component was expanded from three to 10 sessions and reflected a developmentally appropriate strategy for teaching the participants to restructure their thinking. Furthermore, the manuals were written specifically for girls. Thus, the activities included in the treatment program are gender specific. However, the choice of components and sequence of teaching the components is appropriate for boys and girls.

The latest version of the ACTION program was evaluated over 5 years and in a study that included 159 girls ages 9–13 years who reported experiencing a diagnosable depressive disorder. Multiple methods and multiple measures completed by multiple raters were used to assess the presence and severity of depression. In addition, related constructs, including cognitive triad and family functioning, were assessed. The majority of the girls were experiencing major depressive disorder (81%) or dysthymic disorder (15%), whereas a few were experiencing double depression (4%) or depressive disorder not otherwise specified (DDNOS). Although girls were randomly assigned to treatment conditions, more of the girls in the minimal contact control condition had their depressive episode start to remit before beginning treatment (16% vs. 6% CBT and 10% CBT plus parent training [PT]) and they were more likely to be experiencing DDNOS (7% vs. 0% and 0%). Approximately 50% reported at least one additional comorbid condition. Almost 40% of the sample were of Latin descent, 23% were white non-Hispanic, 18% were African American, and 9% were biracial. Participants were not included if they were actively suicidal ($n = 1$) or had a cognitive deficit that prevented them from understanding or being able to complete the measures ($n = 0$).

Participants were identified through a multiple-gate assessment procedure in which parent permission letters were sent home with 7,737 girls from grades 4–7. Permission for participation in screening with the Children's Depression Inventory (CDI) and a brief *Diagnostic and Statistical Manual of Mental Disorders* (fourth edition, text revision; American Psychiatric Association, 2000) symptom interview was received for 3,396 girls. Eight hundred thirteen reported clinically relevant levels of depressive symptoms on the CDI and were interviewed with the DSM symptom interview. Three hundred eighty-three girls reported depressive symptoms consistent with a diagnosable depressive disorder and were interviewed with the K-SADS. One hundred seventy girls received a diagnosis of a depressive disorder and were invited to participate in the evaluation of the treatment. Parent permission was received for 159 girls.

The participants were randomly assigned to CBT, CBT + PT, or a minimal contact control condition. The design was based on the empirical need to determine whether treatment was better than no treatment, a question that had not yet been addressed using a clinically relevant population and a large number of participants. In addition, it was hypothesized that adding a parent training component would produce greater generalization and maintenance of treatment effects relative to child CBT alone. The CBT groups and parent training groups were completed as described previously. To encourage parent participation, transportation, day care, and dinner or snack were provided. An attempt was made to include fathers in treatment; however, the majority did not participate. Graduate students served as the therapists.

Results (Stark, Stapleton, & Fisher, 2009) indicated that the ACTION treatment with and without parent training was more effective than the minimal contact control condition, because girls in both treatment conditions reported significantly lower mean levels of depressive symptoms at posttreatment relative to girls in the minimal contact control condition. The two active treatments were not significantly different from one another. On a clinical level, more than 80% of the girls no longer met criteria for a diagnosis of a depressive disorder (based on child and parent K-SADS-P ratings) after completion of the treatment. In contrast, 47% of the girls in the minimal contact control condition were no longer depressed after treatment. Results of the measure of the cognitive triad indicated that the girls who completed both treatments experienced significantly greater improvement in their sense of self and future on the CTI-C (Kaslow et al., 1992), and that the girls in the CBT-only condition reported significantly more positive sense of self and future relative to girls whose parents also participated in parent training. Perhaps this is due to the girls in the CBT only condition attributing their improvements in depressive symptoms solely to themselves, whereas girls whose parents also participated in treatment attributed change to their parents' participation too. The parent training component also appeared to produce desired changes in the family. Girls whose parents participated in the parent training component reported that their families were significantly more cohesive and communicative after treatment relative to girls who participated in the CBT-only or the minimal contact control condition. Thus, these improvements in the family environment did not translate into any added improvements in severity of depression. It was further hypothesized that the improvements in family environment would lead to greater maintenance of treatment effects. The majority of the girls in both active treatments maintained their improvements in depressive symptoms at 1 year posttreatment. More specifically, 84% of the girls in the CBT + PT condition reported maintaining their improvements and 73% of the girls in the CBT-only condition reported maintaining their improvements. The mean depression severity rating scores were not significantly different. An equal number of girls in all three experimental conditions reported improvement in comorbid anxiety disorders; however, the two active treatments were more effective at preventing the development of additional or new anxiety disorders. More specifically, 27% of the girls in the minimal contact control condition developed an additional anxiety disorder over the course of treatment, whereas none of the girls in the active treatments developed an additional anxiety disorder. Overall, the ACTION treatment is a very effective treatment for 9- to 13-year-old girls who are experiencing clinically relevant depressive disorders. The girls and their parents liked the program and found it to be credible.

RECOMMENDATIONS REGARDING IMPLEMENTATION IN PRACTICE

The ACTION treatment program is easy to implement in clinical practice. However, it is important to note that treatment in the original study was guided by a case conceptualization for each of the participants. This conceptualization served as a road map for treatment and as a guide for how to individualize the group intervention. To develop an accurate case conceptualization, therapists must have an extensive background in CBT and a thorough understanding of depressive disorders among children. It is our belief that the intervention cannot be as effectively implemented by therapists who lack a sophisticated conceptual understanding of depressive disorders and CBT. However, this is a belief that should be empirically evaluated.

The intervention was designed for a group format. With minor modifications in some of the activities that are designed for a group of girls, the intervention is appropriate for use with individual clients. It also can be used with boys with a minimum of change in some of the activities that illustrate the therapeutic concepts. The intervention also appears to be appropriate for use with older adolescents, with some modification of the wording and removal of the "cute" aspects of the treatment materials. A significant difference in the intervention delivered as part of the research protocol and in clinical practice is that the groups met twice a week although most insurance plans only allow for weekly meetings. During piloting, it became clear that the girls were more likely to complete their therapeutic homework and to remember what was covered in previous meetings with twice-weekly meetings. It is not clear whether meeting weekly will have an adverse impact on outcome. It certainly decreases the intensity of the program, which may impact overall effectiveness.

In general, it seems as though the ACTION protocol is easier for adolescents to understand and apply. Thus, although it was designed for 9- to 13-year-old girls, it appears to be even more effective with older adolescents. For this older group, the cognitive restructuring component is expanded to include four questions that guide the process: "What is the worst that could happen? What is the best that could happen? What is most realistic?" "What would you tell your best friend?" The first three questions are used when it is clear that the child's upset is due to an unrealistically negative future expectation. The last question is used when the child's upset is due to unreasonably stringent or harsh self-evaluations. It also is important to note that the protocol includes a significantly larger number of meetings devoted to cognitive restructuring than is typical for CBT protocols. We believe that learning to recognize and then apply cognitive restructuring is a difficult skill that takes much time to learn and effectively apply. Furthermore, changing core beliefs requires greater effort and time because these beliefs represent central assumptions that have been acquired and reinforced over time through count-less learning experiences. In addition, the child has a history and pattern of behavior that supports these beliefs. Thus, core beliefs receive extensive support currently and through past learning experiences. Therefore, it takes many new learning experiences to change these beliefs.

DIRECTIONS FOR RESEARCH

There continues to be a paucity of research into the treatment of depressive disorders in children. It would be interesting to evaluate the efficacy of the ACTION program relative to a selective serotonin reuptake inhibitor or another psychosocial intervention. The ACTION program is a multicomponent treatment that is relatively long in duration. Thus, it would be useful to complete a components analysis to determine whether the program could be shortened without losing efficacy and breadth of applicability. What is the process of change when a child participates in ACTION? Does the treatment work through improvements in core beliefs or some other specific or nonspecific variables? Does the mode of program delivery (group vs. individual) make a difference? Clinical experience suggested that the girls who were developing personality disorders were less likely to benefit from the program. In addition, they appeared to have a negative impact on the overall group. It would be useful to empirically evaluate these observations.

Based on clinical experience, it appears as though it is necessary to treat some comorbid conditions before being able to effectively treat depression. For example, it appears that the depression treatment had to wait for the successful treatment of obsessive–compulsive disorder or posttraumatic stress disorder. Social phobia appeared to be effectively treated within the group format. Elective mutism was a limiting factor to treatment. In general, it would be useful to evaluate the impact of various comorbid conditions on treatment outcome. We are in the process of coding the actual therapy tapes to determine whether the quality and frequency of teaching and use of coping, problem solving, cognitive restructuring, behavioral strategies, and therapist relation-ship variables predict change, thus enabling us to address questions about the process of change. It also was evident that the process of change began as soon as the children were identified as depressed, and that some children began reporting symptom improvement during the weeks preceding treatment. The reasons for these improvements are being investigated by the authors. In another study currently underway, the phenomenon of sudden gains is being evaluated using the ACTION outcome data. Clinical experience suggests that the children who improve the most complete their therapeutic homework. Research is needed to determine whether this observation is true or not.

CONCLUSIONS

The ACTION program has evolved over the years in an attempt to increase its efficacy through addressing more of the therapeutic concerns of depressed youths. For example, problem solving and cognitive restructuring have been added to the treatment program because research indicated that depressed youth experience both problem-solving defi-cits and distortions in their thinking. In addition, clinical experience indicated that there is a reciprocal relationship between all of the skills. For example, a child may believe that she is helpless and thus will not enact coping skills. Thus, cognitive restructuring would have to be used to enable the child to use coping skills. Likewise, if she is experiencing too much unpleasant mood, she will not be able to restructure her beliefs about being helpless. Thus, the therapist commonly has to use both treatment strategies simultaneously. Although the ACTION program is very effective in terms of the number of youths who benefit from it, a substantial percentage of children (20%) continue to report a depressive disorder. Thus, continued work is needed to broaden and deepen the efficacy of the program. The addition of the parent component was an attempt to accomplish this. However, it did not add to the overall efficacy. Perhaps a family therapy component rather than parent training needs to be added. However, it also is possible that a ceiling effect has been achieved in terms of psychosocial interventions, and pharmacological intervention is necessary to produce change in additional participants.

Based on our results, the ACTION treatment program is equally effective for girls from different ethnic and racial groups. In fact, it may be the largest sample of depressed Mexican American girls to complete a treatment outcome study. Although the latest version of the ACTION program was designed for depressed girls, changing the activities that teach the therapeutic concepts makes it appropriate for boys. Based on the earlier research and clinical experience, it appears to be equally effective for boys. It is a multicomponent intervention that targets for change the skills and cognitions that are hypothesized to underlie depressive disorders. Research evaluating whether the process of change is, in fact, the improvement in these skills and cognitions has not been conducted to date. Although it is clear that the ACTION treatment is effective with clinically depressed girls who are experiencing multiple comorbid conditions, it is not clear whether it is more effective than another psychosocial intervention or antidepressant medications. It is also possible that the combination of the ACTION program and an antidepressant may be more effective than either mode of treatment alone.

REFERENCES

Ambrosini, P. J., & Dixon, J. F. (2000). *Schedule for affective disorders & schizophrenia for school age children (6–18 years)—Kiddie-SADS (KSADS) (present state and lifetime version), K-SADS-IVR (revision of K-SADS-IIIR)*. Unpublished manuscript, Eastern Pennsylvania Psychiatric Institute.

American Psychiatric Association. (2000). *Diagnostic and statistical manual of mental disorders* (4th ed., text rev.). Washington, DC: Author.

Angold, A., Erkanli, A., Silberg, J., Eaves, L., & Costello, E. J. (2002). Depression scale scores in 8–17-year olds: Effects of age and gender. *Journal of Child Psychology and Psychiatry and Allied Disciplines, 43*(8), 1052–1063.

Beck, A. T., Rush, A. J., Shaw, B. F., & Emery, G. (1979). *Cognitive theory of depression*. New York: Guilford Press.

Beck, J. S. (2005). *Cognitive therapy for challenging problems: What to do when the basics don't work*. New York: Guilford Press.

Beck, J. S., Beck, A. T., & Jolly, J. B. (2001). *Beck Youth Inventories of Emotional and Social Impairment manual*. New York: Psychological Corporation.

Costello, E. J., Erkanli, A., & Angold, A. (2006). Is there an epidemic of child or adolescent depression? *Journal of Child Psychology and Psychiatry, 47*(12), 1263–1271.

Fuchs, C. Z., & Rehm, L. P. (1977). A self-control behavior therapy program for depression. *Journal of Consulting and Clinical Psychology, 45*, 206–215.

Geller, B., Zimerman, B., Williams, M., Bolhofner, K., & Craney, J. (2001). Bipolar disorder at prospective follow-up of adults who had prepubertal major depressive disorder. *American Journal of Psychiatry, 158*, 125–127.

Hankin, B. L., & Abramson, L. Y. (2001). Development of gender differences in depression: An elaborated cognitive vulnerability-transactional stress theory. *Psychological Bulletin, 127*(6), 773–796.

Hankin, B. L., & Abramson, L. Y. (2002). Measuring cognitive vulnerability to depression in adolescence: Reliability, validity, and gender differences. *Journal of Clinical Child and Adolescent Psychology, 31*(4), 491–504.

Kaslow, N. J., Stark, K. D., Printz, B., Livingston, R., & Tsai, S. (1992). Cognitive Triad Inventory for Children: Development and relationship to depression and anxiety. *Journal of Clinical Child Psychology, 21*, 339–347.

Maydeu-Olivares, A., Rodriguez-Fornells, A., Gomez-Benito, J., & D'Zurilla, T. J. (2000). Psychometric properties of the Spanish adaptation of the SPSI-R. *Personality and Individual Differences, 29*, 699–708.

Stark, K. D. (1990). *Childhood depression: School-based intervention.* New York: Guilford Press.

Stark, K. D., Hargrave, J., Hersh, B., Greenberg, M., Herren, J., & Fisher, M. (2008). Treatment of childhood depression: The ACTION program. In J. R. Z. Abela & B. L. Hankin (Eds.), *Handbook of depression in children and adolescents* (pp. 224–227). New York: Guilford Press.

Stark, K. D., Reynolds, W. M., & Kaslow, N. J. (1987). A comparison of the relative efficacy of self-control therapy and a behavioral problem solving therapy for depression in children. *Journal of Abnormal Child Psychology, 15*, 91–113.

Stark, K. D., Schnoebelen, S., Simpson, J., Hargrave, J., Glenn, R., & Molnar, J. (2006). *Children's workbook for ACTION.* Broadmore, PA: Workbook.

Stark, K. D., Simpson, J., Schnoebelen, S., Hargrave, J., Glenn, R., & Molnar, J. (2006). *Therapist's manual for ACTION.* Broadmore, PA: Workbook.

Stark, K. D., Simpson, J., Yancy, M. & Molnar, J. (2006). *Parents' workbook for ACTION.* Ardmore, PA: Workbook.

Stark, K. D., Stapleton, L., & Fisher, M. (2009). *CBT with and without parent training for the treatment of depressed 9- to 13-year-old girls.* Manuscript in preparation.

Stark, K. D., Yancy, M., Simpson, J., & Molnar, J. (2006). *Treating depressed children: Therapist manual for parent component of "ACTION."* Ardmore, PA: Workbook.

8

Group Cognitive-Behavioral Treatment for Adolescent Depression

GREGORY N. CLARKE and LYNN L. DeBAR

OVERVIEW OF THE TREATMENT MODEL

The Clinical Problem

Adolescent major depressive disorder (MDD) has an estimated point prevalence ranging from 3 to 5% and a cumulative lifetime rate approaching 20% by age 18 (Birmaher et al., 1996). The gender ratio is roughly equal before puberty, but by early adolescence girls are two to three times more likely to be depressed than boys. This often chronic and recurrent illness is associated with significant impairment in family, social, and academic functioning. Depressed youths have an increased risk of suicide, other psychiatric difficulties, and substance abuse and are more likely to experience recurrent lifelong depressive episodes than persons with depression onset later in life. These characteristics support the public health significance of adolescent depression.

Conceptual Model and Assumptions Underlying Treatment

Our treatment program, the Adolescent Coping with Depression (CWDA) course, is based on the social learning model in which depression results from learned maladaptive behaviors and responses, interacting with a biological or inherited risk for depression. Learning new adaptive behaviors is hypothesized to be curative. Consistent with this, the behavioral model (Lewinsohn, Hoberman, Teri, & Hautzinger, 1985) hypothesizes that depression arises from low rates of response-contingent positive reinforcement and high rates of negative reinforcement, implying that depression can be decreased by modifying social behaviors so that they lead to more reward and less punishment. Also hypothesized to underlie depression are largely automatic, highly negative, and unrealistic beliefs (Beck, Rush, Shaw, & Emery, 1979), which lead depression-prone persons to interpret ambiguous situations in a highly negative and pessimistic way. This theory posits that changing beliefs in the more positive and realistic direction will lead to a decrease in depression.

Unifying these and other contributing theories is the multifactorial model of depression (Lewinsohn et al., 1985). Briefly, depression is presumed to be the result of multiple factors acting in combination, including negative cognitions, high rates of negative reinforcement, low rates of positive reinforcement, stressful events, predisposing vulnerabilities or risk factors (e.g., being female), and the absence of protective factors (e.g., coping skills). This model posits multiple pathways into depression, while also implying that people can recover from depression in multiple ways, by addressing one or more etiological or maintaining factors. Interestingly, the model does not necessarily require that the treatments address the same etiological factors that led to the onset of depression; that is, it may not be necessary to know the specific cause in order to match the treatment to this factor. Therefore, many interventions, possibly unrelated to the causal factors, may be curative. The CWDA intervention is guided by the hypothesis that teaching individuals new cognitive and behavioral skills strengthens their repertoire of coping techniques, thereby helping them overcome their depression.

Goals and Main Themes of the Treatment Program

The psychoeducational CWDA course (Clarke, Lewinsohn, & Hops, 1990) treats depressed youths in a group setting. Although we have also created and tested an individual cognitive-behavioral therapy (CBT) variant (Clarke, DeBar, et al., 2005), we nonetheless believe that a group approach may have several therapeutic advantages. First, teenagers are generally comfortable with the group learning model given its similarity to school. The psychoeducational approach makes the group, and depression, less stigmatizing. Of course, we try not to replicate the potentially alienating aspects of school; we do not judge or grade youths answers; participation and attendance are encouraged but voluntary; and topics are highly personal and relevant (i.e., their own feelings and behavior). The psychoeducational approach also facilitates therapist ease of use. Few community- and school-based mental health professionals have extensive training in CBT, which is a barrier to more widespread use of this evidence-based treatment. Our detailed manual and the psychoeducational approach are meant to ease implementation of the CWDA course for novice therapists or those new to CBT. With moderate training, CBT-naïve individuals are able to deliver the prevention and treatment programs based on the CWDA program and obtain clinical benefit. Therapists should have at least a master's degree in a mental health discipline and several years of prior experience working with adolescents. Therapists should be comfortable assessing depression and other comorbidities and addressing any crises that may arise (e.g., suicidality, substance abuse, emergent bipolar disorder).

The CWDA program directly focuses on symptom relief, as do other CBT interventions. The course is divided into specific modules or component skills training sections, each several sessions in length. Each module targets a particular depression symptom or deficit, such as depressive thinking, poor social skills, or low rates of pleasant activities. Each module provides training in skills to specifically address that domain of dysfunction. For example, the behavioral therapy module is meant to address low rates of pleasurable activities. The specific CWDA therapy components and their intended targets are listed in Table 8.1.

Each component could be (and in several cases is) an entire, comprehensive treatment for depression in its own right. Our rationale for this number of treatment components arises out of the multidimensional theoretical background for the CWDA program, reviewed previously. We believe that there are many possible approaches to recovering from depression, any one or more of which might be effective for any given individual. Unfortunately, at present, we cannot optimally match persons to specific treatments, so we have opted to offer several treatments with the hope that group participants will find at least one of these techniques that works for them.

We tell all youths that not every skill or technique will be equally useful for all participants but that we expect at least some group members will find each new skill helpful. We ask that all participants try each new skill and not reject it out of hand before trying it. In practice, of course, this can be a problem. As each new skill is presented, at least one youth inevitably claims that he or she has tried it before and it did nothing for them. In these cases, we ask participants to try the skill again while we provide coaching to overcome barriers to its success. However, if a given teen is adamant that she or he will not benefit from a given skill, we ask them to respect that other youths in the group may want to learn it.

The CWDA course therapist is expected to be active and directive. The therapist introduces each new skill with the rationale and underlying basics. Completely didactic presentations are often dry and boring, so therapists are encouraged to provide frequent opportunities for adolescent participation (e.g., asking questions, soliciting youth examples). Even during later practice and individual problem solving, the therapist is expected to actively assist participants through coaching or hints. Therapists may wish to withhold their own comments when group members are providing feedback and advice to one another. This peer feedback seems to be especially valued by group members because it comes from a peer "who understands my life."

Homework is also a regular component of the CWDA program, and it is encouraged but voluntary. Very early in each session, the therapist and group members review the previous session and the assigned homework. Youths who did not complete their homework between sessions often use this period to complete the forms. Homework is

TABLE 8.1. Adolescent Coping with Depression (CWDA) Therapy Components and Their Intended Targets

CWDA skill modules	Targets
Cognitive restructuring	Irrational or highly negative beliefs; guilt, hopelessness, worthlessness
Behavioral therapy	Social withdrawal, impaired interpersonal interactions, anhedonia
Problem solving, communication, negotiation	Impaired interpersonal interactions, conflict, anger, marital/family problems, poor problem solving
Relaxation training	Tension/anxiety, social anxiety
Goal setting	Identifying short- and long-term life goals and potential barriers to achieving these

meant to increase adolescent generalization of these new skills to their lives outside of the therapy session. If homework is not possible or acceptable, therapists should find other methods of promoting skill generalization. One example would be to encourage skills practice immediately before and after sessions, such as engaging in problem solving with parents in the waiting room immediately after sessions.

Characteristics of the Treatment Program

The original version of the CWDA program (Clarke et al., 1990) is a mixed-gender group consisting of 16 two-hour sessions, typically delivered twice a week over 8 weeks. Group membership is between six and 10 depressed adolescents, ages 13–18. In our research studies, we most often conduct groups with a single therapist. However, for training purposes, we sometimes include a trainee therapist who coleads the group before eventually soloing. The course is described in a therapist manual with scripted sessions and explanatory narrative. A companion youth workbook is provided to each participating teenager and contains relevant exercise and worksheets for acquiring and practicing the CWDA skills.

The adolescent CWDA program is an adaptation of the adult Coping with Depression Course (Lewinsohn, Steinmetz, Antonuccio, & Teri, 1984). We revised the adult program to make it more appropriate for teenagers by simplifying the homework and lectures, using cartoons to illustrate cognitive distortions, adding more participatory exercises, and adding problem-solving, communication, and negotiation skills training to address conflict issues with parents, peers, and other adults such as teachers.

Another developmentally relevant adaptation was the creation of a parallel parent course (Lewinsohn, Rohde, Hops, & Clarke, 1991), designed for the parents or guardians of youths enrolled in the CWDA treatment program. This parent course consists of eight 1-hour sessions offered once a week on one of the same nights as the teen group. A separate parent group therapist leads these sessions, although for some latter sessions the adolescent and parent groups meet together to practice family problem-solving techniques. However, research summarized later (Clarke, Rohde, Lewinsohn, Hops, & Seeley, 1999; Lewinsohn, Clarke, Hops, & Andrews, 1990) suggests that there is little incremental benefit from this parent group over that achieved by the adolescent group alone. This may be due in part to the relatively meager parent participation we have experienced, despite several attempts to schedule the parent group at the most convenient times. The parents who do attend seem to be those who need the program the least, whereas those who have clear family conflict are often unavailable or unmotivated to attend.

Who Is Treated?

In all of our treatment outcome trials, we have enrolled youths who meet *Diagnostic and Statistical Manual* (DSM) criteria for major depression or dysthymia, with or without other comorbidities. However, our impression is that youths with subdiagnostic levels of depression may also benefit. This conclusion is supported by the findings of our two randomized trials of a depression prevention program variant of the CWDA program, enrolling youths with elevated but subdiagnostic depression symptoms (Clarke et al., 1995; Clarke, Hornbrook, Lynch, Polen, Gale, Beardslee, 2001). In our earlier, highly controlled CWDA treatment *efficacy* studies (Clarke et al., 1999; Lewinsohn et al., 1990), we excluded a greater number of comorbid conditions than we did in our prevention studies and our later, more real-world CWDA *effectiveness* trials (Clarke, Hornbrook, et al., 2002; Clarke, DeBar, et al., 2005). In general, however, we always exclude youths with active psychotic disorders and bipolar disorder. We often permit active substance abuse or dependence as long as youths are not intoxicated while attending sessions. We also include youths with disruptive behavior disorders. We enrolled most youths with active suicidal ideation and behavior, with only a very few exceptions when the suicidal risk was judged to be extremely imminent (excluded youths were often hospitalized within days).

Content of Treatment

The CWDA program is multimodal; several distinct skills training modules appear throughout the intervention. Figure 8.1 provides a schematic of these modules, indicating the sessions in which those skills are addressed. The first session orients participants to the course features and summarizes the social learning model of depression as justification for the skills training to come. We also establish ground rules during the first session, including confidentiality and expectations of each other and the group leader.

The CWDA intervention has at its core two main components. The first is behavioral therapy, which aims to increase youth rates of age-appropriate and individually tailored pleasant activities; this is primarily addressed in sessions 2–5. Group leaders help youths select a personalized list of 10–20 fun activities that they would like to do more often; participants then collect baseline information on their rates of these activities and their daily mood. In most cases, youths find a positive relationship between their mood and

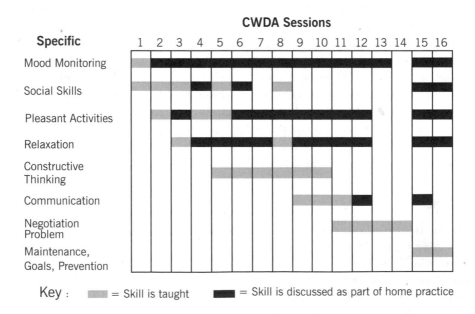

FIGURE 8.1. Timeline of Adolescent Coping with Depression (CWDA) course skills and sessions.

rates of fun activities, further supporting the rationale for increasing the number of fun activities they do each day. A minority of teens will argue that the causal direction of any association between mood and activities is in the other direction; that is, that they only do fun things when they feel good rather than the other (and more therapeutic) way around. We acknowledge that this may be the case but challenge them to test their interpretation by consciously increasing their rate of fun activities and observing the impact this may have on their mood. The latter sessions focus on setting small but achievable goals for increasing their activity level; making a written contract with themselves with small rewards for meeting their goals; and problem-solving solutions to barriers to doing more fun activities, such as chores and homework obligations.

The second main component is an adolescent-appropriate modification of Beck's cognitive therapy (Beck et al., 1979) and the rational emotive therapy approach (Ellis & Harper, 1961). These skills are delivered primarily in sessions 5–10. The group therapist initially introduces the basic concepts of triggering situations (antecedents) that lead to largely unexamined beliefs (beliefs), which, in turn, contribute to the development of feelings (consequences). The early sessions use cartoons such as *Garfield*, *Peanuts*, and *Calvin and Hobbs* to illustrate common beliefs leading to frustration, anger, or depression. By the later sessions, these cartoons fade out as adolescents are asked to provide personal examples of situations, beliefs, and emotional reactions. Adolescents are then taught how to determine whether these beliefs are irrational, unrealistic, or overly negative and judgmental. They are coached through the creation of more realistic, positive counter-thoughts, and then they are asked to rate how their mood changes with their adoption of these new beliefs. Some time may be spent examining family origins of unrealistic thoughts, especially when we have conducted trials with offspring of depressed parents (Clarke, Hornbrook, Lynch, Polen, Gale, Beardslee, et al., 2001; Clarke, Hornbrook, et al., 2002). One constructive feature of the group versions of the CWDA program is that challenges to negative or unrealistic thoughts often come from other adolescents rather than from the adult group leader. This peer feedback is often more palatable and credible to teenagers.

The CWDA program also includes several subsidiary components, including relaxation training (sessions 3 and 8) to cope with tension and social anxiety. Teens are taught progressive muscular relaxation methods and a shorter, more portable deep-breathing technique. Relaxation is valuable in later sessions to overcome social anxiety, which may sabotage other therapy goals such as increasing the frequency of social activities. Another subsidiary component consists of problem solving, negotiation, and communication skills, addressed in sessions 9–14. Adolescents and parents learn and practice the basics of these skills in their separate groups, with a focus on parent–child conflict. In session 14, teens and parents come together in a single, combined group to use their recently acquired skills to problem solve relatively low-intensity family problems. We do not immediately start with the higher intensity problems because feelings about these problems are often so intense that they may derail family negotiations. Families who competently use these skills to address low-intensity conflicts are encouraged to gradually address more contentious problems. Finally, because some depressed adolescents have difficulty making and retaining social connections, rudimentary social skills are taught in sessions 1, 3, 5, and 8. These skills include approaching people and starting conversations, making and maintaining friendships, and practicing positive nonverbal behaviors such as appropriate smiling and eye contact.

Toward the end of the course, the emphasis shifts from specific skills training to reviewing long- and short-term goals in several areas (e.g., social, academic, family, employment), identifying barriers to achieving these goals and problem solving solutions, discussing how to maintain gains by continuing to use the skills learned, learning how to recognize if depression recurs, and creating a personal depression prevention plan, including what to do in an emergency. Part of the final session is spent reviewing individual progress since the beginning of the group, identifying areas of competence and areas still needing work, sharing feelings about the group ending, and discussing what each adolescent might do to replace the support that the group may have provided.

Throughout the group, youths are asked to monitor their daily mood on a 7-point scale. This is meant to provide them with an ongoing measure of their progress, but it is also important for specific exercises that relate to increasing pleasant activities, described previously. In general, we find that orienting adolescents to ongoing self-evaluation contributes to the overall self-change, self-improvement approach of the CWDA group.

Although the specific content and skills training vary by session, the structure and within-session sequencing of activities are similar across most group meetings. The typical group session follows this sequence: (1) review of the agenda for that day's session; (2) review of homework from the previous session, including catch-up for those who did not complete it; (3) presentation of the new skills, emphasizing adolescent examples and participation; (4) practice of the new skills, during which peer and therapist feedback are both important; (5) problem solve solutions to barriers to implementing the new skills; and (6) homework assignment.

Although we would ideally like all teens to acquire and generalize all of the skills taught in the CWDA course, we acknowledge that not every skill will be equally useful for every teen. This approach is meant to relieve perfectionistic pressure for those teens who believe they must master each module and to forestall pessimism and resistance among youths who find the first few modules either too difficult or not pertinent for them. For example, the therapist might say, "Let's see if the next section will be more helpful for you."

How to Determine When Treatment Is "Finished"

The original CWDA program is a group intervention with a fixed duration of 16 two-hour sessions. The acute phase course ends at the same time for all participants regardless of degree of recovery. Therefore, the issue of when treatment is finished is moot. However, recognizing that approximately one-third of youths entering the group may not be fully recovered at the end of the course, we developed and tested a continuation component for the CWDA program that consists of monthly group booster sessions (Clarke et al., 1999). Youths are offered refresher courses in the various skills taught in the acute CWDA program as clinically relevant, most often to address new or ongoing problems for one or more of the group members (e.g., a youth still bothered by unrealistic thoughts of guilt and worthlessness would prompt a review of the cognitive restructuring module). We found that youths who were partially recovered at the end of acute treatment and were assigned to this continuation program continued to improve at higher rates (Clarke et al., 1999).

The original CWDA program is also a fixed membership group. That is, all youths in a given group are enrolled at the very beginning, and no additional youths are added at any later point. Because participating youths need to learn the overall model of depression and the intervention in the early sessions, they may not benefit if they miss this fundamental information by entering the group in later sessions. This restriction sometimes creates difficulty in settings such as inpatient units, where census is highly fluid, and youth presence may be very brief. To address this issue, Paul Rohde and colleagues created a variation of the CWDA program for use with delinquent adolescents with comorbid depression who are held for an average of 30 days in a juvenile detention facility. This version of the program is designed to be used in a circular, endlessly repeating fashion and permits the entry of new group members at the junction between each new skill module. The 16 original CWDA sessions have been divided into three six-session modules consisting of the following skills: (1) social skills, pleasant activities; (2) relaxation, cognitive restructuring; and (3) communication, problem solving, and life goals/maintenance. Each new module begins with a reintroduction of the premise of the group, a review of group norms and guidelines, and instructions on how to monitor daily mood. Group members typically stay in the group for three modules to learn the entire skill repertoire. Although this variant of the CWDA program has not yet been evaluated in outcome studies, our impression is that it offers a good logistical fit with the needs of this setting.

How to Obtain Manuals and Supporting Materials

The CWDA therapist manual and adolescent workbook, and materials for the spin-off individual CBT and prevention programs, are available at *www.kpchr.org/acwd/acwd.html*. All these materials are available free of charge and may be photocopied and used by anyone in any setting. We retain copyright, but we are also open to modification of these materials by other researchers or clinicians to better serve other audiences or target groups as long as these modifications are also made freely available. For example, the CWDA has been translated and culturally adapted into Spanish, French, German, Chinese, Japanese, and Swedish, among other languages.

EVIDENCE FOR THE EFFECTS OF TREATMENT

To date, the original CWDA course has been evaluated in four randomized trials. In all cases, the Children's Schedule for Affective Disorders and Schizophrenia was used to diagnose major depression, dysthymia, and comorbid disorders (Kaufman et al., 1997). Other measures were also administered in these studies but are not reported here.

The first two of these studies (Clarke et al., 1999; Lewinsohn et al., 1990) shared the same basic design. Youths diagnosed with DSM major depression or dysthymia, or both, were randomly assigned to (1) the CWDA course without parent therapy; (2) the CWDA course with parents enrolled in the parallel parent group; or (3) a wait-list control condition. There were 59 youths in the first trial (Lewinsohn et al., 1990) and 123 in the second (Clarke et al., 1999). The principal outcome was recovery from the index DSM depression diagnosis (e.g., at least 8 weeks of no more than one or two residual symptoms with no impairment) at posttreatment and through a 2-year follow-up period. Compared to the wait-list condition, the active treatment conditions resulted in significantly more depression recovery in both studies. The posttreatment depression recovery rate in this first study was 46% for the treatment groups versus 5% for the control condition. The second study found higher depression recovery rates in the treatment groups (67%) than the wait-list condition (48%). However, contrary to expectations, there were few or no significant advantages for parental involvement in either study. Note, however, that these studies were underpowered to detect anything smaller than a medium effect size advantage.

The second CWDA study (Clarke et al., 1999) also included a linked but separate trial of a continuation treatment following the end of the acute CWDA course. The continuation program (described previously) aimed to improve ongoing recovery from depression and minimize relapse. Youths who completed the acute-phase CWDA groups were randomly reassigned to one of three conditions for the remaining 24-month follow-up period: (1) assessments every 4 months with monthly booster sessions, (2) assessments only every 4 months, or (3) assessments only every 12 months. The booster sessions did not reduce the rate of depression recurrence in the follow-up period but did accelerate recovery among depressed youths who were still depressed at the end of the acute CWDA group.

Rohde, Clarke, Mace, Jorgensen, and Seeley (2004) conducted a randomized trial of the CWDA program for depressed, delinquent youths who were recruited through local juvenile justice departments. Ninety-six youth ages 13–17 who met DSM-IV (American Psychiatric Association, 1994) criteria for major depression or dysthymia and conduct disorder were randomized either to the CWDA course or to a life skills tutoring course (the attention-placebo control condition). Depression recovery at posttreatment was 26% in the CWDA condition versus 14% in the life skills condition (odds ratio, 3.4; 95% confidence interval, 1.3–9.3). However, by 12 months posttreatment, there were no differences between conditions for depression outcomes. There were also no differences for overall conduct disorder diagnoses at any time point, although youths in the CWDA condition had lower levels of aggression/rule violation symptoms immediately after acute treatment. Overall, we detected a modest acute treatment advantage for the CWDA program for depression but not conduct disorder; however, this advantage did not persist over the year-long follow-up.

Finally, we have conducted a randomized effectiveness trial of the CWDA course for depressed adolescent offspring of depressed parents (Clarke, Hornbrook, Lynch, Polen, Gale, O'Connor, et al., 2002). Eligible offspring ages 13–18 who met current DSM criteria for major depression or dysthymia were randomized either to usual health maintenance organization care ($n = 47$) or usual care plus the CWDA program ($n = 41$). We were unable to detect any significant advantage for the CBT program over usual care at posttreatment or over the 24-month follow-up for depression or any other outcomes. The reasons why this study failed to find significant benefit for the CWDA program remain unclear. It may be because the comparison condition in the Clarke, Hornbrook, et al. (2002) study was active treatment as usual (TAU) consisting primarily of brief psychotherapy or antidepressant medication or a combination. This was not the case in the three other CWDA trials, in which the comparison condition was either a wait-list or an attention-placebo condition with no focus on depression.

Predictors, Moderators, and Mediators

In a study to identify predictors of depression outcome in the CWDA program (Clarke, Hops, Lewinsohn, & Andrews, 1992), improved depression diagnostic outcomes were associated with a greater number of past psychiatric diagnoses, parent involvement in treatment, and younger age at onset of first depressive episode. Improved depression self-report scores were associated with lower intake depression and anxiety, higher enjoyment and frequency of pleasant activities, and more rational thoughts.

Rohde, Seeley, Kaufman, Clarke, and Stice (2006) examined factors that predicted time to MDD recovery in their CWDA trial of youths with depression and conduct disorder (Rohde, Clarke, et al., 2004). Among all youths irrespective of their study condition, longer time to MDD recovery was predicted by earlier MDD onset, suicidal ideation, presence of attention-deficit/hyperactivity disorder, lower psychosocial functioning, parent report of problem behaviors, higher levels of negative automatic cognitions and hopelessness, poor family cohesion, and low levels of coping skills. This study also found several variables that *moderated* outcome (i.e., predicted significantly different outcome in the study conditions). Youths in CBT had a faster recovery time relative to those in the attention-control treatment if they were of white ethnicity, had recurrent MDD, and had good coping skills.

Using data from this same trial, we examined *mediational* models for change in depression (Kaufman, Rohde, Seeley, Clarke, & Stice, 2005) to identify mechanisms through which CBT might work. Although we were unable to conduct a full test of mediation, we found results consistent with the mechanism that improvements in negative cognitions lead to improved depression outcomes. However, effects for other factors that might explain the mechanisms underlying CBT (i.e., dysfunctional attitudes, pleasant activities, relaxation, social skills, problem solving) were not significant.

Treatment Process and Outcomes

In each of our outcome studies, we have measured therapist fidelity to the CWDA manual using a scale developed for this purpose (Clarke, 1998). Fidelity is typically high, with mean ratings ranging between 78 and 94% compliance with the defined program. However, therapist fidelity in group CWDA is rated for one therapist treating many youths, whereas outcome is recorded for individual youths. All these youths in a given group have highly variable depression recovery but are exposed to the same level of therapist treatment fidelity. Because of this data mismatch between a group therapist and individual outcomes, we have been limited in our ability to examine the relationship between the two (see Clarke, 1998, for more details).

We have also examined the importance of youth adherence with the program. Interestingly, we failed to find any association between degree of between-session homework completion and improved outcome (Clarke et al., 1992). It may be that homework completed between sessions plays no role in improving depression. However, the fact that noncompliant youths have a chance to make up their homework at the beginning of each session may diminish the statistical association between homework completion and outcome. Another aspect of adherence is attendance, which might be seen as a proxy for dose. In two studies (Clarke et al., 1992, 1999), we failed to find an association between number of sessions attended and depression outcomes. In child psychotherapy in general, there have been mixed findings regarding the relationship between psychotherapy dose and outcomes. One complicating factor is that treatment attendance may be at least partly dependent on rapidity of recovery. Those who respond quickly may be more likely to drop out prematurely, having reached a personal level of satisfactory recovery. Conversely, those who are more severely depressed at baseline may be more motivated to stay in treatment longer assuming that this may lead to greater improvement. Both of these nonrandom factors would lead to a pattern of lower doses associated with better outcomes and higher doses associated with poorer outcomes, contrary to the expected dose relationship.

Variants of the CWDA Program

Modifications of the CWDA program include approaches to prevent depression, treat an array of negative emotions in delinquent youths, provide individual (rather than group) CBT for depressed youths either as a monotherapy or as an adjunct to selective serotonin reuptake inhibitor (SSRI) medications, and as an Internet-delivered self-help program. All of these are described next.

Prevention

Although this chapter focuses primarily on the treatment of depression, we have also conducted several studies of a depression prevention program, the Coping With Stress (CWS) course, that is derived from and is closely related to the CWDA intervention but focuses only on a single-skill training module: cognitive restructuring. The CWS program consists of 15 one-hour sessions delivered to small groups of adolescents ages 13–18. We have conducted two trials of this intervention: one with at-risk offspring of depressed parents (Clarke, Hornbrook, Lynch, Polen, Gale, Beardslee, et al., 2001) and another with youths with subdiagnostic depressive symptoms (Clarke et al., 1995). In both randomized trials with high-risk youths, we found significant preventive effects for the CWS program, with significantly fewer prospective cases of major depression among youths participating in the prevention program compared with those in the usual-care control condition. More recently, we and colleagues at three other sites have recently replicated and extended the results of these earlier studies in a large trial ($N = 316$) with offspring of depressed parents, with a significant prevention effect of the program detected at the 8-month follow-up evaluation (Garber et al., 2007).

Negative Emotions and Conduct Disorder

As described earlier, Rohde and colleagues conducted a controlled trial of the original CWDA program with depressed youths with comorbid conduct disorder (Rohde, Clarke, et al., 2004). More recently, Rohde and colleagues modified the CWDA to serve as a general coping and problem-solving skills intervention for incarcerated youths, regardless of depression level. This new intervention, entitled the Coping Course, focused on a broad array of negative emotions, including frustration, boredom, and fear. In a preliminary evaluation of the intervention (Rohde, Jorgensen, Seeley, & Mace, 2004), 76 incarcerated male adolescents were randomly assigned either to the Coping Course ($n = 46$) or usual care ($n = 30$). Significant intervention effects were detected for youth externalizing, suicide proneness, self-esteem, social adjustment, and knowledge regarding CBT skills for mood management.

Individual CBT

As much as we believe that the group format offers many therapeutic benefits, such as peer modeling and acceptance of feedback from peers, we and others have found the logistics of mounting groups to be a barrier. Therefore, in the last decade, we have switched most of our focus from group CBT to individual CBT with and without pharmacotherapy. We are particularly committed to collaborative-care CBT, in which a patient's treatment is comanaged by a mental health specialist and a primary care provider (PCP). Our individual CBT program has a variable duration (five to nine sessions) depending on the degree of youth response at the halfway point. Although this is admittedly abbreviated therapy relative to other youth depression CBT approaches (e.g., Brent et al., 2008), we intentionally kept this program brief to fit best with lean primary care practice parameters, in the hopes of eventually maximizing adoption of this approach in real-world settings should it prove to be effective. The program consists of an initial introductory session, a four-session cognitive restructuring module, and a four-session behavioral activation module. Youths and therapists jointly decide which module to use first, based on each youth's prior therapy experiences and match with each youth's preferred coping strategies. Youths who remain depressed or who have a fragile response after the first half of the program are strongly encouraged to continue for an additional four sessions (for a total of nine), whereas those who are recovered at the fifth session are given two options: either continuing with the remaining skill module to consolidate gains or discontinuing with an option to restart therapy if depression recurs. If youths are also being treated with antidepressants, CBT therapists facilitate greater medication compliance and benefit by monitoring compliance, side effects, benefit or lack thereof, and risk of discontinuation and by conveying relevant information to the prescribing health care provider. All youths receive brief, 10-minute therapist telephone calls periodically during the yearlong continuation period after acute treatment to check for depression recurrence and are provided case management or referrals to address other emergent life events (e.g., pregnancy, family conflict, substance abuse). The therapist manual and youth workbook for individual CBT are similar to the group materials, but they allow greater flexibility regarding ordering of skills, skipping irrelevant sections, and otherwise customizing the content to the presentation, strengths, and deficits of each youth.

We recently conducted a randomized controlled trial (RCT) of this individual CBT variant (Clarke, DeBar, et al., 2005). We enrolled depressed youths ages 12–18 who had been prescribed TAU SSRI medication by their pediatrician PCPs. Consenting youths ($n = 152$) were randomly assigned either to TAU SSRIs delivered by PCPs or to TAU SSRIs plus brief, individual CBT. Unfortunately, no acute treatment CBT advantage was detected for recovery from MDD episodes, although a nonsignificant trend was detected for CBT on self-reported depression symptoms (effect size $d = 0.17$). We also found CBT advantages on the Short Form-12 Mental Component scale and reductions in TAU health care visits and days' supply of medication in the CBT condition. Contributing to the difficulty finding any CBT advantage, 75% of participants in the TAU control condition were recovered from their index depressive episode by the 12-week follow-up. We concluded that the CBT condition was associated with a genuine but modest effect, possibly obscured by a sample that was too small given the very high recovery rate in the TAU condition and attenuated by an unexpected 20% reduction in SSRI pharmacotherapy in the CBT condition.

We are currently conducting another large trial of this same individual CBT program with depressed youths who have recently declined or rapidly discontinued antidepressants; unpublished clinical epidemiology data suggest that up to 75% of youths identified as depressed in primary care fit this description. We are randomizing youths ages 12–18 with major depression into either brief, individual CBT delivered in primary care or a TAU control condition (watchful waiting or alternative, non-CBT psychotherapies or both). Initial outcomes should be available in mid-2010.

Beyond our own projects, the CWDA program was one of the primary source materials for the individual CBT intervention used in the two largest trials of adolescent depression treatment conducted to date: the Treatment of Adolescent Depression Study (TADS; March et al., 2004) and the Treatment of SSRI-Resistant Depression in Adolescents trial (TORDIA; Brent et al., 2008). The TADS study failed to find an advantage of monotherapy CBT over the medication placebo control, although some outcomes favored combination CBT + SSRIs over monotherapy SSRIs. The TORDIA study, conducted with depressed youths who had failed to respond to an initial course of SSRIs, found a significant 15% advantage in response rates of combination CBT + SSRIs over monotherapy SSRIs. Taken together, these two landmark studies have led some to suggest that combination CBT + SSRI treatment should be considered the gold standard for treatment of depression in adolescents. However, uncertainty about this approach has been fueled by another large study that failed to find an advantage for combination CBT + SSRI treatment among youths who remained depressed after an initial exposure to a brief, nonspecific psychosocial "washout" intervention (Goodyer et al., 2007).

Internet Self-Help

Finally, we are in the process of creating an Internet-based self-help variation of the CWDA program for depressed youths. Based on our RCTs of Internet CBT with depressed adults (Clarke, Reid, et al., 2002; Clarke, Eubanks, et al., 2005; Clarke, Kelleher, Hornbrook, DeBar, Dickerson, & Gullion, 2009) the youth web site will ultimately provide online, self-guided training and practice of cognitive and behavioral therapy techniques for adolescents with low-grade depression.

DIRECTIONS FOR RESEARCH

Despite the progress we have made, there are still several unanswered questions about the CWDA course. One principal remaining hurdle is a randomized trial of the CWDA program conducted by researchers other than ourselves in order to get beyond the "founders effect." Another limitation of the extant CWDA research is our reliance on mostly middle-class participants. Three of the CWDA trials were conducted with fairly homogeneous samples of white, middle-class depressed youths with only limited comorbidity. One CWDA study has been conducted with depressed youths with comorbid conduct disorder (Rohde, Clarke, et al., 2004), but these were still predominantly white youths. However, the various translations of the CWDA course into Spanish, German, and other languages will, we hope, lead to evaluation studies in these cultures, if not even full RCTs. We ourselves are attempting to enroll at least 20% Latino participants in our in-progress individual CBT study to examine outcomes separately in that subgroup.

Similar modifications and studies need to be conducted with many other special populations. For example, we have given some thought to variations of the CWDA program for single-gender groups, on the assumption that the dynamics of these groups might enhance outcomes as well as take advantage of emerging knowledge about differences in depression among teenage girls and boys. Jennifer Wisdom has created a version of the CWDA program for girls-only groups (personal communication, December 2001). The revised group includes both discussing the real-world stressors that girls experience within the context of the cognitive and behavioral modules and teaching skills to help girls analyze messages about stereotypes, communicate clearly and assertively, and maintain healthy relationships. This variation has been piloted but has not yet been tested in a randomized trial. Conducting more rigorous evaluations of this and related variations is a high priority.

CONCLUSIONS

In the 18 years since the publication of both the CWDA manual (Clarke et al., 1990) and our first randomized trial (Lewinsohn et al., 1990), we have conducted three additional randomized trials of this program. We have also broadened the target population to include depressed teenagers with comorbid conduct disorder as well as offspring of depressed parents. We and others have created several special purpose variations of the CWDA program for prevention, for individual CBT, and for use with special populations. With one exception (Clarke, Hornbrook, Lynch, Polen, Gale, O'Connor, et al., 2002), all the studies of the CWDA program and its spin-off programs have yielded significant, positive treatment or prevention results (the Clarke, DeBar, et al., 2005, study failed to find an advantage on the primary outcome but CBT advantages were found for several secondary outcomes). Somewhat surprisingly, the addition of a companion parent group has not been shown to significantly improve outcomes. In general, we conclude that the CWDA course has been moderately well tested and is certainly well along the continuum toward becoming an evidence-based treatment. However, we still need to test the benefit of the CWDA program with special populations, particularly minority adolescents, teenagers with greater psychiatric comorbidity, and same-gender groups.

The dissemination and adoption of the CWDA program in practice settings remains a challenge. We developed the original CWDA course as a psychoeducational program in part to facilitate its adoption in practice settings, particularly where groups of adolescents would be easily formed, such as schools and day treatment facilities. The highly scripted therapist manual and youth workbook were meant to provide clear direction for therapists new to CBT. Despite these features, we have heard that it is difficult for providers in many traditional settings (except perhaps schools) to bring together a sufficient number of depressed youths at the same time in order to start a fixed-membership, fixed-duration group. This feedback has led us to develop the circular (endlessly repeating) modification of the CWDA course, and the individual brief (five to nine session) variation. We believe that both adaptations of the CWDA program will ease adoption in practice settings.

REFERENCES

American Psychiatric Association. (1994). *Diagnostic and statistical manual of mental disorders* (4th ed.). Washington, DC: Author.

Beck, A. T., Rush, A. J., Shaw, B. F., & Emery, G. (1979). *Cognitive therapy of depression*. New York: Guilford Press.

Birmaher, B., Ryan, N. D., Williamson, D. E., Brent, D. A., Kaufman, J., Dahl, R. E., et al. (1996). Childhood and adolescent depression: A review of the past 10 years. Part I. *Journal of the American Academy of Child and Adolescent Psychiatry, 35,* 1427–1439.

Brent, D., Emslie, G., Clarke, G., Wagner, K. D., Asarnow, J. R., Keller, M. et al. (2008). Switching to another SSRI or to venlafaxine with or without cognitive behavioral therapy for adolescents with SSRI-resistant depression: The TORDIA randomized controlled trial. *Journal of the American Medical Association, 299,* 901–913.

Clarke, G., DeBar, L. L., Lynch, F. L., Powell, J., Gale, J., O'Connor, E. A., et al. (2005). A randomized effectiveness trial of brief cognitive-behavioral therapy for depressed adolescents receiving anti-depressant medication. *Journal of the American Academy of Child and Adolescent Psychiatry, 44,* 888–898.

Clarke, G., Kelleher, C., Hornbrook, M., DeBar, L., Dickerson, J., & Gullion, C. (2009). Randomized effectiveness trial of an Internet, pure self-help, cognitive behavioral intervention for depressive symptoms in young adults. *Cognitive Behavioural Therapy, 13,* 1–13.

Clarke, G., Reid, E., Eubanks, D., O'Connor, E., DeBar, L. L., Kelleher, C., et al. (2002). Overcoming depression on the Internet (ODIN): A randomized controlled trial of an Internet depression skills intervention program. *Journal of Medical Internet Research, 4,* E14.

Clarke, G. N. (1998). Intervention fidelity in adolescent depression prevention and treatment. *Journal of Prevention and Intervention in the Community, 17,* 19–33.

Clarke, G. N., Eubanks, D., Reid, E., Kelleher, C., O'Connor, E., DeBar, L. L., et al. (2005). Overcoming depression on the Internet (ODIN) (2): A randomized trial of a self-help depression skills program with reminders. *Journal of Medical Internet Research, 7,* e16.

Clarke, G. N., Hawkins, W., Murphy, M., Sheeber, L. B., Lewinsohn, P. M., & Seeley, J. R. (1995). Targeted prevention of unipolar depressive disorder in an at-risk sample of high school adolescents: A randomized trial of a group cognitive intervention. *Journal of the American Academy of Child and Adolescent Psychiatry, 34,* 312–321.

Clarke, G. N., Hops, H., Lewinsohn, P. M., & Andrews, J. (1992). Cognitive-behavioral group treatment of adolescent depression: Prediction of outcome. *Behavior Therapy, 23,* 341–354.

Clarke, G. N., Hornbrook, M., Lynch, F., Polen, M., Gale, J., Beardslee, W., et al. (2001). A randomized trial of a group cognitive intervention for preventing depression in adolescent offspring of depressed parents. *Archives of General Psychiatry, 58,* 1127–1134.

Clarke, G. N., Hornbrook, M., Lynch, F., Polen, M., Gale, J., O'Connor, E. et al. (2002). Group cognitive-behavioral treatment for depressed adolescent offspring of depressed parents in a health maintenance organization. *Journal of the American Academy of Child and Adolescent Psychiatry, 41,* 305–313.

Clarke, G. N., Lewinsohn, P. M., & Hops, H. (1990). *Instructor's manual for the Adolescent Coping with Depression Course.* Portland, OR: Kaiser Permanente Center for Health Research. (Available from *www.kpchr.org/acwd/acwd.html*)

Clarke, G. N., Rohde, P., Lewinsohn, P. M., Hops, H., & Seeley, J. R. (1999). Cognitive-behavioral treatment of adolescent depression: Efficacy of acute group treatment and booster sessions. *Journal of the American Academy of Child and Adolescent Psychiatry, 38,* 272–279.

Ellis, A., & Harper, R. A. (1961). *A guide to rational living.* Hollywood, CA: Wilshire Book.

Garber, J., Brent, D., Clarke, G., Beardslee, W., Weersing, V. R., Gladstone, T. R., et al. (2007, October). *Prevention of depression in at-risk adolescents: Rationale, design, and preliminary results.* Paper presented at the annual conference of the American Academy of Child and Adolescent Psychiatry, Boston, MA.

Goodyer, I., Dubicka, B., Wilkinson, P., Kelvin, R., Roberts, C., Byford, S., et al. (2007). Selective serotonin reuptake inhibitors (SSRIs) and routine specialist care with and without cognitive behaviour therapy in adolescents with major depression: Randomised controlled trial. *British Medical Journal, 335*, 142.

Kaufman, J., Birmaher, B., Brent, D. A., Rao, U., Flynn, C., Moreci, P., et al. (1997). Schedule for Affective Disorders and Schizophrenia for School-Age Children—Present and Lifetime Version (K-SADS-PL): Initial reliability and validity data. *Journal of the American Academy of Child and Adolescent Psychiatry, 36*, 980–988.

Kaufman, N. K., Rohde, P., Seeley, J. R., Clarke, G. N., & Stice, E. (2005). Potential mediators of cognitive-behavioral therapy for adolescents with comorbid major depression and conduct disorder. *Journal of Consulting and Clinical Psychology, 73*, 38–46.

Lewinsohn, P. M., Clarke, G. N., Hops, H., & Andrews, J. A. (1990). Cognitive-behavioral treatment for depressed adolescents. *Behavior Therapy, 21*, 385–401.

Lewinsohn, P. M., Hoberman, H. M., Teri, L., & Hautzinger, M. (1985). An integrative theory of unipolar depression. In S. Reiss & R. R. Bootzin (Eds.), *Theoretical issues in behavioral therapy* (pp. 313–359). New York: Academic Press.

Lewinsohn, P. M., Rohde, P., Hops, H., & Clarke, G. N. (1991). The *Coping With Depression Course—Adolescent version: Instructor's manual for the parent course*. Unpublished manuscript.

Lewinsohn, P. M., Steinmetz, J. L., Antonuccio, D. O., & Teri, L. (1984). A behavioral group therapy approach to the treatment of depression. In D. Upper & S. M. Ross (Eds.), *Handbook of behavioral group therapy* (pp. 303–329). New York: Plenum.

March, J., Silva, S., Petrycki, S., Curry, J., Wells, K., Fairbank, J., et al. (2004). Fluoxetine, cognitive-behavioral therapy, and their combination for adolescents with depression: Treatment for Adolescents With Depression Study (TADS) randomized controlled trial. *Journal of the American Medical Association, 292*, 807–820.

Rohde, P., Clarke, G. N., Mace, D. E., Jorgensen, J., & Seeley, J. R. (2004). An efficacy/effectiveness study of cognitive-behavioral treatment for adolescents with comorbid major depression and conduct disorder. *Journal of the American Academy of Child and Adolescent Psychiatry, 43*, 660–668.

Rohde, P., Jorgensen, J. S., Seeley, J. R., & Mace, D. E. (2004). Pilot evaluation of the Coping Course: A cognitive-behavioral intervention to enhance coping skills in incarcerated youth. *Journal of the American Academy of Child and Adolescent Psychiatry, 43*, 669–676.

Rohde, P., Seeley, J. R., Kaufman, N. K., Clarke, G. N., & Stice, E. (2006). Predicting time to recovery among depressed adolescents treated in two psychosocial group interventions. *Journal of Consulting and Clinical Psychology, 74*, 80–88.

9

Treating Depression in Adolescents Using Individual Cognitive-Behavioral Therapy

V. ROBIN WEERSING and DAVID A. BRENT

OVERVIEW OF THE TREATMENT MODEL

Overview of the Clinical Problem

A growing body of naturalistic studies has documented that depression in youth, particularly during adolescence, is common, of relatively long duration, and recurrent. Specifically, depression has a point prevalence among adolescents of approximately 5%, may produce long-lasting impairments in social and occupational functioning (e.g., Rohde, Lewinsohn, & Seeley, 1994), and substantially increases the risk of early mortality by suicide (e.g., Brent et al., 1993).

In this chapter, we provide an overview of the Pittsburgh program of research on the treatment of depression and suicidality in adolescents. Many of the findings we report are drawn from the original Brent et al. (1997) clinical trial, which tested the effects of cognitive-behavioral therapy (CBT) against an active treatment (systemic-behavioral family treatment [SBFT]) and nonspecific therapy (nondirective supportive treatment [NST]) control. Data from this investigation have been used to evaluate the efficacy of CBT relative to alternate treatments, probe possible mechanisms of CBT action, and delineate moderators of treatment effects. In addition to these core clinical trial findings, we present results from two recent projects: (1) testing the effects of CBT with treatment-resistant youth who have already failed a medication protocol for depression (Brent et al., 2008) and (2) probing the effectiveness of CBT for adolescent depression under conditions approximating real-world clinical practice (Weersing, Iyengar, Kolko, Birmaher, & Brent, 2006).

Conceptual Models Underlying Treatment

Factors implicated in the onset and maintenance of depression among youth fall into two broad, conceptual categories: (1) intraindividual cognitive and biological vulnerabilities (e.g., depressogenic information processing) and (2) interpersonal and environmental factors (e.g., family expressed emotion). CBT for adolescent depression targets both of these broad domains by changing youths' cognitive distortions, encouraging activities that promote positive mood, and teaching teens problem-solving skills to promote better coping with negative life events. We provide a brief overview of the relevant theories and empirical findings related to these treatment targets and the development of the Pittsburgh program.

Cognitive Vulnerability

Several theories of depression fall under the umbrella of the cognitive vulnerability model. The best known of these is cognitive theory of depression developed by Beck and colleagues (Beck, Rush, Shaw, & Emery, 1979). In brief, Beck and colleagues noted that depressed individuals have inaccurate, overly negative views of themselves, the world, and possibilities for the future, a negative cognitive triad of depressogenic beliefs. This cognitive triad is hypothesized to be resistant to disconfirmation by contradictory positive information, in part because of systematic errors in depressed individuals' information processing (e.g., selective abstraction of negative information). At a deeper level, both the cognitive triad and errors in information processing are thought to derive from more stable cognitive structures, or schemata. Schemata are core beliefs and recollections that organize past experience and, when activated by internal or external stimuli, bring that past experience to bear on the current situation. Depressogenic schemata are thought to develop from early negative experiences, to become activated during analogous stressful circumstances in the present, and to predispose the individual to dysfunctional beliefs and errors in processing information and, thus, symptoms of depression. The Beck model was developed to describe and explain adult depression; however, evidence suggests that depressed adolescents display similar patterns of negative beliefs and errors in information processing (see Gladstone & Kaslow, 1995, for a review).

Negative Life Events and Family Conflict

Experiencing negative, uncontrollable events has been linked to helplessness and apathy both in humans and in animals. In adolescents, first-onset and recurrence of depression are often preceded by negative psychosocial events, including family conflict, physical illness, breakup of romantic relationships, and loss of friendships (Lewinsohn, Allen, Seeley, & Gotlib, 1999). Of these, familial stress may play a particularly important role: Parental depression, parent–child conflict, parental divorce, low family cohesion, and high levels of expressed emotion have all been found to significantly increase the risk of depression in adolescents (e.g., Lewinsohn et al., 1994). In CBT, treatment addresses these environmental factors by targeting irrational, overly negative thoughts about these events and by teaching problem-solving and hypothesis-testing skills to enable patients to better cope with and solve life problems.

CHARACTERISTICS OF THE TREATMENT PROGRAM

In this section, we describe the characteristics of the Pittsburgh CBT program as delivered in the original clinical trial (Brent et al., 1997). Study-specific modifications to this original CBT program are described in the same section as the findings for these investigations.

Format and Duration

CBT was delivered individually to depressed adolescents on a weekly schedule. Youth received 12–16 sessions of the active intervention and up to four additional booster treatment sessions. Therapists presented themselves as collaborators and coaches and encouraged teens to take an active role in their own recovery. Occasionally, therapists would be in contact with parents to provide general information about the progress of treatment. However, in the original clinical trial, CBT was to be compared against an explicitly family-based model (SBFT), and family-focused sessions were kept to a minimum.

Content of Treatment

As seen in Figure 9.1, CBT sessions focused primarily on altering the irrational, overly negative cognitions viewed to be at the root of depressive symptomatology. Youth were taught to identify their automatic thoughts, accurately label thoughts as distorted or overly pessimistic, and challenge their depressive thinking about themselves and the world. In addition to focusing on depressogenic cognitions, CBT therapists targeted difficulties in affect regulation and impulsivity, particularly as related to reducing self-injurious, risky, and suicidal behaviors early in the course of treatment. Youths were

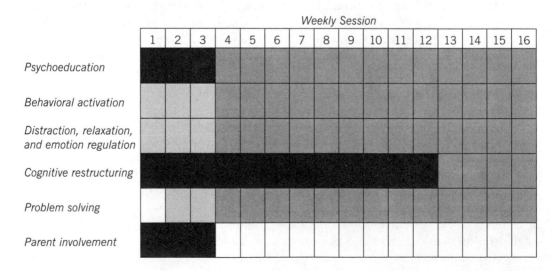

FIGURE 9.1. Content of CBT in the original Pittsburgh clinical trial. Black boxes indicate primary emphasis on technique or scripted use; light gray boxes, typical use; dark gray boxes, optional use, as indicated by the cognitive case conceptualization.

taught how to identify their feelings, use behavioral activities and distraction to regulate mood, and solve problems in a calm, logical manner. These general problem-solving skills were viewed as important (1) for reducing risky behavior and alleviating symptoms in the current depressive episode and (2) for their ability to aid in relapse prevention by helping adolescents to effectively cope with future negative life events and interpersonal difficulties.

Developmental Adaptations

This CBT treatment protocol represented a developmental adaptation of the classic Beck CBT approach. Because adolescents are not autonomous agents, despite their desires to be so, a family psychoeducation component was added to gain parent support for treatment attendance, goals, and completion of homework assignments. The collaborative empiricism of Beck et al. (1979) was articulated to adolescents, often seeking independence from adult authorities, as "I'm going to teach you how to be your own therapist." Because teens frequently do not complete homework, *in vivo* experiences, such as monitoring cognitions associated with in session affective shifts, were used to illustrate and socialize the adolescent to the cognitive model.

Because adolescents present with a wide range of cognitive abilities and prior experience with treatment, it may be necessary to educate adolescent clients to the language and process of psychotherapy. To accomplish this, the CBT therapists summarized, or had the adolescent summarize, frequently in session to be sure that the therapist and young client were indeed speaking the same language. Throughout treatment, the level of abstraction was kept to a minimum, and concrete examples, linked to youths' personal experience, were used whenever possible.

Comparison Treatments

We next briefly describe the comparison treatments from the original clinical trial of CBT (Brent et al., 1997). Many of our later findings on predictors and moderators of outcomes and mechanisms of treatment action rely on an understanding of these comparison groups.

Given the importance of family stress in the development of youth depression, a family therapy treatment was included in the original clinical trial (Brent et al., 1997) as a theoretically interesting comparison condition. The family-based intervention, SBFT, was a combination of two treatments that have been used effectively with dysfunctional families of adolescents. The first phase of SBFT used the methods of functional family therapy. The therapist attempted to clarify the concerns that brought the family to treatment and to redefine the adolescent patient's problem as a problem both for and of the entire family system. In this process, the therapist worked to engage the entire family in solving this problem. Dysfunctional patterns of interaction and inappropriate alliances were identified, and the relationships between these family problems and the patient's symptoms were elucidated. Following this problem definition stage, the second phase of SBFT was more behavioral in focus. Family members were encouraged to try out new patterns of interaction and were given positive practice assignments both within session and for homework. Family members also were coached to improve their communication skills more generally in order to better solve family problems in the future.

In addition, nondirective therapy was included in the clinical trial to control for nonspecific aspects of the therapeutic experience, such as therapist time and attention, the provision of a warm and trusting relationship, and the passage of time. These elements of treatment are common to all forms of therapy, and although they may be necessary for treatment success, they may not be sufficient. In NST, youth were encouraged to explore and express their feelings. Therapists adopted a warm, nonjudgmental, and nondirective stance, offering general support, reflection and clarifications, and messages of hope. Therapists did not provide specific instructions for changing life circumstances or feelings and did not interpret teens' statements or encourage them to adopt a different perspective when evaluating their lives.

Treatment Manuals and Therapist Training

Historically, the Pittsburgh model of CBT has followed a principle-based treatment manual that does not mandate specific didactic exercises or strict order of presentation of skills. The treatment manual stresses developing a cognitive case conceptualization and, as described previously, focuses primarily on cognitive restructuring, with problem-solving/mood regulation and behavioral activation skills applied as adjuncts (see Figure 9.2). Copies of the Pittsburgh CBT manual and manuals for the clinical trial comparison conditions are available from the authors.[1]

In the original clinical trial, all therapists were master's-level clinicians, with a median of 10 years of professional experience treating distressed adolescents. Before participating in the trial, each therapist received six months of intensive treatment-specific training. To be certified for participation, therapists were required to treat two cases with the appropriate treatment manual to criterion. During the clinical trial, therapists were provided with ongoing supervision, and therapy tapes were rated for adherence. As a check on treatment integrity, a random 25% of session tapes were rated by external consultants; analyses of these ratings indicated that the three types of treatment were readily discernible from each other and that sessions within each modality were of acceptable quality or better (over 90% of sessions rated, across all cells).

EVIDENCE ON THE EFFECTS OF TREATMENT

Design of the Original Clinical Trial

Much the of evidence on the effects of the CBT program is drawn from original or follow-up data collection from the Brent et al. (1997) clinical trial. In this study, adolescents largely (two-thirds) were recruited from clinical referral sources, such as inpatient and outpatient units at the academic medical center or referrals from private practitioners. A smaller number (one-third) were recruited directly by self-referral from advertisement. Youth were screened for presence of a Diagnostic and Statistical Manual of Mental Disorders (third edition, revised; American Psychiatric Association, 1987) diagnosis of major depressive disorder (MDD) and high self-report of symptoms (Beck Depression Inventory [BDI]; Beck, Steer, & Garbin, 1988). The sample was predominantly white (85%) and female (75%) and had moderate rates of comorbid anxiety disorder (32%) and dysthymia (22%). A total of 107 youth met entry criteria and were randomly assigned to CBT, SBFT, or NST. As described previously, youth were seen for 12–16 sessions of active treatment and were eligible for up to four follow-up booster appointments. Assessments were conducted at intake, the sixth treatment session, treatment termination, every 3 months in the first year following termination, and 2 years after termination.

Status of the Evidence

Overall Efficacy of CBT

In the original trial, significantly more of the depressed teens receiving CBT (83%) no longer met diagnostic criteria for MDD compared with youth who received NST (58%). Full clinical remission[2] of depression symptoms also was more common in the CBT cell (60%) than in either NST (39%) or SBFT (38%). Additionally, CBT youth experienced improvement in their BDI scores more quickly than those in SBFT, and they improved on interviewer-rated depression symptoms more quickly than youth in SBFT or in NST. Treatments did not differ in their effects on functioning or suicidality, although serious suicidality moderated depression treatment efficacy (discussed further later).

Despite the results favoring CBT at post-treatment, there were no differences in depression between treatment groups at the 2-year follow-up (Birmaher et al., 2000). In terms of current MDD, descriptive data did favor CBT (6%) over SBFT (23%) and NST (26%), although these rates were not significantly different.

Treatment Expectancy and Credibility

In this first trial, parents and youth viewed all three treatments as equally logical and likely to produce positive improvement at intake. Over the course of treatment, parents' positive views of CBT were maintained, whereas their views of the logical basis for and likely outcome of SBFT and NST deteriorated and they became less likely to say they would recommend these treatments to a friend.

Predictors of Treatment Effects and Moderators

Across all of the treatments tested in the original trial, poorer response was predicted by greater cognitive distortion, higher levels of hopelessness, more severe depression at intake, older youth age, and referral from clinical sources rather than newspaper advertisement. For the sample as a whole, intake depression severity predicted failure to recover from depression, a chronic course, and recurrences over the follow-up period (Birmaher et al., 2000). Parent–child conflict, both at intake and over follow-up, similarly predicted lack of recovery, chronicity, and recurrence. Across cells, youth with double depression (comorbid depression and dysthymia) were more likely to withdraw from the study as a result of failure to respond to treatment.

In terms of treatment moderators, CBT appeared to be the best treatment for youth with serious suicidality (attempt or ideation with a plan; Barbe, Bridge, Birmaher, Kolko, & Brent, 2004b). CBT for depression was equally efficacious in those with current or lifetime suicidality as in those without such a history. In contrast, NST did particularly poorly in treating depression among those with current or lifetime suicidality compared with those with no such history (response rate of 26% vs. 64%). This finding was mediated by the differential impact of CBT versus NST on decreasing feelings of hopelessness. In addition, CBT was particularly more efficacious than the other interventions when youth met criteria for a comorbid anxiety disorder (Brent et al., 1998). In contrast, maternal depressive symptoms and history of sexual abuse also moderated treatment efficacy insofar as the presence of these predictors erased the generally superior effect of CBT to comparison conditions (Brent et al., 1998; Barbe, Bridge, Birmaher, Kolko, & Brent, 2004a).

Predictors of Additional Service Use

More than half of the clinical trial participants sought additional services over the 2-year follow-up (Brent, Kolko, Birmaher, Baugher, & Bridge, 1999). Although CBT was the most efficacious intervention in the short term, youth who received CBT were no less likely to seek additional services than those in the comparison treatment conditions. Treatment was most often sought for additional difficulties with depression (62%), but therapy was also obtained for general family problems (33%) and for youth acting-out behavior problems (31%). Given these target complaints, it is not surprising that intake depression severity, comorbid disruptive behavior problems, and family difficulties predicted additional service use across treatment cells.

Mechanisms of Action

Our research group also has conducted investigations to unpack the mechanisms of action in CBT. In the first, Kolko and colleagues investigated the mediating role of cognitive and family process variables in producing the original clinical trial outcomes (Kolko, Brent, Baugher, Bridge, & Birmaher, 2000). As hypothesized, CBT did produce significant, specific changes on a measure of cognitive distortions compared with SBFT and NST. However, CBT was not superior to the comparison treatments in changing feelings of hopelessness.[3] In addition, contrary to hypotheses, CBT was as effective as SBFT in changing general family functioning and was more effective than SBFT in improving marital satisfaction and parents' feelings of behavioral control. Thus, although CBT affected one theoretically specific mechanism of cognitive change, it also produced nonspecific changes in mediators belonging to another theoretical model of intervention (SBFT). Furthermore, these specific changes in cognitive distortions did not statistically mediate the effects of CBT on self-rated depression symptoms.[4]

Additional studies have examined the shape of change in depression symptoms over the course of treatment for clues to mechanisms of therapeutic action. In one investigation, youths were identified who showed a rapid response to treatment, namely an improvement of 50% or more in BDI scores between pretreatment and the second session of therapy (Renaud, Brent, Baugher, Birmaher, Kolko, & Bridge, 1998). These rapid responders had received very little active intervention by the second session of treatment, and the three treatment groups—CBT, SBFT, and NST—did not differ in the number of rapid responders (31% of the sample overall). The timing of this improvement suggests that rapid response to treatment was likely due nonspecific intervention factors, such as therapist warmth. Relevant to our discussion of CBT mechanism, the relationship among nonspecific, rapid response, and treatment outcome varied by intervention. Pairwise comparisons revealed that youth in NST were much less likely to achieve clinical remission of depression if they failed to experience a rapid response to intervention by the second treatment session. This was true for NST youth at posttreatment (21% vs. 100%) and follow-up assessment (55% vs. 88%). Although these data did not shed immediate light on the mechanism of action in CBT, they did imply that our placebo-control intervention, NST, mostly likely operated through nonspecific mechanisms of action, such as remoralization. The data also suggested that the overall effects CBT and SBFT were not solely dependent on a placebo response to treatment

Extension of the Model to Treatment-Resistant Depression

Adolescents with dysthymia comorbid with major depression were significantly more likely to drop out of the Brent et al. (1997) clinical trial, and global severity of depression at intake predicted poor course over the 2-year follow-up period. Data with adult samples support the value of combination treatments—CBT plus antidepressant medication (e.g., selective serotonin reuptake inhibitors [SSRIs])—for chronically and severely depressed individuals (Keller et al., 2000). To address this need, the Pittsburgh group's next major clinical trial of individual CBT tested the efficacy of combination CBT + SSRI treatment for adolescents who had failed a previous community trial of antidepressant medication (Brent et al., 2008).

Manual Modifications

For the Treatment of Resistant Depression in Adolescents (TORDIA) study, the original CBT trial protocol was modified in a number of respects. It seemed likely that a sample of treatment-resistant youth would (1) present with severe and clinically complicated depression, (2) meet criteria for a number of comorbid diagnoses, and (3) have significant mood lability and high levels of suicidality. Accordingly, crisis intervention modules were built into the revised CBT treatment, and greater emphasis was placed on teaching problem-solving and affect regulation skills. The structure of the original treatment manual also was substantially deconstructed. All of the manual components were repackaged as modules rather than as sessions, and therapists thus were given flexibility to spend multiple sessions on critical skills and customize treatment for youths' personalities and life circumstances. Families also were afforded a greater role in treatment than in the original CBT clinical trial, in which family therapy elements were excluded in order to enhance the internal validity of the experimental comparison to SBFT. Given the central role of parent–child conflict in referral, recovery, and treatment of adolescent depression, a CBT approach to family problem solving was included as an explicit part of the revised TORDIA treatment package. The final acute treatment package was designed to be 12 sessions, with three to six sessions involving family contact.

Treatment-Resistant Sample

A total of 334 adolescents with diagnoses of MDD and a previous failed trial of an SSRI were enrolled and randomized to one of four conditions: (1) switch to a second, different SSRI (paroxetine, citalopram, or fluoxetine); (2) switch to a different SSRI plus CBT; (3) switch to venlafaxine; or (4) switch to venlafaxine plus CBT. Participants were recruited for six academic or nonprofit community medical centers; the majority (80%) were referred to the trial from clinical sources rather than self-referred from paid advertisements. Adolescent were generally female (70%) and white (82%) and came from middle-income families. On average, youths had been depressed for almost 2 years before study entry, with 17 weeks of previous SSRI treatment and eight sessions of prior psychotherapy. A high proportion reported clinically significant suicidality (56%), and most (52%) met criteria for at least one comorbid, nonmood disorder. In general, the sample was among the most ill reported in the adolescent depression treatment literature.

Effects of Adjunctive CBT

Overall, results supported the value of the combination of CBT and medication switch. After 12 weeks of care, 55% of youths who received CBT and a new antidepressant showed a substantial clinical response compared with only 41% who responded to medication switch alone; there were no significant differences in response between classes of medication. There were significant effects for time on self-reported depression symptoms, clinician-rated symptoms, suicidality, and functioning. However, there were no significant differential effects of treatment on these outcomes. Notably, sites did differ in the effectiveness of CBT but not in the effectiveness of medication (Spirito et al., 2009). Site effects appeared to be largely driven by differences in sample characteristics at baseline between sites, and the main effect of adjunctive CBT on treatment response was maintained across a variety of sensitivity analyses. The two most robust moderators of CBT response were history of abuse and number of comorbid disorders. Youth *without* a history of abuse showed a better response to combined treatment than to medication alone, whereas the reverse was true for those with a history of abuse (Asarnow et al., 2009). Combination treatment showed the most marked superiority over medication monotherapy as a function of the number of comorbid diagnoses.

Evidence Regarding Implementation in Practice

Results of the Brent et al. (1997) and TORDIA trials suggest that CBT may have the promise of effectiveness in treating clinically complicated youths in real-world outpatient service. To measure the effectiveness of CBT more directly, we assessed the outcomes of adolescents treated in a depression specialty clinic. The Services for Teens at Risk (STAR) Center is an outpatient clinic run by our research group that serves depressed and suicidal adolescents and their families. The STAR Center is housed in the general child outpatient service at Western Psychiatric Institute and Clinic and draws youth from that service as well as youth referred after inpatient care for a suicide attempt. Teens seen at the STAR Center receive combination CBT and medication management, as in TORDIA, although the CBT treatment manual used in STAR is very close in form to the original clinical trial manual. Historically, STAR services have been free to families, as in most clinical trials, but STAR therapy is open ended and the content of therapy sessions is unmonitored. Youth seen at the STAR Center meet criteria for significant mood disorder; however, they also often meet criteria for comorbid diagnoses such as substance abuse. The STAR Center thus shares many features with CBT clinical trials but has a patient base and setting similar to outpatient clinical practice.

Given this blend of research and practice characteristics, we viewed the STAR Center as a natural laboratory in which to begin assessing the effectiveness of CBT under clinically representative conditions. To accomplish this task, we reviewed the medical records of youth treated in the STAR Center between 1995 and 2002 (before recruitment efforts for the TORDIA trial in this setting). In this time span, 80 youths who met criteria for MDD and self-reported significant depression symptoms (BDI score > 12) received a course of individual CBT in STAR. Youths were predominantly white (85%) and female (77%). These teens evidenced a broader range of comorbid diagnoses than youth in the Brent et al. (1997) randomized controlled trial, and 20% of the STAR sample would have been excluded from the clinical trial on the basis of comorbid diagnoses (e.g., substance abuse). In terms of treatment, the content of the CBT intervention in the clinical trial and in STAR was very similar, but the number of sessions in STAR was much more variable, and 75% of STAR youths received concurrent medication treatment. (Note, however, that receipt of medication within the STAR sample did not predict treatment outcome.)

As part of their routine clinical care, youths in STAR completed the BDI each session, and we were able to examine BDI symptom trajectories as an index of treatment effectiveness. Preliminary results indicate that CBT in the STAR Center produced significant improvement in depression symptoms approximately 6 months after intake (i.e., BDI trajectory falling within the normal range; Weersing et al., 2006). This time to recovery is almost twice as long as in the original CBT clinical trial (Brent et al., 1997); however, results of STAR CBT may compare quite favorably to outcomes achieved by eclectic community therapy. In a sample of 67 depressed youths treated in community mental health centers, a similar level of symptom reduction did not occur until 12 months after intake (Weersing & Weisz, 2002). For comparison purposes, BDI trajectories of youths in the STAR Center are plotted alongside data from the original CBT clinical trial as well as from the sample of clinically complicated youths treated with CBT in TORDIA (see Figure 9.2).

Directions for Research

Although our preliminary data from STAR suggest that CBT for depressed adolescents may prove to be effective, there also are reasons to suspect that effects for CBT may be reduced in the context of clinical practice. In addition to differences in youth characteristics, the staff, supervision, and training intensity of community practice are likely quite different from clinical trials and even from the STAR Center. To be feasible for use in general clinical practice, we suspect that CBT protocols may need to be shorter, simpler, and more focused than current clinical trial protocols.

It would be quite helpful to have data on the mechanisms of action of CBT to guide these modifications. Our own efforts to identify core processes of change in youths and core elements of CBT treatment have provided promising leads but no clear answers. CBT appears to impact a wide range of possible change mechanisms but does not seem to function solely as a nonspecific intervention. However, we have not yet been able to identify which CBT techniques (see Figure 9.1) are the most essential for producing outcome and should be the focus of efficient treatment manuals and community training efforts.

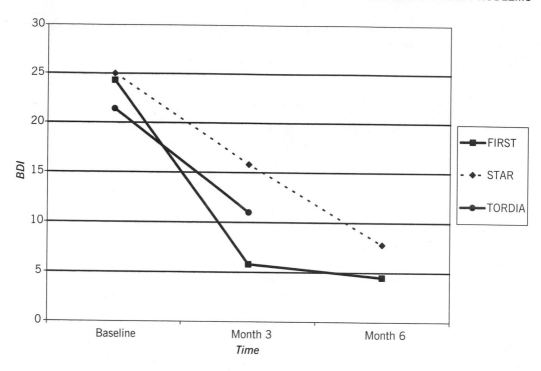

FIGURE 9.2. Trajectories of change on the Beck Depression Inventory (BDI) in the original Pittsburgh cognitive-behavioral therapy (CBT) clinical trial (FIRST; Brent et al., 1997), CBT delivered in a tertiary care clinic (STAR; Weersing et al., 2006), and the CBT intervention adapted for use with treatment-resistant cases (TORDIA; Brent et al., 2008).

Of course, any feasibility modifications to CBT will need to be balanced against possible decrements in efficacy associated with making treatments simpler and shorter. Even in current full-length programs, a substantial portion of adolescents treated with CBT remain symptomatic at acute posttreatment (40%), and the superior effects of CBT relative to alternate interventions appear to dissipate over long-term follow-up. In addition, although CBT has produced substantial changes in depression in the Pittsburgh studies, CBT was no more efficacious than alternate treatments in improving teens' functioning or suicidality in either our original clinical trial or the TORDIA investigation.

Broadly, findings such as these highlight the need for additional research on efficient CBT treatment programs for dissemination into practice; the efficacy of longer term, continuing-care treatment models for treatment-refractory youths; and clinical decision-making tools to prospectively guide youths to the best combination of interventions (e.g., CBT + SSRI) to optimize their long-term recovery from depression.

CONCLUSIONS

In sum, individual CBT appears to be an efficacious short-term intervention for the treatment of depression in adolescents. In the original Brent et al. (1997) clinical trial,

60% of teens treated with CBT experienced clinical remission of depression by posttreatment, a significantly higher percentage than in SBFT (38%) or NST (39%). Outcomes on dimensional measures of depression symptoms, both youth report and interviewer rated, also supported the superiority of CBT. In addition, youth treated with CBT experienced relief from depression more quickly than those in either of the comparison treatments.

The TORDIA investigation reinforces this encouraging view of individual CBT for depressed teens. Adolescents in TORDIA had been depressed for an average of 2 years, experienced significant suicidality and comorbidity, and had previously failed a first-line intervention for depression (i.e., an SSRI). In this sample of seriously depressed youths, a combination of CBT and medication led to substantial clinical improvement for more than half of participants.

There also is evidence that CBT may work well outside of clinical trial contexts under the conditions of real-world clinical care. Data for this conclusion come from two sources. In the original 1997 clinical trial, CBT was more robust to adverse treatment indicators, such as hopelessness, suicidality, and comorbid anxiety, than either SBFT or NST (Brent et al., 1998; Barbe et al., 2004b), and in the TORDIA trial, the value of adding CBT to medication switch was more clear as the number of comorbid diagnoses increased (Asarnow et al., 2009). Additional support for the effectiveness of CBT in practice comes from our investigation of CBT in the STAR Center. In the STAR Center, depressed teens provided with CBT experienced substantial improvement in their depression symptoms in approximately 6 months, twice as long as in the original clinical trial sample but twice as quickly as youth treated with traditional psychotherapy in community clinics (Weersing et al., 2006).

ACKNOWLEDGMENTS

Preparation of this chapter was facilitated by support from the William T. Grant Foundation to V. Robin Weersing. Data collection for this program of work was supported the National Institute of Mental Health (Grant Nos. MH46500, MH18269, MH61835).

NOTES

1. Manuals for the three treatments are available from David A. Brent at Western Psychiatric Institute and Clinic, University of Pittsburgh Medical School, 3811 O'Hara Street, Pittsburgh, Pennsylvania 15213.
2. Remission was defined as the absence of diagnosable MDD and at least three consecutive BDI scores of less than 9. See Birmaher et al. (2000) for a discussion of issues surrounding the definition of remission, recovery, and recurrence of depression.
3. These results held for the sample, and all treatment cells, as a whole. Among youth for whom there were suicidality data, CBT did produce better effects on hopelessness than NST, and these changes in hopelessness mediated the superior efficacy of CBT in treating seriously suicidal youth (Barbe et al., 2004b).
4. This may be due, in part, to missing data. Some youths were missing data on cognitive distortions, and these participants could not be included in the mediational analyses. When these youths were excluded, the previously significant effect of CBT on BDI scores, reported for the sample as a whole, lapsed into marginal significance (see Kolko et al, 2000, for details). Because there was no effect of treatment on outcome (BDI scores), the attempt to search for mediated effects was cut short.

REFERENCES

American Psychiatric Association. (1987). *Diagnostic and statistical manual of mental disorders* (3rd ed., rev.). Washington, DC: Author.

Asarnow, J. R., Emslie, G. J., Clarke, G., Wagner, K. D., Spirito, A., Vitiello, B., et al. (2009). Treatment of SSRI-Resistant Depression in Adolescents (TORDIA): Predictors and moderators of treatment response. *Journal of the American Academy of Child and Adolescent Psychiatry, 48,* 330–339.

Barbe, R. P., Bridge, J. A., Birmaher, B., Kolko, D. J., & Brent, D. A. (2004a). Lifetime history of sexual abuse, clinical presentation, and outcome in a clinical trial for adolescent depression. *Journal of Clinical Psychiatry, 65,* 77–83.

Barbe, R. P., Bridge, J., Birmaher, B., Kolko, D., & Brent, D. A. (2004b). Suicidality and its relationship to treatment outcome in depressed adolescents. *Suicide and Life-Threatening Behavior, 34,* 44–55.

Beck, A. T., Rush, A. J., Shaw, B. F., & Emery, G. (1979). *Cognitive therapy of depression.* New York: Guilford Press.

Beck, A. T., Steer, R. A., & Garbin, M. G. (1988). Psychometric properties of the Beck Depression Inventory: Twenty-five years of evaluation. *Clinical Psychology Review, 8,* 77–100.

Birmaher, B., Brent, D. A., Kolko, D., Baugher, M., Bridge, J., Iyengar, S., et al. (2000). Clinical outcome after short-term psychotherapy for adolescents with major depressive disorder. *Archives of General Psychiatry, 57,* 29–36.

Brent, D., Emslie, G., Clarke, G., Wagner, K. D., Asarnow, J. A., Keller, M., et al. (2008). Switching to another SSRI or to venlafaxine with or without cognitive behavioral therapy for adolescents with SSRI-resistant depression: The TORDIA randomized controlled trial. *Journal of the American Medical Association, 299,* 901–913.

Brent, D. A., Holder, D., Kolko, D., Birmaher, B., Baugher, M., Roth, C., et al. (1997). A clinical psychotherapy trial for adolescent depression comparing cognitive, family, and supportive treatments. *Archives of General Psychiatry, 54,* 877–885.

Brent, D. A., Kolko, D., Birmaher, B., Baugher, M., & Bridge, J. (1999). A clinical trial for adolescent depression: Predictors of additional treatment in the acute and follow-up phase of the trial. *Journal of the American Academy of Child and Adolescent Psychiatry, 38,* 263–271.

Brent, D. A., Kolko, D., Birmaher, B., Baugher, M., Bridge, J., Roth, C., et al. (1998). Predictors of treatment efficacy in a clinical trial of three psychosocial treatments for adolescent depression. *Journal of the American Academy of Child and Adolescent Psychiatry, 37,* 906–914.

Brent, D. A., Perper, J. A., Moritz, G., Allman, C., Roth, C., Schweers, J., et al. (1993). Psychiatric risk factors of adolescent suicide: A case control study. *Journal of the American Academy of Child and Adolescent Psychiatry, 32,* 521–529.

Gladstone, T. R. G., & Kaslow, N. J. (1995). Depression and attributions in children and adolescents: A meta-analytic review. *Journal of Abnormal Child Psychology, 23,* 597–606.

Keller, M. B., McCullough, J. P., Klein, D. N., Arnow, B., Dunner, D. L., Gelenberg, A. J., et al. (2000). A comparison of nefazodone, the cognitive behavioral-analysis system of psychotherapy, and their combination for the treatment of chronic depression. *New England Journal of Medicine, 342,* 1462–1470.

Kolko, D., Brent, D., Baugher, M., Bridge, J., & Birmaher, B. (2000). Cognitive and family therapies for adolescent depression: Treatment specificity, mediation and moderation. *Journal of Consulting and Clinical Psychology, 68,* 603–614.

Lewinsohn, P. M., Allen, N. B., Seeley, J. R., & Gotlib, I. H. (1999). First onset versus recurrence of depression: Differential processes of psychosocial risk. *Journal of Abnormal Psychology, 108,* 483–489.

Lewinsohn, P. M., Roberts, R. E., Seeley, J. R., Rohde, P., Gotlib, I. H., & Hops, H. (1994). Adolescent psychopathology: II. Psychosocial risk factors for depression. *Journal of Abnormal Psychology, 103,* 302–315.

Renaud, J., Brent, D. A., Baugher, M., Birmaher, B., Kolko, D. J., & Bridge, J. (1998). Rapid response to psychosocial treatment for adolescent depression: A two-year follow-up. *Journal of the Ameri can Academy of Child and Adolescent Psychiatry, 37,* 1184–1190.

Rohde, P., Lewinsohn, P. M., & Seeley, J. R. (1994). Are adolescents changed by an episode of major depression? *Journal of the American Academy of Child and Adolescent Psychiatry, 33,* 1289–1298.

Spirito, A., Brent, D., Emslie, G., Clarke, G., Wagner, K., Asarnow, J., et al.. (2009). Site differences and their possible sources in the outcomes of a multi-site clinical trial: The Treatment of SSRI-Resistant Depression in Adolescents (TORDIA) Study. *Journal of Consulting and Clinical Psychology, 77,* 439–450.

Weersing, V. R., Iyengar, S., Kolko, D. J., Birmaher, B., & Brent, D. A. (2006). Effectiveness of cognitive behavioral therapy for adolescent depression: A benchmarking investigation. *Behavior Therapy, 37,* 36–48.

Weersing, V. R., & Weisz, J. R. (2002). Community clinic treatment of depressed youth: Benchmarking usual care against CBT clinical trials. *Journal of Consulting and Clinical Psychology, 70,* 299–310.

10

Treating Adolescent Depression Using Interpersonal Psychotherapy

COLLEEN M. JACOBSON and LAURA MUFSON

OVERVIEW OF THE CLINICAL PROBLEM

Adolescent depression is a prevalent and serious disorder that carries with it substantial impairment across several domains of functioning, including academic, social, and physical aspects of one's life. As described in the *Diagnostic and Statistical Manual of Mental Disorders* (fourth edition [DSM-IV]; American Psychiatric Association, 2000), adolescent depression is characterized by depressed or irritable mood, loss of interest in school and recreational activities, feelings of boredom, sleep and appetite changes, low self-esteem, hopelessness, and, in some cases, thoughts of suicide or engagement in self-injurious behaviors. In contrast to adult depression, adolescent depression is often marked by mood swings, with periods of relative euthymia interspersed with periods of dysphoric mood, in the form of depression or irritability. Perhaps because of hormonal changes that occur with puberty, the rate of depression rises with the onset of adolescence, especially for girls (Costello, Pine, Hammen, March, & Plotsky, 2002). Adolescent depression can interrupt developmental process and lead to social dysfunction.

There is no single cause of depression; it likely results from the combination of biological vulnerability and environmental stressors (which may take many forms and vary from individual to individual). Thus, although not the sole cause of depression, interpersonal conflict is more common among depressed adolescents than their nondepressed peers (e.g., Sheeber, Davis, Leve, Hops, & Tildesley, 2007) and may both precipitate and be a consequence of depression (Allen et al., 2006; Rudolph et al., 2000) in teens. For example, dysfunctional interaction patterns with parents and peers were linked to higher levels of depression 1 year later among a group of adolescents (Allen et al., 2006). Further, some evidence suggests that interpersonal stressors are more strongly linked to depression than noninterpersonal stressors (Rudolph et al., 2000), suggesting that interpersonal relationship issues are an important target for treatment. Problematic relationships with both parents and peers are related to depression in youths. For example, research indicates that conflictual and unsupportive relationships with parents are associated with depressive disorders (Sheeber et al., 2007). In addition, problematic relationships with peers, including peer victimization and lack of connectedness, are associated with elevated depressive symptoms (Brunstein-Klomek, Marrocco, Kleinman, Schonfeld, & Gould, 2007). Thus, although the cause of depression is multifaceted, it is clear that interpersonal conflict plays a significant role in adolescent depression and, therefore, intervention at the interpersonal level is likely to be beneficial.

CONCEPTUAL MODEL

Interpersonal psychotherapy for depressed adolescents (IPT-A; Mufson, Dorta, Moreau, & Weissman, 2004) was adapted from the original treatment, interpersonal psychotherapy (IPT; Klerman, Weissman, Rounsaville, & Chevron, 1984; Weissman, Markowitz, & Klerman, 2007), which was designed for nonpsychotic depressed adults. The model of depression underlying IPT and IPT-A has its roots in the interpersonal theory of depression purported by Sullivan (1953) and by Bowlby's (1978) attachment theory. Sullivan believed that mental health is dependent on experiencing positive interpersonal relationships, and that a lack of positive relationships may have a negative impact on mental well-being. Bowlby contended that humans have an innate drive to form interpersonal bonds, and interruptions or problems within those bonds give rise to emotional distress, including depression. Adolescence is a time during which interpersonal bonds are typically changing as teens desire increased autonomy from parents and become more connected to peers. Teens and parents need to learn to negotiate the pull between increasing independence and maintaining intimacy with one another. Problems within those transitions can lead to conflict, isolation, and eventually depression. IPT-A has been adapted from the adult model to address more specifically the interpersonal issues unique to adolescence, including negotiating peer relationships and peer pressure, the development of initial romantic relationships, and parental separation and divorce.

The theoretical basis of IPT and IPT-A is that clinical depression takes place within an interpersonal context. Specifically, the onset, course, and successful treatment of depression are influenced by the adolescent's interpersonal relationships with significant others. Therefore, intervening within one's interpersonal relationships during a depressive episode can change the course and outcome for that person. Depression is conceptualized as having three components: symptom formation, social functioning, and personality. IPT-A is a brief treatment that focuses predominantly on the present. The therapist intervenes with only the first two components: symptom formation and social functioning. Within IPT-A, depression is conceptualized as a disorder that is caused by a combination of biological predisposition and interpersonal experience. Although acknowledging the important role that biological factors may play, the assumption of IPT-A is that improvement in mood can be achieved with intervention at the interpersonal level. Specifically, IPT-A aims to decrease depressive symptoms and improve interpersonal relationships through psychoeducation and interpersonal skills building and to create a supportive therapeutic relationship that encourages the understanding and expression of affect.

Concurrent treatment with medication may be recommended when there is a lack of improvement after the initial phase or when adolescents appear unable to make use of the therapy given the severity of symptoms. For example, antidepressant medication may be necessary if adolescents' symptoms are not improving during the course of IPT-A. In addition, adolescents with severe neurovegetative symptoms (such as lethargy and anhedonia) may warrant medication to increase their energy and motivation to engage in, and thus learn from, psychotherapy. To date, there are no clinical trials testing the efficacy of the combined use of medication and IPT-A.

The interpersonal content in IPT-A is quite circumscribed, focusing on the problematic relationship that seems most closely related to the depressive symptoms. A primary interpersonal problem area is identified for which the interpersonal skills are tailored, with the intention that those skills will generalize to adolescents' other relationships. For some adolescents, a secondary area may be identified and their therapist facilitates the generalization of interpersonal skills practiced in regard to the primary area to the secondary problem area. There are four problem areas: interpersonal role dispute, role transition, interpersonal deficits, and grief (discussed in more detail later). In general, IPT-A is a time-limited outpatient treatment that is practical and didactic in nature and aims to highlight the interpersonal context of depression.

CHARACTERISTICS OF THE TREATMENT PROGRAM

Indications for IPT-A

IPT-A was initially developed as an individual outpatient treatment for clinical depression, with limited inclusion of parents, for adolescents ages 12–18 years. It is typically delivered over the course of 12 weeks, with a total of 12–15 sessions, depending on whether additional parent sessions are included (Mufson, Weissman, Moreau, & Garfinkel, 1999). IPT-A was adapted to be delivered in school-based health clinics with 12 sessions delivered over 12–16 weeks: the first eight sessions delivered weekly and the remaining four scheduled flexibly over the final 8 weeks. This enables the clinician to shift to a continuation model if the adolescent is doing well or to adapt to the school calendar. As in the adult model, when possible, monthly maintenance sessions are recommended to prevent relapse and recurrence, but formal study of the maintenance sessions with adolescents is needed.

Recently, IPT-A has been adapted for use with groups of depressed adolescents (Mufson, Gallagher, Dorta, & Young, 2004) and as a group-based prevention strategy for adolescents at risk for depression as a result of subsyndromal symptoms (Young, Mufson, & Davies, 2006). The current chapter focuses on the original IPT-A protocol for individual treatment of depressed teens. Although IPT-A was developed for adolescents with depression, it is commonly used with adolescents with comorbidities including anxiety disorders, attention-deficit disorder, and oppositional defiant disorder. IPT-A is not indicated for adolescents who are actively suicidal, are psychotic, have bipolar disorder, are mentally retarded, or are actively abusing substances.

Content of Treatment: General Overview

The three primary components of IPT-A are similar to the primary components of the adult IPT model: education, affect identification, and interpersonal skills building. At the start of treatment and throughout, psychoeducation plays an important role. First, a thorough diagnostic assessment of depression is conducted, and psychoeducation about the disorder of clinical depression, the limited sick role, and their role in treatment is delivered to the child and parent. Throughout the course of treatment, adolescents' symptoms of depression are reviewed so that they have a clear understanding of their progress/improvement.

Affect identification is an extremely important part of IPT-A because many depressed adolescents have difficulty understanding and expressing their feelings. Depressed adolescents typically engage in one of two extreme forms of affect expression, both of which can be problematic: the tendency to keep feelings (especially negative) to oneself and the tendency to express feelings in an impulsive or negative manner, which can exacerbate the problem. For some adolescents, affect identification may be simple, but linking affect to an event may be more difficult. Others may be able to identify problematic relationships but do not see the connection to their emotions. IPT-A therapists assist the adolescents with labeling their emotions; facilitate adolescents' expression of emotions, with themselves and with significant others; and assist adolescents in monitoring their emotions and linking their feelings to problematic relationships. Successful treatment will allow the adolescents to have an improved understanding of the subtleties of different emotions, the types of interpersonal situations that may lead to positive and negative feelings, and how best to communicate their feelings with others.

Directly linked to affect identification is interpersonal skills building. Skills building takes place directly through the adolescent–therapist relationship as therapists model appropriate interpersonal skills and give feedback to the adolescents regarding their style of communication. In addition, specific didactic and experiential techniques are used throughout the course of treatment and are indicated for use with the majority of depressed adolescents regardless of the specific problem area. These techniques include communication analysis, decision analysis, perspective taking, interpersonal problem solving, and role-playing. Finally, more general strategies of IPT-A include involvement of parents as needed, telephone contact between sessions to maintain therapeutic work, and consultation with the school as needed.

The structure of the IPT-A protocol includes three phases: initial (weeks 1–4), middle (weeks 5–9), and termination (weeks 10–12). The initial and termination phases of IPT-A are similar across adolescents; however, the middle phase is tailored to the specific problem area being addressed. The specific steps taken in the initial and termination phases are followed in sequence, whereas the specific techniques implemented in the middle phase are used when indicated based upon the case. In this way, the IPT-A manual is fairly flexible because it is guideline based.

Initial Phase

The initial phase (weeks 1–4) includes seven components: (1) identify and diagnose symptoms, (2) provide psychoeducation about depression, (3) assign the limited sick role, (4) complete the interpersonal inventory, (5) identify the problem area, (6) explain the theory and goals of IPT-A, and (7) set the treatment contract. To confirm a diagnosis of depression—the first step of the IPT-A protocol—it is helpful to use a formal rating scale, such as the Children's Depression Rating Scale-Revised, as a guide. A thorough review of depressive symptoms should be completed in the first session, and a review of the previously endorsed symptoms, in addition to suicidal ideation and behavior, should be completed in each subsequent session. In session 2 and thereafter, the symptom review includes a mood rating (i.e., adolescents rate their mood over the past week on a scale of 1 (*the best ever felt*) to 10 (*the worst ever felt*). The teens are then asked to identify a time during the past week when they felt particularly bad and particularly good and to rate both of those instances on a 1–10 scale. Therapists then assist teens in recalling the specific events that coincided with the moments of feeling good and bad. Improving insight into the link between events and emotions is a first step at overcoming depression.

Psychoeducation about depression in adolescents—step 2 of the initial phase—may include information about rates of depression, common symptoms and co-occurring impairments, impact on functioning, and effective treatment strategies. Then the limited sick role should be explained and assigned (step 3). The limited sick role is adapted from the notion of the sick role in the adult IPT protocol. Therapists explain that depression is similar to an illness such as pneumonia, that it affects the way people function in their daily activities and that, when recovering, patients will gradually start their activities and build back up to their baseline level of performance. Therefore, when depressed, people should not be expected to complete their responsibilities as well as they did before. However, adolescents are encouraged to continue to engage in all activities to the best of their ability because withdrawal from normal activities can worsen depression or hamper recovery. During the explanation of the limited sick role therapists encourage the parents to be less critical and blaming of their adolescents' academic performance and completion of activities while depressed and to recognize that there will be improvements as the depression remits.

The next step in the initial phase is to complete the interpersonal inventory over two to three sessions so that the appropriate problem area can be identified. Therapists ask adolescents to identify the most important people in their life, especially those who they feel most influence their mood. This is done with the aid of the "closeness circle," a visual diagram of four circles within one another (see Figure 10.1). The adolescents identify themselves as the center circle and place people within the different rings depending on how close they view them. Feelings of closeness are not necessarily always positive; a relationship can be seen as very important to teens but currently as problematic because of conflict. Therapists then proceed to ask the adolescents to discuss the four to five people who seem most related to the current depression with the goal of understanding the following components of each relationship: nature of interactions, expectations, positive and negative aspects, desired changes in the relationship, and the depression's impact on the relationship. It is important to ask questions about feelings, events, and facts linked to each relationship. Successful completion of the interpersonal inventory should leave therapists and adolescents with an understanding of which relationship is most closely linked to the adolescents' depressive symptoms. With the information collected from the interpersonal inventory, one of the four target problem areas (grief, role transition, role dispute, interpersonal deficits) is identified as an appropriate focus of treatment.

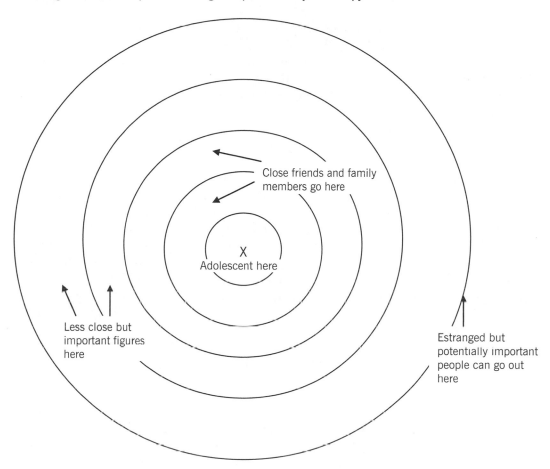

FIGURE 10.1. Closeness circle.

1. *Grief.* The problem area of grief is the focus when teens have experienced the death of a loved one and when that loss is associated with the onset or persistence of depressive symptoms. It is possible that the depression may not have immediately followed the death, so it is important to query about any significant losses when completing the closeness circle.

2. *Role transition.* This is a commonly identified problem area among teens because growing from childhood to adolescence is a challenge in itself. This problem area is applied when the adolescents experience difficulties linked to adjusting to a new role, such as a new developmental phase, gaining a new sibling or parent, becoming a caregiver, or starting a new school. A role transition may lead to a depression or exacerbate an already existing depression.

3. *Role dispute.* This problem area is the target of treatment when teens and significant others have different expectations for their relationship, thus leading to conflict. Disputes between parents and their teens commonly center on independence, sexuality,

money, and intimacy. A role dispute may precipitate or exacerbate depression; irritability and withdrawal may intensify the dispute.

4. *Interpersonal deficits.* The final problem area, interpersonal deficits, is assigned to teens who find themselves lonely and socially isolated because, in part, of a lack of social and communication skills and for whom this deficit in interpersonal skills is the key link to depression. Although mild interpersonal deficits may precede depression, the onset of depression often increases social withdrawal, thus hindering the increase in social relationships and making recovery from the depression more difficult.

One of the four problem areas is chosen as the focus of the next two phases of treatment. If two problem areas seem appropriate, the one that appears most primary is the initial focus, with the possibility of addressing a secondary area if it can be easily linked to the primary problem. For example, if an adolescent lost her mother after a battle with cancer and is having difficulty transitioning to living with her father, a focus on both grief and role transition may seem appropriate. However, a closer examination of the adolescent's current difficulties may clarify that, although she is upset about the loss of her mother, she has mourned the loss, and the problem most affecting her mood is the new rules and boundaries her father is imposing. The therapist would begin by discussing the mother's death and confirming that the teen has mourned the loss adequately and would then shift the discussion to how that loss has led to changes in the patient's relationship with her father and the current specific difficulties she is experiencing.

During the final session of the initial phase, therapists' conceptualization of the case, the problem area, and the relationship most central to the adolescents' depression are discussed. The therapists elicit feedback from the adolescents and amend the conceptualization as necessary. The therapists ask the adolescents to summarize the problem formulation in their own words to ensure that they understand it and feel that it is the correct focus for treatment. It is crucial that the adolescents agree with the case conceptualization for the treatment to be successful. The therapists and adolescents also discuss expectations for treatment, including the number of remaining sessions, parents' expected level of participation and the policy on missed sessions. As mentioned, the IPT-A protocol is typically 12 sessions; therefore, there are typically eight sessions remaining at the conclusion of the initial phase.

Middle Phase

The structure of each session during the middle and termination phases should follow a similar pattern. Each session typically begins with a brief check-in regarding depressive symptoms, the mood rating, and a brief review of the week's activities (with a focus on interpersonal events). The middle part of each session typically includes a review of the adolescents' work at home, discussion of a particular interpersonal event from the past week, and practice of specific skills. It is important for therapists to assist the adolescents in seeing continuity across sessions by placing the work in the sessions in the context of the problem area formulation that links the focus on different interpersonal events and patterns of communication and problem solving. Finally, the therapists summarize the content discussed during the session, and work at home for the upcoming week is planned.

Several techniques are used frequently in IPT-A treatment across each of the specific problem areas: affect identification and expression (through directive and exploratory techniques), communication analysis, decision analysis, role-playing, and work at home. Because the overall goals of IPT-A are to reduce depression and improve interpersonal relationships, the skills used directly target each of these goals.

Affect Identification

First, affect labeling and expression are encouraged. Teens entering therapy want to feel heard and desire a sense of control, but at the same time require structure and direction, so a combination of directive and nondirective techniques should be used. Through such techniques, effort is made to assist the adolescents in linking interpersonal experiences to changes in their mood and understanding their communication style, with the ultimate goal of helping them to experience more interpersonal interactions of the type that will improve their mood. Nondirective techniques include asking open-ended questions, allowing adolescents to discuss an interpersonal event freely, and making supportive statements to allow them to feel validated. Directive techniques, such as keeping the depressed adolescents on task and offering practical advice or specific information, are also used to provide structure and guidance. Specific communication skills have been described for the adolescents on a "Teen Tips" information sheet (Figure 10.2), which can be given to the adolescents in the middle phase of treatment. These skills can be used throughout the course of therapy and even referred to during booster sessions.

Communication Analysis

Communication analysis is indicated for use in many IPT-A cases, most commonly in the role dispute problem area. The goal of the communication analysis, which is a play-by-play review of a specific conversation between the teens and the persons involved in the problematic relationship, is to assist the adolescents to understand (1) the impact of their words on others, (2) the feelings they convey with verbal and nonverbal communications, (3) the feelings that generated the exchange, (4) their ability to modify such exchanges and, therefore, the affect associated with the relationship and, consequently, their general mood. A key interpersonal interaction is identified; this can typically be identified during the check-in period at the beginning of the session and is usually an interaction that is linked to negative affect. To begin, the therapists simply ask the adolescents to retell the conversation in great detail, statement by statement. The therapists may assist the adolescents by saying, "Imagine that you are telling your friend about a scene in a movie that you very much want him to understand; tell me about the [conversation] as if it is a movie being played in slow motion." First, the adolescents should tell the story without interruption. The therapists then ask the adolescents to tell the story again but warn that "this time I may interrupt here and there." During the retelling of the interaction, the therapists interrupt throughout, asking for more detail as needed and gently inquiring about how the teens may have felt when saying a statement, how the other person might have felt in response to the statement, and how it may have impacted on the person's response. Finally, therapists discuss how the adolescents could have responded differently and thus changed the outcome of the interaction, and then practice the revised conversation.

A. AIM FOR GOOD TIMING

1. Make "appointments" with people you need to talk to.

2. Avoid times when those people are tired/upset/etc.

    Example: "Mom, I know you are pretty tired from working so hard today. There's something I want to talk to you about. Can we talk on Saturday after we clean?"

3. Strike when the iron is COLD—Wait until you feel calm to have a discussion about the problem or conflict.

B. GIVE TO GET: START WITH A POSITIVE STATEMENT THAT SHOWS YOU UNDERSTAND HOW THEY FEEL

1. "Dad, I know how much you love me and want nothing to ever happen to me, but . . . "

2. "Mom, I know you worked really hard today and you are probably pretty tired. I understand that, but can I ask you a quick question: Can I use the phone for 20 minutes?"

C. USE "I" STATEMENTS

1. Say how YOU feel about what they do.

    Example: "I feel frustrated and angry when you insist on my being home by 7 P.M. on Saturday nights because it seems like you don't trust ME to be on my own with my friends."

2. People cannot read your mind no matter how it seems. PUT IT IN WORDS!
   Start with "I"

    Example: "Mom, I feel sad when you . . . "; "Dad, I feel you don't trust me . . . "

D. HAVE A FEW SOLUTIONS IN MIND

If you want to work something out, do a little prep work! Come up with three or four compromises to whatever you are arguing about.

Example: "Dad, I know you how much you worry about me when I go out after 7 P.M. on Saturday nights. But I feel really angry when you call me every 5 minutes on my cell phone. I love you, and I don't want to feel this way." Can we talk about some ideas that may make you feel better when I go out?

Solutions: 1. How about if I call you every hour (every 2 hours)?

2. How about if I let you speak with my friend's parents when I go to her house and that I call you if I leave there so you will know where I am?

3. How about if I call you when we get to the movies, and then again when we leave so you will know when to expect me at home? I promise I will call you immediately if we change plans.

E. DON'T GIVE UP!

Remember, it takes a LONG time to teach someone to do something differently. Your parents/friends are used to handling things the way they have for YEARS. KEEP TRYING!

FIGURE 10.2. Teen tips.

Decision Analysis

Decision analysis is used when adolescents are experiencing conflict. The goal of decision analysis is to teach basic problem-solving skills, including compromise and negotiation skills. First, a specific problem is identified, and teens are encouraged to generate many possible solutions, both realistic and perhaps fantastical, to the problem. If teens have difficulty generating the solutions, therapists can assist by saying, for example, "What if your best friend, Jen, were having this problem? What might you suggest she try?" and "What have you tried in the past when you experienced a similar problem?" Once several solutions are identified, therapists and teens evaluate the pros and cons of each possible solution. Teens choose one solution to try over the next week, and the execution of the solution is discussed and rehearsed in detail in the session. Adolescents are then encouraged to try the solution as work at home during the upcoming week. The interaction is reviewed in the next session. The therapists encourage the adolescents to try it during the week so that they will have more information to work with about how to improve the situation, deemphasizing the notion of the attempt succeeding or failing but rather referring to it as an experiment to provide more data about what may or may not be helpful for this relationship problem. If there were difficulties in the experiment that week, an alternative solution may be chosen or the current one revised, and another experiment may be rehearsed and proscribed for the following week.

Role-Playing

Role-playing, a technique common to several therapies, is used frequently in IPT-A because it is effective and typically fun and engaging. Role-playing is engaged with three goals in mind: (1) to give adolescents a safe place to practice newly acquired interpersonal communication skills, (2) to provide an opportunity to receive constructive feedback before testing out a new skill in real life, (3) and to increase the teens' social confidence. Role-playing is an active process; therefore, the therapists and the adolescents need to truly act out a situation, not simply talk about acting it out. It is often helpful to outline the situation first (especially with more anxious teens). It is recommended that the teens play the role they are more comfortable with first, and then the roles can be switched. Also, it is effective to choose a more benign situation to rehearse first to increase the likelihood of a successful experience. As the adolescents gain confidence in trying new skills, more difficult problems or interactions can be addressed.

Work at Home

Finally, a work-at-home plan is used throughout the middle phase of treatment to assist with the reinforcement and generalization of the skills rehearsed in session. The specific work-at-home assignments should develop naturally out of the material discussed during the therapy sessions; specific assignments often arise following a role play or decision analysis discussed in session. To increase the odds that adolescents will complete the work at home, it is crucial to choose a feasible interaction, to provide adequate coaching within the session, to address how to initiate the interaction and barriers to initiation, and to review the assignment during the subsequent session. It is important when developing a work-at-home" plan to pick a circumscribed problem or interaction to change, something with a good likelihood of successful outcome. By starting small with encouraging results, the adolescents will be more confident in attempting to use these skills in more challenging situations. Consistent use of work at home allows the teens to internalize the new skills, gain a sense of mastery independent of their therapists, and, of course, improve important relationships.

Specific Goals of Each Problem Area

The skills just described are used to accomplish the specific goals of the targeted problem area, as also described in the Initial Phase section.

1. *Grief.* Specifically, therapists' treatment goals for adolescents who are experiencing grief are to assist them in mourning appropriately and in reestablishing relationships and interests to substitute for those lost. Specific helpful strategies include encouraging adolescents to speak about the loss in great detail; discussing the sequence of events before, during, and after the death and the associated feelings; and helping teens find ways to meet new people and develop new social relationships to fill the void created by the loss.

2. *Role dispute.* IPT-A therapists have several goals when addressing a role dispute problem area. First, the specific stage of the dispute is identified. The three stages of role dispute include renegotiation, impasse, and dissolution. The renegotiation phase is identified when the adolescents and their significant others are still in communication and both are willing to attempt to pursue conflict resolution. In the impasse stage, the adolescents and significant others have stopped talking completely, but resolution remains a possibility. In the dissolution stage, the adolescents and significant others have determined that the dispute cannot be resolved, and they have chosen to dissolve the relationship. For the renegotiation and the impasse stages, the goal of treatment is to reach a resolution regarding the dispute. The skills of communication analysis, decision analysis, and role play are especially crucial for the role dispute problem area. These skills enable the adolescents to better link their actions to problematic events, analyze their own communication patterns, and practice communication strategies that allow for effective negotiation. For those in the dissolution phase, the task of the therapists is to assist adolescents in ending the relationship, in mourning the loss of the relationship, in gaining an understanding of why the dissolution occurred, and in improving social skills to engage in new relationships in the future.

3. *Role transition.* When presented with a role transition, the goals of the therapists include helping the adolescents find a way to accept and move into the new role with less difficulty, develop new social skills, develop new attachments and social support in the new role, and recognize and accept the positive aspects of the new role. Strategies to accomplish these goals include allowing the adolescents to understand what the change means to them, identifying the demands of the new role that are problematic, assessing what will be gained and what will be lost (from the old role), and mastering new interpersonal skills that will ease the transition. Role-playing is an effective way to practice new ways of communication and interaction that may be helpful in easing the transition.

4. *Interpersonal deficits.* Finally, the interpersonal deficits problem area is assigned to adolescents who do not know how to reenter their social world and establish new

relationships. The goal is to assist adolescents in reducing their isolation by improving social skills, thus strengthening current relationships and making new connections. To achieve this goal, IPT-A therapists should relate the adolescents' depressive symptoms to the problem of social isolation, review in detail past and current relationships in order to assist in identifying problematic and positive communication patterns, and rehearse new social skills for the formation of new relationships and the deepening of existing ones. It is very beneficial for the therapists to initiate a good deal of role-playing to help the adolescents practice new skills in a safe, nonthreatening environment. Additionally, the therapists can use the therapeutic relationship and give interpersonal feedback to the adolescents in a sensitive manner.

Termination Phase

The final phase of IPT-A takes place in sessions 10–12. The goals of the termination phase are to assist the adolescents in transitioning away from reliance on the therapist relationship to independent use of interpersonal skills. To accomplish this, the therapists nurture a sense of competence to enable the teens to deal with their future problems. To facilitate the adolescents' sense of competence, both therapists and adolescents discuss their feelings about the conclusion of treatment, review skills learned and goals accomplished, discuss warning signs of depression and potential future challenges, and discuss how the strategies can be used to more effectively to deal with future situations. Finally, therapists, adolescents, and their parents determine whether there is a need for further treatment. At least one of the final sessions should include the parents. Ideally, the adolescents should explain to their parents in her own words, what they and their therapists have already reviewed regarding effective skills that have been acquired, potential future challenges, and warning signs of relapse. In addition, the therapists should ask the parents how they feel treatment has affected the adolescents and their families, any changes observed in their relationships, and ideas about how to maintain the treatment gains.

Further treatment is indicated if some symptoms of depression remain or impairment in functioning is still evident. In addition, even if depressive symptoms have remitted, further treatment may be necessary for adolescents to address other accompanying problems, such as a history of sexual abuse or other trauma or coping with a chaotic, unstable family environment. The therapists should discuss these options and the possible benefits of additional treatment with the adolescents and parents and assist them in pursuing more treatment if desired.

Manuals and Training

An important benefit of IPT-A is that therapists interested in learning the treatment can easily obtain the treatment manual. The manual, *Interpersonal Psychotherapy for Depressed Adolescents* (second edition; Mufson, Dorta, Moreau, et al., 2004), is available in bookstores and online. Clinicians can read the manual and incorporate the techniques into their clinical practice. To become a formally trained IPT-A therapist, interested clinicians must attend a training workshop and receive supervision by an IPT-A expert on the treatment of several cases, often using audiotapes to assess adherence and competence. Training workshops are offered biyearly at the International Society of Interpersonal

Psychotherapy conferences as well as by several IPT experts at other times. This information is accessed through the website, *www.interpersonaltherapy.org*, which has information about various IPT activities worldwide.

EVIDENCE ON THE EFFECTS OF TREATMENT

Three individual studies have examined the efficacy and effectiveness of individual IPT-A and concluded that IPT-A is more efficacious than treatment as usual (TAU), clinical monitoring, and wait list and as efficacious as CBT (Mufson et al., 1999; Mufson, Dorta, Wickramaratne, et al., 2004; Rosselló & Bernal, 1999). The initial efficacy study completed by Mufson and colleagues (1999) compared 12 weeks of individual IPT-A with clinical monitoring (which included one-to-two 30-minute meetings with a supportive therapist each month) in a randomized clinical trial of 48 clinic-referred adolescents who met criteria for major depressive disorder. The majority of the participants in this study were Hispanic, female, and living in single-parent homes. Results indicated an average effect size of 0.54; 75% of those receiving IPT-A compared with 46% in the control group recovered, achieving a score of ≤ 6 on the Hamilton Rating Scale for Depression (HRSD) at week 12. Both the Beck Depression Inventory and HRSD scores were lower at week 12 (after controlling for baselines scores) for the IPT-A group compared with the clinical monitoring group. The dropout rate in the control condition was greater than in the treatment condition. Further, at week 12, those in the IPT-A condition reported significantly greater improvement in social functioning than those in the control condition after controlling for baseline scores. In addition, those in the IPT-A group reported greater improvement on the Positive Problem-Solving Orientation and Rational Problem-Solving scales of the Interpersonal Problem-Solving Inventory than those in the clinical monitoring group at week 12, whereas no differences were noted on the other subscales of this inventory.

Rosselló and Bernal (1999) conducted an IPT efficacy study using their own adaptation of the original IPT manual (Klerman et al., 1984) for Puerto Rican adolescents. This randomized controlled trial included 71 depressed adolescents (54% female, 12–17 years) randomly assigned to three conditions: 12 weeks of IPT, 12 weeks of CBT, or wait list. Results indicated that both IPT and CBT were superior to wait list in the reduction of depressive symptoms as measured by the Children's Depression Inventory (CDI). Based on the CDI scores, the effect size for IPT compared with wait-list was 0.73 and for CBT compared with wait-list, 0.43. Further, 82% of those who received IPT and 59% of those who received CBT were deemed functional (as indicated by a score of = 17 on the CDI) at week 12. Notably, the IPT group, but not the CBT group, improved on self-esteem and social adaptation significantly more than the wait-list group. There were no significant differences between the CBT group and the IPT group at 3-month follow-up.

In light of the positive findings regarding the efficacy of IPT-A in treating depression, Mufson, Dorta, Wickramaratne, et al. (2004) completed an effectiveness study in which they compared IPT-A with TAU in school-based mental health clinics to determine whether the IPT-A model could be effectively disseminated to school-based settings. Sixty-four adolescents (84% female; 71% Hispanic; age range, 12–18 years) who met study inclusion criteria (HRSD score ≤ 10, Children's Global Assessment Scale [C-GAS] score ≤ 65, and a diagnosis of adjustment disorder with depressed mood, depression disorder not otherwise specified, major depression, or dysthymia) were randomized to IPT-A (12 sessions over a 12- to 16-week period) or TAU. The IPT-A was delivered by school-based clinic mental health clinicians ($N = 7$) who were trained and supervised in IPT-A by treatment experts. TAU was also delivered by school-based clinic mental health counselors ($N = 6$) and included mainly individual supportive psychotherapy. Results indicated an average effect size of 0.50 for IPT-A over TAU. Those in the IPT-A group reported significantly greater decreases in depressive symptoms than those in the TAU group at week 12. Fifty percent of those in the IPT-A group and 34% of those in the TAU group met the recovery criteria (HRSD ≤ 6). Differences on depression indicators between the two groups emerged at week 8 of treatment. Those in the IPT-A group also experienced significantly greater overall improvement in functioning as measured by the CGAS than those in the TAU group. Social functioning on the Social Adjustment Scale–Self-Report was higher at week 12 for the IPT-A group than the TAU group. Two moderators were identified: age and depression severity. Specifically, IPT-A was more effective compared with TAU in older adolescents (15–18 years) and in more severely depressed adolescents. Finally, although those in the IPT group received more therapy hours than those in the TAU group, secondary analyses indicated that the difference in dose did not account for the significant differences in depression among the two groups (Mufson, Gallagher, et al., 2004).

The results of this study are encouraging regarding the ability to disseminate the IPT-A protocol to settings other than research institutions. It also demonstrates that the IPT-A treatment can be effectively taught to school social workers using a fairly low-intensity training program (i.e., reading the IPT-A manual, 1 day of didactics, and ongoing weekly supervision). The parsimony of the IPT-A model may be one reason for the success of the effectiveness study and thus a practical strength of the treatment model.

Overall, IPT-A has demonstrated a moderate to moderately large effect size for effectively improving depression and overall functioning compared with clinical monitoring, wait list, and TAU (Mufson et al., 1999; Mufson, Dorta, Wickramaratne, et al., 2004; Rosselló & Bernal, 1999). The effect sizes reported for IPT-A (0.50–0.73) are comparable to other empirically supported treatments for depression in adolescents, such as CBT, with the exception of one CBT treatment that involved parents (McCarty & Weisz, 2007). There are limitations to the studies that have addressed the efficacy of IPT-A. Each study was conducted among mostly Hispanic, female participants and included relatively small sample sizes. Thus, it is imperative that future studies of IPT-A be conducted with larger, more ethnically and gender-diverse populations. In addition, follow-up data are needed to address the long-term effectiveness of IPT-A.

DIRECTIONS FOR RESEARCH AND ADAPTATIONS OF IPT-A

Because of the success of IPT-A in treating depression among adolescents, there are several adaptations of IPT-A that are have or are currently being evaluated. IPT-A has been adapted for use with groups of depressed adolescents (Mufson, Gallagher, et al., 2004). In addition, IPT-A has been adapted as a preventive intervention for adolescents with subthreshold symptoms: Interpersonal Psychotherapy–Adolescent Skills Training (Young et al., 2006). Compared with those receiving school counseling, those in IPT skills training groups reported significantly fewer depression symptoms and were functioning significantly better overall posttreatment and at follow-up. Given the desire to identify ways to further increase treatment response, IPT-A has been adapted to increase parental involvement to assess whether this might augment treatment outcome, particularly for those adolescents experiencing parent–child conflict, because there is evidence that IPT-A may be more effective for adolescents who are experiencing high levels of interpersonal conflict (Gunlicks-Stoessel, Mufson, & Jekal, 2008). In addition, pilot studies are currently underway to assess the feasibility of adapting IPT-A for use with adolescents with comorbid depression and nonsuicidal self-injury and to assess the effectiveness of delivering a brief model of IPT-A in the pediatric primary care clinics.

CONCLUSIONS

Adolescent depression is a prevalent and impairing disorder. The need for effective and feasible psychosocial interventions for the treatment of this disorder is clear. IPT-A is a brief (12–15 sessions), empirically supported, interpersonally based psychotherapy that can be effectively administered by clinicians of various levels of expertise. IPT-A demonstrates that the course of a depressive episode can be changed with intervention at the interpersonal level. The main components of IPT-A include affect identification, psychoeducation, and interpersonal skills building. A problem area—grief, role transition, role dispute, or interpersonal deficit—is identified. Specific skills taught over the course of treatment are tailored to the individual. These skills focus on improving communication, perspective taking, problem solving, and expressing affect.

Several studies have assessed the efficacy and effectiveness of IPT-A, and more are underway. The research to date supports the identification of IPT-A as a likely efficacious treatment for adolescents reporting a depression of moderate severity and its inclusion as a recommended treatment in the American Academy of Child and Adolescent Psychiatry's Practice Parameters for the Treatment of Adolescent Depression. Most importantly, IPT-A can be learned and delivered with reasonable adherence and competence by community clinicians in school-based health clinics to achieve effective results. More research is needed on the long-term outcomes for adolescents treated with IPT-A and the effectiveness of a continuation and maintenance model in the prevention of relapse and recurrence.

REFERENCES

Allen, J. P., Insabella, G., Porter, M. P., Smith, F. D., Land, D., & Phillips, N. (2006). A social-interactional model of the development of depressive symptoms in adolescence. *Journal of Consulting and Clinical Psychology, 74*(1), 55–65.

American Psychiatric Association. (2000). *Diagnostic and statistical manual of mental disorders* (4th ed., text rev.). Washington, DC: Author.

Bowlby, J. (1978). Attachment theory and its therapeutic implications. *Adolescent Psychiatry, 6,* 5–33.

Brunstein-Klomek, A., Marrocco, F., Kleinman, M., Schonfeld, I., & Gould, M. (2007). Bullying, depression, and suicidal ideation in adolescents. *Journal of the American Academy of Child and Adolescent Psychiatry, 46,* 40–49.

Costello, E. J., Pine, D. S., Hammen, C., March, J. S., & Plotsky, P. M. (2002). Development and natural history of mood disorders. *Biological Psychiatry, 52,* 529–542.

Gunlicks-Stoessel, M. L., Mufson, L., & Jekal, A. (2008). *The impact of interpersonal functioning on treatment for adolescent depression: IPT-A versus treatment as usual in school-based health clinics.* Manuscript in preparation.

Klerman, G. L., Weissman, M. M., Rounsaville, B. J., & Chevron, E. (1984). *Interpersonal psychotherapy for depression.* New York: Basic Books.

McCarty, C. A., & Weisz, J. R. (2007). Effects of psychotherapy for depression in children and adolescents: What we can (and can't) learn from meta-analysis and component profiling. *Journal of the American Academy of Child and Adolescent Psychiatry, 46,* 879–886.

Mufson, L., Dorta, K. P., Moreau, D., & Weissman, M. M. (2004). *Interpersonal psychotherapy for depressed adolescents* (2nd ed.). New York: Guilford Press.

Mufson, L., Dorta, K. P., Wickramaratne, P., Nomura, Y., Olfson, M., & Weissman, M. M. (2004). A randomized effectiveness trial of interpersonal psychotherapy for depressed adolescents. *Archives of General Psychiatry, 61,* 577–584.

Mufson, L., Gallagher, T., Dorta, K. P., & Young, J. (2004). A group adaptation of interpersonal psychotherapy for depressed adolescents. *American Journal of Psychotherapy, 58*(2), 220–238.

Mufson, L., Weissman, M. M., Moreau, D., & Garfinkel, R. (1999). Efficacy of interpersonal psychotherapy for depressed adolescents. *Archives of General Psychiatry, 56,* 573–579.

Rosselló, J., & Bernal, G. (1999). The efficacy of cognitive-behavioral and interpersonal treatments for depression in Puerto Rican adolescents. *Journal of Consulting and Clinical Psychology, 67,* 734–745.

Rudolph, K. D., Hammen, C., Burge, D., Lindberg, N., Herzberg, D., & Daley, S. E. (2000). Toward an interpersonal life-stress model of depression: The developmental context of stress generation. *Development and Psychopathology, 12,* 215–234.

Sheeber, L. B., Davis, B., Leve, C., Hops, H., & Tildesley, E. (2007). Adolescents' relationships with their mothers and fathers: Associations with depressive disorders and subdiagnostic symptomatology. *Journal of Abnormal Psychology, 116 (1),* 144–154.

Sullivan, H. S. (1953). *The interpersonal theory of psychiatry.* New York: Norton.

Weissman, M. M., Markowitz, J. C., & Klerman, G. L. (2007). *Clinician's quick guide to interpersonal psychotherapy.* New York: Oxford University Press.

Young, J. F., Mufson, L., & Davies, M. (2006). Efficacy of interpersonal psychotherapy—Adolescents skills training: An indicated preventive intervention for depression. *Journal of Child Psychology and Psychiatry, 47,* 1254–1262.

B

Externalizing Disorders and Problems

11

Parent Management Training—Oregon Model

An Intervention for Antisocial Behavior in Children and Adolescents

MARION S. FORGATCH and GERALD R. PATTERSON

The study and treatment of antisocial behavior problems have been underway at the Oregon Social Learning Center (OSLC) for more than four decades. The work, initiated by Gerald Patterson, has been conducted by a group of colleagues who have specialized in different aspects of the problem and its treatment. The present chapter provides an overview of the theory-driven intervention practices, processes, and outcomes relevant to the Parent Management Training–Oregon Model (PMTO™), a family of interventions designed to treat and prevent antisocial behavior (ASB) problems in children and adolescents.

A DEVELOPMENTAL MODEL OF ASB

The model underlying PMTO interventions is social interaction learning (SIL), a moniker that reflects the merging of social interaction, social learning, and behavioral perspectives. The social interactional dimension examines the microsocial connections among family members and peers that become patterns of behavior leading to healthy or dysfunctional adjustment. The social learning and behavioral dimensions address the question of how patterns become established through reinforcing contingencies. At a more molar level, the model incorporates contexts impinging on families that influence youngsters' social environments and thereby indirectly affect outcomes. This ecological perspective is tested with analyses of models in which the impact of background contexts on youngsters' adjustment is mediated by processes within the social environment (i.e., parenting practices and peer behaviors). The SIL model has been evaluated with several passive and experimental longitudinal studies using samples of varying clinical indication and risk levels for child ASB problems reviewed later.

The Oregon model of ASB involves a trajectory that begins with relatively innocuous aversive behaviors that become increasingly noxious with youngsters' development. The first problem behaviors to emerge are overt and tend to be shaped by parents, often inadvertently through the use of negative reinforcement. Overt behaviors include excessive noncompliance, temper tantrums, hyperactivity, hitting, biting, fighting, and other direct actions against others. For some children the deviancy process stops there. Others develop a set of covert ASBs that may include lying, stealing, truancy, fire setting, animal abuse, and substance use and abuse. Covert problems may develop as a means of avoiding overly harsh parental discipline practices, and they can be further buttressed by positive reinforcement from peers and siblings. When youngsters learn both forms of ASBs from the distinct social regimens of parents and deviant peers, delinquency can emerge in adolescence or preadolescence. Either form by itself, overt or covert behavior, is presumed *not* to predict adult crime in the Oregon ASB model; rather it is the interaction of the two.

Adverse contexts surrounding social environments can seriously disrupt processes within the social environment and indirectly affect youth outcomes. Challenging contexts can come from diverse sources, including family circumstances (e.g., poverty, family structure transitions, extreme stress), environmental conditions (e.g., high-crime neighborhoods, traumatic events, discrimination), and individual factors (e.g., temperament, physical or mental health, personal resources). The most proximal socializing agents for healthy or deviant youth adjustment trajectories are parents and eventually peers.

Parents affect the child at home, and they determine the amount of time a youngster spends with the peer group, the kinds of settings in which peer interactions will occur, and whether or not the youngsters are supervised by responsible adults. Parents define house rules, establish a safe environment, and set in place routines and structures in which daily living skills are learned. They may also shape overt ASB patterns that generalize to settings outside the home. When youngsters with overt ASB arrive in schools and other community settings, their abrasiveness, lack of social skills, and obdurate noncompliance can quickly lead to academic failure and rejection by normal peers. This failure across social settings can contribute to internalizing problems within the children, a perspective further enhanced by findings that show that problem children and family members engage in a mutual negative attribution process.

In adolescence, youngsters spend more time away from home and the settings in which ASB takes place change, as does the topography of the behavior. Rejected by prosocial peers, the children drift toward deviant peers. What is particularly interesting is that these unsavory social agents use positive reinforcement to shape deviant behavior, a process that is observable both in the playground and in the laboratory. The bulk of this reinforcement is for covert ASB (Snyder et al., 2005). Although the model indicates that peers are important socializing agents, a PMTO intervention based on changing peers has yet to be developed. An early attempt at this led to the discovery of iatrogenic effects inherent in bringing together groups of deviant peers (Dishion & Andrews, 1995).

PMTO: CHARACTERISTICS OF THE TREATMENT PROGRAM

The Oregon ASB model places parenting as an early and proximal mechanism for the development of increasingly serious ASB problems. Within this model, parenting is conceived as a construct comprising coercive and positive parenting practices, as displayed in Figure 11.1. Disruptions in parenting practices are presumed to mediate the relationship between harsh contexts and negative child outcomes starting in childhood.

Coercion takes place when one person uses aversive behavior to control the behavior of another. Temper tantrums and their threat are frequent forms of child coercion; harsh punishment involving either physical or psychological dimensions is a parental form. The coercive sequence begins when one person introduces an aversive behavior into a peaceful social environment. If the other person responds in kind, a conflict bout begins, which ends when one member terminates the negative exchange with a negative behavior, thereby "winning" the bout. This dance includes negative reciprocity and negative reinforcement. Variations incorporate escalation into the sequence, and escalation in intensity or topography of behavior can lead to serious outcomes, such as violence. On public school playgrounds, an aversive event can be observed about once every 3 minutes. In clinical families, conflict bouts occur about once every 16 minutes, and mothers, fathers, and siblings get caught up in the process (Patterson, 1982).

Coercion is functional, and it is stable within and across settings. For example, in one study, the relative rate of reinforcement for coercion observed in the home during 1 week was a predictor for the relative rate of coercive child behavior of the following week. The multiple correlation of .83 between the relative rate of reinforcement and the relative rate of child behavior represents an application of the matching law to the human experience. In a clinical sample, the relative rate of reinforcement observed in the home was a significant predictor for measures of out-of-home placement and police arrest 2 years later. Coercive processes in the family have been identified as early as age

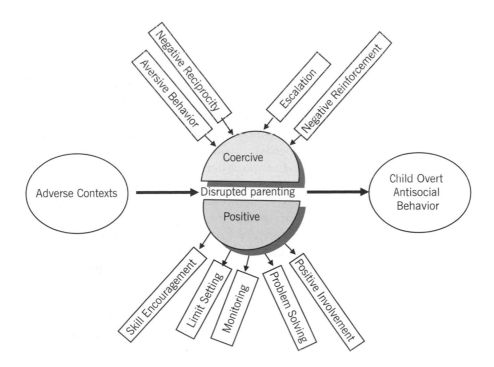

FIGURE 11.1. Parenting practices are complex.

2. The studies describing these coercive processes are cited and reviewed by Dishion and Patterson (2006) and Snyder et al. (2008) as well as in books by Patterson and colleagues (Patterson, 1982; Patterson, Reid, & Dishion, 1992; Reid, Patterson, & Snyder, 2002).

Who Is Seen and in What Formats

Sessions are highly structured, yet there is considerable room to respond to the issues families bring into sessions, introduce and practice new skills, and tailor procedures to each family's needs. In individual family format, sessions are more principle driven than agenda driven. For group-administered treatment, sessions are highly structured, with less room for individual attention. Family sessions generally last 60 minutes and group sessions, 90 minutes. All formats begin with a warm-up phase followed by a review of the home practice assignment, incorporating troubleshooting and adjustment as necessary; the introduction, practice, and tailoring of new material; and close with a new home practice assignment. Depending on the family's needs, severity and duration of the problem, and other factors, most individual treatment consists of 25–30 sessions. In the group format, which follows the same principles, there are 14 sessions. Most families attend weekly.

In the individual format, children are incorporated into the sessions to varying degrees, depending on family and therapist preferences and needs. Each session ends with an assignment to practice some portion of the newly introduced strategy. New sessions begin with a careful debriefing of the home practice assignment. Changes are often needed, and therapists and parents troubleshoot ways to tailor the procedures to specific family circumstances. Midweek phone calls are another standard means of preventing problems, promoting successful application, and maintaining collaborative contact.

Contents of the Treatment

The positive parenting practices shown in Figure 11.1 comprise five dimensions. Skill encouragement involves the use of scaffolding (e.g., breaking complex behaviors into achievable steps and encouraging approximations toward the goal) and positive reinforcement to teach new (prosocial) behavior. Limit setting is framed as another teaching tool, this one to discourage deviant behaviors with contingent small negative sanctions. Monitoring involves parental tracking of youngsters' whereabouts, activities, peers, and behaviors while at home and away from home and their provision of appropriate adult supervision. Problem solving is the basic family skill that involves setting goals, developing strategies to achieve these goals, committing to the decision, trying it out, and making relevant adjustments. Finally, positive involvement includes the many ways that parents show their children love and interest. The intervention moves in a step-by-step basis, with parents learning one skill before adding new strategies to their parenting tool box. The core components have been demonstrated malleable by PMTO and serve as mediators of intervention effects on child outcomes (see Table 11.1).

The positive parenting practices are the sine qua non of PMTO; however, several supporting dimensions provide the healthy foundation on which the intervention stands. These supporting strategies have received little emphasis in our written materials, but

(text resumes on p. 166)

TABLE 11.1. Main Research Evaluating Outcomes, Experimentally Testing Theoretical Models, and Studying Therapy

Study	Sample	Design and objective	Main findings
Patterson (1979)	1972 SA[a]; N = 27; M[b]; MA[c] = 8.7	P/P/FU[d]—12 months	Reduced observed deviant behavior Reduced PDR[e]
	1977 SA; N = 28; M; MA = 7.4	P/P/FU—12 months	Replication achieved; reduced deviant behavior (observed and PDR)
Patterson, Chamberlain, & Reid (1982)	SA; N = 19; M and F[f]; MA = 6.8	RCT[g]: E vs. TAU[h]	Reduced deviant behavior (observed and PDR)
Bank, Marlowe, Reid, Patterson, & Weinrott (1991)	Delinquent adolescents; N = 55; M; MA~14	RCT: E vs. TAU P/P/FU—1, 2, and 3 years	Fewer nonstatus offenses at termination (1 year) Fewer status offenses at FU1 (2 years) Less time incarcerated at termination, FU1, and FU2 Fewer delinquent behaviors (PDR)
Patterson & Forgatch (1985)	Therapy process; N = 6; M and F; MA = 9.9	Single subject ABABA reversal design	Therapist teach, confront, and teach/confront increase client resistance
Patterson & Chamberlain (1988)	Therapy process; N = 50; M and F; MA = 9.5	Direct observation of therapy	Theory specification Struggle work through (early therapy—form relationship; midtherapy—struggle to promote change; late—back off and reach closure)
Stoolmiller, Duncan, Bank, & Patterson (1993)	Therapy process; N = 68; M and F; MA~10	P/P/FU—2 years	Struggle work H supported: negative quadratic shape in resistance (low early, higher mid, less late) predicts fewer OHP[i] and fewer arrests at 2-year FU; baseline (BL) maternal inept discipline and ASB predict chronically high levels of resistance
Chamberlain & Reid (1991)	MTFC[j] state hospital patients; N = 20; M and F; MA~14	RCT: MTFC vs. TAU	Greater frequency placement outside hospital Less time to placement outside hospital Less cost for treatment
Chamberlain & Reid (1998)	MTFC; adjudicated OHP; N = 79; M; MA = 14.9	RCT: MTFC vs. TAU P/P/FU 12 and 48 months	At 12 months: fewer arrests, runaways; less youth-reported delinquency; greater program completion At 48 months: fewer arrests
Chamberlain, Leve, & DeGarmo (2007)	MTFC same as previous but F; N = 81; MA = 15.3	RCT: MTFC or TAU P/P/FU—12 and 24 months	Fewer incarcerations and criminal referrals; less youth-reported delinquency Findings sustained from 12–24 months with increased effect size

(cont.)

TABLE 11.1. *(cont.)*

Study	Sample	Design and objective	Main findings
Chamberlain et al. (2008)	KEEP foster/ kinship families; $N = 700$; M and F; MA = 8.8	RCT: KEEP vs. TAU P/P/FU—5 months	Greater proportion positive reinforcement (PDR and parent interview) Fewer behavior problems (PDR)
Price et al. (2008)	Same as previous	Same as previous	Fewer placement disruptions Greater frequency reunification
Fisher, Gunnar, Dozier, Bruce, & Pears (2006)	MTFC-P; $N = 117$; M and F; MA = 4.4	RCT: MTFC-P vs. RFC[k]; 60 nonmaltreated MCC[l]	Fewer permanent placement failures Increased attachment security Reduced avoidant attachment
Fisher, Stoolmiller, Gunnar, & Burraston (2007)	Same as previous	Same as previous	MTFC-P children became comparable to MCC in cortisol activity; RFC children did not change
Forgatch & DeGarmo (1999, 2002)	Prevention: ODS[m]; $N = 238$; M; MA = 7.8	RCT: PMTO vs. NTC[n]; BL, 6, 12 months	Structured Equation Modeling (SEM) models: Improved observed parenting practices BL–12 months, which, in turn, led to better teacher-rated school adjustment and less observed noncompliance, observed aggression, and DPA[o] at 12 months
DeGarmo, Patterson, & Forgatch (2004)	Same as previous	Same plus assessments at 18, 24, 30, 36 months	SEM mediational models: Improved observed parenting change at 12 months mediated reduced teacher-rated externalizing at 24 months; PMTO reduced slope maternal depression at 30 months, mediated by reduced boy externalizing at 24 months
Forgatch, Patterson, DeGarmo, & Beldavs (2009)	Same as previous	Same as previous plus 6, 7, 8, 9 years post BL	Latent Growth Curve Modeling (LGCM) mediational models: Improved observed parenting practices BL–12 months and reduced deviant peer association 12 months to 8 years mediated intervention effects on reduced growth in police arrests and teacher-reported delinquency over 9 years as H by theoretical model
Forgatch, DeGarmo, & Beldavs (2005)	Prevention: MAPS[p]; $N = 110$; M and F; MA = 7.5	RCT; PMTO vs. NTC; P/P/FU—24 months	SEM models: Intervention improved observed parenting practices for mothers and stepfathers, led to decreased observed noncompliance, reduced parent-reported home problems at 12 months, and reduced teacher-reported school problems at 24 months
Forgatch, Patterson, & DeGarmo (2005)	MAPS; $N = 4$ therapists; M and F; 20 families	Validate fidelity measure	SEM: Observed therapist behavior in session predicted change in observed parenting practices BL–12 months

(cont.)

TABLE 11.1. *(cont.)*

Study	Sample	Design and objective	Main findings
Reid, Eddy, Fetrow, & Stoolmiller (1999)	Prevention: LIFT[q]; N = 671 (310 first graders; 361 fifth graders); M and F	RCT: by schools P/P/FU—12 months	Intervention decreased observed playground aggression, decreased observed maternal coercive behavior toward child, with highest BL aversive behavior having greatest improvement; improved peer relations based on teacher ratings
DeGarmo, Eddy, Reid, & Fetrow (2009)	Fifth-grade sample from above	Same as previous P/P/FU—7 years	Intervention improved family PS[r] and reduced playground aggression from BL to termination; intervention reduced tobacco/illicit drug use, particularly for girls from grades 5–12. Improved PS and reduced playground aggression mediated these effects
DeGarmo & Forgatch (2004)	Fifth-grade LIFT ODS Sample	P/P/FU—3 years P/P/FU—3 years	Improved PS at 6 months reduced problem behaviors at 3 years Improved PS at 1 year reduced problem behaviors at 3 years In both samples PS was the mediator
Dishion & Andrews (1995)	Prevention: ATP[s]; N = 195; M and F; MA~12	RCT: P,[t] T,[u] P and T; SD[v] P/P/FU—12 months	Fewer observed coercive interactions for P and P and T groups vs. T and SD; iatrogenic effects for teen conditions (T and P and T) such that they showed increased teacher-reported externalizing and youth-reported tobacco use
Dishion, Nelson, & Kavanagh (2003)	Prevention: FCU[w] and ATP; N = 71; M and F; MA = grade 7	Multiple-gated RCT: FCU vs. NTC; ATP vs. NTC	Experimental (E) groups: less substance use; less decline in parental monitoring Mediated model: E led to greater parental monitoring and less growth substance use; parental monitoring mediated E effect on growth in substance use
Connell, Dishion, Yasui, & Kavanagh (2007)	Prevention: FCU; N = 998; M and F; MA = grade 6	RCT: FCU vs. matched control; P/P/FU—6 years	Complier Average Causal Effects (CACE) analysis. Engagers compared with nonengagers: more youth-reported family conflict, more biological father absence, more teacher-reported risk factors. FCU yielded less growth substance use, less antisocial behavior by age 17, less arrest by age 18
Dishion et al. (2008)	Prevention: preschool FCU; N = 731; M and F; MA = 28 months	RCT: FCU vs. NTC; P/P/FU—12 and 24 months	At 12 months: Increased observed positive parenting At 24 months: Less parent-reported problem behavior

[a]Socially aggressive; [b]male; [c]mean age; [d]pre/post/follow-up; [e]parent-report deviant behavior—repeated telephone interview; [f]female; [g]randomized controlled trial; [h]treatment as usual; [i]out-of-home placement; [j]Multidimensional Treatment Foster Care; [k]regular foster care; [l]matched community control; [m]Oregon Divorce Study; [n]no-treatment control; [o]deviant peer association; [p]Marriage and Parenting in Stepfamilies; [q]Linking the Interests of Families and Teachers; [r]problem solving; [s]Adolescent Transitions Program; [t]parent; [u]teen; [v]self-directed; [w]Family Check-Up.

they are an integral part of all PMTO training programs. PMTO manuals provide detailed information for the principles defining the PMTO method. In individual family treatment, content order can vary, as can the amount of time spent on each component, depending on particular families.

The goal of PMTO interventions is to empower parents in their use of positive parenting strategies and to reduce their reliance on more coercive approaches. Parents learn to be proactive in settings in which problems are likely to occur (e.g., during the "arsenic hour" before dinner, in the grocery store). An important yet seldom described supporting component for PMTO is the regulation of emotional expression within each of the five positive parenting practices. Role play is used extensively as a teaching tool and helps parents understand situations from differing perspectives by playing their own role or that of their children. Role play also provides practice with a coach (therapist) to ensure generalization of the skills from the therapy room to the home.

For the first several sessions, we are rather strict in adhering to the following sequence: (1) an introduction to change with a focus on strengths; (2) giving effective directions; and (3) teaching through encouragement. Typically, we follow encouragement with limit setting, but in some families a module on emotional regulation is productive before limit setting. Following these components, order of content is more flexible, including monitoring, problem solving (as a general strategy, for couples to promote a united parenting front, and for family meetings), promoting school success (at home and linking with the school setting), and positive involvement. Additional content may be included using methods other than PMTO as necessary. In this chapter, we provide details on the first few content areas.

Sequence of the Sessions

The intervention (treatment and prevention programs) begins with a focus on strengths within the family, the focal child, the parents as individuals and as parents, the couple when appropriate, and the family as a whole. The first home practice assignment is to track and record these strengths. Many parents are surprised with the attention given to positive behavior because the referral is for deviancy, but we explain that all children and families have strengths, and it is on this foundation that we will build the change program. Parents are helped to specify goals, at first general and grandiose and then more specific and achievable. Almost all families have problems with noncompliance (i.e., stubbornness, not listening, not minding, arguing), and this is frequently one of the first behaviors in which we intervene.

The next topic involves introducing a supporting dimension of PMTO: parental use of effective directions (not commands and not requests). Most therapists and parents find that giving children good directions magically leads to improved cooperation, at least temporarily. The training ground for directions is active with extensive use of role play. Therapists model wrong-way and right-way strategies, debriefing each approach with a questioning process that leads parents to identify the specific behaviors (verbal and nonverbal) that make directions more or less effective. Parents are engaged in these minidramas by playing their children and eventually themselves, which provides them with expanded perspectives of the ways in which their behavior affects their children.

There is a specific sequence of steps to follow in the effective directions intervention: (1) identify the goal behavior (what they want the child to do, such as hang up the jacket); (2) calm oneself; (3) get the child's attention (with proximity and physical or eye contact) and state the child's name in a neutral manner; (4) state the goal behavior (what is wanted rather than not wanted) with no extraneous words; (5) add the word "please"; and (6) stand and hold in a neutral manner for 10 seconds after giving the directive. During the series of role plays designed to introduce and practice the procedure, the therapist incorporates as many variations of these steps as possible. Laughter tends to characterize much of this session, and parents often later comment that they hadn't realized how much their own behavior plays a role in their child's reactions. The session ends with a home practice assignment to track the children's cooperative and noncompliant reactions to the parents' effective and ineffective directions. Giving good directions is one of the basic skills that promotes later sessions on skill encouragement and limit setting.

Next in the sequence of therapy is teaching new behavior through encouragement. Following Wesley Becker's early lead, we emphasize that parents are their children's most important teachers, and the most advanced teaching strategies are required for youngsters like their own who have the behavior problems that bring them in for treatment (Becker, 1971). This way of framing the hard work parents are asked to undertake can prevent some of the common resistant phrases we hear (e.g., "Why should we reward them for doing what they ought to be doing in the first place!"; "They KNOW how to do it! They don't need us to teach them."). Given the framework that their children need advanced strategies, the parents feel less like failures and more motivated to work hard to help their children.

Two main approaches are used in the skill encouragement component: incentive charts for routine or complex behaviors (e.g., getting ready for bed, leaving on time for school, cleaning the bedroom) and tokens for behaviors that require management on a moment-by-moment basis (e.g., behavior in public places like the grocery store or neighbors' homes, behavior in the car). Each system emphasizes the use of material rewards. Parents also practice using praise and other social reinforcers paired with material rewards, never with corrective feedback or criticism.

Skill encouragement using contingent positive reinforcement is always taught before limit setting. It may require several sessions before parents become proficient. Parents practice using social reinforcers that are genuinely positive and lack hints of sarcasm, guilt, or other subtle and not-so-subtle elements. Many parents of children with ASB problems are painfully deficient in their ability to use social reinforcement. Some have received little encouragement in their own experience; others are so stressed or depressed that they forget to bathe their children in praise, smiles, hugs, and affectionate gestures. In other families, parents use kind words when they want something or to make up for having been excessively hostile. Youngsters in these families come to regard social reinforcers with suspicion. For these reasons, we use role play to practice giving specific and contingent social reinforcement paired with instrumental rewards (e.g., points, M&Ms, "Scooby loops"). Gradually, the youngsters learn to value social rewards.

Parents learn to use highly structured procedures when setting limits. Time-out (up to 10 minutes) is used for face-to-face situations where disengagement is helpful (e.g., noncompliance, arguing, swearing, sibling warfare). When children refuse time-out, the backup is privilege removal for a longer period of time (e.g., 15–30 minutes depending on the age of the child). Common privileges to withhold include, for example, TV time, videogame time, telephone or cell phone use, outside play, and use of bike or skateboard. Fines can be used for rule violations such as swearing. Extra work chores can be given as a consequence for a variety of covert or serious behavior problems (e.g., lying, stealing, coming home late). The backup for work chores is privilege removal. These seem like old-fashioned commonsensical sanctions, and that is true. However, learning to apply them calmly and consistently requires much practice, and role play is the method of learning. Parents are urged not to use the procedures at home until they and their therapist agree they have a high likelihood of success. The principles related to negative consequences include the following: use to discourage problematic behavior; balance with encouragement (a ratio of five positive to one negative); be calm, yet firm; use small consequences; act immediately; be consistent; don't lecture, argue, or demand promises; maintain appropriate physical distance; and when it's over, let it go.

The time-out sequence begins with 5 minutes, adding 1 minute at a time until 10 minutes is reached. Then a preplanned privilege is specified for removal, usually for about 30 minutes but never more than an hour. Physical restraint is never used unless the child is a preschooler, and then the child is simply taken to the time-out spot. Time-out is a particularly effective consequence for face-to-face behaviors in which escalation is a risk, and we first teach it with reference to noncompliance. For more covert behaviors (e.g., lying, stealing, coming home late), we recommend a strategy called extra work chores. This approach calls for the parents to provide the child with a developmentally appropriate short chore that can be done without adult supervision once a good job description (usually written) is provided. Parents learn to give negative consequences based on the topography of the child's misbehavior, not the parents' emotional state.

In troubled families (as in normal families), parents need considerable practice to regulate their emotions. We role-play the many varieties of negative emotion, including anger, contempt, fear, sadness, and combinations of these. Using a questioning process that guides parents to identify specific nonverbal dimensions relevant to affective expression, parents explore the effects that hostile and friendly approaches to children can have. Instead of encouraging parents to "let it all out," we facilitate the use of neutral and positive expression as well as strategies for managing negative emotions. For children's emotional expression, parents learn to differentiate their own feelings from those of their children and practice ways to engage their youngsters in activities that make it safe to talk about feelings. Parents learn to listen without negative reactions when their children talk about upsetting issues.

EVIDENCE ON THE EFFECTS OF TREATMENT

Over the past four decades, the OSLC group has designed interventions, tested the efficacy and effectiveness of PMTO for ASB problems, refined the theoretical foundation, and studied therapy process to improve outcomes. Focal youngsters have ranged in age from 2–18 years; the intervention has been delivered in various settings (homes, schools, clinics) and in group and individual family formats; and it has used supplementary tools such as books, audio and video recordings, and a variety of parenting materials. Clinical populations have included preadolescents with conduct problems; preadolescents who steal; multiply offending delinquent adolescents; neglected and maltreated children; and delinquent foster care residents, youngsters institutionalized for psychiatric problems, and neglected and maltreated preschoolers. The same principles used in clinical samples have been applied with a wide range of universal, selected, and indicated prevention samples.

The intervention studies are consistent in finding that programs based on the Oregon model of ASB are efficacious. Table 11.1 outlines key programs developed and tested by the OSLC group. Findings are based on multimethod and multiagent assessments to define ASB, family processes, and other outcomes associated with ASB. Assessment methods include in-person interviews; repeated telephone interviews; questionnaires based on parent, child, teacher, and peer report; achievement testing; public records (e.g., police arrests, out-of-home placements, program completion); and direct observation in multiple settings (e.g., home, school, playground, laboratory, therapy session). With the exception of the earliest studies that used replication designs (e.g., Patterson, 1979), methods use random assignment and intention-to-treat (ITT) analyses with outcomes including reduced ASB, depression, deviant peer association, delinquency, incarceration, out-of-home placement, runaways, and police arrests as well as improvements in achievement tests, school functioning, program completion, and out-of-hospital placement.

Using intervention as experimental tests of theory with classic mediational analyses, several of the studies have shown that intervention benefits to parenting and reductions in deviant peer association lead to immediate and long-term reductions in negative youth outcomes. Furthermore, recent studies show that helping parents improve their children's adjustment can further benefit the parents, with reductions in maternal depression, financial stress, and police arrests as well as increased income (DeGarmo, Patterson, & Forgatch, 2004; Forgatch & DeGarmo, 2007).

Both the shape of PMTO and the contexts in which the model has been applied have evolved since the early work of the 1960s and 1970s. To convey this evolution and the associated tests of intervention effects, we present next a developmental history of PMTO.

A DEVELOPMENTAL HISTORY OF THE INTERVENTION

Parent management training emerged in the early 1960s as a potential treatment for young, out-of-control children in response to a crisis in the nation's network of child guidance clinics. A number of studies began to appear suggesting that the clinics were providing treatment that was basically ineffective for aggressive, hyperactive, or out-of-control children. Because these youngsters constituted about three-fourths of all treatment referrals to these clinics, the lack of an effective treatment represented a major crisis. Initially, the intervention was based on a simple operant model in which parents would serve as the treatment agent for the child. The goal was to teach parents to provide positive reinforcement for prosocial skills and mild contingent negative sanctions for deviant behavior. Over the years, new treatment dimensions have been added and considerable attention has been given to how treatment is applied. What follows is a brief review of these developments in PMTO.

1965–1975: A Simple Operant Model

The child guidance crisis sparked the interest of a number of psychologists specializing in child behavior problems, including Robert Wahler (Wahler, Winkle, Peterson, & Morrison, 1965), Constance Hanf (1968), Ivar Lovaas (1978), Sidney Bijou (Bijou & Baer, 1961), and Gerald Patterson (Patterson & Brodsky, 1966). These psychologists ransacked existing learning theories in their search for new ways to treat ASB. Quickly, a consensus emerged on two different issues: (1) children with ASB problems are almost invariably socially unskilled and (2) parental report is an inaccurate accounting of family processes involved in children's behavioral patterns. Methods were developed to collect direct observational data in both natural and laboratory settings. The observational data were used to determine whether or not the new interventions were working. The data were collected in the home, at first on a daily basis. The resulting graphs decorated the walls of the laboratories of these pioneers.

Many specialists adopted an operant strategy that emphasized training parents to use positive contingencies to strengthen prosocial child behavior and negative contingencies to weaken deviant behavior. The intervention was viewed as a simple educative process supported by the assumption that the parents lacked information about effective parenting skills. To fill this gap, books were written for parents to read, techniques like "bug in the ear" were developed so that parent trainers could tell parents what to do during parent–child interactions, and audiotapes and, later, videotapes modeled the procedures. Therapeutic and teaching skills were minimized in importance. One of the staff of our own center actually had his secretary run parent training groups! The early studies were crude but promising, with little or no attention given to clinical sensitivity. The findings from these early studies are reviewed in Patterson (1979). The details of the procedures developed to work with these early cases were described by Patterson, Reid, Jones, and Conger (1975).

1975–Present: Serious Clinical Problems

As the OSLC group became committed to applying PMTO procedures to increasingly more difficult clinical cases, we began weekly clinical meetings to discuss challenges and design innovations. The next two decades were spent adapting the clinical procedures for populations of abused children, children who steal, and samples of preadolescent children with ASB problems. We failed in attempts to follow randomized trial designs with samples of abused children and stealers (e.g., Patterson, 1979). However, we were finally successful in using such a design for a small clinical sample of preadolescent boys with ASB problems. Observation data collected in the home showed clear reductions in ASB for families in the experimental group with families receiving treatment from well-trained professional psychotherapists (Patterson, Chamberlain, & Reid, 1982).

In the early 1980s, we used an ITT design with a sample of chronic offending adolescents referred for delinquency (Bank, Marlowe, Reid, Patterson, & Weinrott, 1991). The data on police arrests showed significant benefits for families in the experimental group compared with community treatment-as-usual group. Although the experiment was a statistical success, most who served as therapists in the project believed that further improvements in PMTO were required.

Patricia Chamberlain applied the lessons learned from the delinquency project and developed the innovative and internationally recognized multidimensional treatment foster care approach for populations of delinquent adolescents (Chamberlain, 2003). In that program, families are recruited and trained to provide specialized foster care for youngsters in their own homes. Foster parents are given extensive training in effective family management practices, with regular phone calls to monitor progress and intervene in problems. The intervention team works with schools, juvenile court, and other relevant community agencies to ensure the youths' success in all domains. The biological family or those who will continue with the child in aftercare receive intervention to enhance the likelihood of continuing success. From Chamberlain's work, several other approaches have been developed for treating youngsters from preschool through adolescence who cannot be helped in the homes of their biological families (Fisher, Gunnar, Dozier, Bruce, & Pears, 2006; Fisher, Stoolmiller, Gunnar, & Burraston, 2007).

1980–Present: A Focus on Therapy Process

As our clinical samples became increasingly complex, we experienced more difficulty in our attempts to help families change. In the best behavioral tradition, we decided to build an observational system to measure therapy process and resistance to change. Patterson and Forgatch spent several months studying therapy tapes from OSLC failure cases and specified key therapist and client behaviors. We based the therapist behaviors on key concepts in the clinical literature (e.g., question, support, teach, reframe, confront). We found many forms of resistance, but four stood out: "I can't," "I won't," "I didn't," and family conflict (verbal arguments among family members). At an international conference in Banff, Canada, where we presented the new work, we were publicly drummed out of the behavioral movement. The transgression was our "mentalistic coding system"!

Fortunately, the focus on therapy was rewarded with a foundation grant, the funds from which enabled us to apply our new microsocial coding system within therapy sessions. The first data to emerge showed that therapist behaviors were associated with increases or decreases in client resistance in the immediate subsequent response. Behaviors such as questioning and support were associated with reduced levels of resistance, but teaching and confronting led to increases. To test experimentally the relationship between teach/confront and resistance, we used an ABAB design. During the A phases, therapists were directed to avoid using teach or confront and to use these behaviors at least 10 times during B phases. Teach or confront produced a threefold increase in parent resistance within the next few seconds. The combination of the two led to an even greater increase. These data suggested a paradox for behavioral therapists, whose primary goal was to teach more effective parenting practices. Direct teaching without attention to sophisticated clinical skills created a context hostile to change (Patterson & Forgatch, 1985).

Other studies in the resistance series showed that parents who were depressed, antisocial, or from low socioeconomic status had higher levels of resistance during therapy. The data also showed that high levels of parent resistance were associated with reduced benefits to child outcomes. Of particular interest was the finding that client resistance was associated with low levels of therapist liking the client. In the process of helping parents change, therapists were being changed. In effect, PMTO represents a transactional process with arrows denoting change pointing in both directions. It became obvious that intervention improvements in families required that we find solutions to the problem of bilateral change. A review of the key resistance studies can be found in Patterson and Chamberlain (1988).

Advances in analytic approaches added new dimensions to our understanding of resistance. Latent growth curve modeling was applied to study the course of resistance during therapy to test the struggle/work-through clinical hypothesis. This complex notion examines the trajectory of resistance over the course of therapy. We posited that early treatment should be devoted to forming a strong therapist–client relationship, with little teach and confront and, therefore, little resistance. During midtherapy, after the relationship is established, the therapist can take a more active teaching role to break homeostasis and advance the change process. Our earlier studies indicated that teach/confront would lead to increased resistance; thus, midtherapy should reflect an increase in resistance, and successful working through of the struggle would be reflected by a reduction in resistance. Stoolmiller, Duncan, Bank, and Patterson (1993) tested the hypothesis and showed that a resistance trajectory that starts low, increases during midtherapy, and reduces by termination does indeed predict improved clinical outcomes, with reductions in out-of-home placements and police arrests 2 years posttermination.

1990–Present: Prevention Programs for Universal and Selected Samples

Three OSLC teams set about adapting the clinical model for prevention approaches based on the same principles in the social interaction learning model and using randomized controlled trials. Reid tested a universal program in schools located in high-crime neighborhoods. Dishion used a series of trials in schools with at-risk adolescents. Later he conducted a study with poor families with preschoolers. Forgatch studied two samples with families at risk because of parental divorce or remarriage.

Reid and colleagues conducted a multipronged universal intervention in first and fifth grades, with parent education groups, classroom and playground programs for the children, and enhanced parent–teacher communication. Findings yielded immediate and longer term effects, with models demonstrating reductions in child aggression, ASB, and tobacco and illicit drug use, and changes in parenting practices were associated, as expected, with the improvements in child outcomes (DeGarmo, Eddy, Reid, & Fetrow, 2009; DeGarmo & Forgatch, 2004; Reid, Eddy, Fetrow, & Stoolmiller, 1999).

Dishion's work has addressed two age groups of at-risk samples: early adolescents and toddlers. The work with adolescents has been implemented in school settings, with advantageous effects when parents are involved in parent education groups. Mediational modeling supports the theoretical model (Connell, Dishion, Yasui, & Kavanagh, 2007; Dishion & Andrews, 1995; Dishion, Nelson, & Kavanagh, 2003). An important discovery in this program of research is that bringing at-risk groups of adolescents together for intervention can have iatrogenic effects (Dishion & Andrews, 1995). Dishion's work with parents of toddlers focuses on families participating in WIC programs and is implemented in community clinics. The findings show increases in positive parenting and decreases in child problem behavior (Dishion et al., 2008). In both the adolescent and toddler samples, Dishion added the family check-up, which is based on motivational interviewing to enhance participant engagement and cooperation.

Forgatch and colleagues conducted prevention programs with divorced families with early elementary school-age children. A program for recently separated single mothers was conducted in parent groups and yielded positive outcomes for mothers and their children, lasting up to 9 years (DeGarmo & Forgatch, 2005; DeGarmo et al., 2004; Forgatch & DeGarmo, 1999, 2002; Forgatch, Patterson, DeGarmo, & Beldavs, 2009). Another program for recently remarried families with stepfathers was conducted in individual family sessions. The positive outcomes for parents and children lasted up to

2 years (Forgatch, DeGarmo, & Beldavs, 2005). Both randomized controlled samples tested models evaluating the theoretical model with supportive findings.

1997–Present: The Implementation Story

During the heyday of behavioral intervention, various groups contacted us with an interest in learning the parent training methods. At the time, we had not developed a training program, although we conducted 3-day workshops as hors d'oeuvres to multicourse meals. Interested parties received manuals or the parent training books. One of these groups was headed by Richard Tremblay from Montreal, Quebec, Canada. Given the lack of a formal PMTO training regimen, the resulting work could hardly be thought of as a PMTO effectiveness trial. However, their 15-year follow-up showed borderline significance for the effect on delinquency reduction and a significant increase in the proportion of youth graduating from high school (Tremblay, Pagani-Kurtz, Mâsse, Vitaro, & Pihl, 1995). Other groups with minimal PMTO training included Earlscourt, a treatment center in Toronto, Ontario, Canada. Earlscourt has maintained coaching contact with us for decades and has published some studies indicating success (Augimeri, Farrington, Koegl, & Day, 2007).

Our real efforts to follow an effectiveness trial design came as a result of a 1997 invitation from Norway's Ministry of Child and Family Welfare, who wanted to establish evidence-based practice for children with conduct problems nationwide. We were asked to design and train a first generation of practitioners who would be able to train their own future generations. We were ill prepared for a venture of this sort, and although the Norwegians recognized our shortcomings, they were impressed by the years of programmatic research and were willing to invest in a collaborative project.

A team headed by Marion Forgatch and bolstered by the expertise of Nancy Knutson (an educational psychologist) and Laura Rains (a social worker), all well trained in PMTO, began to develop the training materials and procedures. We started with our most recent manuals designed for prevention programs with single-mother and stepfather families. We generalized and adapted the materials to incorporate wisdom gleaned from the many clinical samples treated at OSLC over the decades. We decided to train the professionals through a combination of workshops (six workshops in sets of 3 days for a total of 18 days over the course of 18 months) and coaching based on direct observation (through videotapes) of therapy sessions as the training candidates applied the procedures in their home clinics. All candidates saw a minimum of five families: three for training and two for certification.

Of the 36 professionals from child welfare and child mental health treatment centers throughout the nation, 31 (87%) completed the training program with certification. The professionals represented agencies in communities ranging from the farthest northeastern corner bordering on Russia to the western coast, including the city of Bergen, to the southern coastline, and especially the most densely populated regions in the eastern section of the country in and around Oslo. This ambitious nationwide approach called for arsenals of video equipment, teams of translators, extensive use of the Internet, and patience on the part of all. The commitment and leadership of the teams on both sides of the North Pole made our lurch into implementation successful. Today the Norwegians are in the midst of completing the training of their fifth generation of professionals, they have adapted the program for application with immigrant parents (e.g., Somali and

Pakistani groups), and they have conducted a randomized clinical trial demonstrating the effectiveness of PMTO.

The Norway effectiveness trial consisted of 112 children referred for treatment of conduct problems. Families were randomly assigned to PMTO or regular clinical services in two systems (child mental health and child welfare). The trial was conducted nationwide, using multimethod and multiagent assessment, including direct observation of parent–child interactions to define parenting practices and child outcome variables (Ogden & Amlund-Hagen, 2008). The data showed a significant effect for improved parental discipline; those changes, in turn, were significant predictors of reduced child noncompliance, fewer child negative chains, and lower levels of child externalizing problems. This is the first effectiveness trial that is focused solely on the exportability of the PMTO model, one in which the intervention is focused primarily on the parent. Given that several generations of PMTO therapists have now been trained in Norway, a whole new series of clinical studies can be initiated with a primary focus on reducing prevalence of ASB in children in Norway.

One of the questions central to implementation research concerns the fidelity with which an intervention can be transported from a protected environment to the complex practice of clinical agencies. Forgatch and colleagues developed a technique based on direct observation of therapy sessions to score PMTO fidelity. Ratings are based on five dimensions designed to tap competent adherence to the method: knowledge, structure, teaching, process, and overall quality. The Fidelity Implementation Rating System (FIMP) was applied in a randomized trial involving stepfathers. A comparison of baseline to 12-month follow-up showed significant improvements in parenting practices, and these, in turn, predicted improvements in child outcomes. The FIMP ratings were obtained from a sample of five randomly selected cases from each of the four project interventionists. From the 20 cases, two key parenting practices were the focus (i.e., skill encouragement and limit setting). Direct observations of parenting practices were obtained before and after the intervention. FIMP ratings were significant predictors for changes in the observed parenting practices of the mothers and the stepfathers, separately assessed at baseline and 12-month follow-up (Forgatch, Patterson, & DeGarmo, 2005). FIMP data have been applied within the Norwegian study of implementation. The Norwegian therapists trained by OSLC were able to achieve high levels of FIMP scores; even more interesting is the fact that the Norwegian therapists have been able to train the third generation of therapists to FIMP levels as high as those obtained by the first generation. It is clearly the case that PMTO procedures can be taught with negligible drift (Forgatch, 2008).

DIRECTIONS FOR RESEARCH

As the preceding developmental history suggests, PMTO has evolved in multiple directions, with adaptations to fit a number of different contexts and populations. Each adaptation of PMTO is the subject of ongoing research, more than could be described in this focused chapter. However, we can convey a bit about our research directions with two examples.

In one example, we are working to enhance our research by drawing on expertise in family therapy. To study clinical strategies in family therapy, one of the current authors, Marion S. Forgatch, spent a 9-month externship at the Mental Research Institute in

Palo Alto, California, with Dr. Carlos Sluski as her chief mentor. In addition, several members of the Minuchin (1974) group spent a week or more at OSLC introducing the clinical group to a variety of therapy techniques for dealing with resistance. Many of these concepts found their way into what has become PMTO. We learned to get out of our chairs, become more theatrical, and increase our use of standard clinical strategies (e.g., normalize, mirror, paradox, interpret/reframe). In addition to an emphasis on clinical techniques, we learned to become more subtle in our teaching approaches. Role play, effective questioning processes, and problem-solving strategies (especially the use of brainstorming) became standard in our process tool box. Parent training became more playful and productive, with parents changing roles many times in the course of a session and receiving coaching during the practice bouts. Every component in PMTO is now taught with sessions rich in role play and the laughter that accompanies it. These clinical insights have not yet been put to the empirical test, but we intend to do so.

A second example involves extending the implementation work we have done in Norway. Since our initiation with implementation in Norway, we have begun training in other countries (e.g., Iceland, the Netherlands, Mexico) and in the United States. Rather than operate piecemeal, we have limited ourselves to implementing in large-scale systems. Currently, we are working statewide in Michigan within the child mental health system with a supplementary program for the Detroit–Wayne County area. In Detroit, we are also training within the juvenile justice and child welfare systems for parents whose children have been removed for neglect and maltreatment. Each of these venues presents an opportunity for further research on implementation strategies and their effects.

CONCLUSIONS

Studies of the antisocial spectrum from childhood through adolescence with interventions based on the social interaction learning model across clinical and prevention samples have enabled us to improve the theory, measurement, and intervention programs. At the same time, it has taught us humility. Adaptations require sensitivity to variations in culture and context; intervention processes must be conducted with skill and sophistication; intervening at different levels (within systems, agencies, practitioners, parents, children, teachers) is complicated; and keeping up with technological changes can be daunting. Maintaining an iterative process is critical to sustaining a process in which theory, measurement, and practice continue to be refined.

Moving out of the ivory tower and into the community has presented us with new perspectives on the work of the scientist-practitioner. Our implementation team has adopted the phrase "It's elephants all the way down" to describe the PMTO processes we practice at every level. The phrase is based on an ancient Hindu legend that places the four corners of the world on the back of an elephant. That elephant is standing on the back of another, and another, all the way down. For us, SIL theory is the underpinning for our intervention, and it is equally relevant for our implementation procedures. Coercion disrupts and must be kept out of the social environment. Positive practices such as monitoring, skill encouragement, problem solving, positive involvement, and, yes, even limit setting are all relevant for teams of adults who work together to produce short- and long-term change.

When we began implementation in the nationwide Norwegian program, the professionals provided us with a barrage of complaints: Manualized treatments are inhumane and rigid; we don't like behaviorists; what goes on in the therapy room is a private affair; reinforcing children for doing what they ought to do will weaken their character; and punishment is immoral. In Michigan today, much of the resistance is similar, but there are some interesting differences: Manualized interventions (i.e., evidence-based practice) are rigid; behaviorists are still not popular and therapy should be private; reinforcing children for doing what they are supposed to do is silly. But punishment is not seen as immoral. In fact, our style of negative sanctions (small, contingent, consistent) is seen as being too weak and certainly ineffective. What has been interesting in both cultures (Norway and Michigan) is that the therapists seem to resist the approaches more so than the families. And once the families begin to improve, the professionals become enthusiastic proponents of the method.

Decades have been dedicated to the development and testing of effective interventions for children and families with behavior problems. We are in the infancy of learning how to implement programs in real-world settings on a large-scale basis with sustained fidelity. Our group has received decades of support to study the integration of theory and practice. The coming generations of scientist-practitioners must focus on taking evidence-based practices into the field with sustained fidelity and continuing positive outcomes. To do this will require decades of more research.

REFERENCES

Augimeri, L. K., Farrington, D. P., Koegl, C. J., & Day, D. M. (2007). The SNAP Under 12 Outreach Project: Effects of a community based program for children with conduct problems. *Journal of Child and Family Studies, 16,* 799–807.

Bank, L., Marlowe, J. H., Reid, J. B., Patterson, G. R., & Weinrott, M. R. (1991). A comparative evaluation of parent-training interventions of families of chronic delinquents. *Journal of Abnormal Child Psychology, 19,* 15–33.

Becker, W. C. (1971). *Parents are teachers: A child management program.* Champaign, IL: Research Press.

Bijou, S. W., & Baer, D. M. (1961). *Child development: A systematic and empirical theory* (Vol. 1). New York: Appleton-Century-Crofts.

Chamberlain, P. (2003). *Treating chronic juvenile offenders: Advances made through the Oregon multidimensional treatment foster care model.* Washington, DC: American Psychological Association.

Chamberlain, P., Leve, L. D., & DeGarmo, D. S. (2007). Multidimensional treatment foster care for girls in the juvenile justice system: 2–year follow-up. *Journal of Consulting and Clinical Psychology, 75,* 187–193.

Chamberlain, P., Price, J., Leve, L. D., Laurent, H., Landsverk, J. A., & Reid, J. B. (2008). Prevention of behavior problems for children in foster care: Outcomes and mediation effects. *Prevention Science, 9,* 17–27.

Chamberlain, P., & Reid, J. B. (1991). Using a specialized foster care treatment model for children and adolescents leaving the state mental hospital. *Journal of Community Psychology, 19,* 266–276.

Chamberlain, P., & Reid, J. B. (1998). Comparison of two community alternatives to incarceration for chronic juvenile offenders. *Journal of Consulting and Clinical Psychology, 66,* 624–633.

Connell, A. M., Dishion, T. J., Yasui, M., & Kavanagh, K. (2007). An adaptive approach to family intervention: Linking engagement in family-centered intervention to reductions in adolescent problem behavior. *Journal of Consulting and Clinical Psychology, 75,* 568–579.

DeGarmo, D. S., Eddy, J. M., Reid, J. B., & Fetrow, R. A. (2009). Evaluating mediators of the impact of the Linking the Interests of Families and Teachers (LIFT) multimodal preventive intervention on substance use initiation and growth across adolescence. *Prevention Science, 10*, 208–220.

DeGarmo, D. S., & Forgatch, M. S. (2004). Putting problem solving to the test: Replicating experimental interventions for preventing youngsters' problem behaviors. In R. D. Conger, F. O. Lorenz, & K. A. S. Wickrama (Eds.), *Continuity and change in family relations* (pp. 267–290). Mahwah, NJ: Erlbaum.

DeGarmo, D. S., & Forgatch, M. S. (2005). Early development of delinquency within divorced families: Evaluating a randomized preventive intervention trial. *Developmental Science, 8*, 229–239.

DeGarmo, D. S., Patterson, G. R., & Forgatch, M. S. (2004). How do outcomes in a specified parent training intervention maintain or wane over time? *Prevention Science, 5*, 73–89.

Dishion, T. J., & Andrews, D. W. (1995). Preventing escalation in problem behaviors with high-risk young adolescents: Immediate and 1–year outcomes. *Journal of Consulting and Clinical Psychology, 63*, 538–548.

Dishion, T. J., Nelson, S. E., & Kavanagh, K. (2003). The family check-up with high-risk young adolescents: Preventing early-onset substance use by parent monitoring. *Behavior Therapy, 34*, 553–571.

Dishion, T. J., & Patterson, G. R. (2006). The development and ecology of antisocial behavior. In D. Cicchetti & D. Cohen (Eds.), *Developmental psychopathology: Vol. 3. Risk, disorder, and adaptation* (rev. ed., pp. 503–541). New York: Wiley.

Dishion, T. J., Shaw, D., Connell, A., Gardner, F., Weaver, C., & Wilson, M. (2008). The family check-up with high-risk indigent families: Preventing problem behavior by increasing parents' positive behavior support in early childhood. *Child Development, 79*, 1395–1414.

Fisher, P. A., Gunnar, M. R., Dozier, M., Bruce, J., & Pears, K. C. (2006). Effects of therapeutic interventions for foster children on behavioral problems, caregiver attachment, and stress regulatory neural systems. *Annals of the New York Academy of Sciences, 1094*, 215–225.

Fisher, P. A., Stoolmiller, M., Gunnar, M. R., & Burraston, B. O. (2007). Effects of a therapeutic intervention for foster preschoolers on diurnal cortisol activity. *Psychoneuroendocrinology, 32*(8–10), 892–905.

Forgatch, M. S. (2008). *Final report: Implementing parent management training in Norway.* Unpublished manuscript.

Forgatch, M. S., & DeGarmo, D. S. (1999). Parenting through change: An effective prevention program for single mothers. *Journal of Consulting and Clinical Psychology, 67*, 711–724.

Forgatch, M. S., & DeGarmo, D. S. (2002). Extending and testing the social interaction learning model with divorce samples. In J. B. Reid, G. R. Patterson, & J. Snyder (Eds.), *Antisocial behavior in children and adolescents: A developmental analysis and model for intervention* (pp. 235–256). Washington, DC: American Psychological Association.

Forgatch, M. S., & DeGarmo, D. S. (2007). Accelerating recovery from poverty: Prevention effects for recently separated mothers. *Journal of Early and Intensive Behavioral Intervention, 4*, 681–702.

Forgatch, M. S., DeGarmo, D. S., & Beldavs, Z. (2005). An efficacious theory-based intervention for stepfamilies. *Behavior Therapy, 36*, 357–365.

Forgatch, M. S., Patterson, G. R., & DeGarmo, D. S. (2005). Evaluating fidelity: Predictive validity for a measure of competent adherence to the Oregon model of parent management training (PMTO). *Behavior Therapy, 36*, 3–13.

Forgatch, M. S., Patterson, G. R., DeGarmo, D. S., & Beldavs, Z. G. (2009). Testing the Oregon delinquency model with nine-year follow-up of the Oregon Divorce Study. *Development and Psychopathology, 21*, 637–660.

Hanf, C. (1968, November). *Modification of mother child controlling behavior during mother–child interactions in a controlled laboratory setting.* Paper presented at the regional meeting of the Association for the Advancement of Behavior Therapy, Olympia, WA.

Lovaas, O. I. (1978). Parents as therapists. In M. Rutter & E. Schopler (Eds.), *Autism: A reappraisal of concepts and treatment* (pp. 369–378). New York: Plenum Press.

Minuchin, S. (1974). *Families and family therapy*. Cambridge, MA: Harvard University Press.

Ogden, T., & Amlund-Hagen, K. (2008). Treatment effectiveness of parent management training in Norway: A randomized controlled trial of children with conduct problems. *Journal of Consulting and Clinical Psychology, 76*, 607–621.

Patterson, G. R. (1979). Treatment for children with conduct problems: A review of outcome studies. In S. Feshbach & A. Fraczek (Eds.), *Aggression and behavior change: Biological and social process* (pp. 83–132). New York: Praeger.

Patterson, G. R. (1982). *Coercive family process*. Eugene, OR: Castalia.

Patterson, G. R., & Brodsky, G. (1966). A behaviour modification programme for a child with multiple problem behaviours. *Journal of Child Psychology and Psychiatry, 7*, 277–295.

Patterson, G. R., & Chamberlain, P. (1988). Treatment process: A problem at three levels. In L. C. Wynne (Ed.), *The state of the art in family therapy research: Controversies and recommendations* (pp. 189–223). New York: Family Process Press.

Patterson, G. R., Chamberlain, P., & Reid, J. B. (1982). A comparative evaluation of a parent-training program. *Behavior Therapy, 13*, 638–650.

Patterson, G. R., & Forgatch, M. S. (1985). Therapist behavior as a determinant for client noncompliance: A paradox for the behavior modifier. *Journal of Consulting and Clinical Psychology, 53*, 846–851.

Patterson, G. R., Reid, J. B., & Dishion, T. J. (1992). *A social interactional approach: Vol. 4. Antisocial boys*. Eugene, OR: Castalia.

Patterson, G. R., Reid, J. B., Jones, R. R., & Conger, R. (1975). *A social learning approach to family intervention: Families with aggressive children*. Eugene, OR: Castalia.

Price, J. M., Chamberlain, P., Landsverk, J., Reid, J., Leve, L., & Laurent, H. (2008). Effects of a foster parent training intervention on placement changes of children in foster care. *Child Maltreatment, 13*, 64–75.

Reid, J. B., Eddy, J. M., Fetrow, R. A., & Stoolmiller, M. (1999). Description and immediate impacts of a preventive intervention for conduct problems. *American Journal of Community Psychology, 27*, 483–517.

Reid, J. B., Patterson, G. R., & Snyder, J. (2002). *Antisocial behavior in children and adolescents: A developmental analysis and model for intervention*. Washington, DC: American Psychological Association.

Snyder, J., Schrepferman, L., McEachern, A., Barner, S., Johnson, K., & Provines, J. (2008). Peer deviancy training and peer coercion: Dual processes associated with early-onset conduct problems. *Child Development, 79*, 252–268.

Snyder, J., Schrepferman, L., Oeser, J., Patterson, G., Stoolmiller, M., Johnson, K., et al. (2005). Deviancy training and association with deviant peers in young children: Occurrence and contribution to early-onset conduct problems. *Development and Psychopathology, 17*, 397–413.

Stoolmiller, M., Duncan, T. E., Bank, L., & Patterson, G. R. (1993). Some problems and solutions in the study of change: Significant patterns of client resistance. *Journal of Consulting and Clinical Psychology, 61*, 920–928.

Tremblay, R. E., Pagani-Kurtz, L., Mâsse, L. C., Vitaro, F., & Pihl, R. O. (1995). A bimodal preventive intervention for disruptive kindergarten boys: Its impact through mid-adolescence. *Journal of Consulting and Clinical Psychology, 63*, 560–568.

Wahler, R. G., Winkle, G. H., Peterson, R. F., & Morrison, D. C. (1965). Mothers as behavior therapists for their own children. *Behaviour Research and Therapy, 3*, 113–124.

12

Parent–Child Interaction Therapy and the Treatment of Disruptive Behavior Disorders

ALISON ZISSER and SHEILA M. EYBERG

OVERVIEW OF THE CLINICAL PROBLEM

Parent–child interaction therapy (PCIT) is an evidence-based treatment (EBT) for young children with disruptive behavior disorders (DBDs). Disruptive behavior is the most common reason for the referral of young children for mental health services and can vary from relatively minor infractions such as talking back to significant acts of aggression. The DBDs may be classified as oppositional defiant disorder (ODD) or conduct disorder, depending on the severity of the behavior and the nature of the presenting problems. The DBDs often co-occur with attention-deficit/hyperactivity disorder (ADHD). PCIT has been used effectively to treat disruptive behavior across the full range of problem severity.

Untreated DBDs are costly to society. Children with DBDs account for a larger percentage of health care costs than children with chronic health conditions such as epilepsy, asthma, and diabetes (Guevara, Mandell, Rostain, Zhao, & Hadley, 2003). Young children demonstrating persistently high levels of disruptive behavior fail to learn prosocial behavior and are at high risk for antisocial behavior and criminal activity in adolescence and adulthood (Hann & Borek, 2001).

CONCEPTUAL MODEL UNDERLYING PCIT

Based on Baumrind's (1966) developmental theory of parenting, PCIT draws from both attachment and social learning principles to teach authoritative parenting—a combination of nurturance, good communication, and firm control. The authoritative parenting style has been associated with fewer child behavior problems than alternative parenting styles across a diverse range of clinical populations (e.g., Querido, Warner, & Eyberg, 2002).

According to attachment theory, parental warmth and responsiveness to the emotional needs of young children contribute to the development of a secure working model of relationships, which, in turn, leads to greater emotional regulation and enhances the child's desire to please and willingness to comply. Conversely, parents who are unresponsive to their children's emotional expression and needs foster insecure attachment. Maladaptive parent–child attachment has often been linked to children's aggressive behavior, low social competence, poor coping skills, low self-esteem, and poor peer relationships. Moreover, an insecure parent–child attachment is related to increased maternal stress and increased risk of child abuse and neglect.

The specific behavior management techniques taught in PCIT are based on social learning theory, which emphasizes the contingencies that shape dysfunctional interactions between disruptive children and their parents. These interactions are characterized by mutual and escalating aversive behaviors resulting from the attempts of both the parent and child to control the actions (e.g., arguing, criticizing, whining, aggression) of the other. To interrupt this cycle, in our view, parents must change their behavior to incorporate clear limit setting in the context of an authoritative relationship. Thus, the goals of PCIT are to improve both the parent–child relationship and parental behavior management skills.

GOALS OF PCIT

PCIT theory posits that a warm, nurturing relationship is a necessary foundation for establishing effective limit setting and consistency in discipline, which will lead to lasting change in the behaviors of both parent and child. Therefore, in the first phase of PCIT—child-directed interaction (CDI)—parents learn to follow the child's lead in play. The specific goal of CDI is to increase parental responsiveness and establish a secure and nurturing relationship between parent and child. Once parents have mastered the CDI skills (detailed later), the second phase of treatment incorporates parent-directed interaction (PDI), in which parents learn to lead the child's behavior when needed. The goal of PDI is to improve parental limit setting and consistency in discipline in order to reduce the child's noncompliance, aggression, and other negative behaviors. Therapists teach parents problem-solving skills to assist them in applying the principles and skills taught in CDI and PDI to new situations and new problems as they arise.

CHARACTERISTICS OF THE TREATMENT PROGRAM

Family Characteristics

Children and their parents are seen together in PCIT. Most PCIT outcome studies have included children ages 3–6 with DBDs. However, both younger and older children from various clinical populations have been studied. The evidence base for PCIT includes families from diverse ethnic and socioeconomic groups. Study children have been referred by caseworkers, pediatricians, teachers, mental health professionals, and other families. Although most often used to treat children with disruptive behavior, PCIT has also been implemented with physically abusive parents and children with internalizing behavior problems. Treatment may include one or both parents or other significant care-givers in the child's life, such as a grandparent. PCIT was designed for individual fam-ily treatment, but several research teams are examining the efficacy of group PCIT. In group PCIT, the dyadic parent–child coaching component is retained, and group size is typically three to six families per group.

Therapy Structure

Each phase of treatment begins with a teaching session in which the therapist explains, models, and role-plays the CDI or PDI skills with the parents, followed by coaching ses-sions in which parents practice the skills with their child while the therapist coaches them on the new behaviors. Parents complete a short rating scale before each session to monitor child behavior problems at home. The coaching sessions begin with a brief review of the previous week followed by a 5-minute coded observation of the parent–child interaction to determine which skills parents have mastered and which will be important targets for in-session coaching.

Coaching constitutes the majority of session time. Therapists typically coach from an observation room with a one-way mirror into the playroom, using a "bug-in-the-ear" system for communicating to the parents playing with their child. If such a system is unavailable, the therapist may coach the parents from inside the playroom. Coaching consists of frequent, brief statements that give parents immediate feedback on their CDI or PDI skills (e.g., "Nice labeled praise," "Good direct command"), their manner (e.g., "Great enthusiasm," "Good job staying calm"), or their effect (e.g., "He stays on task longer when you describe what he is doing"). The therapist also offers suggestions (e.g., "Praise her as much as you can when she's playing gently like that").

Parents are typically surprised to find how quickly they become comfortable with coaching as they engage with their child, and they often comment on the reassurance it provides. Their comfort likely results from the therapists' training and careful attention to coaching skills. Therapists use brief phrases stated only when neither child nor parent is speaking to prevent parent distraction and to enable parents to concentrate on their child's words and play. Therapists also tailor their coaching to the parents' vocabulary and style of interaction, and they follow coaching guidelines for particular sessions and situations. For example, in the first coaching session, when parent anxiety initially may be high, therapists limit their feedback to reassurance and labeled praise for correct skill application (e.g., "Excellent reflection!"). Children are equally comfortable with coach-ing. Even when the therapists coach from within the playroom, children attend only briefly to the therapists before engaging completely in play with their parents.

At the end of each session, therapists review with parents a summary sheet show-ing how often they used each CDI or PDI skill during the initial 5-minute observation period. Parents can track their weekly skills progress on the summary sheet and decide which skill to focus on most during their daily practice sessions the following week. Ther-apists and parents also review a graph of their children's progress based on the parents' weekly behavior ratings.

CONTENT OF TREATMENT SESSIONS

Child-Directed Interaction

The primary rule for parents during CDI is to follow their child's lead. Parents learn to use specific communication skills (behavior descriptions, reflections, and labeled praise) that give attention to their child's positive behaviors as they play together (see Table 12.1 for further description with examples). Parents also learn not to use specific communications (commands, questions, and criticism) that attempt to lead and can be intrusive in child-led play (see Table 12.1) and to ignore mild negative behaviors that occur. By giving attention only to positive child behaviors in this initial phase of treatment, parents learn to use the technique of *differential social attention* to shape their child's behavior. At the end of the CDI teaching session, therapists provide parents with a handout sum-

TABLE 12.1. Child-Directed Interaction Skills

Skills	Reasons	Examples
"Do" skills		
Labeled praises	• Increases behavior that is praised. • Shows approval. • Increases self-esteem. • Creates positive feelings.	• Good job of cleaning up! • I like how you're building so quietly. • Great idea to make a house. • Thank you for sharing with me.
Reflections	• Lets child lead the conversation. • Shows that you are listening. • Shows that you understand. • Improves speech. • Clarifies ideas.	• Child: I drew a tree. • Parent: Yes, a big tree by the house. • Child: This isn't very easy. • Parent: It's hard to balance that. • Child: I made a choo-choo. • Parent: You *did* make a train.
Behavior descriptions	• Lets child lead activity. • Shows you are interested. • Teaches concepts and builds vocabulary. • Holds child's attention on the task.	• You are building a fort. • You're putting the monkeys where they can watch all the other animals. • You drew six petals on your flower. • Now you're searching for the letters for the next word.
"Don't" skills		
Commands	• Takes lead away from child. • Risks negative interaction.	• Indirect commands: • Let's play with the cars. • Direct commands: • Give me the red car.
Questions	• May be hidden commands. • Suggests you are not listening. • Suggests you disapprove.	• Can you tell me what color this is? • We're building a big house, aren't we? • Child: I want to play with the animals. • Parent: The animals? • You're putting red blocks on the tower?
Critical statements	• Lowers self-esteem. • Creates unpleasant interaction. • Increases the criticized behavior.	• You still have it wrong. • Your tower is crooked. • That's not a good idea. • Stop fidgeting.

marizing the skills and ask parents to practice the skills for 5 minutes each day. On a separate handout, parents record their daily home practice and any problems that arise during home sessions.

In the first CDI coaching session, therapists focus exclusively on reinforcing parents' use of any CDI skill. In subsequent sessions, coaching also targets specific skills that parents find most difficult. For example, a therapist might focus on increasing labeled praise, and whenever the parent gives an unlabeled praise (e.g., "Good job"), the therapist might cue the parent to label it by saying "Good job of what?" or just "Of what?" The therapist also reinforces the parent specifically for each use of labeled praise (e.g., "Great labeling that praise!").

If the child becomes disruptive during a CDI session, parents are coached to ignore the child by looking away and not talking or gesturing to the child. Ignoring negative behavior helps the child understand the difference between the parents' responses to positive and negative behavior. Parents are advised that the ignored behavior may get worse before it gets better, and that the parent must follow through with ignoring until the child's behavior improves. Parents are then coached to return to the positive attention skills when the child begins to behave appropriately again. Parents are also coached to stop the interaction for behaviors that are particularly aggressive or destructive. These behaviors include hitting, biting, or breaking toys or objects. Therapists coach the parent to explain that the child's special time was ended because of the destructive or aggressive behavior (e.g., "Special time has to stop because you [hit]"). Parents are encouraged to reengage in the CDI at a later time when the child is calm.

Therapists continue to guide and coach parents in using the CDI skills until parents meet the minimum criteria for mastery during the initial 5-minute observation: (1) 10 behavioral descriptions; (2) 10 reflective statements; (3) 10 labeled praises; and (4) no more than three total questions, commands, or criticisms. Once parents have met these criteria, they move to the second phase of treatment: PDI. Because the CDI skills form an important foundation for establishing and maintaining effective discipline, however, the therapist continues to observe and code 5 minutes of CDI at the beginning of subsequent therapy sessions. If parents fall below the criterion on any of the CDI skills, the therapist will coach these skills before beginning the PDI coaching in that session. The 5-minute CDI home practice sessions also continue throughout treatment.

Parent-Directed Interaction

Primary goals of PDI include decreasing noncompliance and inappropriate behaviors that do not respond to ignoring or are too severe to ignore (e.g., hitting, destroying toys). Parents continue to give positive attention to appropriate behaviors in PDI. However, rather than exclusively following the child's lead, parents learn to give effective directions and to follow through consistently with calm, predictable responses to their child's behavior. Both parents and children know what consequences will follow the child's obedience or disobedience, which reduces parental anxiety and helps parents feel more in control of their child's behavior.

Therapists teach parents to give their children clear, positively stated, direct commands rather than criticisms (e.g., "Ask me quietly" rather than "Stop yelling") or indirect commands that suggest optional compliance (e.g., "Please sit down" rather than

"How about sitting here by me?"). Parents also learn to explain commands either before they are given ("It is time to leave the playroom. Please put the blocks in the container") or after they are obeyed ("Thank you for minding so quickly! The room is nice and clean for others now"). Parents learn to avoid arguing with the child by ignoring the child's delay tactics (e.g., "Why, Mom?") until the command has been obeyed. In addition to practicing commands during the teaching session, parents receive a handout summarizing the rules to review at home. Table 12.2 lists the eight rules for effective commands that therapists teach parents and includes examples of each.

Next, therapists teach parents specific steps to follow once a command has been given. If the child obeys, the parents give a labeled praise for compliance (e.g., "Thank you for listening!") and then returns to the CDI skills until the next command is needed. If the child disobeys, the parents initiate the time-out sequence. Parents are taught never to ignore noncompliance, because noncompliant behavior is reinforced if the child is permitted to disobey. The time-out procedure provides concrete steps to follow after the child disobeys, with three levels: warning, chair, and room. At each level, the child may choose to obey the parent and end the time-out. The procedure does not end until the child obeys the original command.

The Warning

The warning is given after the child first disobeys a direct command. Before giving the warning, the parent may give the child 5 seconds to begin obeying the command when it is unclear whether the child intends to obey. This 5-second rule is not used when the child clearly disobeys (e.g., after a command to hand the parent the red block, the child throws the block on the floor). The warning is the statement: "If you don't [original command], then you have to go to the time-out chair." If the warning is obeyed, the parent gives the child a labeled praise and the play continues.

The Chair

After the warning, the parent again uses the 5-second rule. If the child has not started to obey the warning within 5 seconds, the parent calmly and quickly takes the child to the time-out chair while saying, "You didn't do what I told you to do, so you have to sit on the time-out chair." This statement reminds the child of the reason for the punishment and reiterates the connection between noncompliance to a direct command and negative consequence. The parent may lead the child to the chair with just a touch or may carry the child from behind, if necessary, with arms under the child's arms and crossed over the child's chest. After placing the child on the chair, the parent says only, "Stay here until I say you can get off." This statement has a very different meaning than, for example, "Stay here until you are ready to behave." It is important for the parent to establish control of the time the child spends on the chair. If a child could get off the chair whenever he or she wished, time-out would be much less effective.

Therapists teach parents to ignore all negative behavior as long as the child stays on the chair. This skill may be difficult for parents because the child will often resort to various forms of emotional manipulation (e.g., "I don't love you anymore," "I want my Daddy," "I'm really really sorry") or, more rarely, negative physical behavior (e.g., taking off clothes). The child must stay on the chair for 3 minutes, plus 5 seconds of quiet at the

TABLE 12.2. Rules for Effective Commands

Rule	Reasons	Examples
Make commands direct rather than indirect.	• Leaves no question that the child is being instructed to do something. • Does not imply a choice or suggest that the parent might do the task for the child. • Reduces confusion for the child.	• Please hand me the car. • Put the block in the box. • Draw a circle. *Instead of* Will you draw a circle? Let's draw a circle.
State commands positively.	• Tells child what to do rather than what not to do. • Avoids criticism of the child's actions. • Provides a clear statement of what the child should do.	• Come sit beside me. *Instead of* Stop running around! • Put your hands in your pockets. *Instead of* Don't touch the glass.
Give commands one at a time.	• Helps child remember the whole command. • Enables parent to determine whether child completed entire command.	• Put the crayons in the box. *Instead of* Put the crayons in the box, put the box in the cupboard, and close the cupboard door. • Put all your shoes in the closet. *Instead of* Clean your room.
Make commands specific rather than vague.	• Tells child exactly what is supposed to be done.	• Get down off the table. *Instead of* Be careful. • Please sit quietly. *Instead of* Behave!
Make commands age appropriate.	• Ensures that child can understand what is expected.	• Put these blue Legos (pointing) back in their box. *Instead of* Put the navy pieces in the proper container. • Draw a square. *Instead of* Draw a cube.
Give commands politely and respectfully.	• Prevents child from learning to obey only if yelled at. • Teaches child to obey polite and respectful commands. • Prepares child for school.	• Child: (banging block) Parent: (in normal voice) Please give me the block. *Instead of* Parent: (loudly) Stop banging and give me that block now!
Explain commands only before they are given or after they are obeyed.	• Explanations before commands help orient the child to the task. • Explanations after commands are obeyed are "heard" and meaningful. • Explanations after the command is given but before it is obeyed reinforce dawdling and often are not "heard."	• Parent: It is just about time for dinner. Please wash your hands. Child: Why? Parent: (ignores). Child: (obeys). Parent: Thank you for washing your hands before dinner. Clean hands keep germs away from your food so you won't get sick.
Use direct (effective) commands only when they are truly necessary.	• If a task is optional, it is better to use an indirect (optional) command or none at all. • If commands are reserved for important tasks, children will be less likely to "test" them.	• (Child is running around room.) Parent: Please sit in this chair. (Good time to use this command.) *Instead of* Please get me a tissue. (Not a good time to give this command, and important to consider whether this command is necessary.)

end of 3 minutes. These 5 seconds of quiet ensure that the child does not leave the chair with the impression that whatever he or she said or did on the chair immediately before the end of time-out caused the parent to end time-out.

Once the child's time on the chair is up, the parent is instructed to walk over to the child and say, "You are sitting quietly on the chair. Are you ready to [original command]?" If the child says "No," begins to argue, or ignores the parent, the parent says, "Then stay on the chair until I say you can get off." The parent then walks away and begins the 3-minute time period again. If the child indicates that he or she is ready, either by saying "Yes" or by getting off the chair in a compliant manner, the parent walks the child back to the task. The parent then indicates that the child should obey the original command (e.g., pointing to the block that the child was originally instructed to hand to the parent). A child rarely refuses to obey at this point, but if the child did disobey, the parent would say again, "You didn't do what I told you to do, so you have to sit on the time-out chair" and then follow through as before.

When the child does obey the original command, the parent gives only a brief acknowledgment, such as "Fine." The parent does not give the child extensive labeled praise at this point because the child did not comply until he or she was sent to time-out. Instead, the parent immediately gives the child another similar but very simple command. The child is also likely to obey this command, and at this point the parent gives the child highly enthusiastic labeled praise for minding and returns to CDI. This way, the child begins to distinguish between the positive responses that follow immediate compliance and the less reinforcing responses that follow compliance that requires time-out.

The Room

When time-out is necessary, the time-out chair alone may not be sufficient if the child gets off the chair without permission. For this reason, parents are taught to use a time-out room as a backup to teach their child to stay on the chair. Parents rarely need to use the time-out room after the first 2 or 3 weeks of PDI because generally children quickly learn to stay on the time-out chair once they realize they will have to go to the time-out room if they get up without permission.

When a child gets off the time-out chair without permission, the parent leads or carries the child to the time-out room while saying, "You got off the chair before I said you could, so you have to go to the time-out room." Once the child is in the time-out room, the parent stays just outside the door and keeps close track of the time. The child stays in the room for 1 minute plus 5 seconds of quiet. The parent then leads the child back to the time-out chair and says, "Stay on the chair until I say you can get off." The child's 3-minute time-out on the chair then starts over. This process may need to be repeated several times during the first time-out, so it is essential that the parent and therapist allow adequate time to follow through until the child learns that the parent is not going to concede.

The time-out room used in PCIT sessions should be easily accessible from the playroom and should be empty or contain only heavy furniture that the child cannot move. Ideally, this room would be constructed with a Dutch door, a half-door just high enough to prevent a child from climbing over it. The room should also have an observation window or a video camera through which the therapist can monitor the child's behavior. The time-out room selected for use in the child's home must be at least 5 x 5 square feet in size and well lit. Although the time-out room will need to be used for only a short time, it is important that it is well prepared so that it is both safe and effective. Some families have utility rooms that can be emptied for a few weeks. Use of a bathroom as a time-out room requires careful discussion of safety requirements, such as removing all cleaning solutions and medicines from cabinets and turning down the water temperature or disconnecting the water supply to a spare bathroom. Some families clear the child's bedroom of all but basic furniture for use as a time-out room during the first few weeks of PDI.

A child will often escalate his or her negative reactions (crying, yelling, kicking) when parents do not give in during the time-out procedure. Coaching time-out during the first and second PDI sessions allows therapists to support parents during the emotionally difficult process of learning consistency so that they do not give up, and it gives therapists many opportunities to teach parents about their own and their child's behavior. Therapists can convey accurate attributions about the reasons for the child's behavior and can provide behavioral interpretations of the change as it is occurring. They can coach parents in relaxation or anger-control techniques *in vivo*, if indicated. Additionally, if the child makes many journeys between the time-out chair and time-out room, the therapist can assure parents that their child does understand the process, is choosing time-out over obeying, but will complete the procedure and obey the original command within the session. Further information on the treatment protocol may be found in the PCIT treatment manual, accessible at *www.pcit.org*.

Measuring Therapy Progress

The therapist assesses the family's progress through PCIT in several ways. First, the observation and coding of parent–child interactions at the start of each session are used both to select the skills to target during the session and to determine when parents have met the criteria for moving from one phase of treatment to the next and for completing treatment. Before each session, parents also complete the Intensity scale of the Eyberg Child Behavior Inventory (ECBI), which measures the child's current frequency of disruptive behavior at home. The therapist graphs the score each week to monitor the child's progress and at various points in treatment shares this graph with the parents. One criterion for treatment termination is an ECBI Intensity score within 0.5 *SD* of the normal mean (raw score = 114, *T* score = 55 or lower). Finally, in addition to these criteria, treatment does not end until parents express confidence in their ability to manage their child's behavior and feel ready for treatment to end. Thus, PCIT is performance based rather than time limited, and the number of treatment sessions varies widely. The average length of treatment is 15 sessions, although completion in the range of 10–20 sessions is not uncommon. The dropout rate is about 35%, which compares favorably to the 40–60% commonly cited for child psychotherapy (Wierzbicki & Pekarik, 1993).

EVIDENCE ON THE EFFECTS OF PCIT

In the first randomized controlled trial (RCT) of PCIT, families receiving PCIT were compared with wait-list controls (WL; Schuhmann, Foote, Eyberg, Boggs, & Algina, 1998). Following initial assessment, 64 clinic-referred families were randomly assigned to an immediate treatment (IT) or WL condition. After treatment, parents in the IT condition interacted more positively with their child and reported clinically and statistically significant improvements in their child's behavior. These parents also reported less parenting stress and a more internal locus of control than WL parents.

In a second RCT investigating the efficacy of PCIT for treating disruptive behaviors of young children with mental retardation and comorbid ODD, mothers interacted more positively with their children, and their children were more compliant and less disruptive following treatment than WL children (Bagner & Eyberg, 2007). Mediational analyses revealed that increases in positive parenting behavior (i.e., praises, reflections, behavior descriptions) and decreases in negative parenting behavior during child-led play (i.e., questions, commands, criticisms) accounted for the changes in children's behavior after treatment (Bagner & Eyberg, 2007).

Maintenance of Treatment Gains

Several follow-up studies have demonstrated maintenance of treatment effects after PCIT. In the first long-term follow-up study of PCIT, decreases in parent and child negative behaviors and increases in positive behaviors and child compliance from baseline to 2-year follow-up showed moderate to large effect sizes for the 13 families who completed the follow-up (Eyberg et al., 2001). Parent ratings of child behavior problems, child activity level, and parenting stress also remained similar to posttreatment levels, and most of the children remained free of disruptive behavior diagnoses after 2 years (Eyberg et al., 2001).

A second study compared longitudinal outcomes of 23 treatment completers and 23 treatment dropouts at 1- to 3-year follow-up (Boggs et al., 2004). Families who completed treatment continued to show significant positive changes in ratings of their child's disruptive behavior and their own parenting stress, whereas families who dropped out of treatment indicated little change from baseline in their ratings (Boggs et al., 2004). At 3- to 6-year follow-up, 23 treatment completers continued to show behavioral gains with time (Hood & Eyberg, 2003). Maternal parenting confidence was also maintained over the 3- to 6-year follow-up period.

Although longitudinal follow-up has been encouraging, with group-level analyses demonstrating maintenance of treatment gains, continued research is needed to evaluate individual differences that affect maintenance. Three to 6 years after treatment, 75% of children showed clinically significant change, but 25% did not maintain their posttreatment gains (Hood & Eyberg, 2003). It is important to understand factors that place families at risk for relapse. It is possible that at-risk families require a period of consolidation (i.e., a few additional sessions after treatment goals have been met) to achieve durable treatment effects. Alternatively, DBDs or maladaptive parenting styles may be chronic conditions for some families, who require ongoing monitoring and treatment. Families who have previously demonstrated the commitment to succeed in treatment may rally quickly with timely booster treatment.

Treatment Attrition

Attrition from PCIT is about 35% (Fernandez & Eyberg, 2009; Werba, Eyberg, Boggs, & Algina, 2006). Several factors that affect successful completion of PCIT have been identified. Because treatment is performance based and continues until the treatment goals are met, the only way a family cannot succeed, theoretically, is by dropping out. In reality, most families complete PCIT in 16 or fewer sessions (Werba et al., 2006), and families who drop out after 20 sessions may not have succeeded with further treatment. Nevertheless, families who meet the criteria for treatment completion are successful treatment completers, and PCIT dropouts are treatment failures (Boggs et al., 2004).

Studies investigating predictors of attrition from PCIT have identified maternal praise and criticism of the child during parent–child interactions and lower socioeconomic status as pretreatment predictors of dropout (Fernandez & Eyberg, 2009). The most common reason cited by parents for dropping out is disagreement with the treatment approach; other commonly cited reasons are being too busy to participate and having additional stressors that interfere with participation (Fernandez & Eyberg, 2009). Preventing treatment attrition continues to be a challenge in PCIT research and treatment.

Moderators of Outcome

Most PCIT outcome studies have been conducted in psychology clinics at major metropolitan medical centers using culturally heterogeneous samples of referred boys and girls with disruptive behavior. Despite this demographic diversity, few studies have investigated results separately for demographic groups. One study examined outcomes for 18 African American families drawn from earlier studies and found that attrition was high in this group (56%), with most families dropping out after the pretreatment assessment but before treatment began. For the treatment completers, however, there was significant improvement in parent-reported child behavior problems, with an effect size of $d = 0.97$ (Fernandez, Butler, & Eyberg, 2009). Studies have also examined treatment effects within particular cultural groups (e.g., McCabe & Yeh, in press), but formal tests of treatment moderation have not, to our knowledge, been conducted. Research on moderators of outcome may reveal ways to refine treatment to improve retention.

Application to New Populations

PCIT has been used clinically to treat behavior problems associated with an array of primary diagnoses beyond the DBDs, including neurological impairments, developmental disorders, and chronic medical conditions (Bagner et al., in press; Brinkmeyer & Eyberg, 2003). Successful completion of PCIT has resulted in significant reduction of internalizing behaviors as well as disruptive behaviors among children with problems in both domains (Chase & Eyberg, 2008). The behavioral principles and skills parents learn in PCIT are not problem specific but apply to classes of behaviors parents wish to either increase or decrease. For example, the positive reinforcement of parental attention will increase positive child behavior, whether that behavior reflects assertiveness or cooperation (Chase & Eyberg, 2008).

PCIT has also been implemented in treatment with abusive families, where the identified patient is typically the parent. Coercive parent–child relationships that characterize families of disruptive children are central to physically abusive families. Further, because abusive families tend to experience few positive interactions, they seem to benefit greatly from coaching in positive parenting skills that facilitate warm, enjoyable family experiences. An RCT conducted by Chaffin et al. (2004) found that physically abusive parents who underwent PCIT were significantly less likely to be reported again for child abuse than parents assigned to a standard community treatment condition. The greater reduction of coercive parent–child interactions in the PCIT condition was shown to mediate the re-abuse outcome.

Clinically significant changes in disruptive child behaviors and parenting stress and competence after PCIT have been documented in studies across cultural groups, including an RCT with Mexican American families (McCabe & Yeh, in press), a pre–post comparison study with Puerto Rican families (Matos, Torres, Santiago, Jurado, & Rodriguez, 2006), a quasi-experimental study with Chinese families (Leung, Tsang, Heung, & Yiu, in press), and both an RCT (Nixon, Sweeny, Erickson, & Touyz, 2003) and a pre–post comparison study (Phillips, Morgan, Cawthorne, & Barnett, 2008) with Australian families. The Phillips et al. (2008) study was notable for its highly successful implementation by community providers in a large mental health clinic.

Successful implementation of PCIT in diverse populations necessitates careful consideration of the cultural factors related to mental health utilization, family structure, discipline norms, and language. As PCIT has been investigated in different cultural groups, the protocol has been adapted to strengthen treatment acceptance and success. When PCIT was introduced to Puerto Rican families, for example, the assessment and treatment materials were translated into Spanish (Matos et al., 2006). Cultural norms were also addressed in several ways in a Mexican American adaptation of PCIT by McCabe and Yeh (in press). They presented the program as an educational/skill-building intervention to reduce the stigma associated with seeking mental health services among the Mexican American community. The Mexican American adaptation also extended the length of treatment sessions to permit more time for social exchanges deemed important to rapport in that culture. As PCIT has been studied around the world, treatment teams have remained in close contact with PCIT experts in the United States to ensure that protocol changes do not compromise treatment integrity.

DIRECTIONS FOR RESEARCH

Studies of PCIT have been presented describing treatment efficacy and generalization of effects across cultures, settings, and time for the majority of families who enter treatment. However, the high prevalence of young children with disruptive behavior as well as children in abusive family situations, combined with the poor long-term prognosis for these children if not treated, highlights the significant need for access to EBTs in real-world settings. Increasing demands within mental health agencies and institutes worldwide to use EBTs requires training of service providers outside traditional graduate training programs. Yet to date, there have been no RCTs of PCIT conducted in community settings by real-world clinicians. It is essential to learn whether PCIT can translate to practice without losing effectiveness.

Therapist training is key to broad dissemination of PCIT. PCIT delivery assumes a broad background of clinical knowledge and skills. Skills specific to PCIT are also necessary for coding parent–child interactions and conducting ongoing functional analyses of parent and child behaviors during coaching to guide parent skills training and determine when to move from one step in treatment to the next. A recent study suggested these therapist skills cannot be learned from reading or didactic course work alone but require some degree of experiential training followed by case supervision (Herschell et al., 2009). Training guidelines for PCIT have been developed (PCIT Committee on Training, 2009), but much more study is needed to delineate the parameters of training and qualifications of clinicians necessary for effective implementation of PCIT.

Cost-effectiveness studies are also needed. As health care costs rise for the average family, and community providers struggle to find funding to serve more children, examining ways to boost time- and cost-effectiveness of treatment without diminishing outcome effects is increasingly important. In one study, we are comparing the cost-effectiveness of group versus individual PCIT for children with a primary diagnosis of ADHD. This study also examines the role of comorbid child and parent psychopathology in moderating outcomes for these two formats of treatment. In other studies with families presenting less severe psychopathology, we are exploring effects of a self-administered version of PCIT as well as an intensive form of PCIT delivered over the course of a week. Consideration of family characteristics may determine the optimal format of PCIT to maximize cost-effectiveness without compromising efficacy or maintenance of treatment gains.

CONCLUSIONS

This chapter describes parent–child interaction therapy for young children with DBDs and their families. Key elements of the treatment are illustrated, including involvement of the parents and child together in treatment, use of assessment to guide the family's progress, active coaching of parents in relationship and behavior change skills, and continuation of treatment until parents have mastered the skills and their child's behavior is within the normal range. These features of PCIT draw on both attachment and social learning principles to produce lasting improvements in the parent–child relationship and lasting reductions in the child's disruptive behavior.

Designated an EBT by the *Journal of Clinical Child and Adolescent Psychology* (Silverman & Hinshaw, 2008) and deemed a "best practice" in the field of child abuse treatment by the Kauffman Best Practices Project (Chadwick Center for Children and Families, 2004), PCIT is effective within a relatively brief period of time. Although sometimes criticized for its strict adherence to a manualized treatment protocol, PCIT has considerable flexibility for individualizing treatment to each family's unique needs.

Since its inception more than 30 years ago, PCIT has been empirically studied and refined based on results from scientific investigations. Although many studies have demonstrated the efficacy of PCIT, many research questions remain. Future study with diverse populations and in new settings will provide guidelines for tailoring or adapting PCIT within real-world settings to provide optimal care for children with disruptive behavior and their families.

REFERENCES

Bagner, D. M., & Eyberg, S. M. (2007). Parent–child interaction therapy for disruptive behavior in children with mental retardation: A randomized controlled trial. *Journal of Clinical Child and Adolescent Psychology, 36*, 418–429.

Bagner, D. M., Sheinkopf, S. J., Miller-Loncar, C. L., Vohr, B. R., Hinckley, M., Eyberg, S. M., et al. (in press). Parent–child interaction therapy for children born premature: A case study and illustration of vagal tone as a physiological measure of treatment outcome. *Journal of Cognitive and Behavioral Practice.*

Baumrind, D. (1966). Effects of authoritative control on child behavior. *Child Development, 37,* 887–907.

Boggs, S.R., Eyberg, S. M., Edwards, D., Rayfield, A., Jacobs, J., Bagner, D., et al. (2004). Outcomes of parent–child interaction therapy: A comparison of dropouts and treatment completers one to three years after treatment. *Child and Family Behavior Therapy, 26,* 1–22.

Brinkmeyer, M., & Eyberg, S. M. (2003). Parent–child interaction therapy for oppositional children. In A. E. Kazdin & J. R. Weisz (Eds.), *Evidence-based psychotherapies for children and adolescents* (pp. 204–223). New York: Guilford Press.

Chadwick Center for Children and Families. (2004). *Closing the quality chasm in child abuse treatment: Identifying and disseminating best practices. The findings of the Kauffman Best Practices Project to help children heal from child abuse.* San Diego, CA: Children's Hospital San Diego, Chadwick Center for Children and Families.

Chaffin, M., Silovsky, J. F., Funderburk, B., Valle, L. A., Brestan, E. V., Balachova, T., et al. (2004). Parent–child interaction therapy with physically abusive parents: Efficacy for reducing future abuse reports. *Journal of Consulting and Clinical Psychology, 72,* 500–510.

Chase, R. M., & Eyberg, S. M. (2008). Clinical presentation and treatment outcome for children with comorbid externalizing and internalizing symptoms. *Journal of Anxiety Disorders, 22,* 273–282.

Eyberg, S. M., Funderburk, B. W., Hembree-Kigin, T. L., McNeil, C. B., Querido, J. G., & Hood, K. (2001). Parent–child interaction therapy with behavior problem children: One and two year maintenance of treatment effects in the family. *Child and Family Behavior Therapy, 23,* 1–20.

Fernandez, M. A., Butler, A., & Eyberg, S. M. (2009). *Treatment outcome for African American families in parent–child interaction therapy: A pilot study.* Manuscript submitted for publication.

Fernandez, M. A., & Eyberg, S. M. (2009). Predicting treatment and follow-up attrition in parent–child interaction therapy. *Journal of Abnormal Child Psychology, 37,* 431–441.

Guevara, J. P., Mandell, D. S., Rostain, A. L., Zhao, H., & Hadley, T. R. (2003). National estimates of health services expenditures for children with behavioral disorders: An analysis of the Medical Expenditure Panel survey. *Pediatrics, 112,* e440–e446.

Hann, D. M., & Borek, N. (2001). *Taking stock of risk factors for child/youth externalizing behavior problems.* Washington, DC: Department of Health and Human Services, Public Health Service, National Institute of Mental Health.

Herschell, A. D., McNeil, C. B., Urquiza, A. J., McGrath, J. M., Zebell, N. M., Timmer, S. G., et al. (2009). Evaluation of a treatment manual and workshops for disseminating parent–child interaction therapy. *Administration and Policy in Mental Health, 36,* 63–81.

Hood, K., & Eyberg, S. M. (2003). Outcomes of parent–child interaction therapy: Mothers' reports on maintenance three to six years after treatment. *Journal of Clinical Child and Adolescent Psychology, 32,* 419–429.

Leung, C., Tsang, S., Heung, K., & Yiu, I. (in press). Effectiveness of parent child interaction therapy (PCIT) among Chinese families. *Research on Social Work Practice.*

Matos, M., Torres, R., Santiago, R., Jurado, M., & Rodriguez, I. (2006). Adaptation of parent–child interaction therapy for Puerto Rican families: A preliminary study. *Family Process, 45,* 205–222.

McCabe, K., & Yeh, M. (in press). Parent–child interaction therapy for Mexican Americans: A randomized clinical trial. *Journal of Clinical Child and Adolescent Psychology.*

Nixon, R. D. V., Sweeny, L., Erickson, D. B., & Touyz, S. W. (2003). Parent–child interaction therapy: A comparison of standard and abbreviated treatments for oppositional defiant preschoolers. *Journal of Consulting and Clinical Psychology, 71,* 251–260.

PCIT Committee on Training. (2008). *Training guidelines for parent–child interaction therapy.* Retrieved March 10, 2009, from *www.pcit.org.*

Phillips, J., Morgan, S., Cawthorne, K., & Barnett, B. (2008). Pilot evaluation of parent–child interaction therapy delivered in an Australian community early childhood clinic setting. *Australian and New Zealand Journal of Psychiatry, 42,* 712–719.

Querido, J. G., Warner, T. D., & Eyberg, S. M. (2002). The cultural context of parenting: An assessment of parenting styles in African-American families. *Journal of Clinical Child and Adolescent Psychology, 31,* 272–277.

Schuhmann, E. M., Foote, R., Eyberg, S. M., Boggs, S., & Algina, J. (1998). Parent–child interaction therapy: Interim report of a randomized trial with short-term maintenance. *Journal of Clinical Child Psychology, 27,* 34–45.

Silverman, W. K., & Hinshaw, S. P. (2008). The second special issue on evidence-based psychosocial treatments for children and adolescents: A 10-year update. *Journal of Clinical Child and Adolescent Psychology, 37,* 1–7.

Werba, B. E., Eyberg, S. M., Boggs, S., & Algina, J. (2006). Predicting outcome in parent–child interaction therapy: Success and attrition. *Behavior Modification, 30,* 618–646.

Wierzbicki, M., & Pekarik, G. (1993). A meta-analysis of psychotherapy dropout. *Professional Psychology: Research and Practice, 24,* 190–195.

13

The Incredible Years Parents, Teachers, and Children Training Series

A Multifaceted Treatment Approach for Young Children with Conduct Disorders

CAROLYN WEBSTER-STRATTON and M. JAMILA REID

OVERVIEW OF THE CLINICAL PROBLEM

The incidence of oppositional defiant disorder (ODD) and conduct disorder (CD) in children is alarmingly high, with reported rates of early-onset conduct problems in young preschool children ranging from 4–6% (Egger & Angold, 2006) and as high as 35% for low-income families (Webster-Stratton & Hammond, 1998). Developmental theorists have suggested that, compared with typical children, early-starter delinquents—that is, those who first exhibit ODD symptoms in the preschool years—have a two- to threefold risk of becoming tomorrow's serious violent and chronic juvenile offenders (Loeber et al., 1993; Patterson, Capaldi, & Bank, 1991; Snyder, 2001; Tremblay et al., 2000). These children with early-onset CD also account for a disproportionate share of delinquent acts in adulthood, including interpersonal violence, substance abuse, and property crimes. Indeed, the primary developmental pathway for serious CDs in adolescence and adulthood appears to be established during the preschool period.

Risk factors from a number of different areas contribute to child conduct problems, including ineffective parenting (Jaffee, Caspi, Moffitt, & Taylor, 2004), family mental health and criminal risk factors (Knutson, DeGarmo, Koeppl, & Reid, 2005), child biological and developmental risk factors (e.g., attention-deficit disorders, learning disabilities, language delays), school risk factors (Hawkins, Catalano, Kosterman, Abbott, & Hill, 1999), and peer and community risk factors (e.g., poverty and gangs) (Collins, Maccoby, Steinberg, Hetherington, & Bornstein, 2000; Hawkins et al., 2008). Treatment–outcome studies suggest that interventions for CD are of limited effect when offered in adolescence, after delinquent and aggressive behaviors are entrenched and secondary risk factors such as academic failure, school absence, and the formation of deviant peer groups have developed (Dishion & Piehler, 2007; Offord & Bennet, 1994). In fact, group-based interventions targeting adolescents with CD may result in worsening of symptoms through exposure to delinquent peers (Dishion, McCord, & Poulin, 1999)

This increased treatment resistance in older CD probands results in part from delinquent behaviors becoming embedded in a broader array of reinforcement systems, including those at the family, school, peer group, neighborhood, and community levels (Lynam et al., 2000). In contrast, there is evidence that the younger a child is at the time of intervention, the more positive the behavioral adjustment at home and at school. For these reasons, The Incredible Years treatment programs were designed to thwart and treat behavior problems when they first begin (infant/toddler through elementary school age) and to intervene in multiple areas through parent, teacher, and child training. It is our belief that early intervention can counteract risk factors and strengthen protective factors, thereby helping to prevent a developmental trajectory to increasingly aggressive and violent behaviors.

CHARACTERISTICS OF THE TREATMENT PROGRAM

To address the parenting, family, child, and school risk factors, we have developed three complementary training curricula, known as The Incredible Years Training Series, targeted at parents, teachers, and children (ages 0–13 years). This chapter reviews these training programs and their associated research.

The Incredible Years Parent Interventions

Goals of the Parent Programs

Goals of the parent programs are to promote parent competencies and strengthen families by

- Increasing positive parenting, self-confidence, and parent–child bonding.
- Teaching parents to coach children's academic and verbal skills, persistence and sustained attention, and social and emotional development.
- Decreasing harsh discipline and increasing positive strategies such as ignoring, logical consequences, redirecting, monitoring, and problem solving.
- Improving parents' problem solving, anger management, and communication.
- Increasing family support networks and school involvement/bonding.
- Helping parents and teachers work collaboratively.
- Increasing parents' involvement in children's academic-related activities at home.

Content of the BASIC Parent Training Treatment Program

In 1980, we developed an interactive, videotape-based parent intervention (BASIC) for parents of children ages 2–7. More recently, we revised and updated this program to include four separate age range BASIC programs: infant (0–1 years), toddler (1–3 years), preschool (3–6 years), and school age (6–13 years). Each of these revised programs includes age-appropriate examples of more culturally diverse families, children with varying temperaments, and added emphases on social and emotional coaching, problem solving, establishing predictable routines, and supporting children's academic success. The baby program is eight to nine weekly 2-hour sessions with parents and infants. The BASIC toddler–parent training program is usually completed in 12 weekly 2-hour sessions while the preschool and school-age programs are 18–20 weekly sessions. The foundation of the therapist-led program is video vignettes of modeled parenting skills (more than 300 vignettes, each lasting approximately 1–3 minutes) shown to groups of eight to 12 parents. The videos demonstrate social learning and child development principles and serve as the stimulus for focused discussions, problem solving, and collaborative learning. The program is also designed to help parents understand typical child development and temperaments.

The BASIC program begins with a focus on enhancing positive parent–child relationships by teaching parents to use child-directed interactive play, academic and persistence coaching, social and emotional coaching, praise, and incentive programs. Next, parents learn how to set up predicable home routines and rules, followed by learning a specific set of nonviolent discipline techniques, including monitoring, ignoring, commands, natural and logical consequences, and ways to use time-out to teach children to calm down. Finally, parents are taught how they can teach their children problem-solving skills.

Content of the ADVANCE Parent Training Treatment Program

In addition to parenting behavior per se, other aspects of parents' behavior and personal lives constitute risk factors for child conduct problems. Researchers have demonstrated that personal and interpersonal risk factors such as parental depression, marital discord, lack of social support, poor problem-solving ability, and environmental stressors disrupt parenting behavior and contribute to coercive parent–child interactions and relapses subsequent to parent training. This evidence led us to expand our theoretical and causal model concerning conduct problems, and in 1989 we developed the ADVANCE treatment program, updated in 2008. We theorized that a broader based training model (i.e., one involving helping parents with conflict management issues) would help mediate the negative influences of these personal and interpersonal factors on parenting skills and promote increased maintenance and generalizability of treatment effects.

The content of this 10- to 12-session video program (more than 90 vignettes), which is offered after the completion of the BASIC training program, involves five components:

1. *Personal self-control.* Parents learn to substitute positive self-talk for depressive, angry, and blaming self-talk. Parents learn specific anger management techniques.
2. *Communication skills.* Parents are taught to identify blocks to communication and to learn effective communication skills for dealing with conflict.
3. *Problem-solving skills for adults.* Parents are taught effective strategies for cop-

ing with conflict with spouses, employers, extended family members, and teachers.

4. *Teaching children problem solving.* Parents learn to use problem-solving strategies with their children. Parents of older children learn to conduct family meetings.

5. *Strengthening social support and self-care.* Group members learn to ask for support when necessary and to give support to others.

The content of both the BASIC and ADVANCE programs is also provided in the text that parents use for the program: *The Incredible Years: A Trouble-Shooting Guide for Parents of Children Aged 3–8* (Webster-Stratton, 2006).

Content of the SCHOOL Parent Training Treatment

In follow-up interviews with parents who completed our parent training programs, 58% requested guidance on school-related issues such as homework, communication with teachers, school behavior problems, and schoolwork. These data suggested a need for teaching parents to access schools, collaborate with teachers, and supervise children's peer relationships. In addition, 40% of teachers reported problems with children's compliance and aggression in the classroom. Clearly, integrating interventions across home and school settings to target school and family risk factors fosters greater between-environment consistency and offers the best chance for long-term reduction of antisocial behavior.

In 1990 we developed an interactive video modeling academic skills training intervention (SCHOOL) as an adjunct to our school-age BASIC program and a school readiness intervention as an adjunct to our preschool BASIC program. These two interventions consist of four to six additional sessions that are offered to parents after completing the BASIC program. For parents of school-age children, these sessions focus on parent–teacher collaboration, ways to foster children's academic readiness and school success through parental involvement in school activities and homework, and the importance of after-school and peer monitoring. For parents of preschool children, the sessions focus on interactive reading skills and ways to promote children's social, emotional, self-regulation, and cognitive skills. Program components include:

1. *Promoting children's self-confidence.* Parents lay the foundation for school success by helping children feel confident about their own ideas and ability to learn.

2. *Promoting children's school readiness, academic success.* Parents prepare their young children for school by facilitating language and reading skills. Parents of school-age children establish a predictable homework routine and learn strategies to support homework success.

3. *Dealing with children's discouragement and learning difficulties.* Parents think about realistic goals for their children, help them persist with difficult tasks, tailor learning tasks to their children's abilities, and use praise, tangible rewards, and academic coaching to motivate and reinforce learning progress at home.

4. *Using teacher–parent conferences to advocate for children.* Parents learn to collaborate with teachers to develop behavior plans that address school difficulties, such as inattention, impulsiveness, noncompliance, social problems, and aggression.

The Incredible Years Teacher Training Intervention

Once children with behavior problems enter school, negative academic and social experiences escalate the development of conduct problems. Aggressive, disruptive children quickly become socially excluded, which leads to fewer opportunities to interact socially and learn appropriate friendship skills. Evidence suggests that peer rejection eventually leads to association with deviant peers. Once children have formed deviant peer groups, the risk for drug abuse and antisocial behavior is even higher.

Furthermore, teacher behaviors and school characteristics, such as low emphasis on teaching social and emotional competence, low rates of praise, and high student–teacher ratio are associated with classroom aggression, delinquency, and poor academic performance. Aggressive children frequently develop poor relationships with teachers and are often expelled from classrooms. In our own studies of children ages 3–7 with conduct problems, more than 50% of the children had been asked to leave three or more classrooms by second grade. Lack of teacher support and exclusion from the classroom exacerbate social problems and academic difficulties, contributing to the likelihood of school dropout.

Goals of the Teacher Training Programs

The goals are to promote teacher competencies and strengthen home–school connections by

- Strengthening teachers' effective classroom management skills.
- Strengthening teachers' use of academic, persistence, social, and emotional coaching with students.
- Strengthening positive relationships between teachers and students.
- Increasing teachers' use of effective discipline strategies.
- Increasing teachers' collaborative efforts with parents.
- Increasing teachers' ability to teach social skills, anger management, and problem-solving skills in the classroom.
- Decreasing levels of classroom aggression.

Content of Teacher Training Intervention

The teacher training intervention is a 6-day (or 42-hour) group-format program for teachers, school counselors, and psychologists. Training targets teachers' use of effective classroom management strategies for dealing with misbehavior; promoting positive relationships with difficult students; strengthening social skills and emotional regulation in the classroom, on the playground, on the bus, and in the lunchroom; and strengthening teachers' collaborative process and positive communication with parents (e.g., the importance of positive home communication, home visits, and successful parent conferences). Teachers, parents, and group facilitators jointly develop transition plans that detail successful classroom strategies for children with conduct problems; characteristics, interests, and motivators for the children; and ways parents would like to be contacted by teachers. This information follows the children each year, being passed along to each teacher at the new grade level. In addition, teachers learn to prevent peer rejection by helping aggressive children learn appropriate problem-solving strategies and helping their peers to respond appropriately to aggression. Teachers are encouraged to be sensitive to developmental differences and biological deficits among the children and the relevance of these differences for enhanced teaching efforts that are positive, accepting, and consistent. Physical aggression is targeted for close monitoring, teaching, and incentive programs. A complete description of the content included in this curriculum is described in the book that teachers use for the course: *How to Promote Children's Social and Emotional Competence* (Webster-Stratton, 2000).

The Incredible Years Child Training Intervention (Dinosaur School)

Research has indicated that some abnormal aspects of children's internal organization at the physiological, neurological, or neuropsychological level are linked to the development of CDs, particularly for children with a chronic history of early behavioral problems. Children with conduct problems are more likely to have certain temperamental characteristics such as inattentiveness, impulsivity, and attention-deficit/hyperactivity disorder (ADHD). Other child factors have also been implicated in early-onset CD. For example, deficits in social-cognitive skills and negative attributions contribute to poor emotional regulation and aggressive peer interactions. In addition, studies indicate that children with conduct problems have significant delays in their peer-play skills, in particular difficulty with reciprocal play, cooperative skills, taking turns, waiting, and giving suggestions. Finally, reading, learning, and language delays are also associated with conduct problems, particularly for "early life course persisters." The relationship between academic performance and ODD/CD is bidirectional. Academic difficulties may cause disengagement, increased frustration, and lower self-esteem, which contribute to behavior problems. At the same time, noncompliance, aggression, elevated activity levels, and poor attention limit children's ability to engage in learning and to achieve academically. Thus, a cycle is created in which one problem exacerbates the other. This combination of academic delays and conduct problems appears to contribute to the development of more severe CD and school failure.

These data suggest that children with conduct problems and ADHD require additional structure, monitoring, and overteaching (i.e., repeated learning trials) to learn to inhibit undesirable behaviors and to manage emotion. Parents and teachers need to use predictable routines; consistent, clear, specific limit setting; simple and calm language; concrete cues; and frequent reminders and redirections. In addition, this information suggests the need for direct intervention with children, focusing on their particular social learning needs, such as problem solving, perspective taking, and play skills as well as literacy and special academic needs.

Goals of the Child Training Programs

The goals are to promote children's competencies and reduce aggressive and noncompliant behaviors by

- Strengthening children's social skills and appropriate play skills.
- Promoting children's use of self-control and self-regulation strategies.

- Increasing emotional awareness by labeling feelings, recognizing the differing views of oneself and others, and enhancing perspective taking.
- Promoting children's ability to persist with and attend to difficult tasks.
- Boosting academic success, reading, and school readiness.
- Reducing defiance, aggression, noncompliance, peer rejection, bullying, stealing, and lying and promoting compliance with teachers and peers.
- Decreasing negative attributions and conflict management approaches.
- Increasing self-esteem and self-confidence.

Content of Child Training Treatment

In 1990 we developed a video modeling a treatment program for children with conduct problems (ages 3–8). This 22-week program consists of a series of DVD programs (more than 180 vignettes) that teach children problem-solving and social skills. Organized to dovetail with the content of the parent training program, the program consists of seven main components: (1) introduction and rules, (2) empathy and emotion, (3) problem solving, (4) anger control, (5) friendship skills, (6) communication skills, and (7) school skills. The children meet weekly in small groups of six for 2 hours.

Group Process and Methods Used in Parent, Teacher, and Child Training Programs

All three treatment approaches rely on performance training methods, including videotape modeling, role play, practice activities, and live feedback from the therapist and other group members. In accordance with modeling and self-efficacy theories of learning, parents, teachers, and children using the program develop their skills by watching (and modeling) video examples of key management and interpersonal skills. We theorized that video examples provide a more flexible method of training than didactic verbal instruction or sole reliance on role play; that is, we could portray a wide variety of models and situations. We hypothesized that this flexible modeling approach would result in better generalization of the training content and, therefore, better long-term maintenance. Further, it would be a better method of learning for less verbally oriented learners. Finally, such a method has the advantage not only of low individual training cost when used in groups but also of possible mass dissemination. Heavily guided by the modeling literature, each program aims to promote modeling effects for participants by creating positive feelings about the video models. For example, the video vignettes show parents, teachers, and children of differing ages, cultures, socioeconomic backgrounds, and temperaments so that participants will perceive at least some of the models as similar to themselves and will, therefore, accept the vignettes as relevant. Whenever possible, vignettes show models (unrehearsed) in natural situations "doing it effectively" and "doing it less effectively" in order to demystify the notion that there is "perfect parenting or teaching" and to illustrate how one can learn from one's mistakes. This approach also emphasizes our belief in a coping and interactive model of learning (Webster-Stratton & Herbert, 1994); that is, participants view a vignette of a situation and then discuss and role-play how the character might have handled the interaction more effectively. Thus, participants improve on the interactions they see in the vignettes. This approach enhances participants' confidence in their own ideas and develops their ability to analyze interpersonal situations and select an appropriate response. In this respect, our training differs from some other training programs in which the therapist provides the analysis and recommends a particular strategy.

The video vignettes demonstrate behavioral principles and serve as the stimulus for discussions, problem solving, and collaborative learning. After each vignette, the therapist solicits ideas from the group and involves them in the process of problem solving, sharing, and discussing ideas and reactions. The therapist's role is to support group members by teaching, leading, reframing, predicting, and role-playing, always within a collaborative context. The collaborative context is designed to ensure that the intervention is sensitive to participants' cultural differences and personal values. The program is tailored to each teacher, parent, or child's individual needs and personal goals as well as to each child's personality and behavior problems.

This program also implies a commitment to group members' self-management. We believe that this approach is empowering in that it restores the dignity, respect, and self-control of parents, teachers, and children, who are often seeking help at time of low self-confidence and feelings of self-blame. The group format is more cost-effective than individual intervention and also addresses an important risk factor for children with conduct problems: the family's isolation and stigmatization. The parent groups provide that support and become a model for parent support networks. (For details of therapeutic processes, please see Webster-Stratton & Herbert, 1994.) The child groups provide children with conduct problems some of their first positive social experiences with peers. Moreover, it was theorized that the group approach would provide more social and emotional support and decrease feelings of isolation for teachers as well as parents and children.

The child program video vignettes show children of differing ages, sexes, and cultures interacting with adults (parents or teachers) or with peers. After viewing the vignettes, children discuss feelings, generate ideas for more effective responses, and role-play alternative scenarios. In addition to the interactive video vignettes, the therapists use life-size puppets to model appropriate behavior and thinking processes for the children. The use of puppets appeals to children on the fantasy level so predominant in this preoperational age group. Because young children are more vulnerable to distraction, are less able to organize their thoughts, and have poorer memories, we use a number of strategies for reviewing and organizing the material, such as (1) playing "copycat" to review skills learned; (2) using many video examples of the same concept in different situations and settings; (3) using cartoon pictures and specially designed stickers as cues to remind children of key concepts; (4) role-playing with puppets and other children to provide practice opportunities; (5) reenacting video scenes; (6) rehearsing skills with play, art, and game activities; (7) assigning homework so children can practice key skills with parents; and (8) distributing letters to parents and teachers that explain the key concepts children are learning and asking them to reinforce these behaviors.

EVIDENCE FOR THE EFFECTS OF TREATMENT

Effects of Parent Training Program

The efficacy of The Incredible Years BASIC parent treatment program for children (ages 3–8) diagnosed with ODD/CD has been demonstrated in numerous published randomized control group trials (RCT) by the program developer and colleagues at the

University of Washington Parenting Clinic (Reid, Webster-Stratton, & Hammond, 2007; Webster-Stratton, 1981, 1982, 1984, 1990a, 1992, 1994, 1998; Webster-Stratton & Hammond, 1997; Webster-Stratton, Hollinsworth, & Kolpacoff, 1989; Webster-Stratton, Kolpacoff, & Hollinsworth, 1988; Webster-Stratton, Reid, & Hammond, 2004). In all of these studies, the BASIC program has been shown to improve parental attitudes and parent–child interactions and reduce harsh discipline and child conduct problems compared with both wait-list control groups. A treatment component analysis indicated that the combination of group discussion, trained therapist, and video modeling produced the most lasting results compared with treatment that involved only one training component (Webster-Stratton, Kolpacoff, & Hollinsworth, 1988; Webster-Stratton, Hollinsworth, & Kolpacoff, 1989). In addition, the BASIC program has been replicated in five projects by independent investigators in mental health clinics with families of children diagnosed with conduct problems (Drugli & Larsson, 2006; Larsson, Fossum, Clifford, Drugli, Handigard, & Morch, 2008; Lavigne et al., 2008; Scott, Spender, Doolan, Jacobs, & Aspland, 2001; Spaccarelli, Cotler, & Penman, 1992; Taylor, Schmidt, Pepler, & Hodgins, 1998) as well as with indicated populations (children with symptoms) and high-risk populations (families in poverty; Gardner, Burton, & Klimes, 2006; Gross et al., 2003; Hutchings et al., 2007; Miller Brotman et al., 2003). These replications were effectiveness trials done in applied mental health settings, not a university research clinic, and the therapists were typical therapists at the centers. Three of the replications were conducted in the United States, two in the United Kingdom, and one in Norway. This illustrates the transportability of the BASIC parenting program to other cultures. See Table 13.1 for summary of all studies of The Incredible Years programs.

In our fourth study (Webster-Stratton, 1994), we examined the effects of adding the ADVANCE intervention component to the BASIC intervention by randomly assigning families to either BASIC parent training or BASIC plus ADVANCE training. Both treatment groups showed improvements in child adjustment and parent–child interactions and a decrease in parent distress and child behavior problems. These changes were maintained at follow-up. ADVANCE children showed significantly greater increases in the number of prosocial solutions generated during problem solving in comparison to those whose parents received only the BASIC program. Observations of parents' marital interactions indicated significantly greater improvements in ADVANCE parents' communication, problem solving, and collaboration skills compared with parents who did not receive ADVANCE.

Overall, these results suggest that focusing on helping families to manage personal distress and interpersonal marital issues through a video modeling group discussion treatment (ADVANCE) added to treatment outcomes for our BASIC program. Consequently, a 20- to 24-week program that combines BASIC plus ADVANCE has become our core treatment for parents with children with conduct problems.

In our sixth and seventh studies (Webster-Stratton & Hammond, 1997; and Webster-Stratton, Reid, & Hammond, 2004, respectively), we examined the additive effects of combining our child training intervention (Classroom Dinosaur School) and teacher training with the parent training program (BASIC plus ADVANCE). Both studies replicated our results from the prior ADVANCE study and provided data on the advantages of training children and teachers as well as parents. (See a description of these study results in the Effects of Child and Teacher Training Programs section.)

TABLE 13.1. Summary of Treatment Results for Studies Evaluating The Incredible Years Programs

Study information

Program evaluated	Number of Studies[a]	Investigator: Program developer or independent replication	Population: Prevention or treatment
Parent	6	Developer	Treatment
Parent	4	Developer	Prevention
Child	2	Developer	Treatment
Child	1	Developer	Prevention
Teacher	1	Developer	Treatment
Teacher	2	Developer	Prevention
Parent	5	Replication	Treatment
Parent	5	Replication	Prevention
Child	1	Replication	Treatment
Child	1	Replication	Prevention
Teacher	2	Replication	Prevention

Outcomes

Variable measured (observation and report)	Effect Size[b] (Cohen's d)	Most effective program
Positive parenting increased	0.46–0.51	Parent
Harsh parenting decreased	0.74–0.81	Parent
Child home behavior problems decreased	0.41–0.67	Parent
Child social competence	0.69–0.79	Child
School readiness and engagement	0.82–2.87	Child and teacher
Child school behavior problems	0.71–1.23	Child and teacher
Parent–school bonding	0.57	Teacher
Teacher positive management	1.24	Teacher
Teacher critical teaching	0.32–1.37	Teacher

[a]All studies used a randomized control group design and are cited in the reference list.
[b]Effect sizes include both treatment and prevention studies conducted by the program developer. The range of effect sizes represents the range for a particular outcome across all studies that included that outcome measure. The information to calculate effect sizes for independent replications was not available.

Parent Training Treatment: Who Benefits and Who Does Not?

We have monitored families longitudinally (1, 2, and 3 years posttreatment), and for study 3 (Webster-Stratton, 1994) we have completed a 10- to 15-year follow-up. We have assessed both the statistical significance and the "clinical significance" of treatment effects. In assessing the clinical significance, we looked at the extent to which parent and teacher reports indicated that the children were within the normal or the nonclinical range of functioning or showed a 30% improvement if there were no established normative data and whether families requested further therapy for their children's behavior problems at the follow-up assessments. In our 3-year follow-up of 83 families treated with the BASIC program, we found that although approximately two-thirds of children showed behavior improvements, 25 to 46% of parents and 26% of teachers still reported child behavior problems (Webster-Stratton, 1990b). We also found that the families whose children had continuing externalizing problems (according to teacher and parent reports) at our 3-year follow-up assessments were more likely to be characterized by maritally distressed or single-parent status, increased maternal depression, lower social class, high levels of negative life stressors, and family histories of alcoholism, drug abuse, and spouse abuse (Webster-Stratton, 1990b; Webster-Stratton & Hammond, 1990).

Hartman, Stage, and Webster-Stratton (2003) examined whether child ADHD symptoms (i.e., inattention, impulsivity, and hyperactivity) predicted poorer treatment results with the parent training intervention (BASIC). Contrary to Hartman et al.'s hypothesis, analyses suggested that the children with ODD/CD who had higher levels of attention problems showed greater reductions in conduct problems than children with no attention problems. Similar findings for children with ADHD were reported in the UK study (Scott et al., 2001). Currently, a study is underway by the developer to evaluate the parent and child treatments for young children with a primary diagnosis of ADHD.

Rinaldi (2001) conducted an 8- to 12-year follow-up of families who were in the ADVANCE study in which she interviewed 83.5% of the original study parents and adolescents (ages 12–19). Results indicated that 75% of the teenagers were typically adjusted with minimal behavioral and emotional problems. Furthermore, parenting skills taught in the intervention had lasting effects. Predictors of long-term outcome were mothers' posttreatment level of critical statements and fathers' use of praise. In addition, the level of coercion between children and mothers immediately posttreatment was a predictor of later teen involvement in the criminal justice system (Webster-Stratton, Rinaldi, & Reid, 2009).

In the past decade, we have also evaluated the parent programs as a selective prevention program with multiethnic, socioeconomically disadvantaged families in two randomized studies with Head Start families as well as with families referred by child welfare for abuse and neglect. Results of these studies suggest the program's effectiveness in promoting more positive parenting and preventing the development of conduct problems and strengthening social competence among preschool children (Webster-Stratton, 1998; Webster-Stratton, Reid, & Hammond, 2001). Reid et al. (2001) evaluated the effects of the parent intervention with an indicated, culturally diverse population of elementary school-age children. Those who received the intervention showed fewer externalizing problems, better emotion regulation, and stronger parent–child bonding than control children. Mothers in the intervention group showed more supportive and less coercive parenting than those in the control group. Similar results with selective and indicated populations were reported by independent investigators (Gardner et al., 2006; Gross et al., 2003; Hutchings, Gardner, et al., 2007; Linares, Montalto, MinMin & Vikash, 2006; Miller Brotman et al., 2003).

Effects of Child and Teacher Training Programs

To date, the developer has conducted two randomized studies evaluating the effectiveness of the child training program for reducing conduct problems and promoting social competence in children diagnosed with ODD/CD. In the first study, children and their parents were randomly assigned to one of four groups: parent training treatment (PT), child training treatment (CT), child and parent treatment (CT + PT), or a wait-list control group. Posttreatment assessments indicated that all three treatment conditions resulted in improvements in parent and child behaviors compared with controls. Children who received CT showed significantly greater improvements in problem solving and conflict management skills compared with those in the PT condition. On measures of parent and child behavior at home, PT and CT + PT parents and children had significantly more positive interactions compared with CT parents and children.

One-year follow-up assessments indicated that all the significant changes noted immediately posttreatment were maintained over time. Moreover, child conduct problems at home had decreased over time. Analyses of the clinical significance of the results suggested that the combined CT + PT condition produced the most improvements in child behavior at 1-year follow-up. However, children from all three treatment conditions showed increases in behavior problems at school 1 year later, as measured by teacher reports (Webster-Stratton & Hammond, 1997).

The second study tested the effects of different combinations of parent, child, and teacher training. Families with a child diagnosed with ODD were randomly assigned to one of six groups: (1) parent training only (BASIC + ADVANCE); (2) child training only (Dina Dinosaur curriculum); (3) parent training, academic skills training, and teacher training (BASIC + ADVANCE + SCHOOL + TEACHER); (4) parent training, academic skills training, teacher training, and child training (BASIC + ADVANCE + SCHOOL + TEACHER + CHILD); (5) child training and teacher training (CHILD + TEACHER); and (6) wait-list control group. Results indicated that, as expected, trained teachers were rated as less critical, harsh, and inconsistent and more nurturing than control teachers. Parents in all three conditions who received parent training were significantly less negative and more positive than those who did not receive training. Children in all five treatment conditions showed significantly greater reductions in aggressive behaviors with mothers at home and with peers and teachers at school compared with controls. Greater treatment effects for children's positive social skills with peers were found in the three conditions with child training compared with the control condition. Most treatment effects were maintained at 1-year follow-up. In summary, short-term results replicate our previous findings on the effectiveness of the parent and child training programs and indicate that teacher training teachers' classroom management skills and improves children's classroom aggressive behavior. In addition, treatment combinations that added either child training or teacher training to the parent training were most effective.

A randomized control group study by the developer (Webster-Stratton et al., 2001) and a study by an independent evaluator evaluated the teacher training curriculum in prevention settings with Head Start teachers (Raver et al., 2008). In the first study, parent–teacher bonding was higher for experimental conditions than for controls. Children in the experimental group showed fewer conduct problems at school than controls, and trained teachers showed better classroom management than control teachers. In the second study, Head Start classes in the treatment condition had higher levels of positive classroom climate, teacher sensitivity, and behavior management than those in the control condition.

Last, a recent RCT study by Webster-Stratton, Reid, and Stoolmiller (2008) evaluated The Incredible Years teacher training and Classroom Dinosaur School curriculum with Head Start and schools that have high numbers of economically disadvantaged children serving as controls. Results showed significantly greater improvements in conduct problems, self-regulation, and social competence for the intervention group compared with the control groups. Effect size comparing treatment versus control groups at postassessment showed that the intervention had small to moderate effects on children whose baseline behavior was in the average range but large effects on children with high initial levels of conduct problems.

Who Benefits from Small Group Dinosaur Child Treatment Program?

Families of 99 children with ODD/CD ages 4–8 years who were randomly assigned to either the small-group child training treatment group or a control group were assessed on multiple risk factors (child hyperactivity, parenting style, and family stress). These risk factors were examined in relation to children's responses to the child treatment. The hyperactivity or family stress risk factors did not impact children's ability to benefit from the treatment program. Negative parenting, on the other hand, did have a negative impact on children's treatment outcome. Fewer children who had parents with one of the negative parenting risk factors (high levels of criticism or physical spanking) showed improvements compared with children who did not have a negative parenting risk factor. Thus, for children whose parents exhibit harsh and coercive parenting styles, it may be necessary to offer a parenting intervention in addition to a child intervention (Webster-Stratton et al., 2001). Our studies also suggest that child training enhances the effectiveness of parent training treatment for children with pervasive conduct problems (home and school settings).

WHO BENEFITS FROM TREATMENT AND HOW?

Beauchaine, Webster-Stratton, and Reid (2005) examined mediators, moderators, and predictors of treatment effects by combining data from six randomized controlled trials of The Incredible Years (including 514 children ages 3–9). Families in these trials received parent training, child training, teacher training, or a combination. Marital adjustment, maternal depression, paternal substance abuse, and child comorbid anxiety, depression, and attention problems were treatment moderators. In most cases, analyses of these treatment moderators showed that intervention combinations that included parent training were generally more effective than those that did not. For example, children of mothers who were maritally distressed fared better if treatment included parent training. Indeed, parent training exerted the most consistent effects across different moderating variables, and there were no instances in which interventions without parent training were more effective than interventions with parent training. However, the addition of teacher training seemed to be important for impulsive children. Finally, despite these moderating effects, more treatment components (parent, child, and teacher training) were associated with steeper reductions in mother-reported externalizing slopes as well as internalizing problems (Webster-Stratton & Herman, 2008). This suggests that, all things being equal, more treatment is better than less. Harsh parenting practices both mediated and predicted treatment success; in other words, the best treatment responses were observed among children of parents who scored relatively low on verbal criticism and harsh parenting at baseline but nevertheless improved during treatment.

In a prevention study that included socioeconomically disadvantaged children with and without conduct problems (Reid, Webster-Stratton, & Baydar, 2004), we found that child change was related to maternal engagement in the parenting program and to maternal reduction of critical parenting. In this study, maternal engagement was highest for highly critical mothers and for mothers of children who had the highest levels of conduct problems. A second study analyzing these same prevention data (Baydar, Reid, & Webster-Stratton, 2003) showed that although mothers with mental health risk factors (i.e., depression, anger, history of abuse as a child, substance abuse) exhibited poorer parenting at baseline than mothers without these risk factors, they were engaged in and benefited from the parenting training program at comparable levels. Recent research with children with ADHD and ODD also showed that dosage of intervention was related to treatment outcome: Mothers who attended 8–20 sessions showed significantly more change in parenting and child outcome than those who attended 8–10 sessions (Webster-Stratton, 2009). A similar independent finding regarding dose effects, with greater improvement for those receiving more treatment sessions, was also found in a study treating children with ODD in a primary care setting (Lavigne, LeBailly, Gouze, Cicchetti, Pochyly, Arend, et al., 2008). This argues for the importance of not abbreviating intervention.

DIRECTIONS FOR FUTURE RESEARCH

In recent years, The Incredible Years parent programs have been extended to include older children (8–13 years) as well as infants and toddlers (0–3 years). Current studies are in progress to evaluate their effectiveness. A recent study (Hutchings, Bywater, Williams, Shakespeare, & Whitaker, 2009) using the 8–12-year-old version of the School Age version of the IY parenting program has shown significantly improved parent reports of child behavior problems, as well as significant improvements in parental depression and parenting skills. Other research is evaluating The Incredible Years programs with new populations, including neglectful and abusive families referred by child protective service agencies, children with ADHD, and families from many different countries and regions including Russia, Turkey, Australia, and Scandinavia.

Although our programs were first designed and evaluated to be used as clinic-based treatments for diagnosed children, our recent work has extended our clinic-based treatment model to school settings and has targeted high-risk populations. As more is known about the type, timing, and dosage of interventions needed to prevent and treat children's conduct problems, we can further target children and families to offer treatment and support at strategic points. By providing a continuum of prevention and treatment services, we believe we will be able to prevent the further development of conduct disorders, delinquency, and violence.

ACKNOWLEDGMENTS

This research was supported by the National Institutes of Health National Center for Nursing Research Grant No. 5 R01 NR01075 and the National Institute of Mental Health Research Scientist Development Award No. MH00988.

The first author has disclosed a potential conflict of interest due to the fact that she provides training and instructional materials for these treatment programs and therefore stands to gain financially from a positive review. This interest has been disclosed to the university and is managed consistent with federal and university policy.

REFERENCES

Baydar, N., Reid, M. J., & Webster-Stratton, C. (2003). The role of mental health factors and program engagement in the effectiveness of a preventive parenting program for Head Start mothers. *Child Development, 74*(5), 1433–1453.

Beauchaine, T. P., Webster-Stratton, C., & Reid, M. J. (2005). Mediators, moderators, and predictors of one-year outcomes among children treated for early-onset conduct problems: A latent growth curve analysis. *Journal of Consulting and Clinical Psychology, 73*(3), 371–388.

Collins, W. A., Maccoby, E. E., Steinberg, L., Hetherington, E. M., & Bornstein, M. H. (2000). Contemporary research on parenting: The case for nurture and nature. *American Psychologist, 55,* 218–232.

Dishion, T. J., McCord, J., & Poulin, F. (1999). When interventions harm: Peer groups and problem behavior. *American Psychologist, 54,* 755–764.

Dishion, T. J., & Piehler, T. F. (2007). Peer dynamics in the development and change of child and adolescent problem behavior. In A. S. Masten (Ed.), *Multilevel dynamics in development psychopathology: Pathways to the future* (pp. 151–180). Mahwah, NJ: Erlbaum.

Drugli, M. B., & Larsson, B. (2006). Children aged 4–8 years treated with parent training and child therapy because of conduct problems: Generalisation effects to day-care and school settings. *European Child and Adolescent Psychiatry, 15,* 392–399.

Egger, H. L., & Angold, A. (2006). Common emotional and behavioral disorders in preschool children: Presentation, nosology, and epidemiology. *Journal of Child Psychology and Psychiatry, 47,* 313–337.

Gardner, F., Burton, J., & Klimes, I. (2006). Randomized controlled trial of a parenting intervention in the voluntary sector for reducing conduct problems in children: Outcomes and mechanisms of change. *Journal of Child Psychology and Psychiatry, 47,* 1123–1132.

Gross, D., Fogg, L., Webster-Stratton, C., Garvey, C., Julian, W., & Grady, J. (2003). Parent training with families of toddlers in day care in low-income urban communities. *Journal of Consulting and Clinical Psychology, 71*(2), 261–278.

Hartman, R. R., Stage, S., & Webster-Stratton, C. (2003). A growth curve analysis of parent training outcomes: Examining the influence of child factors (inattention, impulsivity, and hyperactivity problems), parental and family risk factors. *The Child Psychology and Psychiatry Journal, 44*(3), 388–398.

Hawkins, J. D., Brown, E. C., Oesterle, S., Arthur, M. W., Abbott, R. D., & Catalano, R. F. (2008). Early effects of Communities That Care on targeted risks and initiation of delinquent behavior and substance abuse. *Journal of Adolescent Health, 43*(1), 15–22.

Hawkins, J. D., Catalano, R. F., Kosterman, R., Abbott, R., & Hill, K. G. (1999). Preventing adolescent health-risk behaviors by strengthening protection during childhood. *Archives of Pediatrics and Adolescent Medicine, 153,* 226–234.

Hutchings, J., Bywater, T., Williams, M. E., Shakespeare, M. K., & Whitaker, C. (2009). *Evidence for the extended School Age Incredible Years parent programme with parents of high-risk 8– to 16–year-olds.* Unpublished manuscript, Bangor University, Bangor, UK.

Hutchings, J., Gardner, F., Bywater, T., Daley, D., Whitaker, C., Jones, K., et al. (2007). Parenting intervention in Sure Start services for children at risk of developing conduct disorder: Pragmatic randomized controlled trial. *British Medical Journal, 334*(7595), 1–7.

Jaffee, S. R., Caspi, A., Moffitt, T. E., & Taylor, A. (2004). Physical maltreatment victim to antisocial child: Evidence of environmentally mediated process. *Journal of Abnormal Psychology, 113,* 44–55.

Knutson, J. F., DeGarmo, D., Koeppl, G., & Reid, J. B. (2005). Care neglect, supervisory neglect and harsh parenting in the development of children's aggression: A replication and extension. *Child Maltreatment, 10,* 92–107.

Larsson, B., Fossum, B., Clifford, G., Drugli, M., Handegard, B., & Morch, W. (2008). Treatment of oppositional defiant and conduct problems in young Norwegian children: Results of a randomized controlled trial. *European Child Adolescent Psychiatry, 18*(1), 42–52.

Lavigne, J. V., LeBailly, S. A., Gouze, K. R., Cicchetti, C., Pochyly, J., Arend, R., et al. (2008). Treating oppositional defiant disorder in primary care: A comparison of three models. *Journal of Pediatric Psychology, 33*(5), 449–461.

Linares, L. O., Montalto, D., MinMin, L., & Vikash, S. O. (2006). A promising parent intervention in foster care. *Journal of Consulting and Clinical Psychology, 74*(1), 32–41.

Loeber, R., Wung, P., Keenan, K., Giroux, B., Stouthamer-Loeber, M., Van Kammen, W. B., et al. (1993). Developmental pathways in disruptive child behavior. *Development Psychopathology, 5,* 103–133.

Lynam, D. R., Caspi, A., Moffitt, T. E., Wikstrom, P. H., Loeber, R., & Novak, S. (2000). The interaction between impulsivity and neighborhood context on offending: The effects of impulsivity are stronger in poorer neighborhoods. *Journal of Abnormal Child Psychology, 109,* 563–574.

Miller Brotman, L., Klein, R. G., Kamboukos, D., Brown, E. J., Coard, S., & Sosinsky, L. S. (2003). Preventive intervention for urban, low-income preschoolers at familial risk for conduct problems: A randomized pilot study. *Journal of Child Psychology and Psychiatry, 32*(2), 246–257.

Offord, D. R., & Bennet, K. J. (1994). Conduct disorder: Long term outcomes and intervention effectiveness. *Journal of the American Academy of Child and Adolescent Psychiatry, 33,* 1069–1078.

Patterson, G. R., Capaldi, D., & Bank, L. (1991). An early starter model for predicting delinquency. In D. J. Pepler & K. H. Rubin (Eds.), *The development and treatment of childhood aggression* (pp. 139–168). Hillsdale, NJ: Erlbaum.

Raver, C. C., Jones, S. M., Li-Grining, C. P., Metzger, M., Champion, K. M., & Sardin, L. (2008). Improving preschool classroom processes: Preliminary findings from a randomized trial implemented in Head Start settings. *Early Childhood Research Quarterly, 23,* 10–26.

Reid, M. J., Webster-Stratton, C., & Baydar, N. (2004). Halting the development of externalizing behaviors in Head Start children: The effects of parenting training. *Journal of Clinical Child and Adolescent Psychology, 33*(2), 279–291.

Reid, M. J., Webster-Stratton, C., & Hammond, M. (2007). Enhancing a classroom social competence and problem-solving curriculum by offering parent training to families of moderate-to-high-risk elementary school children. *Journal of Clinical Child and Adolescent Psychology, 36*(5), 605–620.

Rinaldi, J. (2001). Long-term outcomes of parent training and predictors of adolescent adjustment. *Dissertation Abstracts International, 62*(05), 2498 (UMI No. 3014016).

Scott, S., Spender, Q., Doolan, M., Jacobs, B., & Aspland, H. (2001). Multicentre controlled trial of parenting groups for child antisocial behaviour in clinical practice. *British Medical Journal, 323*(28), 1–5.

Snyder, H. (2001). Epidemiology of official offending. In R. Loeber & D. Farrington (Eds.), *Child delinquents: Development, intervention and service needs* (pp. 25–46). Thousand Oaks, CA: Sage.

Spaccarelli, S., Cotler, S., & Penman, D. (1992). Problem-solving skills training as a supplement to behavioral parent training. *Cognitive Therapy and Research, 16,* 1–18.

Taylor, T. K., Schmidt, F., Pepler, D., & Hodgins, H. (1998). A comparison of eclectic treatment with Webster-Stratton's Parents and Children Series in a children's mental health center: A randomized controlled trial. *Behavior Therapy, 29,* 221–240.

Tremblay, R. E., Japel, C., Perusse, D., Boivin, M., Zoccolillo, M., Montplaisir, J., et al. (2000). The search for the age of "onset" of physical aggression: Rousseau and Bandura revisited. *Criminal Behavior and Mental Health, 24*(2), 129–141.

Webster-Stratton, C. (1981). Modification of mothers' behaviors and attitudes through videotape modeling group discussion program. *Behavior Therapy, 12,* 634–642.

Webster-Stratton, C. (1982). Teaching mothers through videotape modeling to change their children's behaviors. *Journal of Pediatric Psychology, 7*(3), 279–294.

Webster-Stratton, C. (1984). Randomized trial of two parent-training programs for families with conduct-disordered children. *Journal of Consulting and Clinical Psychology, 52*(4), 666–678.

Webster-Stratton, C. (1990a). Enhancing the effectiveness of self-administered videotape parent training for families with conduct-problem children. *Journal of Abnormal Child Psychology, 18*, 479–492.

Webster-Stratton, C. (1990b). Long-term follow-up of families with young conduct problem children: From preschool to grade school. *Journal of Clinical Child Psychology, 19*(2), 144–149.

Webster-Stratton, C. (1992). Individually administered videotape parent training: "Who benefits?" *Cognitive Therapy and Research, 16*(1), 31–35.

Webster-Stratton, C. (1994). Advancing videotape parent training: A comparison study. *Journal of Consulting and Clinical Psychology, 62*(3), 583–593.

Webster-Stratton, C. (1998). Preventing conduct problems in Head Start children: Strengthening parenting competencies. *Journal of Consulting and Clinical Psychology, 66*(5), 715–730.

Webster-Stratton, C. (2000). *How to promote children's social and emotional competence.* London, UK: Sage.

Webster-Stratton, C. (2006). *The Incredible Years: A trouble-shooting guide for parents of children aged 3–8.* Seattle, WA: Incredible Years Press.

Webster-Stratton, C., & Hammond, M. (1990). Predictors of treatment outcome in parent training for families with conduct problem children. *Behavior Therapy, 21*, 319–337.

Webster-Stratton, C., & Hammond, M. (1997). Treating children with early-onset conduct problems: A comparison of child and parent training interventions. *Journal of Consulting and Clinical Psychology, 65*(1), 93–109.

Webster-Stratton, C., & Hammond, M. (1998). Conduct problems and level of social competence in Head Start children: Prevalence, pervasiveness and associated risk factors. *Clinical Child Psychology and Family Psychology Review, 1*(2), 101–124.

Webster-Stratton, C., & Herbert, M. (1994). *Troubled families—Problem children: Working with parents: A collaborative process.* Chichester, UK: Wiley.

Webster-Stratton, C., & Herman, K. (2008). The impact of parent behavior-management training on child depressive symptoms. *Journal of Counseling Psychology, 55*(4), 473–484.

Webster-Stratton, C., Hollinsworth, T., & Kolpacoff, M. (1989). The long-term effectiveness and clinical significance of three cost-effective training programs for families with conduct-problem children. *Journal of Consulting and Clinical Psychology, 57*(4), 550–553.

Webster-Stratton, C., Kolpacoff, M., & Hollinsworth, T. (1988). Self-administered videotape therapy for families with conduct-problem children: Comparison with two cost-effective treatments and a control group. *Journal of Consulting and Clinical Psychology, 56*(4), 558–566.

Webster-Stratton, C., Reid, M. J., & Hammond, M. (2001). Preventing conduct problems, promoting social competence: A parent and teacher training partnership in Head Start. *Journal of Clinical Child Psychology, 30*(3), 283–302.

Webster-Stratton, C., Reid, M. J., & Hammond, M. (2004). Treating children with early-onset conduct problems: Intervention outcomes for parent, child, and teacher training. *Journal of Clinical Child and Adolescent Psychology, 33*(1), 105–124.

Webster-Stratton, C., Reid, M. J., & Stoolmiller, M. (2008). Preventing conduct problems and improving school readiness: Evaluation of The Incredible Years teacher and child training programs in high-risk schools. *Journal of Child Psychology and Psychiatry, 49*(5), 471–488.

Webster-Stratton, C., Rinaldi, J., & Reid, M. J. (2009). *Long-term outcomes of Incredible Years Parenting Program: Predictors of adolescent adjustment.* Unpublished manuscript.

14

Problem-Solving Skills Training and Parent Management Training for Oppositional Defiant Disorder and Conduct Disorder

ALAN E. KAZDIN

OVERVIEW

Clinical Focus

Oppositional defiant disorder (ODD) and conduct disorder (CD) refer to patterns of disruptive behavior that can have broad implications for child functioning at home, at school, and in the community. ODD encompasses primarily stubbornness, disobedience, and tantrums. CD includes these but also much more severe behaviors such as bullying, fighting, fire setting, using a weapon, stealing, and running away from home. Each disorder has an untoward long-term prognosis in terms of adjustment in everyday life (e.g., interpersonal relations, employment) and high rates of other psychiatric disorders.

Cases of either diagnosis invariably are associated with other (comorbid) conditions. Moreover, child symptoms often are embedded in parent, family, and contextual factors that influence both the administration and impact of interventions. In all likelihood, multiple paths lead to ODD and CD given the broad range of risk factors and the diversity of symptom patterns among those who meet a given diagnosis. For example, over 32,000 combinations of the requisite symptoms can meet the formal psychiatric diagnosis of CD (*Diagnostic and Statistical Manual of Mental Disorders* [DSM]). At this point, several evidence-based interventions are available and can exert significant impact on the problems that children with ODD or CD present.

Conceptual Model

The treatments we provide include cognitive problem-solving skills training (PSST) and parent management training (PMT). Originally, our treatment of choice was PMT because of the evidence supporting the use of basic techniques with many different populations. However, in our early work, occasionally no parent was available to participate in treatment as a result of, for example, mental illness, substance abuse, incarceration, mental retardation, or simple refusal, and for such cases, treatment for the child was especially important. Therefore, we continued to examine both treatments, separately and combined, even when we moved to outpatient treatment and when parents were available.

PSST focuses on cognitive processes, a broad class of constructs that pertain to how the individual perceives, codes, and experiences the world. Individuals who engage in conduct problem behaviors, particularly aggression, show distortions and deficiencies in various cognitive processes. Examples include generating alternative solutions to interpersonal problems (e.g., different ways of handling social situations); identifying the means to obtain particular ends (e.g., making friends) or consequences of one's actions (e.g., what could happen after a particular behavior); making attributions to others of the motivation for their own actions; perceiving how others feel; and identifying expectations of the effects of one's own actions. Deficits and distortions among these processes relate to teacher ratings of disruptive behavior, peer evaluations, and direct assessment of overt behavior. Our program drew heavily on the pioneering work of Shure and Spivack (e.g., Shure, 1992; Spivack & Shure, 1982).

PMT focuses on parent–child interactions and child behavior at home, at school, and in the community. The intervention draws on two lines of influence: (1) the seminal conceptual and empirical work of Patterson and colleagues, which focused on sequences of parent–child interactions in the home and how they can be altered (Patterson, 1982; Patterson, Reid, & Dishion, 1992); and (2) advances in applied behavior analysis on how to foster behavior (e.g., establishing operations, functional analysis, differential reinforcement). These lines of work can be translated into multiple techniques to alter both parent and child behavior.

PSST and PMT emphasize changing how the child responds in interpersonal situations at home, at school, and in the community and with teachers, parents, peers, siblings, and others. Both treatments use learning-based procedures to develop behavior, including modeling, prompting and fading, shaping, positive reinforcement, practice and repeated rehearsal, extinction, and mild punishment (e.g., time-out from reinforcement, response cost). For both interventions, most of the treatment is conducted outside of the sessions. The sessions serve to develop or practice new skills and check on those that have been learned in prior sessions.

CHARACTERISTICS OF THE TREATMENT PROGRAM

Who Is Seen in Treatment

Our program began with an exclusive focus on CD among children ages 5–12 referred for inpatient care (Child Psychiatric Intensive Care Service, University of Pittsburgh School of Medicine).[1] The program expanded to outpatient treatment, which has been the focus for more than 20 years. We have seen a few thousand children. Our current program, the Yale Parenting Center and Child Conduct Clinic (*www.yale.edu/childcon-ductclinic*) provides services for both children and families. Over the years, the range of diagnoses has expanded, as has the age range. Originally, we limited the upper age range to 12 years because, with adolescence, new issues routinely emerge (e.g., substance use, contact with the courts, extensive sexual activity, stronger peer influences, longer periods spent outside the home), and although none of these precludes effective treatment or application of our procedures, we decided to retain our focus based on practical (many cases available) and methodological (reduce variability resulting from a broader age range and from additional variants of treatment) grounds. Over the years, however, because of pleas to take cases, we extended the upper limit to 14 years, although these older patients remain exceptions.

We continue to focus on CD. However, referrals have increased among children (< 5 years) who are more likely to be referred for ODD. All of the children are referred for oppositional, aggressive, and antisocial behavior and usually meet criteria for a primary diagnosis (using DSM criteria) of CD or ODD. Approximately 70% of the children meet criteria for two or more disorders (range, 0–5). Most youths fall within the normal range of intelligence (e.g., mean full-scale IQ, 100–105; range, 60–140 on the Wechsler Intelligence Scale for Children—Revised). The families are primarily European American (~60%), African American (~30%), and Hispanic American (~5%); most of the remainder are biracial. Approximately 50% of our patients come from two-parent families. All socioeconomic–occupational levels are represented, although there is a slight skew toward lower socioeconomic classes.

The manner in which we apply our treatment varies with child age. Generally, for children ages 6 and younger, we have used PMT as our stand-alone treatment. In our outpatient work, there is a parent or guardian available, unlike our original work on the inpatient service. For children ages 7 and older, we have applied and evaluated PSST and PMT alone and in combination. The combined treatment requires two therapists so the parent (for PMT) and the child (PSST) can be seen during the same clinic visit.

Content of the Sessions

Problem-Solving Skills Training

PSST consists of weekly (30- to 50-minute) sessions with the child. The core program (12 sessions; see Table 14.1) may be supplemented with optional sessions if the child requires additional assistance in grasping the problem-solving steps (early in treatment) or their application in everyday situations (later in treatment). Few cases (< 5%) draw on these sessions.

Central to treatment is teaching the *problem-solving steps*, which serve as verbal prompts that the children use to engage in thoughts and actions that guide behavior. The steps or self-statements include the following: (1) What am I supposed to do?, (2–3) I need to figure out what to DO and what would HAPPEN, (4) I need to make a choice, and (5) I need to find out how I did. Combining steps 2 and 3 requires the child to identify a solution (what to do) and then the consequence (what would happen) and to do this with three or more solutions before proceeding to step 4. The steps are taught

TABLE 14.1. Problem-Solving Skills Training: Overview of the Core Sessions

1. *Introduction and learning the steps.* This initial session teaches the problem-solving steps in a game-like fashion in which the therapist and child take turns learning the individual steps and placing them together in a sequence.

2. and 3. *Applying the steps.* The child applies the steps to simple problem situations presented in a board game in which the therapist and child alternate turns. A series of "supersolvers" (homework assignments) begins at this point, in which the steps are used in increasingly more difficult and clinically relevant situations as treatment continues.

4. *Applying the steps and role-playing.* The child applies the steps to identify solutions and consequences in multiple problem situations. Then the preferred solution, based on the likely consequences, is selected and then enacted through repeated role-plays.

5. *Parent–child contact.* The parents, therapist, and child are seen in the session. The child enacts the steps to solve problems. The parents learn more about the steps and are trained to provide attention and contingent praise for the child's use of the steps and for selecting and enacting prosocial solutions.

6.–11. *Continued applications to real-life situations.* The child uses the problem-solving steps to generate prosocial solutions to provocative interpersonal problems or situations. Each session concentrates on a different category of social interaction that the child might realistically encounter (i.e., peers, parents, siblings, teachers). Real-life situations, generated by the child, parent, or from contacts with teachers and others, are enacted; hypothetical situations are also presented to elaborate themes and problem areas of the child (e.g., responding to provocation, fighting, being excluded socially, being encouraged by peers to engage in antisocial behavior). The child's supersolvers also become a more integral part of each session; they are reenacted with the therapist beginning in session in order to better evaluate how the child is transferring skills to his or her daily environment.

12. *Wrap up and role reversal.* This "wrap-up" session is included (1) to help the therapist generally assess what the child has learned in the session, (2) to clear up any remaining confusions the child may have concerning the use of the steps, and (3) to provide a final summary for the child of what has been covered in the meetings. The final session is based on role reversal in which the child plays the role of the therapist and the therapist plays the role of a child learning and applying the steps.

through modeling; the therapist and child alternate turns using and applying the steps and each helps the other. The problems and solutions and use of the steps are practiced extensively in the session through role play between the therapist and child and eventually involve the parents as well. Over the course of treatment, the steps progress from being overt statements (said aloud) to covert statements (silent, internal), and by the end of treatment, use of the steps is not visible.

The early sessions use simple tasks and games to teach the problem-solving steps, to help to deter impulsive responding, and to introduce the reward system and response cost contingencies, noted later. The treatment focuses on the child's use of the problem-solving steps to generate and apply prosocial solutions to a range of interpersonal problems or situations. Role play is used extensively to give the child the opportunity to enact what he or she would do in a situation, thus making these interactions similar to real-life exchanges. Sessions concentrate on situations the child actually encounters (i.e., with peers, parents, siblings, teachers, and others) across multiple stimulus characteristics and conditions in an effort to promote generalization and maintenance. Throughout sessions, the therapist prompts the child verbally and nonverbally to guide performance, provides a rich schedule of contingent social reinforcement, delivers concrete feedback for performance, and models improved ways of performing.

As an illustration, a typical situation might be where a child is being teased or threat-ened by a peer at school. In the session, the therapist presents the problem to the child and the child is asked to use her steps. The child asks herself, "What am I supposed to do?" (step 1), arrives at an answer ("I am supposed to solve this problem without hitting or getting into any trouble."), and then proceeds to the other steps. At step 2, the child identifies one alternative (e.g., "I could ignore the person and walk away") and immedi-ately goes to step 3 to note the likely effect of that action ("That might work because the person might stop teasing, and I would not get into a fight"). She then returns to steps 2 and 3 for another solution and consequence (e.g., "I could go to the teacher; she could help stop it and know that I was being picked on and did not do anything"). This process continues for at least three prosocial solutions. The child proceeds to step 4 to make a choice and explains her selection. (There might be a choice among good solutions and hence no necessary argument about one being the only choice.) Then the child moves to the final step assessing how she did ("I used the steps, I came up with good solutions, the one I chose did not get me into trouble; I did great!). The therapist provides effusive praise also, noting specifically the components of the process that were done well. Any further suggestions for improvements are noted and practiced. When the sequence is practiced, it is enacted in "real life" (i.e., role-playing using the selected solution).

Children begin each session with tokens (small plastic chips) that can be exchanged for small prizes at a "store" after each session. During the session, children can lose chips (response cost) for misusing or failing to use the steps or gain a few additional chips, although this rarely occurs. Social reinforcement and extinction are relied on more than token reinforcement to alter child behavior. The chips present opportunities to address special issues or problems, such as encouraging a particular type of prosocial solution that the child might find difficult.

In vivo practice, referred to as *supersolvers*, consists of systematically programmed assignments designed to extend the child's use and application of problem-solving skills to everyday situations. Parents are brought into sessions over the course of treatment to learn the steps and practice joint supersolver assignments that will be carried out at home. The therapist uses prompting, shaping, and praise to develop the parents' behav-ior. Over time, the child and parent supersolvers increase in complexity and encompass problem domains that led to the child's referral to treatment.

Parent Management Training

PMT is conducted primarily with the parents who directly implement several procedures at home. Usually there is no direct intervention of the therapist with the child. The treatment sessions cover such techniques as positive reinforcement (e.g., use of social praise and tokens or points for prosocial behavior), prompting, setting events, shaping, and mild punishment (e.g., use of time-out from reinforcement, loss of privileges). The sessions provide opportunities for parents to see and practice how the techniques are implemented and to review the behavior-change programs in the home.

The core treatment consists of 12 weekly sessions, each typically lasting 45–60 min-utes (see Table 14.2). As with the child therapy, optional sessions are interspersed as needed to convey the approach, to develop the procedures or ensure they are being implemented at home and at school, and to alter specific behavior-change programs, but such sessions are infrequent.

TABLE 14.2. Parent Management Training Sessions: Overview of the Core Sessions

1. *Introduction and overview.* This session provides the parents with an overview of the program and outlines the demands placed on them and the focus of the intervention.

2. *Defining and observing.* This session trains parents to pinpoint, define, and observe behavior. The parents and trainer define specific problems that can be observed and develop a specific plan to begin observations.

3. *Positive reinforcement (point chart and praise).* This session focuses on learning the concept of positive reinforcement, factors that contribute to the effective application, and rehearsal of applications in relation to the target child. An incentive (token/point) chart is devised, and the delivery praise of the parent is developed through modeling, prompting, feedback, and praise by the therapist.

4. *Time-out from reinforcement.* Parents learn about time-out and the factors related to its effective application. Delivery of time-out is extensively role-played and practiced.

5. *Attending and ignoring.* Parents learn about attending and ignoring and chose undesirable behavior that they will ignore and a positive opposite behavior to which they will attend. These procedures are practiced within the session.

6. *Shaping/school intervention.* Parents are trained to develop behaviors by reinforcement of successive approximations and to use prompts and fading of prompts to develop terminal behaviors. Also, in this session, plans are made to implement a home-based reinforcement program to develop school-related behaviors based on consultation of the therapist with the school.

7. *Review of the program.* Observations of the previous week as well as application of the reinforcement program are reviewed. Details about the administration of praise, points, and backup reinforcers are discussed and enacted so the therapist can identify how to improve parent performance. The parent practices designing programs for a set of hypothetical problems.

8. *Family meeting.* At this meeting, the child and parents are bought into the session. The programs are discussed along with any problems. Revisions are made as needed to correct misunderstandings or improve implementation.

9. and 10. *Negotiating, contracting, and compromising.* The child and parents meet together to negotiate new behavioral programs and to place these in contractual form. The therapist shapes negotiating skills in the parents and child, reinforces compromise, and provides less and less guidance as more difficult situations are presented.

11. *Reprimands and consequences for low-rate behaviors.* Parents are trained in effective use of reprimands and how to deal with low-rate behaviors such as fire setting, stealing, or truancy.

12. and 13. *Review, problem solving, practice, and role reversal.* Parents practice designing new programs, revising ailing programs, and responding to a complex array of situations in which principles and practices discussed in prior sessions are reviewed. Also, parents pretend to be the therapist and "train" the therapist pretending to be a parent.

Note. The complete manual and supporting materials are provided elsewhere (Kazdin, 2005).

The general purpose of the individual sessions is to convey content, teach specific skills, and develop use of the skill in the home. Thus, the session usually begins by discussing the general concept (e.g., positive reinforcement) and how it is to be implemented. Programs in the home consider special features of the family situation (others in the home, schedules), target child behaviors (e.g., noncompliance, fighting), available incentives, and parameters that are required for effective implementation (e.g., rich reinforcement schedule, shaping, immediate and contingent consequences). Most of the treatment session consists of modeling by the therapist and role-playing and rehearsal by the parent of such tasks as presenting the program to the child, providing prompts, and delivering consequences.

For example, in a session on attending and ignoring, parents will engage in several role plays with the therapist. Parents and the therapist may alternate playing role of the child and the parent. The "child's behavior" is modeled by the therapist who is demanding something. After being told "no," the therapist whines, follows the parent, who is walking away, and demands to be heard, hoping the parent will tire and give in. The parent ignores the behavior. Once the therapist as child calms down or begins to ask nicely, the parent attends to him or her and, depending on the behavior, may even praise the child for calming down quickly. This is rehearsed multiple times to help the parent practice ignoring and walking away and then returning calmly to reinforce child behavior that is more appropriate. Many different skills are taught in this fashion throughout the course of training.

A token reinforcement or point system is implemented in the home to provide parents with a structured way of implementing the reinforcement contingencies. The tokens, paired with praise, are contingent on specific child behaviors. Among the many advantages, tokens or a point chart serve a prompting function for the parents to reinforce and praise child behavior. Also, tokens facilitate tracking of reinforcement exchanges between parent and child (earning and spending the tokens).

Teachers are contacted to discuss individual problem areas, including deportment, grades, and homework completion. A home-based reinforcement system is devised in which child performance at school is monitored, with consequences provided at home by the parents. Teachers may also implement programs in the classroom. The school program is monitored through phone contact with the teachers as well as in discussions with parents in the treatment sessions.

Over the course of treatment, the child is brought into the PMT sessions to review the program and focus on concrete examples of what was done by and to whom and with what consequences. An effort is made to identify how parent and child behavior can be improved, to practice and provide feedback to the parents, and to refine or alter programs as needed. Modeling, rehearsal, and role play are used here as well.

Sessions with the parents or child are designed to train in specific everyday skills and activities. The "treatment" is not in the session. The skills are practiced in the sessions and are implemented in the settings and contexts in which the problems are occurring. Thus, from our perspective, the treatment is carried out by the parents (PMT) and children (PSST) and monitored by the parents and therapist.

Manuals and Supporting Materials

Both PSST and PMT are manualized but also individualized. There is a core set of themes and skill domains for each treatment and treatment session. Within the core sessions, child, parent, and family circumstances, including problem areas, domains of dysfunction, special family conditions (e.g., living arrangements, custody issues, presence of extended family members), are accommodated.

Our PMT manual, with dialogue and supporting materials for each session is available for professionals (Kazdin, 2005; *www.oup.com/us/pmt*). Also, a parent manual, *The Kazdin Method for Parenting the Defiant Child* (Kazdin & Rotella, 2008), translates key procedures to handle common child-rearing challenges in the home (e.g., toilet training, minor tantrums, teen "attitude" problem); a DVD is also available (*www.alankazdin.com*). As for PSST, there are many manuals available (e.g., Horne & Sayger, 1990; Larson & Lochman, 2002; Shure, 1992). Our manual has yet to be published, although a more detailed description is available from the author.

EVIDENCE ON THE EFFECTS OF TREATMENT

Status of the Evidence

The measures to evaluate our program cover descriptive intake information; child, parent, and family functioning; treatment process measures; and other treatment-related measures (see Table 14.3). Our key findings can be highlighted by noting the following five interrelated domains of our work; details of the key studies related to outcome are provided in Table 14.4. (text resumes on p. 222)

TABLE 14.3. Primary Measures Related to Treatment Evaluation

Measures	Domain assessed
Intake	
General information sheet	Subject and demographic characteristics
Research Diagnostic Interview	Child DSM diagnosis, number of conduct disorder symptoms, total number of symptoms
Risk Factor Interview	Child, parent, family, and contextual factors related to conduct disorder
Child functioning	
Wechsler Intelligence Scale for Children (Revised)	Verbal and Performance scores, overall IQ
Wide Range Achievement Test	Reading ability
Interview for Antisocial Behavior	Child aggressive and antisocial behavior
Self-Report Delinquency Checklist	Child delinquent acts
Children's Action Tendency Scale	Child aggressiveness, assertiveness, submissiveness
Parent Daily Report	Parent evaluation of problems at home
Child Behavior Checklist (Parent)	Diverse behavior problems and social competence
Child Behavior Checklist—TRF (Teacher)	Diverse behavior problems and adaptive functioning
Peer Involvement Inventory	How well child gets along with peers in school
Parent and family functioning	
Dyadic Adjustment Scale	Perceived quality of marital relation
Family Environment Scale	Domains of family functioning
Parenting Stress Index	Perceived parental stress and life events
Beck Depression Inventory	Parent depression
Hopkins Symptom Checklist	Overall parent impairment
Quality of Life Inventory	Parent evaluation of quality of life
Treatment process	
Child–therapist Alliance	Alliance of the child and therapist (separate versions for the child and the therapist)
Parent–therapist Alliance	Alliance of the parent and the therapist (separate versions for the parent and the therapist)
Treatment related	
Parent Expectancies for Child Therapy	Parents' expectancies of treatment, their role, and child improvement
Barriers to Participation in Treatment	Barriers, obstacles, stressors that parents experience specifically in relation to treatment
Child, Parent, and Therapist Evaluation Inventories	Acceptability of and progress in treatment

TABLE 14.4. Main Studies to Evaluate Treatment Outcome and Therapeutic Change

Investigation	Sample	Design and objective	Main Findings
Kazdin et al. (1987a)	Inpatient children (ages 7–13, $N = 56$)	Randomized controlled trial (RCT); PSST, relationship therapy, and treatment-contact control	PSST led to significantly greater decreases than the other treatment and control conditions in externalizing and other behavioral problems at home and at school and greater increases in prosocial behavior; the effects remained at 1-year follow-up.
Kazdin et al. (1987b)	Inpatient children (ages 7–12, $N = 40$)	RCT; PSST + PMT and treatment-contact control (where both parents and child were seen as in the combined treatment)	Combined treatment showed significantly greater improvements in externalizing and prosocial behaviors; as in the prior study, effects were maintained at 1-year follow-up.
Kazdin et al. (1989)	Inpatient and outpatient children (ages 7–13, $N = 112$)	RCT; compared PSST, PSST with *in vivo* practice, and relationship therapy	Both PSST conditions showed significant changes on measures of problem and prosocial behavior compared with relationship therapy; PSST with *in vivo* practice led to greater improvements in behaviors at school than PSST alone, but these differences were no longer evident at 1-year follow-up.
Kazdin, Siegel, & Bass (1992)	Outpatient children (ages 7–13, $N = 97$)	RCT; evaluated effects of PSST, PMT, and PSST + PMT combined	All treatments improved child functioning on measures of externalizing symptoms and prosocial behavior; combined treatment led to significantly greater changes immediately after treatment and at 1-year follow-up and placed more children within the nonclinic (normative range) in levels of functioning.
Kazdin, Mazurick, & Siegel (1994)	Outpatient children (ages 4–13, $N = 75$)	Evaluated therapeutic change of completers and dropouts and factors that account for their different outcomes	At the end of treatment, children who terminated prematurely showed greater impairment at home, at school, and in the community compared with those who completed treatment. However, primarily severity of impairment at pretreatment rather than less treatment accounted for these differences.
Kazdin (1995)	Outpatient children (ages 7–13, $N = 105$)	Evaluated moderators of change among families who received PMT or PSST + PMT	Child severity and scope of dysfunction, parent stress, and family dysfunction predicted symptoms and prosocial functioning at end of treatment, but effects varied by outcome (at home or at school). The proposed moderators, even when significant, were not strongly related to outcome.
Kazdin & Crowley (1997)	Outpatient children (ages 7–13, $N = 120$)	Examined relation of intellectual functioning and severity of symptoms on responsiveness to PSST	Children more deficient in cognitive/academic skills and more severely impaired improved significantly with treatment but not as much as their less impaired counterparts.

(cont.)

219

TABLE 14.4. (cont.)

Investigation	Sample	Design and objective	Main Findings
Kazdin & Wassell (1998)	Outpatient children (ages 3–13, $N = 304$)	Examined the relation of treatment completion and therapeutic change among children who received PSST, PMT, or PSST + PMT	Treatment completion was strongly related to therapeutic change, with greater change among those who completed treatment. However, 34% of early dropouts made significant improvement compared with 78% of those who remained in treatment. Predictors of improvement did not vary as a function of whether individuals dropped out or completed treatment.
Kazdin & Wassell (1999)	Outpatient children (ages 3–13, $N = 200$)	Examined predictors of therapeutic change	Perceived barriers to treatment participation was related to therapeutic changes in children. Greater barriers were associated with less change; the findings could not be explained by several child, parent, and family variables.
Kazdin & Wassell (2000a)	Outpatient children (ages 2–14, $N = 169$)	Examined relation of parent psychopathology and quality of life as moderators of therapeutic change in children who received PSST, PMT, or PSST + PMT	Greater parent psychopathology and lower quality of life at pretreatment predicted therapeutic changes, controlling for SES and child severity of dysfunction. Greater perceived barriers to treatment by parents were associated with less therapeutic change in children.
Kazdin & Wassell (2000b)	Outpatient children (ages 2–14, $N = 250$)	Examined therapeutic changes in children, parents, and families and the predictors of these changes among children who received PSST, PMT, or PSST + PMT	Child, parent, and family functioning improved over the course of treatment. Moderators of treatment varied as a function of child, parent, and family outcomes.
Kazdin & Whitley (2003)	Outpatient children (ages 6–14, $N = 127$)	RCT: All families received PSST + PMT; half were assigned to receive a supplementary component to address parental stress	Treatment with the component to address parental stress was associated with greater therapeutic change among children and reduced barriers to treatment perceived by parents.

220

Kazdin, Marciano, & Whitley (2005)	Outpatient children (ages 3–14, N = 138)	Evaluated child–therapist and parent–therapist alliance as a predictor of therapeutic change among families who received PMT alone or PSST + PMT	A more positive therapeutic alliance (for either child or parent) was associated with greater therapeutic change, fewer barriers to treatment, and greater acceptability of treatment. SES, parent dysfunction and stress, and pretreatment child dysfunction did not account for findings.
Kazdin, Whitley, & Marciano (2006)	Outpatient children (ages 6–14, N = 77)	Evaluated child–therapist and parent–therapist alliance as a predictor of therapeutic change among families who received PSST + PMT	Both alliances predicted therapeutic change in children. Parent–therapist alliance predicted improvements in parenting practices in the home; effects were not explained by SES, parent and child dysfunction, and/or parental stress.
Kazdin & Whitley (2006a)	Outpatient children (ages 2–14, N = 218)	Evaluated parent–therapist alliance, pretreatment parent social relations, and parenting practices developed with PMT among families who received PMT alone or PSST + PMT	Alliance predicted parent improvements over the course of treatment; alliance was partially mediated by pretreatment parent social relations.
Kazdin & Whitley (2006b)	Outpatient children (ages 3–14) who met criteria for ODD or CD (N = 315)	Evaluated comorbidity (0, 1, or ≥ 2 comorbid disorders separately for ODD and CD cases) and case complexity (SES, scope of child dysfunction, parent and family stress and dysfunction, barriers to treatment); children received PSST, PMT, or PSST + PMT	Children were not different in outcomes as a function of comorbidity or case complexity; greater change (pre–post) was associated with more dysfunction (multiple comorbidities and greater family complexity) but the end points (post) were not different. Barriers to treatment moderated outcome: Greater barriers were associated with less change in children.

Note. PSST, problem-solving skills training; PMT, parent management training; SES, socioeconomic status; ODD, oppositional defiant disorder; CD, conduct disorder.

Outcome Effects

PSST and PMT alone or in combination produce reliable and significant reductions in oppositional, aggressive, and antisocial behavior and increases in prosocial behavior among children. The combined treatment (PSST + PMT) tends to be more effective than either treatment alone. The effects of treatment extend beyond multiple outcomes of the child. Parent dysfunction and stress decline and family relations improve (Kazdin, Esveldt-Dawson, French, & Unis, 1987a, 1987b; Kazdin, Bass, Siegel, & Thomas, 1989; Kazdin, Siegel, & Bass, 1992).

Experimental Interventions to Improve Outcome

The effects of PSST can be enhanced by including *in vivo* practice (homework assignments) as part of treatment. The effects of PMT can be enhanced by providing supplementary sessions that focus on parent sources of stress. Also, a motivational enhancement intervention can improve parent motivation for and adherence to treatment and session attendance (Kazdin et al., 1989; Kazdin & Whitley, 2003; Nock & Kazdin, 2005).

The Therapeutic Alliance

The child–therapist and parent–therapist alliances relate to several outcomes. The more positive the child–therapist and parent–therapist alliances are during treatment, the greater the therapeutic change of the child and improvement of parents in parenting practices, the fewer barriers that parents experience during the course of treatment, and the more favorably parents rate the acceptability of the treatment (Kazdin, Marciano, & Whitley, 2005; Kazdin & Whitley, 2006b; Kazdin, Whitley, & Marciano, 2006).

Other Moderators of Treatment

Several parent and child characteristics moderate therapeutic change, including, among others, severity of child dysfunction, child IQ, parent stress, and parent psychopathology. The relations are not always what might be expected. For example, severity of child dysfunction (comorbid diagnoses and total number of symptoms) and severity of parent and family impairment are positively related to outcome. More severe cases change more over the course of treatment (regression related), and their end point is no different from less severe cases. The most robust moderator of our treatment has been parental report of barriers to participation in treatment. The greater the perceived barriers, the smaller the therapeutic change among the children, although changes among parents high in barriers are still large (effect size > 1.00). This relationship is not accounted for by such other factors as severity of parent or child dysfunction, stress in the home, or parent attendance to treatment (Kazdin, 1995; Kazdin & Crowley, 1997; Kazdin, Holland, & Crowley, 1997; Kazdin, Holland, Crowley, & Breton, 1997; Kazdin & Wassell, 1999, 2000a, 2000b; Kazdin & Whitley, 2006a).

Participation in Treatment

Parent dysfunction, family stress, and barriers to participation in treatment are among the more robust predictors of session cancellation or failure to attend and early dropout.

Interestingly, early dropout is not indicative of treatment failure. Of those who drop out very early, 34% report large improvements in the behavior of their children. Because we work closely with and know the families, teachers, and others involved with the child, we have ongoing knowledge of how well treatment is working and when child improvements serve as a key consideration for dropping out. In such cases, parents often tell us that they see no reason to continue given the child's improvements (Kazdin, 1990; Kazdin & Mazurick, 1994; Kazdin, Mazurick, & Bass, 1993; Kazdin, Mazurick, & Siegel, 1994; Kazdin, Stolar, & Marciano, 1995; Kazdin & Wassell, 1998).

Overall, our work has shown that PSST and PMT can effect significant change in severely disturbed children and children with multiple psychiatric disorders in both inpatient and outpatient settings. The effects of treatment are evident in performance at home, at school, and in the community both immediately after treatment and up to a 1-year follow-up assessment. Child improvements have been documented using rating scales and direct behavioral measures across settings; the magnitude of the changes is relatively large (e.g., effect sizes > 1.00), and symptom levels at the end of treatment often fall within a sex- and age-based normative range. Relationship-based therapy and treatment-contact control conditions in our studies have not led to reliable changes.

Implementation in Clinical Practice

There are obstacles in transferring interventions to broader applications. First and perhaps most salient, there are few adequate training opportunities for mental health professionals to learn these techniques. Although many treatment manuals and workshops are available, they only a beginning and not sufficient training for providing PMT or PSST.

Second, extension of effective treatments to clinical practice requires better assessment in clinical work. Even if evidence-based treatments were used routinely in clinical work, the treatment is not likely to be effective or optimally effective for all cases. Some monitoring procedures are needed to evaluate progress during treatment and to provide the basis for decision making about continuing, changing, or ending treatment. Ultimately, the quality of clinical work will depend not only on using evidence-based techniques but also systematically examining their impact with individual children and families.

DIRECTIONS FOR RESEARCH

Multiple lines of research can be identified that pertain to PSST and PMT but include evidence-based treatments more generally. First, long-term follow-up data are needed. There are too few demonstrations that adolescents and adults are better off as a result of receiving evidence-based treatments in childhood. Our work has evaluated follow-up of only 1 to 2 years.

Second, a high priority ought to be given to understanding the mechanisms of change (i.e., processes that produce the change and how these unfold to improve child functioning). Mediators reflect constructs that may statistically explain, in varying degrees, the connection between intervention and outcome and hence provide leads. However, mechanism has a greater level of specificity in conveying precisely what has changed and how the change leads to the outcome. Promising work in PMT has identified parenting practices as critical to producing changes in the child (e.g., Patterson et al., 1992; Reid, Patterson, & Snyder, 2002).

Third, considerable research has been conducted on moderators of therapeutic change (i.e., factors that influence the direction or magnitude of therapeutic change). Much of the work, including ours, has not been very useful as a way of translating findings to clinical care. A research priority must be identifying of moderators that influence outcome and evaluating them in a way that could inform clinical decision making. Perhaps a moderator that attenuates the impact of one treatment would have a pervasive effect and operate similarly across all treatments. Alternatively, the hope would be that the moderator is specific to a particular treatment so that other interventions are likely to be more effective. The effectiveness of treatment can be improved by more effective interventions as well as by better triage that directs patients to treatments from which they are likely to profit.

Finally, systematic work on ethnicity and culture as moderators of treatment is needed. Perhaps one should not assume that treatments developed primarily with one or two cultural or ethnic groups will be inapplicable or less applicable to other groups without modification. However, the topic requires more empirical attention. In the case of PMT, demands are made on families about how to interact and rear children. Many parent-child interactions and child-rearing practices are deeply woven into religious teachings and cultural beliefs and customs (e.g., type of punishment, how and what demands are made on the children). It is reasonable to expect ethnicity and culture to moderate intervention effects.

CONCLUSIONS

Our program is devoted to the treatment of ODD and CD among children. We have used cognitive-behavioral procedures to focus on interpersonal cognitive processes of the child and parent–child interactions. Treatment–outcome studies, our own and those of others, have indicated that clinically referred patients improve with PSST and PMT. Several moderators of treatment have been identified and include characteristics of the children, parents, and families.

CD, more than ODD, represents a special treatment challenge, given the multiple domains of functioning that are routinely affected. Indeed, we consider CD a pervasive developmental disorder not to group this with autism but rather to convey the scope of dysfunction children present. Even this characterization is inadequate in the context of clinical work, because broader influences (parental, familial, and contextual) often must be considered in treatment. These influences have a demonstrated relation to child oppositional, aggressive, and antisocial behavior, to participation and completion of treatment, and to therapeutic change. In the process of developing and evaluating treatment, we have been drawn into other areas as part of our research because of their strong connections to dysfunction and change.

ACKNOWLEDGMENTS

Research reported in this chapter was facilitated by support from a Research Scientist Development Award and Research Scientist Award (No. MH00353), a MERIT Award (No. MH35408), and an R01 grant (No. MH59029) from the National Institute of Mental Health, and by support from the Leon Lowenstein Foundation, the William T. Grant Foundation (No. 98-1872-98), and Yale University. No less essential to the work has been the remarkable staff that has served at the Yale Parenting Center and Child Conduct Clinic.

NOTE

1. The Yale Parenting Center and Child Conduct Clinic and the research reported in this chapter initially began at the Western Psychiatric Institute and Clinic, University of Pittsburgh School of Medicine (1981–1989, inpatient and outpatient services) and continued at Yale University (1989–present, outpatient only).

REFERENCES

Horne, A. M., & Sayger, T. V. (1990). *Treating conduct and oppositional disorders in children*. Elmsford, NY: Pergamon Press.

Kazdin, A. E. (1990). Premature termination from treatment among children referred for antisocial behavior. *Journal of Child Psychology and Psychiatry, 3*, 415–425.

Kazdin, A. E. (1995). Child, parent, and family dysfunction as predictors of outcome in cognitive-behavioral treatment of antisocial children. *Behaviour Research and Therapy, 33*, 271–281.

Kazdin, A. E. (2005). *Parent management training: Treatment for oppositional, aggressive, and antisocial behavior in children and adolescents*. New York: Oxford University Press.

Kazdin, A. E., Bass, D., Siegel, T., & Thomas, C. (1989). Cognitive-behavioral treatment and relationship therapy in the treatment of children referred for antisocial behavior. *Journal of Consulting and Clinical Psychology, 57*, 522–535.

Kazdin, A. E., & Crowley, M. (1997). Moderators of treatment outcome in cognitively based treatment of antisocial behavior. *Cognitive Therapy and Research, 21*, 185–207.

Kazdin, A. E., Esveldt-Dawson, K., French, N. H., & Unis, A. S. (1987a). The effects of parent management training and problem-solving skills training combined in the treatment of antisocial child behavior. *Journal of the American Academy of Child and Adolescent Psychiatry, 26*, 416–424.

Kazdin, A. E., Esveldt-Dawson, K., French, N. H., & Unis, A. S. (1987b). Problem-solving skills training and relationship therapy in the treatment of antisocial child behavior. *Journal of Consulting and Clinical Psychology, 55*, 76–85.

Kazdin, A. E., Holland, L., & Crowley, M. (1997). Family experience of barriers to treatment and premature termination from child therapy. *Journal of Consulting and Clinical Psychology, 65*, 453–463.

Kazdin, A. E., Holland, L., Crowley, M., & Breton, S. (1997). Barriers to Participation in Treatment Scale: Evaluation and validation in the context of child outpatient treatment. *Journal of Child Psychology and Psychiatry, 38*, 1051–1062.

Kazdin, A. E., Marciano, P. L., & Whitley, M. (2005). The therapeutic alliance in cognitive-behavioral treatment of children referred for oppositional, aggressive, and antisocial behavior. *Journal of Consulting and Clinical Psychology, 73*, 726–730.

Kazdin, A. E., & Mazurick, J. L. (1994). Dropping out of child psychotherapy: Distinguishing early and late dropouts over the course of treatment. *Journal of Consulting and Clinical Psychology, 62*, 1069–1074.

Kazdin, A. E., Mazurick, J. L., & Bass, D. (1993). Risk for attrition in treatment of antisocial children and families. *Journal of Clinical Child Psychology, 22*, 2–16.

Kazdin, A. E., Mazurick, J. L., & Siegel, T. C. (1994). Treatment outcome among children with externalizing disorder who terminate prematurely versus those who complete psychotherapy. *Journal of the American Academy of Child and Adolescent Psychiatry, 33*, 549–557.

Kazdin, A. E., & Rotella, C. (2008). *The Kazdin Method for parenting the defiant child: With no pills, no therapy, no contest of wills*. Boston: Houghton Mifflin.

Kazdin, A. E., Siegel, T., & Bass, D. (1992). Cognitive problem-solving skills training and parent management training in the treatment of antisocial behavior in children. *Journal of Consulting and Clinical Psychology, 60,* 733–747.

Kazdin, A. E., Stolar, M. J., & Marciano, P. L. (1995). Risk factors for dropping out of treatment among white and black families. *Journal of Family Psychology, 9,* 402–417.

Kazdin, A. E., & Wassell, G. (1998). Treatment completion and therapeutic change among children referred for outpatient therapy. *Professional Psychology: Research and Practice, 29,* 332–340.

Kazdin, A. E., & Wassell, G. (1999). Barriers to treatment participation and therapeutic change among children referred for conduct disorder. *Journal of Clinical Child Psychology, 28,* 160–172.

Kazdin, A. E., & Wassell, G. (2000a). Predictors of barriers to treatment and therapeutic change in outpatient therapy for antisocial children and their families. *Mental Health Services Research, 2,* 27–40.

Kazdin, A. E., & Wassell, G. (2000b). Therapeutic changes in children, parents, and families resulting from treatment of children with conduct problems. *Journal of the American Academy of Child and Adolescent Psychiatry, 39,* 414–420.

Kazdin, A. E., & Whitley, M. K. (2003). Treatment of parental stress to enhance therapeutic change among children referred for aggressive and antisocial behavior. *Journal of Consulting and Clinical Psychology, 71,* 504–515.

Kazdin, A. E., & Whitley, M. K. (2006a). Comorbidity, case complexity, and effects of evidence-based treatment for children referred for disruptive behavior. *Journal of Consulting and Clinical Psychology, 74,* 455–467.

Kazdin, A. E., & Whitley, M. K. (2006b). Pretreatment social relations, therapeutic alliance, and improvements in parenting practices in parent management training. *Journal of Consulting and Clinical Psychology, 74,* 346–355.

Kazdin, A. E., Whitley, M., & Marciano, P. L. (2006). Child-therapist and parent-therapist alliance and therapeutic change in the treatment of children referred for oppositional, aggressive, and antisocial behavior. *Journal of Child Psychology and Psychiatry, 47,* 436–445.

Larson, J., & Lochman, J. E. (2002). *Helping school children cope with anger: A cognitive-behavioral intervention.* New York: Guilford Press.

Nock, M. K., & Kazdin, A. E. (2005). Randomized controlled trial of a brief intervention for increasing participation in parent management training. *Journal of Consulting and Clinical Psychology, 75,* 872–879.

Patterson, G. R. (1982). *Coercive family process.* Eugene, OR: Castalia.

Patterson, G. R., Reid, J. B., & Dishion, T. J. (1992). *Antisocial boys.* Eugene, OR: Castalia.

Reid, J. B., Patterson, G. R., & Snyder, J. (Eds.). (2002). *Antisocial behavior in children and adolescents: A developmental analysis and model for intervention.* Washington, DC: American Psychological Association.

Shure, M. B. (1992). *I can problem solve (ICPS): An interpersonal cognitive problem solving program.* Champaign, IL: Research Press.

Spivack, G., & Shure, M. B. (1982). The cognition of social adjustment: Interpersonal cognitive problem solving thinking. In B. B. Lahey & A. E. Kazdin (Eds.), *Advances in clinical child psychology* (Vol. 5, pp. 323–372). New York: Plenum.

15

Anger Control Training for Aggressive Youths

JOHN E. LOCHMAN, CAROLINE L. BOXMEYER, NICOLE P. POWELL,
TAMMY D. BARRY, and DUSTIN A. PARDINI

OVERVIEW OF THE TREATMENT MODEL

Childhood aggression has become a central focus of many prevention and treatment efforts because of its relative stability over time and consistent linkage with a variety of negative outcomes, including delinquency, substance use, conduct problems, academic difficulties, and poor adjustment. Early hostile behavior has also received considerable attention because youths who engage in the most persistent, severe, and violent antisocial behavior are most likely to initiate their deviant behavior in childhood rather than adolescence. As a result, childhood aggression is often viewed as an indication of a broader based syndrome characterized by various norm-violating behaviors in adolescence. Although there is no commonly accepted definition of aggressive behavior, various conceptualizations have included behaviors such as arguing, bullying, use of strong-arm tactics, threatening, striking in anger, and engaging in physical fights. The diversity of these aggressive activities, as well as the tendency for some children to exhibit only certain types of combative behavior, has prompted researchers to devise classification systems aimed at identifying clinically meaningful subgroups of aggressive children. These complexities aside, aggressive behavior has an aversive effect on others, leading children who exhibit this behavior to develop poor relations with their peers, parents, and teachers.

Contextual Social-Cognitive Model of Prevention

The development of adolescent antisocial behavior is often conceptualized as the result of a set of familial and personal factors, with children's aggressive behavior representing a substantial part of that developmental course. Poor parenting practices may contribute to children's aggressive behavior, and as these aggressive behavior patterns become entrenched, they may lead to the development of substance abuse and conduct disorder. In early to middle childhood, increasingly oppositional children can experience highly negative reactions from teachers and peers and develop impaired social-cognitive processes. As their academic progress and social bond to school weaken, they become more susceptible to deviant peer group influences. By adolescence, this trajectory results in a heightened risk of substance use, delinquent acts, and academic failure. Thus, the contextual social-cognitive model of prevention presented here focuses on two relevant sets of potential mediators of adolescent antisocial behavior: (1) child-level factors, including lack of social competence and poor social-cognitive skills, and (2) parent-level contextual factors, including poor caregiver involvement and discipline of the child.

Children's Social-Cognitive Processes

The Anger Coping Program model (see Larson & Lochman, 2002) stresses the cognitive processes that occur as children respond to interpersonal conflicts or frustrations with environmental obstacles. This first stage of cognitive processing consists of the children's perceptions and attributions of the problem event, which, in turn, influence subsequent anger. The second stage of processing consists of the children's cognitive plan for their response to the perceived threat or provocation. The anger arousal model proposes that children's cognitive and emotional processing of the problem and their planned response lead to their behavioral response (ranging from aggression to assertion, passive acceptance, or withdrawal).

The more recent development of the Coping Power Program, which is an extension of the Anger Coping Program, was influenced by research supporting the six-stage model of social information processing (SIP). In the first three stages (Lochman, FitzGerald, & Whidby, 1999), children encode relevant details in the immediate environment, generate interpretations about the nature of the situation, and then formulate a social goal that will influence their response to the situation (e.g., gaining revenge, avoiding conflict). During the encoding stage, aggressive children are more likely to attend to hostile cues, remember fewer cues, and attend only to the most recent cues in comparison to their nonaggressive peers. Higher levels of aggression are associated with an increased tendency to view others' actions as hostile, suggesting that aggressive children have problems interpreting the information they have encoded. When generating interpersonal goals, aggressive children also tend to endorse goals associated with dominance, disruption, and troublemaking more often than their peers, even in fairly benign conflict situations.

The final three stages of the SIP model involve generating a mental list of possible behavioral responses, systematically evaluating the quality of each response, and then enacting the chosen response. Aggressive children have been shown to have problems at each of these stages (Lochman & Dodge, 1994). When asked to generate solutions to interpersonal conflicts, aggressive children demonstrate deficiencies in the overall number and quality of solutions generated and produce fewer verbal solutions and more direct-action solutions involving physical aggression. Youths exhibiting deviant behavior are also more confident that aggressive solutions will produce positive outcomes and less likely to believe that negative consequences will result from hostile actions. Even when aggressive children choose to enact positive responses, evidence suggests that they are less adept at carrying them out. The entire process is said to be circular in nature because the outcome of the enacted response often influences future response choices.

Contextual Parenting Behaviors

Childhood aggressive behavior may arise out of early contextual experiences with parents who provide harsh or irritable discipline, poor problem solving, vague commands, and poor monitoring of child behavior. Parental risk factors such as lack of maternal involvement and inconsistent discipline have been linked to childhood aggression and the development of adolescent antisocial behavior. There is also evidence suggesting that parents who use irritable and ineffective discipline are more likely to have children who exhibit overt (oppositional behavior, physical aggression) and covert (stealing, lying, truancy) antisocial behavior. These results suggest that parent factors can exert a direct effect on adolescent antisocial behavior and an indirect effect via their association with factors such as childhood aggression, poor social competence, and academic failure. The relation between poor parenting and children's aggressive behavior is also viewed as bidirectional, with poor parenting stimulating children's negative behavior and deteriorating in response to increasingly negative child behaviors.

Goals of Anger Coping and Coping Power Programs

Using the contextual social-cognitive model as a guide, the Anger Coping and Coping Power Programs are designed to prevent the development of antisocial behavior in adolescence by modifying maladaptive parenting practices and child social information-processing problems that have been associated with childhood aggression. The child components of the Anger Coping and Coping Power Program include group sessions addressing issues such as anger management, perspective taking, social problem solving, emotional awareness, relaxation training, social skills enhancement, positive social and personal goals, and dealing with peer pressure. The Coping Power Program also has a parent component, with group sessions designed to address issues such as social reinforcement and positive attention, importance of clear house rules, behavioral expectations and monitoring procedures, use of appropriate and effective discipline strategies, family communication, positive connection to school, and stress management. During parent group meetings, parents are also informed of the skills their children are working on during their sessions and are encouraged to reinforce their children for using these new skills at home and school.

CHARACTERISTICS OF THE TREATMENT PROGRAM

Anger Coping Program

Format and Clients

The Anger Coping Program is designed for five to seven children in a group format; however, the content can be delivered in individual sessions as well. A group format has several advantages over individual sessions: It provides opportunities to address children's difficulties with social competence through modeling, role-playing, group problem solving, and feedback/reinforcement of children's social behavior with peers and adult group leaders. The program has been successfully implemented in both school and clinical settings.

Ideally, each group has two coleaders, who alternate between leading specific group activities and monitoring children's behaviors. This minimizes the behavioral management difficulties that can arise with an aggressive population and allows for frequent feedback, redirection, and reinforcement. The program consists of 18 sessions and groups generally meet weekly for 60–90 minutes. Research findings suggest that specific client characteristics are associated with greater improvement following involvement in the Anger Coping Program. Specifically, aggressive children who are extremely poor social problem solvers, have lower perceived levels of hostility, and are more rejected by their peers tend to exhibit better treatment-related outcomes (Lochman et al., 1999). Likewise, children with a more internalized attributional style and higher levels of anxiety symptoms and somatic complaints tend to benefit more from the intervention. The most successful groups will include children who have some level of understanding that their aggressive behavior is problematic and have some desire to change this behavior.

Sequence and Content of Therapy Sessions

The main goals of the Anger Coping Program (Larson & Lochman, 2002; Lochman et al., 1999) are outlined for each session in Table 15.1. Leaders are encouraged to implement the structured program in a flexible manner so that the agenda can be shifted to address specific problems and issues that arise. Nevertheless, it is important that the overall objectives of the program and the specific objectives of each session are completed to ensure that the social-cognitive difficulties of aggressive children are impacted.

TABLE 15.1. Sessions for the Anger Coping Program

Session	Title
Session 1	Introduction and Group Rules
Session 2	Understanding and Writing Goals
Session 3	Anger Management: Puppet Self-Control Task
Session 4	Using Self-Instruction
Session 5	Perspective Taking
Session 6	Looking at Anger
Session 7	What Does Anger Feel Like?
Session 8	Choices and Consequences
Session 9	Steps for Problem Solving
Session 10	Problem Solving in Action
Sessions 11–18	Video Productions I–VIII and Review

Common Elements of Anger Coping Sessions

Review Main Points from Previous Session. Beginning with session 2, the first portion of each session is used to review information from the previous session in a group discussion format. Each group member is asked to recall one point from the previous session, and group leaders use reminders and encouragement to shape the discussion.

Review Goals. Beginning with session 3, each child's goal sheet (see later discussion of session 2) from the previous week is reviewed and a point is awarded if the goal has been met. Leaders help members discuss what led to their success or, for those who were not successful, problem solve ways to reach their goal.

Positive Feedback and Optional Free Time. Although each session has certain objectives, all 18 sessions end with positive feedback and free time. During positive feedback, group members are asked to identify one positive thing about themselves and one positive thing about another group member. Leaders should shape comments to focus on positive behaviors and good use of problem-solving skills rather than vague compliments or concrete statements about physical characteristics. At this time, points earned during group are tallied and added to the total, and children have the option of using their points to purchase a prize from the prize box.

Free play is optional (if time allows). Leaders should monitor the children's activities and encourage "problem solving in action" if conflict arises (i.e., identify the problem, discuss choices and consequences, select a solution, and plan ways to avoid the problem in the future). Free play also provides an opportunity for leaders to reinforce prosocial behavior (e.g., sharing, following group rules).

Content of Anger Coping Sessions

Session 1. Leaders explain the purpose of the intervention and set the group structure, including developing group rules with input from the students and establishing a contingency system for behavior management. Students also participate in a group activity designed to foster group cohesion. The final goal of the first session is to heighten students' awareness of individual perceptual processes. Toward this end, students participate in an activity in which they individually audio record their thoughts about an ambiguous stimulus picture and then, as a group, listen to the various descriptions and identify similarities and differences.

Session 2. The main objective is to introduce the concept of setting and realizing goals. The overall goal of the program is reviewed (i.e., to learn problem-solving and anger coping skills) and the program goal sheets are introduced. Goal sheets require each member to generate a behavioral goal related to anger coping or self-control to work toward during the following week (e.g., "ignoring Billy's teasing in the lunchroom" and "keeping my hands and feet to myself in the classroom"). Using the goal sheets, teachers provide daily feedback to students regarding their progress toward the goal. Group leaders assist students in identifying goals that are observable, relevant, and challenging but attainable. A level of performance needed to reach the goal is determined and written on the sheet (e.g., 3 of 5 days). Leaders explain that members can each earn a point for meeting their goal, and points may be used for individual or group rewards.

Session 3. The two main purposes of this session are to assess students' problem-solving skills and to introduce the role of thoughts in helping to control strong feelings such as anger. Problem-solving skills are assessed informally, with leaders instructing each child to obtain a puppet from a box purposely containing one fewer puppet than the number of students. Following a discussion of the students' attempts to solve this shortage problem, the concepts of self-talk, distraction techniques, and relaxation methods are introduced as ways to manage feelings and reactions. To illustrate, one of the leaders uses a puppet to model self-talk and distraction techniques while being teased by the other coleader. Each member then uses a puppet to practice self-talk while his or her puppet is being teased by other group members.

Session 4. Practice of self-instruction techniques to manage anger continues in session 4. The activities are designed to elicit mild to moderate levels of anger so that students can actually practice anger control strategies. The first activity focuses on distraction. Members try to remember the numbers on 10 playing cards in 5 seconds while being teased by others in the group. The member with the most correct numbers is deemed the winner, and group members discuss how difficult or easy it was to keep their attention focused on the cards while being teased. In the next activity, students practice using self-talk to manage anger while building a domino tower with only one hand, again while being teased by other group members. Students then discuss their experience during the activity and how the self-talk technique worked for them. Finally, a group leader models the use of self-talk while being directly teased by the coleader. Each group member then has a turn to practice using self-talk while being teased by other students. Feelings and coping techniques for this activity are discussed, with an emphasis on self-talk that helps members "stay cool."

Session 5. The main goal is to assist students in taking the perspective of another person. After being shown a picture of an ambiguous situation, students are asked to come up with their own interpretation. Differences in interpretations are then discussed. In a second activity, students are shown another picture of an ambiguous situation and are asked to role-play the scene. A group leader then "interviews" each student about his or her perspective about the problem. Differences in perspectives are discussed, with an emphasis on the fact that it is often difficult to interpret others' intentions.

Session 6. Additional activities are presented to address perspective taking. Leaders expand on the concept by introducing the role of anger in social problem situations. Students perform several role plays similar to the activity in session 5, taking on different roles and demonstrating angry reactions in their portrayals. The session concludes with a discussion of anger and its effects on social situations.

Session 7. Students learn to recognize the physiological cues that serve as early warning signs of their anger. Group members view a videotape that demonstrates physiological aspccts of anger arousal and discuss their own individual bodily changes that occur when they are angry. Next, through a videotape presentation and discussion, students learn to recognize maladaptive thoughts that accompany their anger and identify alternative self-statements that can help them to control their anger.

Session 8. This session begins to address the problem-solving deficiencies demonstrated by aggressive children. Leaders assist students in generating multiple alternatives (both positive and negative) to a social problem situation, and students determine whether each choice involves anger coping or self-control. Next, the concept of consequences is established. Students identify the potential consequences for each choice listed in the previous activity and rate each consequence as good or bad.

Session 9. The steps of the problem-solving model are presented and include the following: (1) What is the problem? (2) What are my feelings? (3) What are my choices? (4) What will happen? and (5) What will I do? Leaders elicit real-life problems from students and go through the steps to demonstrate use of the model.

Session 10. The main goal of session 10, and all subsequent sessions, is the creation of a videotape demonstrating the problem-solving model. In this session, students view a sample video depicting a problem situation and three alternative solutions. Students discuss the alternatives and identify the best choice.

Session 11. Students identify a school-related problem involving anger arousal to depict in their video. Leaders assist students in using the problem-solving model to determine thrcc or four choices (involving both good and poor anger control) for solving the problem and the consequences that might follow.

Session 12. Students portray the problem situation for audio or video recording, demonstrating an initial inappropriate, aggressive action with a negative consequence for the aggressive child. Leaders then assist students in assigning roles and outlining the content of the alternative solutions. Students act out the solution choice that demonstrates lack of anger control.

Session 13. Students review the problem stem recorded during the previous session and then act out the alternative choices that involve anger control and the associated consequences.

Sessions 14–18. During the final sessions, concepts presented during the previous sessions are reviewed and techniques are applied to group members' real-life situations. Goal sheets and the point system continue throughout the remainder of the program. Time permitting, students produce videotapes of other problems, alternatives, and consequences or create a cartoon scenario or comic book for a problem-solving situation. As the intervention concludes, the steps of the social problem-solving model are reviewed, and leaders discuss how students might cope with setbacks. Leaders summarize students' progress and hold a "graduation" ceremony.

Treatment Skills, Accomplishments, and Duration

With a focus on anger arousal and social-cognitive processes, the Anger Coping Program targets the development of several skills found to be poorly developed in aggressive children. Such skills include awareness of negative feelings, use of self-talk and distraction techniques to decrease anger arousal, and perspective-taking, goal-setting, and problem-solving skills. The concepts presented in session 8 are the most critical components of the anger coping model in terms of behavior change. Given their predisposition to believe that angry behaviors lead to desired outcomes, members must come to view anger as a problem with which they need to cope and begin to look at alternative solutions that will lead to better consequences. Use of weekly goal sheets promotes generalization of skills learned in group sessions to other environments such as the classroom.

The Anger Coping Program is designed to include 18 weekly sessions. Ideally, following treatment, group members will show improvements in the targeted skills, as outlined previously. An individual child's improvements can be tracked across his or her weekly goal sheets and can be observed through the child's behavior in group (e.g., the ability to generate nonaggressive solutions to problems). In addition, assessment instruments used to collect data before group can be readministered to determine individual change following the intervention. Approximately one-third of children in clinical settings may require some follow-up, including booster sessions, regular individual sessions for several months to reinforce the content of the Anger Coping Program, or parent management training to continue improvements or to maintain gains. The related Coping Power Program addresses several of these needs by including a longer course of child therapy and concurrent parent management training.

The Coping Power Program—Child and Parent Components

The Coping Power Program (Lochman, Wells, & Lenhart, 2008; Wells, Lochman, & Lenhart, 2008) is an extension of the Anger Coping Program and includes 34 child sessions delivered over a 15-month period as well as a 16-session parent component delivered during the same period. The additional child group sessions allow for coverage of other problem areas associated with aggression, such as advanced emotional awareness skills, relaxation training, and positive social and personal goals. Likewise, the additional sessions focus on the enhancement of social skills, including methods of entering new peer groups, using positive peer networks, and coping with peer pressure. In addition, the group sessions are augmented with regular individual meetings (at least monthly) to aid in the generalization of skills.

Parent group sessions address the use of social learning techniques, such as identifying prosocial and disruptive behavioral targets for children using specific operational terms, rewarding and attending to appropriate child behaviors, giving effective instructions and establishing age-appropriate rules and expectations for children in the home, and applying effective consequences to negative child behaviors. Parents also learn ways to manage child behavior outside the home and to establish ongoing family communication structures. In addition to these standard skills, parents learn additional techniques that support the social-cognitive and problem-solving skills that their children learn in the child component. For example, parents learn techniques to manage sibling conflict in the home and to apply the problem-solving model to family problem solving. Finally, the parent component includes sessions on stress management for parents. Part of the rationale for this is to help parents learn to remain calm and in control during stressful or irritating disciplinary interactions with their children.

EVIDENCE ON THE EFFECTS OF TREATMENTS

The Anger Coping Program has been evaluated in two studies that included random assignment of children to either an anger coping condition or an untreated control condition (Lochman, Burch, Curry, & Lampron, 1984; Lochman, Lampron, Gemmer, Harris, & Wyckoff, 1989). In addition, Lochman et al. (1999) compared two versions of the program using random assignment and in a separate study used a quasi-experimental design to compare different treatment lengths. Two studies examined follow-up effects of the program (Lochman, 1992; see Lochman et al., 1999), and another examined moderator variables (Lochman, Lampron, Burch, & Curry, 1985). Variants of the Anger Coping Program, which have included an enhanced focus on social relations training (Lochman, Coie, Underwood, & Terry, 1993), and the Coping Power Program described previously have been studied with randomized designs. Treatment effects have been evaluated, in different studies, with behavioral checklists completed by teachers and by parents, by behavioral observations of children's behaviors in classrooms, by peer sociometric ratings, and by measures of the child and parent processes that were the targets of the intervention. An overview of the results of these studies follows.

Anger Coping Outcome Effects

After an initial within-group pilot study indicated that second- and third-grade children had reduced aggression following involvement in an anger control program (see Larson & Lochman, 2002), identified as aggressive based on teacher ratings 76 boys were randomly assigned to anger coping (AC), goal setting (GS), AC + GS, or untreated control cells (Lochman et al., 1984). The boys were in fourth through sixth grades, and 53% were African American and 47% were Caucasian. They participated in 12 weekly school-based anger coping group sessions, based on the Anger Coping Program. Groups were co-led by university-based project staff (psychologists, social workers, psychology interns) and by counselors based at each school. Goal setting was conceptualized as a minimal treatment condition and included eight group sessions in which boys set weekly goals for classroom behaviors and received contingent reinforcements for goal attainment. In comparison to the untreated control and GS conditions, aggressive boys in the AC cells (AC, AC + GS) displayed less parent-reported aggressive behavior and had lower rates of independent observers' time-sampled ratings of disruptive classroom behavior. The addition of a goal-setting component in the AC + GS cell tended to enhance the treatment effects of the program (Lochman et al., 1984).

In the quasi-experimental study by Lochman et al. (1999), Anger Coping Program effects have been found to be augmented with the use of an 18 session version compared with a 12-session version. In this study, 22 teacher-identified aggressive boys (55% African American, 45% Caucasian; mean age, 10 years 4 months) received an 18-session version of the Anger Coping Program (with more emphasis on perspective taking, role playing, and more problem solving about anger-provoking situations). The results were compared with those of the Lochman et al.'s (1984) 12-session program study. Aggressive boys in the longer 18-session program displayed significantly greater improvement in on-task behavior and greater reduction in passive off-task behavior that did not involve interactions with others (e.g., not paying attention to classroom work), illustrating the need for longer intervention periods for children with chronic acting-out behavior problems.

However, in two other studies of the effects of variations in delivery of the Anger Coping Program, the addition of a five-session teacher consultation component (Lochman et al., 1989) and a self-instruction training component focusing on academic tasks did not enhance intervention effects. Lochman et al. (1989) had randomly assigned 32 boys (31% African American, 69% Caucasian; mean age, 11 years 0 months) to AC, AC plus teacher consultation, or an untreated control condition. The school-based groups lasted for 18 weekly sessions, and the boys in both intervention conditions displayed greater reductions in teacher-rated aggression, improvements in perceived social competence and in self-esteem, and reductions in off-task classroom behavior than did boys in the untreated control condition (Lochman et al., 1989).

Two other studies have examined the follow-up effects of the Anger Coping Program. A partial follow-up was conducted of the Lochman et al. (1984) sample in four of the eight schools (Lochman & Lampron, 1988). This follow-up study included 21 boys who had received the Anger Coping Program and 10 who had been in the untreated control condition (39% African American, 61% Caucasian; mean age, 11 years 7 months). When their classroom behavior was examined at a 7-month follow-up, the Anger Coping Program boys had significantly improved levels of independently observed on-task classroom behavior and significant reductions in passive off-task behavior compared with those in the control condition. At a 3-year follow-up, when the boys were a mean of 15 years old, the Anger Coping Program group ($N = 31$) exhibited lower levels of marijuana, drug, and alcohol use and maintained increases in self-esteem and problem-solving skills (Lochman, 1992) compared with the untreated control group ($N = 52$). Boys who were followed up were highly similar on baseline peer aggression nominations and social status ratings to boys who were not available for follow-up. These results indicate the Anger Coping Program produced long-term maintenance of social-cognitive gains and important prevention effects in relation to adolescent substance use. The Anger Coping Program boys' functioning in these domains was within the range of a nonaggressive comparison group ($N = 62$), indicating the clinical significance of these positive effects. However, the Anger Coping Program boys did not have significant reductions in delinquent behavior at follow-up, and the reductions in independently observed off-task behavior and parent-rated aggression were maintained only for a subset of Anger Coping Program boys who had received a brief six-session booster intervention for themselves and their parents the year after their initial Anger Coping Program treatment. Thus, across multiple controlled intervention studies, this child-centered cognitive-behavioral intervention reduced children's disruptive behaviors immediately after treatment and reduced the risk of later adolescent substance use.

Moderation of Anger Coping Program Effects

Boys in the Anger Coping Program who had the greatest reductions in parent-rated aggression in the Lochman et al. (1984) study initially had higher levels of peer rejection, more comorbid internalizing symptoms, and the poorest problem-solving skills (Lochman et al., 1985). The latter variable was a particularly important predictor of treatment effectiveness because boys with the poorest social problem-solving skills in the untreated control condition were likely to have increasingly higher levels of aggressive behavior by the end of the school year.

In another study of child characteristics that predict intervention outcomes, Lochman and colleagues (1993) evaluated a social relations program that included the Anger Coping Program components addressing anger management and social problem-solving skills as well as additional social skill training components (e.g., social skill training sessions on entering new groups of peers and on negotiating when experiencing interpersonal conflict on a task). These specific areas of social skill training have been incorporated into the social problem-solving sessions in the related Coping Power Program. In the study involving fourth-grade African American inner-city children, Lochman et al. (1993) found that the Anger Coping Program enhanced with social relations training had a significant impact for aggressive-rejected children at postintervention and a 1-year-follow-up but not for rejected-only children. Relative to control conditions, the intervention aggressive-rejected children had reductions in peer-rated and teacher-rated aggressive behavior.

Coping Power Program Outcome Effects

A number of studies have examined the efficacy and effectiveness of the Coping Power Program, as well as factors affecting program dissemination. In the first study (Lochman & Wells, 2004), 183 boys (61% African American, 39% Caucasian) who had high rates of teacher rated aggression in fourth or fifth grades were randomly assigned to a school-based Coping Power Program child component, a combination of Coping Power Program child and parent components, or an untreated control condition. Intervention took place over two academic years (fourth and fifth grades for some children, fifth and sixth grades for others). Outcome analyses indicated that both Coping Power Program conditions produced lower rates of delinquent behavior and parent-rated substance use at a 1-year follow-up than the control cell, and these intervention effects were most apparent for the combined treatment condition. Boys also displayed teacher-rated behavioral improvements in school during in follow-up year, and these effects were evident in both intervention conditions and appeared to be primarily influenced by the Coping Power Program child component. The intervention effect on substance use was stronger for boys from moderate-income versus low-income families, and the intervention-produced improvements in school behavior were more apparent for Caucasians than for African American. Normative comparison analyses with a nonrisk sample of 63 boys from the same schools indicate that the intervention moved at-risk boys into normative ranges for substance use, delinquency, and school behavior in contrast to at-risk control boys, who differed significantly from the normative group on the latter two outcomes.

Path analyses indicate that the intervention effects were at least partly mediated by changes in boys' social-cognitive processes, schemas, and parenting processes (Lochman & Wells, 2002). Changes in social-cognitive appraisal processes, involving hostile attributions and resulting anger, and decision-making processes, involving reductions in the expectations that aggressive behavior would lead to good outcomes, reduced the risk for antisocial behavior. Similarly, changes in boys' schemas involving beliefs about their degree of internal control over successful outcomes and the complexity of their internal representations of others and changes in their perceptions of the consistency of their parents' discipline efforts were found to mediate reductions in delinquency, substance use, and school behavioral problems. Consistent with the assumptions of the contextual social-cognitive model, boys' engagement in serious problem behavior in the year after their involvement in the Coping Power Program intervention was affected in part by changes in the way that they perceived and processed their social world and in their expectations of more consistent and predictable responses from their parents.

Another study examined whether the effects of the Coping Power Program, offered as an indicated prevention intervention for high-risk aggressive children, could be enhanced by adding a universal prevention component (Lochman & Wells, 2003). The universal intervention consisted of in-service training for teachers and large-scale meetings for all parents of children in the universal intervention classrooms. The sample consisted of 245 aggressive fourth-grade male (66%) and female (34%) students (78% African American, 20% Caucasian, 2% other), who were randomly assigned to one of four conditions: indicated intervention plus universal intervention (II + UI), indicated intervention plus universal control (II + UC), indicated control plus universal intervention (IC + UI), and indicated control plus universal control (IC + UC). The universal intervention was randomly offered to half of the fifth-grade teachers. Intervention began in the fall of the fifth-grade year and continued midway through the following year. Analyses of postintervention effects (see Lochman et al., 2008) comparing intervention with control conditions indicate that II + UI treatment produced lower rates of self-reported substance use, lower teacher-rated aggression, higher perceived social competence, and greater teacher-rated behavioral improvement, indicating the value of nesting the Coping Power Program within a universal prevention program. The Coping Power Program intervention by itself produced reduced ratings of parent-rated proactive aggression, lower activity level by children, better teacher-rated peer acceptance of target children, and increased parental supportiveness. At 1-year follow-up, all intervention cells produced reductions in substance use and delinquency in comparison to the control condition, and the reduction in delinquency was most apparent for children who had received the combined II + UI interventions (Lochman & Wells, 2003).

Two randomized controlled trials have examined outcomes of an abbreviated version of the Coping Power Program that can be implemented in one school year (with 24 child sessions and 10 parent sessions). In a study of 240 at-risk aggressive fifth graders, the program produced significant reductions in teacher-rated externalizing behavior for children who had a caregiver attend at least one parent session (Lochman, Boxmeyer, Powell, Roth, & Windle, 2006) in comparison to randomly assigned control children. In a randomized controlled trial with 119 students, an independent investigative team found that the 24-session Coping Power Program child component alone produced significant teacher-rated behavioral improvements (Peterson, Hamilton, & Russell, 2008) in comparison to the control condition. The Coping Power Program has also been adapted effectively for use with aggressive hearing-impaired children (Lochman et al., 2001): Children assigned to a Coping Power Program condition had improved problem-solving skills, compared with randomly assigned controls.

The Coping Power Program has also been adapted for use with clinic populations. A briefer Dutch version was evaluated in a study in which children with disruptive behavior disorders (N = 77) were randomly assigned to the Coping Power Program or to clinic treatment as usual (TAU). Both groups improved significantly on disruptiveness post-treatment and at a 6-month follow-up, but the Coping Power Program group had significantly greater reductions in overt aggression by posttreatment (van de Wiel et al., 2007) compared with the TAU group. Coping Power Program clinicians had significantly less experience than TAU therapists, indicating that the Coping Power Program was more cost-effective in producing similar effect sizes (van de Wiel, 2003). At a later 4-year follow-up of this sample, the TAU children had significantly lower marijuana and tobacco use than the TAU children, although the groups did not differ in alcohol use (Zonnevylle-Bender, Matthys, van de Wiel, & Lochman, 2007). The Coping Power Program children were using marijuana and tobacco within the range of a normative comparison group at the time of this long-term follow-up, indicating long-lasting, preventive effects of the intervention (Zonnevyille-Bender et al., 2007).

Overall Evaluation of the Anger Coping and Coping Power Programs

This series of research studies indicates that a cognitive-behavioral intervention using the Anger Coping Program framework can have immediate effects at postintervention on children's aggressive behavior at home and at school, according to parent, teacher, and independent observer ratings. The effect sizes are typically in the moderate range, and moderators such as initial levels of problem-solving skills and family income level can impact the intervention effects, indicating that not all children respond to this form of intervention. The Anger Coping Program can have lasting preventive effects on children's later substance used up to 3 years following intervention completion—but an adjunctive parent intervention component appears necessary to achieve longer term effects on delinquency. The results emphasize that this form of cognitive-behavioral intervention can be useful not only for short-term treatment purposes but also for longer term prevention purposes and that the program can be effectively delivered in school and clinic settings.

Dissemination Study of the Coping Power Program

A controlled dissemination study of the Coping Power Program was recently conducted in 57 schools in five Alabama systems. School counselors (N = 531) were randomly assigned to implement Coping Power Program training for implementation with high-risk aggressive fourth- and fifth-grade students or to a TAU control condition (N = 531). The intensity of training had a notable impact on child outcomes. In comparison to the control condition, significant reductions in child externalizing behavior (based on teacher, parent, and child ratings) and improvements in social and academic behaviors only occurred when a more intensive form of training was provided (i.e., when counselors received immediate supervisory feedback based on recorded sessions; Lochman et al., 2009). School-level factors and counselor traits were associated with quality of program implementation, with agreeable and conscientious counselors demonstrating the best program implementation. Counselors rated high on cynicism and from schools with low levels of staff autonomy and high levels of managerial control had particularly poor implementation and child and parent engagement levels (Lochman et al., in press).

DIRECTIONS FOR RESEARCH

A strength of cognitive-behavioral interventions for children's aggressive behavior such as the Anger Coping and Coping Power Programs is that they are based on a clear conceptual model of the mutable mediating processes. However, despite interesting recent findings, further research is needed to examine whether these interventions have any immediate proximal effects on an array of social-cognitive and parenting practices and, if so, whether these effects lead to distal reductions in conduct disorder, delinquency, and substance abuse and improve participants' long-term adjustment in adolescence and adulthood. It will also be necessary to consider how larger contextual factors, such as the degree of neighborhood violence and crime, impact intervention effects. A critical goal will be to identify the dissemination and training process characteristics, as well as organizational and provider characteristics, that promote effective and sustained use of the Anger Coping and Coping Power Program interventions in school and service settings.

CONCLUSIONS

The Anger Coping and Coping Power Programs provide a theoretically and empirically based framework for preventing and treating child's aggressive behavior. Next steps for development and research include a focus on identification of the intervention characteristics and mediating factors that are most strongly associated with long-term behavioral improvements and on methods for addressing children's broader contextual risk factors and identifying the processes that lead to successful program implementation and dissemination.

A key challenge in disseminating interventions such as the Anger Coping and Coping Power Programs to naturalistic settings is ensuring that the core features are implemented with fidelity while providing sufficient flexibility to maximize the use of clinical expertise and to address diverse setting, provider, and client characteristics. The next generation of research should examine methods for training practitioners to utilize the Anger Coping and Coping Power Program intervention manuals as a framework for targeting the mediating factors underlying children's aggressive behavior, including child social-cognitive difficulties and parenting behaviors. Provision of ongoing training and consultation during program implementation appears to be critical to this process (Lochman et al., 2009).

Although group-based interventions can provide valuable opportunities for *in vivo* practice of emotional coping and social problem-solving skills and for peer modeling and reinforcement of prosocial strategies, they also carry the risk of peer reinforcement of deviant attitudes and behaviors. In our research on the Anger Coping and Coping Power Programs group interventions, we have not found iatrogenic effects. However, deviant peer effects in the groups may have limited the degree of behavioral gains for some children. Thus, an important next line of research is to identify the structural intervention components and leader behaviors that help generate and maintain a positive group process. Key group leader behaviors may include the ability to monitor disruptive and deviant behaviors in a group, to restructure and refocus a group to other tasks to divert the members from reinforcing deviant behaviors, and to provide clear, consistent consequences within the group (such as loss of group rules points). In current ongoing research, the Coping Power Program has been adapted for individual administration, and this research will include a direct comparison of group versus individual administration and the identification of leader behaviors associated with effective outcomes. Moving forward, emphasis will be placed on examining implementation, dissemination, and training processes with scientific rigor.

ACKNOWLEDGMENTS

The intervention research on the Anger Coping and Coping Power Programs has been supported by grants from the National Institute on Drug Abuse (Nos. R01DA023156, R01DA016135, R01DA008453), Center for Substance Abuse Prevention (Nos. KDISP08633, UR65907956), Centers for Disease Control and Prevention (No. R49/CCR418569), Department of Justice (Nos. 2006JLFX0232, 2000CKWX0091), and National Institute of Mental Health (No. R01MH039989).

REFERENCES

Larson, J., & Lochman, J. E. (2002). *Helping school children cope with anger: A cognitive-behavioral intervention.* New York: Guilford Press.

Lochman, J. E. (1992). Cognitive-behavioral interventions with aggressive boys: Three-year follow-up and preventive effects. *Journal of Consulting and Clinical Psychology, 60,* 426–432.

Lochman, J. E., Boxmeyer, C. L., Powell, N. P., Qu, L., Wells, K. C., & Windle, M. (2009). Dissemination of the Coping Power Program: Importance of intensity of counselor training. *Journal of Consulting and Clinical Psychology, 77,* 397–409.

Lochman, J. E., Boxmeyer, C. L., Powell, N. P., Roth, D., & Windle, M. (2006). Masked intervention effects: Analytic methods for addressing low dosage of intervention. *New Directions for Evaluation, 110,* 19–32.

Lochman, J. E., Burch, P. P., Curry, J. F., & Lampron, L. B. (1984). Treatment and generalization effects of cognitive-behavioral and goal setting interventions with aggressive boys. *Journal of Consulting and Clinical Psychology, 52,* 915–916.

Lochman, J. F., Coie, J. D., Underwood, M., & Terry, R. (1993). Effectiveness of a social relations intervention program for aggressive and nonaggressive rejected children. *Journal of Consulting and Clinical Psychology, 61,* 1053–1058.

Lochman, J. E., & Dodge, K. A. (1994). Social-cognitive processes of severely violent, moderately aggressive and nonaggressive boys. *Journal of Consulting and Clinical Psychology, 62,* 366–374.

Lochman, J. E., FitzGerald, D. P., Gage, S. M., Kannaly, M. K., Whidby, J. M., Barry, T. D., et al. (2001). Effects of social-cognitive intervention for aggressive deaf children: The Coping Power Program. *Journal of the American Deafness and Rehabilitation Association, 35,* 39–61.

Lochman, J. E., FitzGerald, D. P., & Whidby, J. M. (1999). Anger management with aggressive children. In C. Schaefer (Ed.), *Short-term psychotherapy groups for children* (pp. 301–349). Northvale, NJ: Jason Aronson.

Lochman, J. E., & Lampron, L. B. (1988). Cognitive behavioral interventions for aggressive boys: Seven month follow-up effects. *Journal of Child and Adolescent Psychotherapy, 5,* 15–23.

Lochman, J. E., Lampron, L. B., Burch, P. R., & Curry, J. E. (1985). Client characteristics associated with behavior change for treated and untreated boys. *Journal of Abnormal Child Psychology, 13,* 527–538.

Lochman, J. E., Lampron, L. B., Gemmer, T. C., Harris, S. R., & Wyckoff, G. M. (1989). Teacher consultation and cognitive-behavioral interventions with aggressive boys. *Psychology in the Schools, 26,* 179–188.

Lochman, J. E., Powell, N. P., Boxmeyer, C. L., Qu, L., Wells, K. C., & Windle, M. (in press). Implementation of a school-based prevention program: Effects of counselor and school characteristics. *Professional Psychology: Research & Practice.*

Lochman, J. E., & Wells, K. C. (2002). Contextual social-cognitive mediators and child outcome: A test of the theoretical model in the Coping Power Program. *Development and Psychopathology, 14,* 971–993.

Lochman, J. E., & Wells, K. C. (2003). Effectiveness study of Coping Power and classroom intervention with aggressive children: Outcomes at a one-year follow-up. *Behavior Therapy, 34,* 493–515.

Lochman, J. E., & Wells, K. C. (2004). The Coping Power Program for preadolescent aggressive boys and their parents: Outcome effects at the one-year follow-up. *Journal of Consulting and Clinical Psychology, 72,* 571–578.

Lochman, J. E., Wells, K. C., & Lenhart, L. (2008). *Coping Power: Child group facilitators' guide.* New York: Oxford University Press.

Peterson, M. A., Hamilton, E. B., & Russell, A. D. (2008). *Starting well: Evidenced-based treatment facilitates the middle school transition.* Manuscript submitted for publication.

van de Wiel, N. M. H., Matthys, W., Cohen-Kettenis, P. T., Maassen, G. H., Lochman, J. E., & van Engeland, H. (2007). The effectiveness of an experimental treatment when compared with care as usual depends on the type of care as usual. *Behavior Modification, 31,* 298–312.

van de Wiel, N. M. H., Matthys, W., Cohen-Kettenis, P. T., & van Engeland, H. (2003). Application of the Utrecht Coping Power Program and care as usual to children with disruptive behavior disorders: A comparative study of cost and course of treatment. *Behavior Therapy, 34,* 421–436.

Wells, K. C., Lochman, J. E., & Lenhart, L. (2008). *Coping Power: Parent group facilitators' guide.* New York: Oxford University Press.

Zonnevylle-Bender, M. J. S., Matthys, W., van de Wiel, N. M. H., & Lochman, J. (2007). Preventive effects of treatment of disruptive behavior disorder in middle childhood on substance use and delinquent behavior. *Journal of the American Academy of Child and Adolescent Psychiatry, 46,* 33–39.

16

Multidimensional Treatment Foster Care for Adolescents
Processes and Outcomes

DANA K. SMITH and PATRICIA CHAMBERLAIN

OVERVIEW

Researchers have identified myriad risk factors associated with conduct problem behavior, including childhood trauma and maltreatment, poor parenting practices, parent criminality and psychopathology, delinquent peer associations, and low IQ. The results from previous work have helped to identify possible pathways to delinquency, have suggested that child and family factors independently contribute to the onset of delinquency (Leve & Chamberlain, 2004), and have highlighted risks associated with childhood conduct problems. Youths with conduct problems have been shown to be at high risk for a cascading host of additional problems as they age, including severe and persistent physical and mental health problems, incarceration, and early death. Despite substantial progress in understanding the developmental course of conduct problems and antisocial behavior, few evidence-based treatment options exist. Effective programs for youths with severe and chronic conduct problems are particularly limited.

In settings where youths with severe delinquency are typically placed and treated (e.g., state training schools and residential care centers), treatment programs generally lack empirical support and are often expensive to operate. In addition, some researchers have demonstrated the negative outcomes of congregating youths with conduct problems in treatment settings (Dishion, McCord, & Poulin, 1999). Despite research on the iatrogenic effects of group care and the high cost of operating residential care facilities, these treatment approaches are common for youths with severe conduct problems. In this chapter, we describe a community-based model for treating youths with severe and chronic delinquency and conduct problems, highlight the outcomes from three random-ized clinical trials with adolescents referred from the juvenile justice system, and discuss adaptations to the model and future directions.

ORIGINS AND DEVELOPMENT OF MULTIDIMENSIONAL TREATMENT FOSTER CARE

Multidimensional treatment foster care (MTFC; Chamberlain, 2003) was developed in 1983 in response to a state of Oregon request for proposals for community-based alternatives to incarceration and placement in residential/group care settings. MTFC is a community-based treatment model based on more than 40 years of longitudinal research on the development and treatment of antisocial behavior. Although MTFC was originally designed as an alternative to group home placement or commitment to state training facilities for severely delinquent boys, it has since been adapted to treat girls with chronic delinquency problems (Chamberlain, Leve, & DeGarmo, 2007) and youths and their families referred from mental health and child welfare systems because of severe emotional and mental health problems (Chamberlain et al., 2008; Chamberlain & Reid, 1991; Fisher, Burraston, & Pears, 2005).

OVERVIEW OF THE MTFC MODEL

The underpinnings of the MTFC model are founded in social learning theory. From a social learning theory perspective, conduct problem behavior can be characterized as a process of inadvertently reinforced negative behavior that grows in severity and complexity over time. The coercive processes that sustain these negative behaviors are often reciprocal and transactional: Parent–child interactions influence parenting prac-tices, which are simultaneously influenced by environmental and contextual factors. For example, a child's temperamental difficulties at various stages of development might elicit frustrated and helpless responses from the parents, which can contribute to par-ents' feelings of ineffectiveness or inadequacy. Feelings of parental ineptitude and frus-tration have been shown to be related to aversive responses and withdrawal in response to child noncompliance, which can then elicit further challenging behaviors from the child. Contextual influences such as parental stress might further reinforce coercive family processes to the extent that such stress increases marital conflict or disrupts con-sistent and thoughtful parenting practices. Once coercive processes are in place, they tend to be maintained with very little reinforcement. The good news, however, is that coercive processes, regardless of severity or duration, can be interrupted at any point in the developmental process by improving parenting practices. Parenting plays a central role in the development, maintenance, and treatment of antisocial behavior. The results from research on the MTFC model have helped to identify specific parenting practices that serve as key variables in the development and treatment of antisocial behavior and delinquency.

According to social learning theory, new behaviors are most effectively taught and generalized in naturally occurring settings (e.g., the family). In the MTFC model, which was designed with this in mind, youths are kept in the community, and the foster fam-ily setting is used to teach, practice, and reinforce adaptive youth responses to everyday compliance demands. The MTFC model has been designed to capitalize on the powerful social role that parents play in the lives of their children and on the family as the change agent. Using a community-based family environment to teach and reinforce desired behaviors provides a closer approximation to the real-world experiences that youths encounter and thus provides a greater chance for successful generalization of desired behaviors.

MTFC Basics

There are two primary goals of MTFC: (1) to create opportunities for youths to live successfully in their communities while providing them with intensive supervision, support, and skill development and (2) to simultaneously prepare the youths' biological parents (or other aftercare resources) to provide effective parenting that will interrupt coercive family processes and increase the chance for positive reintegration into the family after treatment. The MTFC model involves working simultaneously with youths, biological parents (or other aftercare resources), and trained foster parents using a series of well-coordinated, multicomponent, multilevel interventions that occur in family, school, and community settings. Youths are placed one per MTFC home for 6–9 months and are provided with intensive interventions that span seamlessly across multiple settings via a comprehensive individualized behavior management program and consistent case management. Youths are provided with close supervision and frequent reinforcement for learning and practicing adaptive interpersonal skills. Each youth receives weekly individual therapy and skills training, academic support, and psychiatric consultation as needed. Parents (or other aftercare resources) receive weekly family therapy that is based on the parent management training treatment model. Family therapy focuses on implementing effective parenting strategies and techniques, such as monitoring the adolescent's whereabouts and peer associations, reinforcing positive and normative behavior and activities, and setting limits.

The MTFC Treatment Team

The MTFC model includes a core team of clinicians and staff. As is seen in Figure 16.1, the MTFC treatment team is composed of a program supervisor, who is responsible for leading the team; the MTFC foster parents; a family therapist for the biological/aftercare family; an individual therapist for the youth; a skills trainer for the youth; and an on-site consulting psychiatrist. A MTFC recruiter/trainer participates in the recruitment and training of new MTFC parents and conducts short (7–10 minutes) daily telephone calls with MTFC parents to measure youth behaviors and MTFC parent stress levels.

Program Supervisors

The program supervisors have small caseloads (10 families each) so that they can provide intensive, personal case management for each family. They are responsible for coordinating all aspects each youth's treatment plan: supervising the MTFC parents and the treatment team and ensuring that all interventions are well thought out and seamless across settings (i.e., multiple interventions do not conflict with each other). The program supervisor is the liaison between all of the youth's environments and is responsible

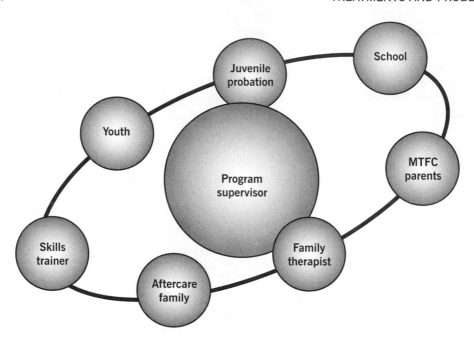

FIGURE 16.1. Multidimensional treatment foster care (MTFC) model.

for providing clear communication and consultation with biological family members, school personnel, and community service providers. The daily school cards, which track attendance, behavior, and class work completion and are carried by each youth, facilitate consistent communication between the school and the program supervisor. The program supervisor is responsible for maintaining daily contact with the MTFC parents to collect data on youth adjustment and for providing ongoing consultation, support, and 24-hour crisis intervention. The program supervisor provides ongoing training and support to the MTFC parents via mandatory weekly meetings and is the "go-to" person for decision making for the biological parents (or other aftercare resource). The program supervisor also conducts weekly phone or in-person meetings with probation/parole officers to discuss each youth's progress.

Because of the complexities involved in designing multisetting interventions, balancing the unique needs of each case, and the staff supervision responsibilities, the program supervisors are the most skilled clinical member of the MTFC team. Each must hold a master's degree in psychology or a related field (with training in social learning theory, developmental psychology, and behavioral treatment approaches) and receive weekly supervision by the MTFC program director.

MTFC Foster Parents

Potential foster parents receive 20 hours of preservice training from the foster parent recruiter/trainer and the MTFC staff before becoming state certified. The MTFC parents are trained according to social learning and behavioral approaches, in which modeling, role-playing, and reinforcement are strongly emphasized. The MTFC parents are seen as the central change agents. They are taught to pay close attention to youths' strengths, to reinforce positive and adaptive behaviors at a high rate, to turn daily experiences into teaching opportunities, and to create opportunities for youths to observe and practice prosocial responses to challenging situations.

The MTFC parents are taught to implement a daily behavior management system that is focused on providing feedback to youths about their daily behaviors in a nonreactive way. This system consists of three levels that use contingencies to reinforce positive behaviors over the course of treatment. As is seen in Figure 16.2, this system involves typical daily expectations for adolescents. The youths earn points for completing each behavior and lose points for maladaptive or noncompliant behaviors. All positive behaviors are reinforced via the point system, which includes the opportunity to exchange points for a standard list of privileges in the MTFC program (Figure 16.3). According to this system, youths need to budget their points to access to the number and types of privileges they desire. Data on emotional and behavioral problems for each youth in the program are collected each weekday using the Parent Daily Report (PDR; see Figure 16.4; Chamberlain & Reid, 1987) to identify possible ongoing problems and to monitor MTFC parent stress levels. Using these data, the program supervisor tracks each youth's progress daily. The behavior management system is constructed so that privilege removal in response to negative behavior occurs for a short duration (1 day) so that youths are taught to recover quickly from maladaptive behaviors. Work chores and interventions from probation/

MTFC LEVEL II POINTS		
Name:	Date:	
BEHAVIOR	DESCRIPTION	POINTS
UP ON TIME	Out of bed	10
READY IN MORNING	Showered, teeth brushed, hair combed, wearing clean clothes, and eating breakfast	10
MORNING CLEAN UP	Bed made, dirty clothes put away, room neat, bath towel and wash rag put away, and dishes placed in sink	10
GO TO SCHOOL	On time for the bus and attending each class with no tardiness	5
CARRY SCHOOL CARD	Carrying school card to each class and having teacher sign it	2/class
BEHAVIOR IN CLASS	Paying attention to tasks in class, cooperating with teacher, and handing homework in on time	5/class
READ AND STUDY	50 minutes reading/writing each day (not including letter writing)	20
SCHOOL CARD BONUS	Getting all signatures and having no overdue homework, no tardies, and good behavior	10
CHORE	To be explained each day	10
ATTITUDE/MATURITY	Being helpful, taking criticism well, being pleasant, not pushing limits, not being moody, and accepting "No"	15 A.M. 15 P.M.
VOLUNTEERING	Volunteering to do extra tasks (parent will decide on points)	2–10
EXTRA CHORE	Optional (must be approved by parent)	5–50
BED ON TIME	If you can buy BASICS (minimum of 50 points): 9:30 P.M. If you can't buy BASICS: 8:30 P.M.	10

FIGURE 16.2. Behavior management system: level II behaviors. (MTFC, multidimensional treatment foster care.)

MTFC LEVEL II PRIVILEGES		
Name: Date:		
PRIVILEGE	DESCRIPTION	COST IN POINTS
BASICS*	Using telephone for 15 minutes once a day, listening to radio in room, or 9:30 P.M. bedtime	350
TV	Watch TV after homework and chores are completed	100
LATER BEDTIME	11:00 P.M. bedtime: Fridays, Saturdays, and holidays	40
EXTRA TELEPHONE TIME	One 20-minute phone call (not long distance)	25
ACTIVITY TIME	With prior permission and approval, plan to go to a friend's house, sport event, or school activity or go for a walk, bike ride, etc. Overnight activities are to be negotiated. Plans must be made 24 hour in advance Having a friend over	½ point/min Maximum 2 hrs activity time/ week) ¼ point/min
PERSONAL PURCHASES	$10.00/week: must have receipts for all purchases	200
BONDS	1 bond costs 100 points 6 bonds needed to advance to Level III	50/week max toward bonds

*BASICS must be purchased before you are eligible for other privileges.

FIGURE 16.3. Behavior management system: level II privileges. (MTFC, multidimensional treatment foster care.)

parole officers are reserved for larger behavior violations (e.g., substance use and skipping school).

Aside from the MTFC training, the MTFC parents are not required to have any formal education. However, several commonalities have been found among successful MTFC parents: flexibility and interest in working closely with the treatment team, a general interest in and compassion for teaching and guiding youths as they grow and change, and a sense of humor. Each of these characteristics is helpful in implementing the MTFC model, providing support for fellow MTFC parents, and working with the often unpredictable nature of adolescents.

Family Therapists

The ultimate goal of MTFC is to successfully reunite youths with their biological parents (or other relatives or aftercare resources). As such, family therapy is a central focus of the MTFC model and begins immediately upon a youth's placement in the program. The family therapist meets weekly with the biological parents (or other aftercare resources) to provide parent training and to problem solve difficulties with parent management. During weekly family therapy sessions with their child, parents are taught to implement the MTFC behavior management system, which is a series of core parent management strategies that include effective supervision and monitoring techniques, effective contingency management strategies, and effective strategies for setting clear limits while avoiding power struggles with the child. As the youth progresses in the program, home visits grow in length, providing the biological parents (or other aftercare resources) greater

BEHAVIORS	Sun	Mon	Tues	Wed	Thurs
Arguing					
Back talking					
Bedwetting					
Competitiveness					
Complaining					
Defiance					
Destructive/vandalism					
Encopresis					
Fighting					
Irritability					
Lying					
Negativism					
Boisterous/rowdy					
Not minding					
Staying out late					
Skipping meals					
Running away					
Swearing/obscene language					
Tease/provoke					
Depression/sadness					
Sluggish					
Jealous					
Truant					
Stealing					
Nervous/jittery					
Short attention span					
Daydreaming					
Irresponsibility					
Marijuana/drugs					
Alcohol					
School problem					

MTFC Parent Daily Report — Youth, PDR Caller, Foster Parent, Phone, Week of.

FIGURE 16.4. Multidimensional treatment foster care (MTFC) Parent Daily Report (PDR).

opportunities to successfully implement these new parenting skills. The visits typically begin as short day visits (4 hours) and progress to weekly overnights by the end of the program.

After several sessions of meeting alone with the parents, the family therapy sessions begin to include the youth. The initial joint family therapy sessions include the youth for 10–15 minutes to focus on the introduction of a new parenting skill that has been practiced during the previous family therapy sessions, for example, the presentation of a clearly defined set of house rules to be implemented during home visits (as guided by the family therapist during the previous family therapy sessions). The focus of such a session is on the presentation and explanation of the rules by the parents and on the acceptance of the rules by the youth. The family therapist carefully avoids focusing on processing the parents' feelings or reactions related to the introduction of a new skill in the presence of the youth. Strict attention is paid to timing so that parents are confident in successfully implementing each new skill. An individual therapist (described later) often attends the joint therapy sessions to support the youth and coach him or her on the expected behaviors.

In concert with the program supervisor, the family therapist provides on-call support to parents throughout the course of treatment, so that supportive interventions can occur in the moment, when the youth is being noncompliant rather than after the fact. This provides the opportunity for parents to practice new, more effective parenting skills during real-life experiences and allows for immediate reinforcement by the family therapist of the parents' use of a new skill. In the MTFC model, the foster parents are not expected or encouraged to provide therapy or support for the biological parents; rather, this is the role of the family therapist. This avoids potential strained relationships between the two families and allows both the foster and the biological parents to focus directly and specifically on working with the youth without giving him or her an opportunity to play the adults off each other. The family therapist continues meeting with parents for up to 3 months after reunification to increase the likelihood of a successful transition to the home setting. The family therapist attends the weekly MTFC clinical meetings, is supervised by the program supervisor, and typically holds a master's degree.

Individual Therapists

Individual therapists serve as the primary support for MTFC youths, are introduced as an ally at the start of the placement, and meet weekly with youths throughout the course of treatment. The focus of the weekly individual therapy sessions is to assist youths in adjusting to the demands of MTFC: prosocial skills reinforcement, social skill development, problem solving, emotion management, and the development of educational or occupational plans. The work of individual therapists is carefully integrated into the overall treatment plan so that behavioral targets are well thought out and reinforcement occurs across settings. For example, youths with conduct problems often have difficulty receiving direction from parents or other authority figures. Support from individual therapists during moments of noncompliance can help youths to manage frustration *in vivo* and possibly to implement effective problem-solving or emotion management skills. The youths are able to contact individual therapists by phone for support as needed between weekly sessions. It is also common for the program supervisors to orchestrate support from individual therapists (e.g., after learning of a difficult or challenging situation for a youth in the foster home). The individual therapists are taught to focus on problem-solving and role-playing adaptive responses rather than on processing feelings to avoid inadvertently reinforcing maladaptive youth behaviors such as arguing.

Individual therapists provide on-call support to youths throughout the course of treatment and continue meeting with them for up to 3 months after reunification to increase the likelihood of a successful transition to the home setting. The individual therapists attend the weekly MTFC clinical meetings, are supervised by the program supervisor, and typically hold a master's degree.

Skills Trainers

The skills trainers also serve as supports for MTFC youths. The skills training sessions occur one to two times per week and focus on skill development in community settings via the modeling, teaching, practicing, and reinforcing of prosocial and adaptive behaviors during one-on-one sessions in common community environments (e.g., restaurant, library, community center, school). The behavioral targets and accompanying interventions are discussed during the weekly MTFC clinical team meetings. The skills training sessions have a coaching style, in which the skills trainers take a supportive, friendly, and encouraging approach to provide a more relaxed teaching atmosphere. For example, a skills training session targeting good sportsmanship might take place at a bowling alley, where the youth is provided the opportunity to practice winning and losing in a positive way. A skills training session might also be used for youths to practice such skills as gathering information or researching a topic of interest at a local library or ordering a meal in a restaurant. The skills training sessions differ from individual therapy sessions in that they tend to focus on the development and reinforcement of social skills that are common to typically developing adolescents rather than on behavioral targets that are central to conduct problems, although the skills training sessions are also commonly used to support and reinforce skills that have been practiced during individual therapy sessions. For example, an individual therapist for a youth who has trouble not arguing might focus an individual therapy session on role-playing how to accept feedback without commenting, and the skills trainer might simply reinforce the youth for prosocially accepting feedback from adults in the community.

The skills trainers continue to meet with youths for up to 3 months after reunification to offer support and skill building during the transition home. They attend the weekly MTFC clinical meetings, are supervised by the program supervisors, and typically hold bachelor's-level degrees or are undergraduate students.

MTFC Recruiter/Trainers

The MTFC recruiter/trainers participate in the recruitment and training of the MTFC parents and conduct the daily PDR interviews with the MTFC parents. The purpose of PDR interviews is to catch behaviors when they are small and to provide daily support to the MTFC parents. The MTFC recruiter/trainers are typically paraprofessionals who know the MTFC model well (e.g., a former MTFC parent who has firsthand experience implementing the MTFC model). The MTFC recruiter/trainers attend the weekly foster parent support meetings, provide backup to the program supervisors, and are supervised by the MTFC program supervisors.

Consulting Psychiatrist

A consulting psychiatrist conducts psychiatric evaluations of the youths and coordinates medication management. MTFC youths often have multiple diagnoses and are taking multiple medications at the time of placement; however, the medications are typically decreased or discontinued after the MTFC program. The consulting psychiatrist is experienced in treating conduct problems and comorbid conditions and is cognizant of the basic MTFC treatment model. To facilitate communication and coordination, it is ideal for the consulting psychiatrist to conduct youth evaluations and ongoing medication management meetings on-site.

Role Differentiation

Careful adherence to the specific roles of each treatment team member is a necessary component of the MTFC program. Clearly defined roles are needed for two primary reasons. First, the youths and families are less likely to become confused or overwhelmed when interfacing with numerous treatment team members if communications are well coordinated. Families referred to MTFC often have complex treatment needs that require a clear and orderly approach. Receiving treatment information from multiple sources complicates and diffuses the treatment. Therefore, the program supervisor and the family therapist are the only treatment team members who interact with the family in a therapeutic manner. Although other treatment team members (e.g., individual therapist, skills trainers, MTFC parents) interact with families in a positive, friendly, and encouraging manner as they come and go from meetings, visits, and therapy sessions, these interactions do not incorporate any behavioral or therapeutic interventions.

Second, youths with severe behavioral and emotional problems often have complex reactions to challenging situations, and adverse reactions are more likely to occur when circumstances are unpredictable. Responding to the youths and families in an orderly and predictable manner can help to avoid problems and ease treatment implementation. For example, the program supervisor is identified from the outset of each placement as the head of the MTFC program. The program supervisor outlines the expectations for the youths and sets clear limits throughout the course of treatment. The individual therapist is introduced as an ally for the youths. It is essential that each program supervisor maintains a limit-setting role and that each individual therapist maintains a supportive role with the youths. Similarly, an extra degree of freedom is often helpful to the MTFC parents. Youths with conduct problems often have difficulty receiving feedback or limits from authority figures. Allowing each program supervisor to be the primary limit setter provides MTFC parents with the ability to play a supportive and encouraging role with their youths.

EVIDENCE ON THE EFFECTS OF TREATMENT

The results from several outcome evaluations have demonstrated the effectiveness of MTFC in treating youths with conduct problems. Three clinical efficacy trials have shown that MTFC is effective in decreasing delinquency in adolescent boys (Chamberlain & Reid, 1998) and girls (Chamberlain et al., 2007) compared with group care. The effectiveness of MTFC in treating children and adolescents with severe mental health problems has also been demonstrated via randomized clinical trials with youths from a state mental hospital (Chamberlain & Reid, 1991) and the child welfare system (Chamberlain, Moreland, & Reid, 1992). The following data focus on MTFC outcomes for youths who were referred to out-of-home care from the juvenile justice system.

MTFC Effects on Outcomes among Juvenile Justice Boys

Examinations of the MTFC model applied to the treatment of adolescent boys with chronic delinquency problems have yielded positive results across several emotional and behavioral domains. In a randomized trial of 79 boys (ages 12–17) referred to out-of-home care as a result of chronic delinquency, outcomes were examined at 12 and 24 months postbaseline using a multimethod, multi-informant assessment strategy (e.g., youth, parent, probation/parole, teacher/school, official records).

Delinquency

The results showed the MTFC model to be effective in reducing arrest rates, with boys in MTFC showing larger decreases in official criminal referrals compared with boys in group care. These findings concurred with the MTFC boys' self-reports of delinquent behavior using the Elliott Behavior Checklist, including the General Delinquency, Index Offenses, and Felony Assaults subscales, which were significantly lower compared with self-reports of boys in group care. The MTFC boys spent significantly more time in their intended placements, less time incarcerated, and less time running away. The MTFC boys were also significantly less likely to commit violent offenses compared with boys treated with more traditional intervention models, even when preplacement risk factors were considered (e.g., age at first arrest, age at placement; Eddy, Bridges Whaley, & Chamberlain, 2004).

Mediation of Treatment Outcomes

To better understand what key factors accounted for differences in outcomes, we examined whether the hypothesized treatment components (e.g., family management, deviant peer associations) mediated the relative impact of MTFC. The effect of group assignment on subsequent criminal referrals (i.e., from time of placement to 1 year posttreatment) was examined using path models. Family management skills (i.e., supervision, discipline, and positive adult–youth relationship) and deviant peer association mediated the effects in the treatment condition and accounted for 32% of the variance in subsequent antisocial behavior (see Figure 16.5; Eddy & Chamberlain, 2000).

MTFC Effects on Outcomes among Juvenile Justice Girls

Positive results have also been found for the MTFC model when applied to the treatment of adolescent girls with serious delinquency problems. The intervention effects across a number of emotional and behavioral domains at 12 and 24 months postbaseline are outlined next (Chamberlain et al., 2007).

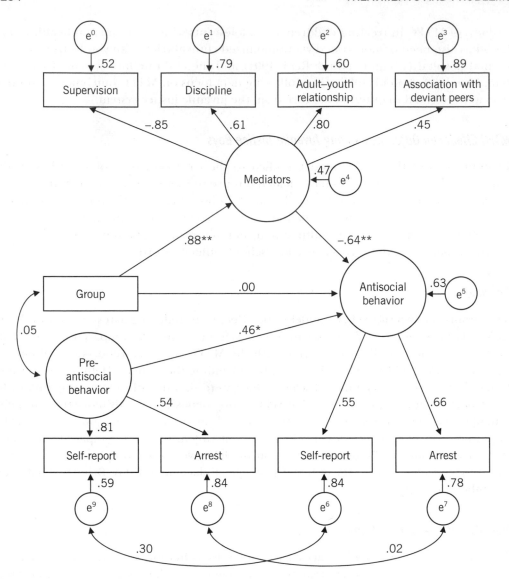

FIGURE 16.5. Multidimensional treatment foster care mediation model. $?^2(22) = 21.802$, $p = .472$, goodness-of-fit index = .920, adjusted goodness-of-fit index = .837, $N = 53$. *$p < .05$; **$p < .01$; ***$p < .001$.

Delinquency

Overall, MTFC demonstrated efficacy above and beyond group care in reducing girls' delinquency at both follow-up assessments. At 12 months postbaseline, the MTFC girls had spent fewer days in locked settings. In addition, there was a trend for the MTFC girls (compared with the group care girls) to have had significantly fewer criminal referrals by the 12-month assessment and a significant effect of MTFC on caregiver-reported delinquency levels on the Child Behavior Checklist. At 24 months postbaseline, we confirmed that the 12-month outcomes had persisted and that the MTFC girls showed a significantly greater rate of reduction in delinquent behavior over time. These findings also suggest the potential for the MTFC intervention to impact costly public service utilization outcomes. For example, the MTFC girls (compared with the group care girls) had spent more than 100 fewer days in locked settings at the 24-month follow-up assessment.

Deviant Peer Associations

Based on prior work demonstrating a strong positive relationship between deviant peer associations and the development and maintenance of adolescent delinquency, reducing deviant peer associations is one of the key aims of the MTFC intervention. Using multimethod constructs (i.e., self- and caregiver reports), we examined whether MTFC reduced rates of deviant peer associations for girls during the course of treatment and whether this reduction mediated the effect of the intervention on deviant peer associations measured at 12 months postbaseline. As hypothesized, MTFC was found to be more effective than group care in reducing delinquent peer associations during treatment, and this reduction fully mediated the intervention effect on 12-month delinquent peer association (Leve & Chamberlain, 2005).

School Engagement

We also examined the impact of MTFC on increasing girls' prosocial and adaptive behaviors. The results from the school outcome (e.g., attendance and homework completion) analyses indicated that the MTFC girls had significantly higher rates of homework completion during treatment and attended school at a higher rate compared with the group care girls at 12 months postbaseline. We also confirmed that homework completion during the intervention mediated the effects on girls' time spent in locked settings at 12 months postbaseline (see Figure 16.6). These results suggest that the implementation of relatively simple daily routines (e.g., homework time) plays a powerful role in changing the negative trajectory of delinquency (Leve & Chamberlain, 2007).

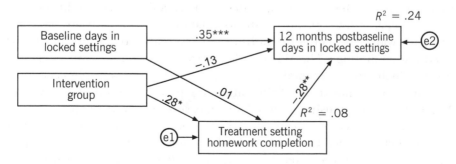

FIGURE 16.6. Mediating effects of homework completion on treatment. Note. $\chi^2(1) = .513$, $p = .474$, comparative fit index = 1.000, root mean square error of approximation = .000. $*p < .05$; $**p < .01$; $***p < .001$.

Pregnancy Rates

Reducing rates of health-risking sexual behavior is another key outcome of MTFC. We examined the effects of MTFC on girls' pregnancy rates at 24 months postbaseline. The results from the logistic regression analyses indicated fewer pregnancies for MTFC girls (26.9%) compared with group care girls (45.7%). This effect persisted after controlling for significant effects of baseline criminal referrals and pregnancy history (Kerr, Leve, & Chamberlain, 2009).

Summary

Overall, MTFC has demonstrated efficacy in reducing girls' delinquency, associations with deviant peers, and pregnancy rates. MTFC has also been shown to be associated with more positive school performance, with a significant mediated effect found: Completing homework during treatment mediated the effects of MTFC on time spent in locked settings. These results suggest that MTFC effectively decreases health-risking sexual behavior and conduct problems and increases positive and adaptive behaviors. Based on the randomized controlled trials conducted, MTFC has received national attention as a cost-effective alternative to institutional and residential care. The results from a series of independent cost–benefit analyses from the Washington State Public Policy group and from three randomized trials led the MTFC model to be selected as one of 10 evidence-based National Model Programs (The Blueprints Programs) by the Office of Juvenile Justice and Delinquency Prevention and as one of nine National Exemplary Safe, Disciplined, and Drug Free Schools Model Programs. The MTFC model was also highlighted in two U.S. Surgeon General reports and was selected by the Center for Substance Abuse Prevention and the Office of Juvenile Justice and Delinquency Prevention as an Exemplary I program for Strengthening America's Families. However, despite the positive outcomes for the MTFC girls, most outcomes examined to date have been behavioral in nature and have not addressed issues related to the complex psychological presentation typical of girls with co-occurring trauma and conduct problems.

ADAPTATIONS TO THE MTFC MODEL

Because prior research has shown high rates of childhood adversity and trauma in juvenile justice populations, we examined the association between early adversity and conduct problems with multimethod data from our juvenile justice studies with girls and discovered similar findings. The MTFC girls had experienced a wide array of childhood adversity and high rates of mental health symptoms (e.g., rates of physical and sexual abuse are up to 300 times those of the national population; Smith, Leve, & Chamberlain, 2006). Additionally, using a cumulative measure of adverse experiences derived from eight unique indicators, we predicted rates of adolescent offending and health-risking sexual behavior (Smith et al., 2006). The results from our analyses also indicated that childhood adversity predicted higher levels of drug use particularly cocaine and methamphetamine, for juvenile justice girls (Smith, Chamberlain, & Leve, 2008). These findings highlight the importance of examining the role of early adversity in the development of later constellations of problem behaviors.

In an effort to improve MTFC outcomes, we adapted the MTFC model for the specific treatment of co-occurring trauma and delinquency in girls. This adapted MTFC intervention was piloted in a small-scale randomized trial with MTFC girls, and results suggest that the adapted MTFC intervention is effective in improving trauma-related mental health symptoms and delinquency outcomes.

DIRECTIONS FOR RESEARCH

In future MTFC research, issues related to the differential impact of the intervention, tailoring the model to address the needs of specific populations, and factors and mechanisms that optimize the ability of community service providers to implement MTFC will be examined. A critical research area is the integration of the MTFC model into usual care or routine practice settings. Although the MTFC model was developed *in situ* in community juvenile justice and mental health clinic settings, whether the model can be imported with comparable effectiveness to that found in the Oregon-based randomized trials is an open question. Currently, randomized trials are being conducted in Sweden by Kjell Hansson and colleagues at Lund University (Westermark, Hansson, & Vinnerljung, 2007) and in the United Kingdom as part of their countrywide implementation of MTFC for Looked After children (*www.hackney.gov.uk/fostering-MTFC.htm*). The results of these trials and others that examine outcomes within the context of a variety of child and family public service systems will yield much needed information about the translatability of the model and will lead to future generations of research questions.

CONCLUSIONS

Over the past several years, community-based interventions such as MTFC have become more widely accepted for the treatment of serious emotional and behavioral problems. MTFC appeals to clinicians and policymakers because, compared with residential treatment, it is less intrusive and expensive and has been shown to produce greater behavioral improvements. Thus, the MTFC model is being implemented at 69 sites across the United States, Canada, Britain, Sweden, Ireland, and the Netherlands. In addition, the MTFC model is being implemented as part of a randomized trial in up to 40 California counties to examine what factors at the county, agency/organizational, and practitioner levels predict the successful implementation of MTFC (e.g., how to effectively engage and support public agencies in adopting, implementing, and sustaining the MTFC model). In the experimental condition for the California study, community development teams are used to promote peer-to-peer exchanges and support among key stakeholders. The community development team model is a theory-driven intervention designed to engage and support evidence-based practices and is being contrasted with the traditional MTFC model.

Results from the research to date have demonstrated the effectiveness of MTFC with the following treatment groups: adolescents in the juvenile justice system who have severe delinquency and children and adolescents in the child welfare system and adolescents in the state mental hospital who have emotional and behavioral problems. The results from recent studies on MTFC adaptations and dissemination are promising and suggest that MTFC might be a widely accepted, cost-effective intervention for treating youths with complex emotional and behavioral problems.

REFERENCES

Chamberlain, P. (2003). *Treating chronic juvenile offenders: Advances made through the Oregon multidimensional treatment foster care model.* Washington, DC: American Psychological Association.

Chamberlain, P., Leve, L. D., & DeGarmo, D. S. (2007). Multidimensional treatment foster care for girls in the juvenile justice system: 2-year follow-up of a randomized clinical trial. *Journal of Consulting and Clinical Psychology, 75,* 187–193.

Chamberlain, P., Moreland, S., & Reid, K. (1992). Enhanced services and stipends for foster parents: Effects on retention rates and outcomes for children. *Child Welfare, 5,* 387–401.

Chamberlain, P., Price, J., Leve, L. D., Laurent, H., Landsverk, J. A., & Reid, J. B. (2008). Prevention of behavior problems for children in foster care: Outcomes and mediation effects. *Prevention Science, 9,* 17–27.

Chamberlain, P., & Reid, J. B. (1987). Parent observation and report of child symptoms. *Behavioral Assessment, 9,* 97–109.

Chamberlain, P., & Reid, J. B. (1991). Using a specialized foster care community treatment model for children and adolescents leaving the state mental hospital. *Journal of Community Psychology, 19,* 266–276.

Chamberlain, P., & Reid, J. B. (1998). Comparison of two community alternatives to incarceration for chronic juvenile offenders. *Journal of Consulting and Clinical Psychology, 66,* 624–633.

Dishion, T. J., McCord, J., & Poulin, F. (1999). When interventions harm: Peer groups and problem behavior. *American Psychologist, 54,* 755–764.

Eddy, J. M., Bridges Whaley, R., & Chamberlain, P. (2004). The prevention of violent behavior by chronic and serious male juvenile offenders: A 2-year follow-up of a randomized clinical trial. *Journal of Emotional and Behavioral Disorders, 12,* 2–8.

Eddy, J. M., & Chamberlain, P. (2000). Family management and deviant peer association as mediators of the impact of treatment condition on youth antisocial behavior. *Journal of Consulting and Clinical Psychology, 5,* 857–863.

Fisher, P. A., Burraston, B., & Pears, K. C. (2005). The Early Intervention Foster Care Program: Permanent placement outcomes from a randomized trial. *Child Maltreatment, 10,* 61–71.

Kerr, D. C. R., Leve, L. D., & Chamberlain, P. (2009). Pregnancy rates among juvenile justice girls in two randomized controlled trials of multidimensional treatment foster care. *Journal of Consulting and Clinical Psychology, 77,* 588–593.

Leve, L. D., & Chamberlain, P. (2004). Female juvenile offenders: Defining an early-onset pathway for delinquency. *Journal of Child and Family Studies, 13,* 439–452.

Leve, L. D., & Chamberlain, P. (2005). Association with delinquent peers: Intervention effects for youth in the juvenile justice system. *Journal of Abnormal Child Psychology, 33,* 339–347.

Leve, L. D., & Chamberlain, P. (2007). A randomized evaluation of multidimensional treatment foster care: Effects on school attendance and homework completion in juvenile justice girls. *Research on Social Work Practice, 17,* 657–663.

Smith, D. K., Chamberlain, P., & Leve, L. D. (2008). *Trauma and delinquency: Predicting substance use for girls in the juvenile justice system.* Manuscript submitted for publication.

Smith, D. K., Leve, L. D., & Chamberlain, P. (2006). Adolescent girls' offending and health-risking sexual behavior: The predictive role of trauma. *Child Maltreatment, 11,* 346–353.

Westermark, P. K., Hansson, K., & Vinnerljung, B. (2007). Foster parents in multidimensional treatment foster care: How do they deal with implementing standardized treatment components? *Children and Youth Services Review, 29,* 442–459.

17

Treating Serious Antisocial Behavior Using Multisystemic Therapy

SCOTT W. HENGGELER and CINDY SCHAEFFER

OVERVIEW

Multisystemic therapy (MST; Henggeler, Schoenwald, Borduin, Rowland, & Cunningham, 2009) is a comprehensive and empirically supported treatment for youths with severe antisocial behavior and their families. Because of its relative intensity, MST is most appropriate and cost-effective for youths with serious and chronic patterns of offending and at high risk for out-of-home placement (e.g., incarceration, residential treatment). Such youths often incur significant long-term social and economic costs to themselves, their families, and their communities. Thus, the provision of effective treatment for this population can provide many benefits for themselves (e.g., healthier and more successful lives) and society (e.g., reduced crime and associated costs). MST is also appropriate for youths with substance abuse disorders or problem sexual behavior separately or in conjunction with juvenile offending. In addition, clinical trials of adapted versions of MST for other serious child and adolescent clinical problems (e.g., serious emotional disturbance, chronic pediatric health conditions) have been conducted, and dissemination efforts for these adaptations are underway.

CHARACTERISTICS OF THE MST MODEL

The development of MST began in the late 1970s, with the first clinical trial published in 1986. At that time, existing treatments for juvenile offenders were office or institution based, rarely focused on the known risk factors for antisocial behavior in adolescents, were narrow in their problem conceptualization, and had little empirical support. Hence, as explicated by Henggeler and his colleagues (Henggeler, 1982), it seemed reasonable to argue that in order to be effective, treatments for delinquency must be capable of attenuating a comprehensive array of risk factors, with the family viewed as the primary factor. Moreover, in light of the extremely low rates of treatment attendance for families of delinquents, it was also clear that strategies had to be developed to overcome barriers to treatment delivery. These circumstances set the stage for the next 30 years of MST development and research.

Theoretical Framework

MST was designed to address the multiple risk factors associated with juvenile offending that have been identified through decades of basic research on the causes and correlates of antisocial behavior. Because these risk factors exist and interact within and across multiple domains of a person's life, Bronfenbrenner's (1979) social ecological model provides a useful organizing framework for MST. The social-ecological model maintains that youth behavior is largely determined by the functioning of the multiple systems (i.e., family, school, peer, and neighborhood) in which the youth is embedded and the reciprocal interplay between these systems (e.g., contacts between caregivers and school personnel). Moreover, the youth's key systems are themselves embedded in larger contexts (e.g., the caregiver's workplace, the school system) that also indirectly affect youth functioning through their impact on more proximal systems (e.g., stress in the caregiver's workplace interferes with parenting, zero-tolerance policy decided by the school board results in expulsion). Thus, the social-ecological model asserts that all adolescent behavior is determined by multiple direct and indirect factors, and that these factors exert their influences in individualized ways based on each youth's unique social context.

In light of the social-ecological model and research on the determinants of antisocial behavior in adolescents, MST contends that for treatment of serious antisocial behavior to be effective, interventions must have the capacity to target known risk factors at multiple levels, including individual (e.g., cognitive biases, attention problems), family (e.g., lax parental supervision, caregiver substance abuse), peer (e.g., association with deviant peers), school (e.g., poor achievement, low bonding to school), and neighborhood (e.g., few opportunities for prosocial activities, availability of drugs). Similarly, interventions must have the capacity to address difficulties between systemic levels (e.g., caregiver interactions with the youth's peers and teachers). Factors in the broader ecology (e.g., caregiver work hours, lack of prosocial activities in neighborhood) that create barriers to the effective functioning of proximal systems (e.g., caregiver's ability to supervise and set limits) also must be addressed for positive change to occur.

The social-ecological perspective, therefore, emphasizes the importance of understanding behavior within its naturally occurring context, which has very important implications for the design of MST interventions. MST uses a home-based service delivery model that emphasizes ecological validity in the assessment and delivery of interventions. Ecologically valid assessments require that the clinician understand the youth's functioning in a variety of real-world settings (e.g., at home, in the classroom, during community activities), and that such understanding come from firsthand sources (e.g., caregivers, siblings, extended family, teachers, coaches) as much as possible. Similarly, therapeutic interventions are provided where problems occur—in homes, schools, and community locations—and, whenever possible, are delivered to the youth by key ecology members such as caregivers and teachers.

MST Theory of Change

In MST, caregivers are viewed as the main conduits of change, and interventions focus on empowering them with the resources and skills needed to be more effective with their children. Then, as caregiver effectiveness increases, the therapist guides caregiver efforts to, for example, disengage their teenagers from deviant peers and enhance school performance. Thus, the family is viewed as critical to achieving and sustaining decreased adolescent antisocial behavior and improved functioning. Importantly, the emphasis of MST on improved parenting and decreased youth association with deviant peers as central vehicles for change has been supported in studies that assessed mediators of change in MST (e.g., Henggeler, Letourneau, Chapman, Borduin, Schewe, & McCart, 2009; Huey, Henggeler, Brondino, & Pickrel, 2000).

From a more clinical perspective, the therapist collaborates with the family, using family strengths (e.g., love for the adolescent, indigenous social support) to overcome barriers to caregiver effectiveness (e.g., caregiver substance abuse, debilitating stress, hopelessness). As caregiver effectiveness increases (e.g., ability to monitor, supervise, and support the child), the therapist helps the caregivers design and implement interventions aimed at decreasing youth antisocial behavior and improving youth functioning across family, peer, school, and community contexts. The ultimate aim is to surround the youth with a context that supports prosocial behavior (e.g., prosocial peers, involved and effective caregivers, supportive school), replacing the context that is conducive to antisocial behavior. Similarly, treatment aims to surround the caregivers with indigenous (i.e., extended family, friends, neighbors) support to help sustain the changes achieved during treatment.

CHARACTERISTICS OF MST TREATMENT

Treatment Delivery

MST is provided by full-time master's-level therapists, who each carry caseloads of four to six families. Two to four therapists work within a team, and each team is supervised by an advanced master's- or doctoral-level supervisor, who devotes at least 50% of time to the team. Team members usually work for private service provider organizations contracted by public juvenile justice, child welfare, and mental health authorities. Teams also receive weekly consultation from an expert MST consultant, who helps facilitate model adherence.

MST clinicians provide 24-hour/7-day a week availability, which allows sessions to occur at times convenient for families and enables therapists to react quickly to crises that might threaten goal attainment (e.g., caregiver needs evening support to address an adolescent's drug relapse). Although the duration of treatment is relatively brief (3–5 months), the intervention process is intensive and often involves 60 hours or more of direct contact between the therapist and the family as well as others in the youth's ecosystem. As noted previously, MST uses a home- and community-based (e.g., schools, workplaces) model of service delivery, which, in addition to enhancing the ecological validity of assessments and interventions, also decreases barriers to service access, supports therapeutic engagement, and promotes generalization of therapeutic gains.

Treatment Principles

Because of its highly individualized nature, MST does not follow a rigid manualized plan for treatment. Rather, nine treatment principles provide the underlying structure and framework on which therapists build their interventions. In addition to principles that stem from the social-ecological model, interventions are designed to be intensive (i.e., daily or weekly effort by family members), developmentally appropriate, present focused, and action oriented. Interventions also must aim to encourage responsible behavior by all parties and are designed from the beginning to promote the generalization and long-term maintenance of therapeutic gains. Thus, for example, while grounding an adolescent for 6 months might decrease antisocial behavior, such extended isolation will not likely meet the adolescent's developmental need for peer interaction, provide opportunities for the youth to demonstrate responsible behavior (e.g., coming home before curfew), or allow the caregiver to practice important new skills that will be essential for ongoing success (e.g., monitoring the youth's whereabouts and associations).

An overriding treatment principle is that all aspects of MST must be strength based and that ecological strengths are used as levers for change. An optimistic perspective is communicated clearly to the family and other members of the youth's social network throughout the assessment and treatment process. Therapists look for potential strengths within the various ecological contexts, investigating factors pertaining to the child (e.g., competencies, attractiveness), caregivers and extended family (e.g., affective bonds, social support), peers (e.g., prosocial activities, achievement orientation), the school (e.g., management practices, course offerings), and the neighborhood/community (e.g., neighbor concern, recreational opportunities). Identified strengths then are leveraged in interventions. For example, a neighbor or extended family member might be enlisted to assist with monitoring the youth after school until the caregiver gets home from work. Clinicians are trained to incorporate this strength-based approach throughout their work. For example, supervisors assist clinicians in identifying barriers to treatment success rather than perceiving clients as being resistant to change.

Clinical Procedures and Interventions

Clinical interventions adhere to the nine treatment principles and are applied using a standardized analytical/decision-making process that structures the treatment plan, its implementation, and the evaluation of its effectiveness. Specific goals for treatment are set at individual, family, peer, and social network levels. However, as noted previously, the adolescent's caregivers are viewed as key to achieving desired outcomes and as crucial for the generalizability and sustainability of treatment gains.

At the beginning of treatment, the problem behaviors to be targeted are specified clearly from the perspectives of key stakeholders (e.g., family members, teachers, juvenile justice authorities) and ecological strengths are identified. Then, based on multiple perspectives, the ecological factors that seem to be driving each problem are organized into a coherent conceptual framework (e.g., the youth's marijuana use seems to be associated with a lack of caregiver monitoring, association with substance-using peers, and poor school performance). Next, the MST therapist, with support from other team members (other therapists, supervisor, consultant), designs specific intervention strategies to target those "drivers." Strategies incorporate interventions from empirically supported, pragmatic, problem-focused treatments such as structural/strategic and behavioral family therapies, behavioral parent training, cognitive-behavioral therapy, and motivational interviewing. In addition, when evidence indicates biological contributors to identified problems, evidence-based psychopharmacological interventions are incorporated into treatment.

A critical feature of MST, however, is that these empirically supported interventions are highly integrated, so that all treatment components focus on meeting the overarching goals of treatment. Such integration is achieved primarily through the use of a single therapist, who understands and responds to the needs and desires of family members and external stakeholders. An MST therapist, for example, might teach anger management techniques (e.g., relaxation) to an aggressive adolescent while simultaneously working with the caregivers to implement a comprehensive behavior plan that includes rewards for the successful use of these techniques. Moreover, such interventions might occur in conjunction with family therapy interventions to enhance positive communications and problem-solving skills as well as with individual adult sessions to address anxiety symptoms the caregiver experiences when attempting to discipline the youth. Importantly, these integrated services are delivered in conjunction with select interventions that address other pertinent drivers of the identified problems in the youth's social ecology (e.g., supporting caregivers in advocating for more appropriate school services, connecting caregivers with the parents of the youth's peers) and barriers to treatment participation (e.g., meeting with families on weekends to accommodate the caregiver work schedules).

The MST approach contrasts with brokered services (e.g., case manager, the wraparound approach), in which a care coordinator links family members to various component interventions (e.g., a youth anger management group, family therapy, parent training classes) and attempts to ensure the integration of the efforts of separate providers. Although likely more beneficial than uncoordinated community or residential care, the case management or wraparound approach cannot guarantee the quality of services that families receive (i.e., existing community services are unlikely to be empirically supported) or the necessary degree of collaboration and cooperation among providers. In addition, case management and wraparound services usually require that the family work with multiple agencies and in disparate settings, which can create significant logistical challenges for caregivers (e.g., transportation, time off of work) that reduce treatment attendance and compliance. Indeed, in a recent study of youth with serious emotional disturbances and at risk for out-of-home placement, MST was superior to wraparound services in decreasing youth symptomatology and improving adaptive functioning (Stambaugh et al., 2007).

Recursive Clinical Decision Making

As MST interventions are implemented, their effectiveness is monitored continuously from multiple perspectives. Using a recursive feedback process (Figure 17.1), identified drivers are reconceptualized when interventions are ineffective, and modifications are made until an effective strategy is developed. For example, if a youth's substance abuse

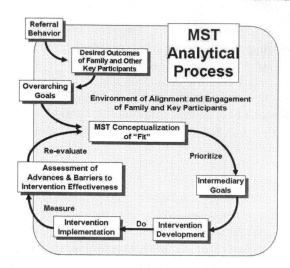

FIGURE 17.1. The MST recursive feedback process.

was conceptualized as stemming primarily from his or her association with drug-abusing peers, interventions would be developed to eliminate or reduce the youth's association with such peers while concomitantly building relations with more prosocial peers. However, if these peer interventions were successful but the youth was still using drugs (e.g., as evidenced by results of random urine screens), the fit of the youth's substance abuse would need to be reconceptualized (e.g., perhaps he or she is using drugs primarily for anxiety reduction), and interventions redesigned and implemented accordingly (e.g., relaxation training, a self-management plan for coping with cravings). The outcomes of these interventions would be evaluated again and implementation plans revised or not, accordingly.

This reiterative process reinforces two important features of the MST model. First, MST teams strive to never give up on youth and families, doing whatever it takes to help families reach treatment goals. Second, when interventions are not successful, the failure is the team's rather than the family's. In other words, when the team develops accurate hypotheses of the drivers, identifies barriers to implementation success, and delivers corresponding interventions appropriately, families tend to achieve their goals, and youth antisocial behavior usually diminishes.

Training, Supervision, and Ongoing Quality Assurance

As discussed more extensively in Schoenwald's Chapter 34 (this volume), several processes and structures are set up within the MST model to support treatment fidelity and help therapists attain desired clinical outcomes. New therapists participate in a 5-day orientation training that provides initial grounding in MST, and all team members participate in quarterly booster trainings. The majority of MST clinical learning, however, occurs as therapists work with families and receive weekly structured supervision and feedback both from the on-site MST team supervisor and the off-site MST consultant. The MST team meets weekly with the supervisor as a group, and the supervisor follows a specified protocol for reviewing and addressing the issues in each case with the team.

The entire team, in turn, discusses cases with an MST expert consultant once a week to obtain additional feedback and direction as needed.

MST training, supervision, and consultation take place within a comprehensive quality assurance/quality improvement (QA/QI) system designed to help ensure that the dissemination of MST occurs with fidelity to the key aspects of the model that are essential in attaining youth and family outcomes. The process underlying this system has been worked out through more than 15 years of experience assisting community-based agencies in developing and maintaining sustainable MST teams. Indeed, 17,000 youth and families are treated annually through MST programs in more than 30 states and 10 nations. In addition to the well-specified initial and ongoing training, supervision, and consultation protocols, key components of the QA/QI system include validated measures of implementation adherence at all levels (therapists, supervisors, and consultants) and a web-based implementation tracking system to provide teams and provider organizations with ongoing team-specific feedback about adherence and youth outcomes. Importantly, many aspects of the QA/QI system have been validated in ongoing research, and findings suggest that there are significant associations between program (e.g., therapist, supervisor, consultant) fidelity and favorable youth outcomes (see Schoenwald's Chapter 34, this volume).

In addition to supporting practitioner implementation of MST on a case-by-case basis, MST consultants provide extensive organizational support to communities and provider organizations who are interested in establishing MST programs. Initially, this support involves conducting a community assessment to determine whether the needs that prompted stakeholder interest in MST are likely to be met by an MST program, determining whether an MST program is viable in a specific practice context (e.g., mechanisms are in place to reimburse therapists for mileage used to travel to families' homes), and cultivating stakeholder buy-in and commitment to the success of the program. Once MST has been implemented in a community, ongoing organizational support involves semiannual program reviews, problem solving of organizational and stakeholder barriers to implementation, and support for program directors. More information regarding the development and sustainability of MST programs is available from Henggeler et al. (2009) and the MST Services website *www.mstservices.com.*

EVIDENCE ON THE EFFECTS OF MST

As described in Henggeler et al. (2009), more than 20 groups of prestigious independent reviewers have supported the promise and effectiveness of MST in treating serious antisocial behavior in adolescents. These groups include leading researchers, entities charged with evaluating research (e.g., National Institute on Drug Abuse, U.S. Public Health Service), and consumer advocates (e.g., National Alliance on Mental Illness). Such conclusions were based on the 15 published randomized clinical trials and two published quasi-experimental trials of MST, most of which have examined outcomes with adolescents presenting with serious antisocial behavior. A relatively comprehensive overview of the samples (N = almost 2,000 youth and families), designs, and outcomes of these trials is presented in Table 17.1. The following text summarizes these results.

(text resumes on p. 269)

TABLE 17.1. Published Multisystemic Therapy (MST) Outcome Studies

Study	Population	Comparison	Follow-up	Treatment effects[a]
Henggeler et al. (1986)	Delinquents $N = 57$[b]	Diversion services	Posttreatment	• Improved family relations • Decreased behavior problems • Decreased association with deviant peers
Brunk, Henggeler, & Whelan (1987)	Maltreating families $N = 33$	Behavioral parent training	Posttreatment	• Improved parent–child interactions • Behavioral parent training improved caregiver social problems
Borduin, Henggeler, Blaske, & Stein (1990)	Adolescent sexual offenders $N = 16$	Individual counseling	3 years	• Reduced sexual offending • Reduced other criminal offending
Henggeler et al. (1991)[c]	Serious juvenile offenders	Individual counseling Usual community services	3 years	• Reduced alcohol and marijuana use • Decreased drug-related arrests
Henggeler, Melton, & Smith (1992)	Violent and chronic juvenile offenders $N = 84$	Usual community services—high rates of incarceration	59 weeks	• Improved family relations • Improved peer relations • Decreased recidivism (43%) • Decreased out-of-home placement (64%)
Henggeler et al. (1993)	Same sample		2.4 years	• Decreased recidivism (doubled survival rate)
Borduin et al. (1995)	Violent and chronic juvenile offenders $N = 176$	Individual counseling	4 years	• Improved family relations • Decreased psychiatric symptomatology • Decreased recidivism (69%)
Schaeffer & Borduin (2005)	Same sample		13.7 years	• Decreased rearrests (54%) • Decreased days incarcerated (57%)
Henggeler et al. (1997)	Violent and chronic juvenile offenders $N = 155$	Juvenile probation services—high rates of incarceration	1.7 years	• Decreased psychiatric symptomatology • Decreased days in out-of-home placement (50%) • Decreased recidivism (26%, nonsignificant) • Treatment adherence linked with long-term outcomes
Henggeler, Rowland, et al. (1999)	Youths presenting psychiatric emergencies ($N = 116$, final $N = 156$)	Psychiatric hospitalization	4 months postrecruitment	• Decreased externalizing problems (CBCL) • Improved family relations • Increased school attendance • Higher consumer satisfaction • Increased self-concept for youths in hospitalization condition

(cont.)

TABLE 17.1. *(cont.)*

Study	Population	Comparison	Follow-up	Treatment effects[a]
Schoenwald et al. (2000)	Same sample		4 months postrecruitment	• 75% reduction in days hospitalized • 50% reduction in days in other out-of-home placements
Huey et al. (2004)	Same sample		16 months postrecruitment	• Decreased rates of attempted suicide
Henggeler et al. (2003)	Same sample		16 months postrecruitment	• Favorable 4-month outcomes, noted above, dissipated
Sheidow et al. (2004)	Same sample		16 months postrecruitment	• MST cost benefits at 4 months, but equivalent costs at 16 months
Henggeler, Pickrel, & Brondino (1999)	Substance-abusing and substance-dependent delinquents (N = 118)	Usual community services	1 year	• Decreased drug use at posttreatment • Decreased days in out-of-home placement (50%) • Decreased recidivism (26%, nonsignificant) • Treatment adherence linked with decreased drug use
Henggeler, Pickrel, Brondino, & Crouch (1996)	Same sample			• 98% rate of treatment completion
Schoenwald et al. (1996)	Same sample		1 year	• Incremental cost of MST nearly offset by between-groups differences in out-of-home placement
Brown et al. (1999)	Same sample		6 months	• Increased attendance in regular school settings
Henggeler, Clingempeel, et al. (2002)	Same sample		4 years	• Decreased violent crime • Increased marijuana abstinence
Borduin & Schaeffer (2001)—preliminary report Borduin, Schaeffer, & Heiblum (2009)—full report	Juvenile sexual offenders (N = 48)	Usual community services	9 years	• Decreased behavior problems and symptoms • Improved family relations, peer relations, and academic performance • Decreased caregiver distress • Decreased sex offender recidivism (83%) • Decreased recidivism for other crimes (50%) • Decreased days incarcerated (80%)

(cont.)

TABLE 17.1. *(cont.)*

Study	Population	Comparison	Follow-up	Treatment effects[a]
Ogden & Halliday-Boykins (2004)	Norwegian youths with serious antisocial behavior ($N = 100$)	Usual child welfare services	6 months postrecruitment	• Decreased externalizing and internalizing symptoms • Decreased out-of-home placements • Increased social competence • Increased consumer satisfaction
Ogden & Hagen (2006a)	Same sample		24 months postrecruitment	• Decreased externalizing and internalizing symptoms • Decreased out-of-home placements
Ellis et al. (2005b)	Inner-city adolescents with chronically poorly controlled type 1 diabetes ($N = 127$)	Standard diabetes care	7 months postrecruitment	• Increased blood glucose testing • Decreased inpatient admissions • Improved metabolic control
Ellis et al. (2005)	Same sample		7 months postrecruitment	• Decreased medical charges and direct care costs
Ellis et al. (2005a)	Same sample		7 months postrecruitment	• Decreased diabetes stress
Ellis et al. (2007)	Same sample		13 months postrecruitment	• Decreased inpatient admissions sustained • Favorable metabolic control outcomes dissipated
Rowland et al. (2005)	Youths with serious emotional disturbance ($N = 31$)	Hawaii's intensive continuum of care	6 months postrecruitment	• Decreased symptoms • Decreased minor crimes • Decreased days in out-of-home placement (68%)
Timmons-Mitchell et al. (2006)	Juvenile offenders (felons) at imminent risk of placement ($N = 93$)	Usual community services	18-month follow-up	• Improved youth functioning • Decreased substance use problems • Decreased rearrests (37%)
Henggeler, Halliday-Boykins, et al. (2006)	Substance-abusing and substance-dependent offenders in juvenile drug court ($N = 161$)	Four treatment conditions, including family court with usual services and drug court with usual services	12 months postrecruitment	• MST enhanced substance use outcomes • Drug court was more effective than family court in decreasing self-reported substance use and criminal activity

(cont.)

TABLE 17.1. *(cont.)*

Study	Population	Comparison	Follow-up	Treatment effects[a]
Rowland, Chapman, & Henggeler (2008)	Nearest-age siblings (*N* = 70)		18 months postrecruitment	• Evidence-based treatment decreased sibling substance use
Stambaugh et al. (2007)[b]	Youths with serious emotional disturbance at risk for out-of-home placement (*N* = 267)	Wraparound	18-month follow-up	• Decreased symptoms • Decreased out-of-home placements (54%)
Sundell et al. (2008)	Youths met diagnostic criteria for conduct disorder (*N* = 156)	Usual child welfare services in Sweden	7 months postrecruitment	• No outcomes favoring either treatment condition • Low treatment fidelity
Letourneau et al. (2009)	Juvenile sexual offenders (*N* = 127)	Usual sex offender-specific treatment	12 months postrecruitment	• Decreased sexual behavior problems • Decreased delinquency, substance use, externalizing symptoms • Reduced out-of-home placements

Note. CBCL, Child Behavior Checklist.
[a]All treatment effects pertain to MST unless otherwise noted.
[b]Quasi-experimental design (groups matched on demographic characteristics); all other studies are randomized.
[c]Based on participants in Henggeler et al. (1992) and Borduin et al. (1995).

Early Efficacy Trials

As is typical in treatment development research, early MST outcome studies were conducted in ways that optimized the probability that the new treatment would achieve favorable outcomes, assuming that it was actually efficacious. Thus, for example, Henggeler and Borduin provided close supervision of therapists, who were highly motivated doctoral students, and the MST program was sheltered from the many challenges of implementation in real-world (i.e., community-based clinics) settings. These studies (i.e., Borduin et al., 1995; Borduin, Henggeler, Blaske, & Stein, 1990; Brunk, Henggeler, & Whelan, 1987; Henggeler et al., 1986) demonstrated many favorable effects for MST with juvenile offenders and their families (e.g., reduced rearrest and incarceration, improved family functioning), some of which have been sustained for 14 years posttreatment (Schaeffer & Borduin, 2005).

Effectiveness Trials

The favorable results in the aforementioned efficacy trials led to studies of MST conducted in collaboration with community mental health centers and using public sector practitioners. Results from these studies (i.e., Henggeler, Melton, Brondino, Scherer, & Hanley, 1997; Henggeler, Melton, & Smith, 1992; Letourneau et al., 2009) further supported the capacity of MST to improve family functioning and decrease the rearrest and incarceration rates of serious juvenile offenders. Importantly, this work also highlighted the critical role that treatment fidelity plays in achieving favorable outcomes. For example, Henggeler et al. (1997) found that higher therapist treatment fidelity was significantly associated with better long-term youth outcomes. Similarly, meta-analyses have shown that the effect sizes in MST effectiveness trials were, on average, lower than those in MST efficacy trials (Curtis, Ronan, & Borduin, 2004), suggesting increased challenges in moving this evidence-based treatment into real-world contexts. Together, these findings have led to extensive efforts to develop effective strategies for transporting MST to community settings and to research evaluating the success of these efforts (see Schoenwald's Chapter 34, this volume).

Trials for Juvenile Offenders with Substance Use Disorders

In light of favorable reductions in substance use achieved in early trials of MST with juvenile offenders (Henggeler et al., 1991), two subsequent trials were conducted with juvenile offenders meeting diagnostic criteria for substance abuse or dependence. The first study (Henggeler, Pickrel, & Brondino, 1999; Henggeler, Clingempeel, Brondino, & Pickrel, 2002) demonstrated favorable MST effects in several areas, including the reduction of substance use. The second study (Henggeler, Halliday-Boykins, et al., 2006) showed that MST enhanced the favorable effects of juvenile drug court intervention in reducing substance use and criminal behavior. Sheidow and Henggeler (2008) provide a detailed overview of substance-related MST outcome research.

Independent Transportability Trials

With the transport of MST programs to many states and nations, several independent groups of researchers have published rigorous evaluations of MST with antisocial youth. In a randomized trial conducted in Norway, Ogden and colleagues (Ogden & Hagen, 2006a; Ogden & Halliday-Boykins, 2004) replicated favorable outcomes of MST in earlier studies (e.g., decreased youth symptoms and out-of-home placement, high consumer satisfaction). Similarly, Timmons-Mitchell, Bender, Kishna, and Mitchell (2006) provided the first independent replication with serious juvenile offenders in the United States. MST improved youth functioning, decreased recidivism, and decreased substance use problems. On the other hand, Sundell et al. (2008) failed to support the greater effectiveness of MST in treating Swedish youth with conduct disorder. This failure might have been due to the low therapist adherence observed in this study or the relatively high quality of services provided in the comparison condition. Nevertheless, across the 12 efficacy, effectiveness, and transportability trials of MST with youth presenting with serious antisocial behavior and their families, MST has achieved relatively consistent outcomes, including

- Reduced short- and long-term (up to 14 years) rates of criminal offending.
- Reduced rates of out-of-home placements.
- Decreased substance use.

- Decreased behavioral and mental health problems.
- Improved family functioning.
- Cost savings in comparison with usual mental health and juvenile justice services.

Finally, although many independent reviewers and organizations have supported the promise or effectiveness of MST (see Henggeler et al., 2009, for citations), at least one review has disagreed. Littell, Popa, and Forsythe (2005) concluded in their meta-analysis that MST was not significantly more effective than other services. This review, however, had many methodological anomalies (see critiques by Henggeler, Schoenwald, Borduin, & Swenson, 2006; Ogden & Hagen, 2006b) and has not been replicated in other meta-analyses of MST (Aos, Miller, & Drake, 2006; Curtis et al., 2004).

Adaptations to the Basic MST Model

Several groups of investigators have adapted the basic MST model (e.g., focus on serious clinical problems with multiple causes, intervention design guided by treatment principles, home-based model of service delivery, strong quality assurance system, integration of evidence-based treatment techniques, and the view that caregivers are the key to long-term outcomes) to address other types of serious clinical problems presented by youths and their families and have evaluated the effectiveness of these adaptations.

Sexual Offending

Three randomized trials of MST with juvenile sexual offenders (Borduin et al., 1990; Borduin, Schaeffer, & Heiblum, 2009; Letourneau et al., 2009) present strong evidence of the short- and long-term effectiveness of MST with juvenile sexual offenders.

Serious Emotional Disturbance

Three published trials (two randomized, one quasi-experimental) have adapted MST to treat youths with serious emotional disturbance. In the first (Henggeler, Rowland, et al., 1999), MST was effective in reducing symptomatology and out-of-home placements for youths in psychiatric crisis. The second (Rowland et al., 2005) replicated these findings in the context of an effectiveness trial. The third (Stambaugh et al., 2007) was an independent transportability trial that demonstrated more favorable outcomes for MST versus wraparound, which is a widely disseminated family-based intervention.

Chronic Pediatric Health Care Conditions

Ellis, Naar-King, and their colleagues have taken the lead in adapting and evaluating the use of MST for improving the health outcomes of youths with challenging and costly health care problems. In a randomized clinical trial, these investigators demonstrated the capacity of MST to improve the health status of adolescents with type 1 diabetes who had chronically poor metabolic control (Ellis et al., 2005a, 2005b). This research group has also successfully pilot tested adaptations of the MST model for other challenging health problems such as HIV (Cunningham, Naar-King, Ellis, Pejuan, & Secord, 2006; Ellis, Naar-King, Cunningham, & Secord, 2006).

New Adaptation Pilots

Several other MST adaptations are in their pilot stages. For example, the Building Stronger Families project (Swenson, Schaeffer, Tuerk, Henggeler, Tuten, Panzarella, et al., 2009) integrates an MST adaptation for child maltreatment with reinforcement-based therapy (Jones, Wong, Tuten, & Stitzer, 2005) to treat co-occurring caregiver substance abuse and child maltreatment. Another example is provided by Trupin, Kerns, Walker, and Lee (in press), who have integrated MST with other evidence-based treatments to address the current and postrelease needs of incarcerated juvenile offenders with co-occurring mental health disorders.

DIRECTIONS FOR RESEARCH

At the present point in the development, validation, and dissemination of MST, key issues for future research range from micro- to macroprocesses. At the microlevel, published research has not yet examined the MST "black box." Although MST has achieved a range of favorable clinical outcomes, the exact nature of the types of therapist–family interactions that contribute to these outcomes has not been examined. Specification of such processes might be used to increase the efficiency of MST as well as to inform the emphases of other intervention approaches for juvenile offenders and their families.

Two additional suggestions for future research pertain to the more macrolevel. In light of the worldwide transport of MST (and other evidence-based treatments), a pressing need has emerged for the development and validation of effective and efficient strategies for recruiting, training, and retaining therapists, supervisors, and consultants. MST and other evidence-based treatments represent significant departures from traditional mental health practices, and the field knows little about how to retool the workforce to support the implementation of these innovations. Similarly, as also noted by Schoenwald (Chapter 34, this volume), increased research is needed on the organizational and service system factors that are critical for the sustainability of high-quality MST programs. Therapists work in complicated ecological contexts (e.g., including supervisors, administrators, colleagues, organizational mandates and constraints, fiscal challenges), and it seems likely that various aspects of these contexts can attenuate or enhance therapist capacity to implement evidence-based practices with the fidelity needed to achieve desired results.

CONCLUSIONS

As suggested in this chapter, MST has become an extensively validated and widely disseminated evidence-based treatment of antisocial behavior in adolescents. Consistent with research and dissemination findings regarding other evidence-based treatments of antisocial behavior in adolescents, several conclusions can be drawn for the field. Effective interventions must

- Address known risk factors comprehensively.
- Focus on the family as the key change agent.
- Provide services in community settings, not in restrictive settings.
- Incorporate pragmatic, behaviorally oriented intervention techniques.
- Include well-conceived quality assurance protocols to support treatment fidelity and youth outcomes.

MST has followed these principles faithfully, and the evidence suggests that its beneficial effects have been substantial. MST has been found to be effective in reducing antisocial behavior in multiple forms and with youths treated in multiple contexts. Despite the good news about MST effects in so many trials, much remains to be learned about the nature of therapist–family interactions within the black box of MST treatment, what kinds of interactions are most helpful, and what other factors—internal and external to the treatment process—influence treatment effectiveness. This suggests real potential for productive research and improved treatment in the years ahead.

REFERENCES

Aos, S., Miller, M., & Drake, E. (2006). *Evidence-based public policy options to reduce future prison construction, criminal justice costs, and crime rates.* Olympia: Washington State Institute for Public Policy.

Borduin, C. M., Henggeler, S. W., Blaske, D. M., & Stein, R. (1990). Multisystemic treatment of adolescent sexual offenders. *International Journal of Offender Therapy and Comparative Criminology, 35,* 105–114.

Borduin, C. M., Mann, B. J., Cone, L. T., Henggeler, S. W., Fucci, B. R., Blaske, D. M., et al. (1995). Multisystemic treatment of serious juvenile offenders: Long-term prevention of criminality and violence. *Journal of Consulting and Clinical Psychology, 63,* 569–578.

Borduin, C. M., & Schaeffer, C. M. (2001). Multisystemic treatment of juvenile sexual offenders: A progress report. *Journal of Psychology and Human Sexuality, 13,* 25–42.

Borduin, C. M., Schaeffer, C. M., & Heiblum, N. (2009). A randomized clinical trial of multisystemic therapy with juvenile sexual offenders: Effects on youth social ecology and criminal activity. *Journal of Consulting and Clinical Psychology, 77,* 26–37.

Bronfenbrenner, U. (1979). *The ecology of human development: Experiments by design and nature.* Cambridge, MA: Harvard University Press.

Brown, T. L., Henggeler, S. W., Schoenwald, S. K., Brondino, M. J., & Pickrel, S. G. (1999). Multisystemic treatment of substance abusing and dependent juvenile delinquents: Effects on school attendance at posttreatment and 6–month follow-up. *Children's Services: Social Policy, Research, and Practice, 2,* 81–93.

Brunk, M., Henggeler, S. W., & Whelan, J. P. (1987). A comparison of multisystemic therapy and parent training in the brief treatment of child abuse and neglect. *Journal of Consulting and Clinical Psychology, 55,* 311–318.

Cunningham, P. B., Naar-King, S., Ellis, D. A., Pejuan, S., & Secord, E. (2006). Achieving adherence to antiretroviral medications for pediatric HIV disease using an empirically supported treatment: A case report. *Journal of Developmental and Behavioral Pediatric, 27,* 44–50.

Curtis, N. M., Ronan, K. R., & Borduin, C. M. (2004). Multisystemic treatment: A meta-analysis of outcome studies. *Journal of Family Psychology, 18,* 411–419.

Ellis, D. A., Frey, M. A., Naar-King, S., Templin, T., Cunningham, P. B., & Cakan, N. (2005a). The effects of multisystemic therapy on diabetes stress in adolescents with chronically poorly controlled type 1 diabetes: Findings from a randomized controlled trial. *Pediatrics, 116,* e826–e832.

Ellis, D. A., Frey, M. A., Naar-King, S., Templin, T., Cunningham, P. B., & Cakan, N. (2005b). Use of multisystemic therapy to improve regimen adherence among adolescents with type 1 diabetes in chronic poor metabolic control: A randomized controlled trial. *Diabetes Care, 28,* 1604–1610.

Ellis, D. A., Naar-King, S., Cunningham, P. B., & Secord, E. (2006). Use of multisystemic therapy to improve antiretroviral adherence and health outcomes in HIV-infected pediatric patients: Evaluation of a pilot program. *AIDS Patient Care and STDs, 20,* 112–121.

Ellis, D. A., Naar-King, S., Frey, M. A., Templin, T., Rowland, M., & Cakan, N. (2005). Multisystemic treatment of poorly controlled type 1 diabetes: Effects on medical resource utilization. *Journal of Pediatric Psychology, 30,* 656–666.

Ellis, D. A., Templin, T., Naar-King, S., Frey, M. A., Cunningham, P. B., Podolski, C., et al. (2007). Multisystemic therapy for adolescents with poorly controlled type I diabetes: Stability of treatment effects in a randomized controlled trial. *Journal of Consulting and Clinical Psychology, 75,* 168–174.

Henggeler, S. W. (Ed.). (1982). *Delinquency and adolescent psychopathology: A family-ecological systems approach.* Littleton, MA: John Wright-PSG.

Henggeler, S. W., Borduin, C. M., Melton, G. B., Mann, B. J., Smith, L., Hall, J. A., et al. (1991). Effects of multisystemic therapy on drug use and abuse in serious juvenile offenders: A progress report from two outcome studies. *Family Dynamics of Addiction Quarterly, 1,* 40–51.

Henggeler, S. W., Clingempeel, W. G., Brondino, M. J., & Pickrel, S. G. (2002). Four-year follow-up of multisystemic therapy with substance abusing and dependent juvenile offenders. *Journal of the American Academy of Child and Adolescent Psychiatry, 41,* 868–874.

Henggeler, S. W., Halliday-Boykins, C. A., Cunningham, P. B., Randall, J., Shapiro, S. B., & Chapman, J. E. (2006). Juvenile drug court: Enhancing outcomes by integrating evidence-based treatments. *Journal of Consulting and Clinical Psychology, 74,* 42–54.

Henggeler, S. W., Letourneau, E. J., Chapman, J. E., Borduin, C. M., Schewe, P. A., & McCart, M. R. (2009). Mediators of change for multisystemic therapy with juvenile sexual offenders. *Journal of Consulting and Clinical Psychology, 77,* 451–462.

Henggeler, S. W., Melton, G. B., Brondino, M. J., Scherer, D. G., & Hanley, J. H. (1997). Multisystemic therapy with violent and chronic juvenile offenders and their families: The role of treatment fidelity in successful dissemination. *Journal of Consulting and Clinical Psychology, 65,* 821–833.

Henggeler, S. W., Melton, G. B., & Smith, L. A. (1992). Family preservation using multisystemic therapy: An effective alternative to incarcerating serious juvenile offenders. *Journal of Consulting and Clinical Psychology, 60,* 953–961.

Henggeler, S. W., Melton, G. B., Smith, L. A., Schoenwald, S. K., & Hanley, J. H. (1993). Family preservation using multisystemic treatment: Long-term follow-up to a clinical trial with serious juvenile offenders. *Journal of Child and Family Studies, 2,* 283–293.

Henggeler, S. W., Pickrel, S. G., & Brondino, M. J. (1999). Multisystemic treatment of substance abusing and dependent delinquents: Outcomes, treatment fidelity, and transportability. *Mental Health Services Research, 1,* 171–184.

Henggeler, S. W., Pickrel, S. G., Brondino, M. J., & Crouch, J. L. (1996). Eliminating (almost) treatment dropout of substance abusing or dependent delinquents through home-based multisystemic therapy. *American Journal of Psychiatry, 153,* 427–428.

Henggeler, S. W., Rodick, J. D., Borduin, C. M., Hanson, C. L., Watson, S. M., & Urey, J. R. (1986). Multisystemic treatment of juvenile offenders: Effects on adolescent behavior and family interactions. *Developmental Psychology, 22,* 132–141.

Henggeler, S. W., Rowland, M. D., Halliday-Boykins, C., Sheidow, A. J., Ward, D. M., Randall, J., et al. (2003). One-year follow-up of multisystemic therapy as an alternative to the hospitalization of youths in psychiatric crisis. *Journal of the American Academy of Child and Adolescent Psychiatry, 42,* 543–551.

Henggeler, S. W., Rowland, M. R., Randall, J., Ward, D., Pickrel, S. G., Cunningham, P. B., et al. (1999). Home-based multisystemic therapy as an alternative to the hospitalization of youth in psychiatric crisis: Clinical outcomes. *Journal of the American Academy of Child and Adolescent Psychiatry, 38,* 1331–1339.

Henggeler, S. W., Schoenwald, S. K., Borduin, C. M., Rowland, M. D., & Cunningham, P. B. (2009). *Multisystemic therapy for antisocial behavior in children and adolescents* (2nd ed.). New York: Guilford Press.

Henggeler, S. W., Schoenwald, S. K., Borduin, C. M., & Swenson, C. C. (2006). Methodological critique and meta-analysis as Trojan horse. *Children and Youth Services Review, 28,* 447–457.

Huey, S. J., Henggeler, S. W., Brondino, M. J., & Pickrel, S. G. (2000). Mechanisms of change in multisystemic therapy: Reducing delinquent behavior through therapist adherence and improved family and peer functioning. *Journal of Consulting and Clinical Psychology, 68,* 451–467.

Huey, S. J., Jr., Henggeler, S. W., Rowland, M. D., Halliday-Boykins, C. A., Cunningham, P. B., Pickrel, S. G., et al. (2004). Multisystemic therapy effects on attempted suicide by youth presenting psychiatric emergencies. *Journal of the American Academy of Child and Adolescent Psychiatry, 43,* 183–190.

Jones, H. E., Wong, C. J., Tuten, M., & Stitzer, M. L. (2005). Reinforcement-based therapy: 12–month evaluation of an outpatient drug-free treatment for heroin abusers. *Drug and Alcohol Dependence, 79,* 119–128.

Letourneau, E. J., Henggeler, S. W., Borduin, C. M., Schewe, P. A., McCart, M. R., Chapman, J. E., et al. (2009). Multisystemic therapy for juvenile sexual offenders: 1–year results from a randomized effectiveness trial. *Journal of Family Psychology, 23,* 89–102.

Littell, J. H., Popa, M., & Forsythe, B. (2005). *Multisystemic therapy for social, emotional, and behavioral problems in youth aged 10–17* (Campbell Collaborative Library, Issue 4). New York: Wiley.

Ogden, T., & Hagen, K. A. (2006a). Multisystemic therapy of serious behaviour problems in youth: Sustainability of therapy effectiveness two years after intake. *Journal of Child and Adolescent Mental Health, 11,* 142–149.

Ogden, T., & Hagen, K. A. (2006b). Virker MST?: Kommentarer til en systematisk forskningsoversikt og meta-analyse av MST [Does MST work. Comments on a systemic review and meta-analysis of MST]. *Nordisk Sosialt Arbeid, 26,* 222–233.

Ogden, T., & Halliday-Boykins, C. A. (2004). Multisystemic treatment of antisocial adolescents in Norway: Replication of clinical outcomes outside of the US. *Child and Adolescent Mental Health, 9*(9), 77–83.

Rowland, M. R., Chapman, J. E., & Henggeler, S. W. (2008). Sibling outcomes from a randomized trial of evidence-based treatments with substance abusing juvenile offenders. *Journal of Child and Adolescent Substance Abuse, 17,* 11–26.

Rowland, M. R., Halliday-Boykins, C. A., Henggeler, S. W., Cunningham, P. B., Lee, T. G., Kruesi, M. J. P., et al. (2005). A randomized trial of multisystemic therapy with Hawaii's Felix Class youths. *Journal of Emotional and Behavioral Disorders, 13,* 13–23.

Schaeffer, C. M., & Borduin, C. M. (2005). Long-term follow-up to a randomized clinical trial of multisystemic therapy with serious and violent juvenile offenders. *Journal of Consulting and Clinical Psychology, 73*(3), 445–453.

Schoenwald, S. K., Ward, D. M., Henggeler, S. W., Pickrel, S. G., & Patel, H. (1996). MST treatment of substance abusing or dependent adolescent offenders: Costs of reducing incarceration, inpatient, and residential placement. *Journal of Child and Family Studies, 5,* 431–444.

Schoenwald, S. K., Ward, D. M., Henggeler, S. W., & Rowland, M. D. (2000). MST vs. hospitalization for crisis stabilization of youth: Placement outcomes 4 months post-referral. *Mental Health Services Research, 2,* 3–12.

Sheidow, A. J., Bradford, W. D., Henggeler, S. W., Rowland, M. D., Halliday-Boykins, C., Schoenwald, S. K., et al. (2004). Treatment costs for youths in psychiatric crisis: Multisystemic therapy versus hospitalization. *Psychiatric Services, 55,* 548–554.

Sheidow, A. J., & Henggeler, S. W. (2008). Multisystemic therapy with substance using adolescents: A synthesis of research. In A. Stevens (Ed.), *Crossing frontiers: International developments in the treatment of drug dependence* (pp. 11–33). Brighton, UK: Pavilion.

Stambaugh, L. F., Mustillo, S. A., Burns, B. J., Stephens, R. L., Baxter, B., Edwards, D., et al. (2007). Outcomes from wraparound and multisystemic therapy in a center for mental health services system-of-care demonstration site. *Journal of Emotional and Behavioral Disorders, 15,* 143–155.

Sundell, K., Hansson, K., Lofholm, C. A., Olsson, T., Gustle, L. H., & Kadesjo, C. (2008). The transportability of MST to Sweden: Short-term results from a randomized trial of conduct disordered youth. *Journal of Family Psychology, 22,* 550–560.

Swenson, C. C., Schaeffer, C. M., Tuerk, E., Henggeler, S. W., Tuten, M., Panzarella, P., et al. (2009). Adapting multisystemic therapy for co-occurring child maltreatment and parental substance abuse: The Building Stronger Families project. *Journal of Emotional and Behavioral Disorders, 17,* 3–8.

Timmons-Mitchell, J., Bender, M. B., Kishna, M. A., & Mitchell, C. C. (2006). An independent effectiveness trial of multisystemic therapy with juvenile justice youth. *Journal of Clinical Child and Adolescent Psychology, 35,* 227–236.

Trupin, E., Kerns, S., Walker, S., & Lee, T. (in press). Family Integrated Transitions: A promising program for juvenile offenders with co-occurring disorders. *Psychiatric Services.*

18

Summer Treatment Programs for Attention-Deficit/Hyperactivity Disorder

WILLIAM E. PELHAM, JR., ELIZABETH M. GNAGY, ANDREW R. GREINER, DANIEL A. WASCHBUSCH, GREGORY A. FABIANO, and LISA BURROWS-MacLEAN

OVERVIEW OF THE TREATMENT MODEL

Children with attention-deficit/hyperactivity disorder (ADHD) have serious problems in daily life functioning, including classroom functioning and achievement, peer relationships, and family relationships. It has become increasingly evident that ADHD should be viewed as a chronic disorder, and that models of treatment should be those pertinent to a chronic disease. ADHD results in considerable financial costs to society and has poor long-term outcomes. Thus, interventions need to be effective, implemented across settings, and structured so that they can be conducted for years (Pelham & Fabiano, 2008). Two interventions have been repeatedly documented as solidly evidence-based for ADHD in short-term studies: CNS stimulants and behavioral interventions (Pelham & Fabiano, 2008).

The most common form of treatment for ADHD is medication with CNS stimulants. They have an extensive evidence base and often result in large short-term improvements, but these medications have limitations, among them that (1) parents prefer nonpharmacological interventions, (2) medication has limited impact on key domains of functioning, (3) medication is insufficient to normalize functioning for many children, (4) long-term compliance with medication is poor, (5) medication used alone does not result in improved long-term outcomes (Molina et al., 2009), and (6) the long-term safety of stimulant medications has not been established (see Pelham, 2008, for a discussion of these limitations).

The second most common treatment for ADHD is behavior modification in the form of parent training and school interventions. Behavior modification has a large evidence

277

base and has extensively documented short-term efficacy (Fabiano et al., 2009; Pelham & Fabiano, 2008). Unlike medication, behavioral interventions teach skills to parents, teachers, and children that overcome some of the key functional impairments associated with ADHD. At the same time, there is increasing evidence that, when implemented at a level typical of clinical practice (e.g., a dozen sessions of group parent training, in-clinic social skills groups, and a brief teacher consultation), behavioral interventions are not effectively improving acute functioning. Arguably, relatively more intensive psychosocial treatment programs are necessary to produce substantive, lasting behavioral changes in these children (Pelham & Fabiano, 2008).

We have argued elsewhere that various domains of functional impairment are far more important to both short- and long-term functioning in ADHD than symptoms and should be foremost among treatment targets (Pelham, Fabiano, & Massetti, 2005). It has long been known that impairments in three domains—peer relationships, parenting, and academic/school functioning—predict a variety of negative long-term outcomes in children with a variety of psychopathologies and are thought to mediate these outcomes. Therefore, effective treatment must focus on these problems in daily life functioning.

First, with regard to peer relations, standard treatments such as clinic-based social skills training have *not* proven efficacious (Pelham & Fabiano, 2008). One reason for this failure is that it is difficult to work on peer relationships in the office or in the regular education classroom. However, peer relationships can be targeted in recreational settings in which children can be directly observed interacting with peers and taught not only appropriate behavior and social skills but also sports knowledge, teamwork, and appropriate sportsmanship.

Second, ADHD commonly co-occurs with learning problems, and stimulant medication alone has not been shown to produce long-term gains in achievement (Loe & Feldman, 2007). It has long been argued that children, particularly those at risk for achievement problems, *lose* academic skills during summer breaks, and attendance at traditional summer school is modest at best. Arguably, combining academic instruction with recreational activities increases children's attendance and, therefore, produces greater benefit from summer academic programming.

Finally, deficits in parenting skills and parent–child relationships have long been known to predict dysfunctional outcomes for children. Behavioral parent training targeted at parenting skills is one of the most well-documented interventions for children with ADHD and other disruptive behavior disorders (Pelham & Fabiano, 2008), but it is infrequently provided in community mental health settings. Combining evening parent training with intensive daytime work with children is an ideal way to begin generalizing treatment effects to the home setting. Working with parents during the summer months also provides important opportunities to prepare them for the transition to the school year.

In summary, the summer is an opportune time to focus on the domains of impairment that are most critical to children with ADHD. These children are likely to experience failure in traditional summer camps and in their own neighborhoods, where they are often dismissed for their disruptive behavior or rejected by other children. If treatment provided in traditional settings is interrupted during the summer, gains made during the school year may be lost. Given a chronic care model, year-round intervention is critical for ADHD children.

Our comprehensive treatment model for ADHD has long included intervention in a camp-like setting in which children engage in a variety of activities with peers and academic instruction, supplemented by parent training. In the fall following summer break, parents are encouraged to attend monthly booster parent training sessions and consultations are held with the child's teacher to establish school–home daily report cards (DRCs; *ccf.buffalo.edu*) to maximize generalization of treatment gains. This chapter describes the summer treatment program (STP) and presents information on its efficacy, social validity, and exportability.

Goals of Treatment

Program goals are to improve the children's peer relationships (e.g., social skills, problem solving skills), interactions with adults (e.g., compliance to requests), academic performance (e.g., classroom productivity) and self-efficacy (e.g., competence in sports) while concurrently training parents in behavior management. Notably lacking is a focus on *Diagnostic and Statistical Manual of Mental Disorders* (DSM) symptoms of ADHD. Instead, children's functional impairments are identified and explicitly targeted in treatment. Using a social learning theoretical approach, our intervention is a package of age-appropriate, evidence-based operant and cognitive-behavioral treatments, adding a psychostimulant medication regimen that is evaluated in a controlled assessment when necessary. If the standard STP treatment package does not produce the desired behavior change, staff members conduct a functional analysis and develop individualized programs that target children's unique problems in daily life functioning.

CHARACTERISTICS OF THE TREATMENT PROGRAM

The STP is a weekday program for children and adolescents ages 5–15 years with ADHD and related disorders. Programs typically run for 7–8 weeks, 8–9 hours per day, although programs lasting 5 weeks for 6 hours/day have been used in community settings (Pelham, Fabiano, Gnagy, Greiner, & Hoza, 2005). In addition, an adapted program in Japan that lasts 3 weeks has proven efficacious (Yamashita et al., in press). Children are placed in age-matched groups of 12–16, and four to five college student interns implement treatments. Groups stay together throughout the summer, so that children receive intensive experience in group functioning, in making friends, and in interacting appropriately with adults. Each group spends 2 to 3 hours daily in classroom sessions conducted by teachers and aides. The remainder of each day consists of recreationally based group activities (e.g., sports, swimming). Parent training is held weekly. A treatment manual and supporting documents (e.g., forms necessary for implementing treatments, fidelity/integrity manual) describe the program in detail (Pelham, Greiner, & Gnagy, 1997).

Point System

Using a systematic response–reward cost program, children earn points or tokens for appropriate behavior and lose points or tokens for inappropriate behavior throughout the day. Such programs have an extensive history in behavior modification and have large, acute effects on children's behavior. The behaviors included in the STP point system are those that are commonly targeted for development (e.g., following rules, ignoring provocation, good sportsmanship, paying attention) and elimination (e.g., teasing, noncompliance, aggression) in children with ADHD, oppositional defiant disorder, and conduct disorder. Children exchange points for privileges (i.e., field trips), social honors, and camp-based (e.g., daily recess) and parent-administered rewards.

Social Reinforcement and Appropriate Commands

Social reinforcement in the form of praise and public recognition is ubiquitously used to provide a positive, supportive atmosphere. Counselors systematically praise the children for appropriate behavior, modeling appropriate social reinforcement for the parents during drop-offs and pickups. Children are informed about point losses in a neutral, nonadmonishing tone. In addition, staff members shape appropriate behavior by issuing commands with characteristics (e.g., brevity, specificity) that have been shown to maximize compliance.

Peer Interventions

Social skills training is provided in daily 10-minute group sessions in which the social skill of the day is reviewed. Sessions include instruction, modeling, role-playing, and review. Children also engage in group tasks (e.g., group art projects) that are designed to promote cooperation and contribute to cohesive peer relationships. What sets the STP apart from traditional social skills training is that children's implementation of the skills taught is continually prompted and reinforced using the point system throughout the daily engagement in recreational activities. Combining a reward–cost program with social skills training has been shown to be necessary to effect the development of positive peer skills in children with externalizing disorders. Blending these components with parent training may be critical to enhancing change and generalization to the natural environment.

Children also learn group problem-solving skills. This procedure is the basis for individual social problem solving that has long been applied in work with aggressive boys with and without ADHD.

Daily Report Cards

DRCs to parents have documented effectiveness in the treatment of ADHD. In the STP, DRCs include individualized target behaviors across all settings. Target behaviors and criteria for meeting goals are set and revised in an ongoing manner to ensure that they are appropriately challenge the child but enable success most of the time. Parents provide home-based rewards for reaching STP DRC goals and are taught to establish home-based DRCs (see later discussion). At the end of the day, each child's counselor meets briefly with the child and parents to give feedback about the day and to model for parents how to respond to positive and negative performance on DRC goals.

Sports Skills Training

Children with ADHD typically do not follow game rules and have poor motor skills, deficits that contribute to their social rejection and low self-esteem. Involvement in sports is thought to enhance self-efficacy, which, in turn, is believed to play a role in behavior change. Thus, 4 hours each day are devoted to small-group skills training and play in age-appropriate sports and games. Techniques designed to optimize skill training and practice for children are used. The intensive practice and time necessary to improve sports skills highlight the value of the STP setting for this program component. Figure 18.1 shows a typical recreational hour in the STP.

Time Out

"Prudent punishment" (e.g., appropriate verbal reprimands, privilege loss, time-out) is necessary for effective intervention with children with ADHD. Children are disciplined for certain behaviors (i.e., intentional aggression, intentional destruction of property, repeated noncompliance), with discipline taking the form of loss of privileges (e.g., loss of recess time) or time-out from positive reinforcement (Fabiano et al., 2004).

Classrooms

Children spend 2 hours daily in a classroom modeled after an academic special education classroom, and they spend a third hour in an art class. Behavior is managed using a simplified point system that includes earning points for work completion and accuracy and losing points for rule violations. Public recognition and praise are given for assignment completion and accuracy. The behavior management system can be implemented by a single teacher and a classroom aide and is, therefore, generalizable to regular school settings.

During classroom periods, children engage in a variety of structured academic activities. First, they complete individualized seatwork assignments in major academic

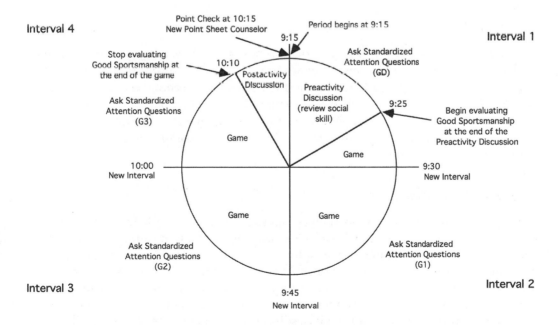

FIGURE 18.1. Timeline of a typical summer treatment program recreational period.

areas (e.g., arithmetic, reading comprehension) based on their needs and abilities. Second, children are paired for cooperative peer reading tasks (see Lyon, Fletcher, Fuchs, & Chhabra, 2006). Third, they work on individualized academic skills using a variety of computer-based instruction software. For young children at risk for reading disabilities, phonemic awareness training may be incorporated (see Lyon et al., 2006).

In the art class, children work on a variety of individual and cooperative group projects. Given that many children with ADHD have behavioral difficulties in less structured special areas in school, this class affords a unique opportunity to assess their problems and build skills for transfer to the regular school setting.

Modification for Adolescents

Age-appropriate adaptations have been made for adolescents with ADHD. These include a modified set of point system categories and a modified feedback delivery system, behavioral contracting, supervised "job" training (e.g., serving as a junior counselor), conducting a group "business" (selling pizza to families on parent training evenings), parent–teen negotiation, and classroom interventions such as note-taking and organizational skills.

Parent Involvement

As described, parents have daily contact with staff members at the beginning and end of each day. Parents also participate in weekly group parent training sessions. The parent training packages that we have used (e.g., Cunningham, Bremner, & Secord-Gilbert, 1998) have been validated as effective with children with externalizing disorders. Parents who have previously completed a course of parent training may participate in an advanced class incorporating *in vivo* training situations.

Medication Assessment

The STP provides the opportunity for parents and physicians to obtain placebo-controlled evaluations of stimulant medication. Data gathered routinely in the STP are evaluated, in addition to daily records of side effects, to determine whether medication was helpful or beyond the effects of concurrent behavioral interventions. If medication benefited the child in the areas of daily life functioning that are most important for him or her without adverse effects, then medication may be recommended as an adjunct to follow-up behavioral intervention.

Monitoring Treatment Response

Information on each child's treatment response is gathered daily from the point system; academic assignments; and counselor, teacher, and parent ratings, and is entered daily into a customized database. The information is immediately available to staff members and supervisors to monitor children's response to treatment and to make necessary modifications for individual children. In addition, staff and parents complete ratings of improvement at the end of the summer across a wide range of functional domains (e.g., compliance, peer relations, sports skills, self-esteem, academic productivity). These ratings have been shown to be sensitive to treatment effects (Pelham, Fabiano & Massetti, 2005).

Treatment Fidelity: Training, Supervision, Manuals, and Materials

The STP is extensively manualized and highly structured to facilitate implementation and fidelity (Pelham et al., 1997). The 425-page treatment manual provides comprehensive information on the intervention. An intensive 4- to 7-day staff training regimen has been developed and implemented at two sites annually over the past 15 years. Training requires preparatory reading of the treatment manual, a written test, and 9-hour days of description, supervised practice, and checkout activities.

After training and throughout the treatment period, an extensive set of documented procedures is implemented daily to monitor and ensure treatment fidelity. Integrity materials cover every treatment component and include both lists of procedures and quality ratings. Supervisory or independent staff observe groups regularly to document adherence to the treatment protocol. Staff members meet regularly to receive structured feedback from supervisors, and if necessary, remedial activities are given. Documentation of program knowledge is evaluated by weekly written tests.

EVIDENCE ON THE EFFECTS OF TREATMENT

How Is Treatment Evaluated?

The STP has been designed from the outset to facilitate clinical research. In contrast to traditional outcome studies that focus on DSM symptom ratings, the STP provides a wealth of objective information on children's behavior in the very settings in which impairment is most evident (e.g., in the classroom, playing baseball with peers). Clinical records have been developed to have such sufficient fidelity, reliability, and validity that they double as dependent measures in studies. Clinical observations generate research ideas, and results of empirical studies are used to modify subsequent treatment protocols. As of summer 2008, nearly 100 empirical STP studies have been conducted. These studies have added to our knowledge base of ADHD, addressing a wide variety of questions regarding the nature and treatment of ADHD, including studies of medication, behavioral treatments, and combined interventions and their impact on cognition and behavior. In addition to the large number of treatment component studies conducted within the context of the STP, the STP treatment package as a whole has a substantial and growing evidence base.

The treatment program has been evaluated using a variety of sources. Primary among these are the treatment records of the children's behavior. Daily records from the point system, classroom work productivity, classroom rule violations, and DRCs provide objective data on which children's response to the treatment is measured. Counselor, teacher, and parent ratings of child behavior supplement these measures and include assessments of improvement in daily life functioning. Parent ratings of satisfaction with the treatment provide an important social validity measure for program effectiveness. Finally, treatment integrity and fidelity measures ensure fidelity and demonstrate that the program can be implemented faithfully across different groups, years, and sites.

Status of the Evidence

A series of studies have demonstrated that STP treatment and its components produce large, clinically meaningful changes in child behavior. As detailed later, in many of these studies the effects of the STP behavioral interventions have been compared with medication with a CNS stimulant, which is a well-established intervention for ADHD, and the obtained effects have been comparable. Selected recent references are included herein, and a more extensive list can be found in Pelham, Fabiano, et al. (2005), Pelham and Fabiano (2008), and Fabiano, Pelham, et al. (2009).

A number of studies have provided evidence for the efficacy of the STP treatment package compared with a no-treatment condition (Chronis et al., 2004, Fabiano et al., 2007; Pelham, Fabiano, & Massetti, 2005; Pelham et al., 2008a, 2008b). In a BAB evaluation of the STP treatment package (i.e., treatment implemented, withdrawn, and then reinstated; Chronis et al., 2004), the withdrawal of treatment produced immediate and highly significant deterioration in behavior with very large effect sizes, regardless of whether or not children were receiving a concurrent medication regimen. A subsequent investigation removed the behavioral treatment in a BABAB design (Pelham, Burrows-MacLean, et al., 2005) and again showed large and significant effects of STP treatment. The latter study compared the STP treatment package with moderate to high doses of stimulant medication (methylphenidate) and showed that the effects were comparable. Notably, on a measure of probability of reaching children's individualized daily goals, the behavioral treatment package produced far greater incremental improvement than medication alone. In other studies with a medication comparison condition, the impact of the STP treatment package is routinely found to be comparable to that of moderate to high doses of stimulant medication (e.g., Fabiano et al., 2007; Pelham et al., 2008a, 2008b).

These results from crossover studies have also been replicated in a recent randomized trial with 152 children with ADHD (see complete description later) in which no behavioral treatment, standard STP treatment, and a lower intensity, modified version of the STP package (i.e.., behavioral feedback without points, DRC with daily and weekly contingencies, sit-outs rather than escalating/deescalating time-outs, no individualized programming, weekly rather than daily parental rewards, weekly rather than daily social skills training) were compared for 3 weeks (random assignment to treatment groups). Patients who received the STP treatment, both the standard and the lower intensity conditions, were significantly superior to those who did not receive behavioral intervention on a large number of objective indexes of functioning, and the effect sizes were large (Pelham et al., 2008a). The standard treatment package was modestly superior to the reduced intensity package; larger differences between the two conditions were apparent in the absence of medication. Thus, the between-groups findings from this study replicate the within-subjects findings from this and previous studies in the context of the STP and demonstrate large effect sizes of the treatment relative to no treatment. Further, consistent with previous studies, the behavioral conditions were comparable to the moderate- (low-intensity STP) and high- (standard STP) dose stimulant conditions.

Studies have also evaluated the incremental contributions of individual treatment components of the STP (see Pelham, Fabiano, et al., 2005, for complete list and further discussion of component studies). One such study investigated the incremental benefit of including time-out in the treatment package (Fabiano et al., 2004) and found that the use of time-out resulted in significant reductions of aggressive and noncompliant behavior. The classroom-based components of the STP have also been evaluated (e.g., Fabiano et al., 2007). In three studies, the classroom behavioral components resulted in clinically and statistically significant improvements compared with control conditions across a variety of measures (e.g., disruptive behavior, teacher ratings, classroom rule violations), with moderate to large effect sizes. These studies included a stimulant medication comparison condition and showed that the behavioral package produced effects comparable to those of moderate doses of methylphenidate (e.g., 0.3 mg/kg/dose). In the recreational (nonclassroom) setting, one explicit goal of the STP is to increase children's knowledge of sports rules and improve sports skills, and children are encouraged to exhibit appropriate sportsmanship. The success of this approach is demonstrated by findings of improved sports skills, increased attention to game situations, and decreased unsportsmanlike behaviors in the context of the STP (e.g., Chronis et al., 2004; Pelham et al., 2008b), again with effects comparable to those produced by medication (e.g., see Figure 18.2).

Additional uncontrolled studies across many STPs and numerous clinical sites have provided support for the effectiveness of STP. In a pretreatment–posttreatment evaluation, Pelham and Hoza (1996) reported on 258 boys with ADHD who participated in STPs over a 6-year period. From pre- to post-STP, significant improvements were found in parent and staff (counselor and teacher) ratings of ADHD and associated symptoms, impairment, and global improvement as well as improvement in multiple functional domains and child ratings of self-perception. Results were consistent across a variety of demographic, diagnostic, and socioeconomic moderators (e.g., comorbid aggression, single- vs. two-parent household, family socioeconomic status [SES]). Because these variables often moderate (typically reduce) the impact of psychosocial treatment, the fact that they did not moderate response to the STP is noteworthy. Similar results were obtained across a variety of domains and measures in the STPs conducted as part of the Multimodal Treatment Study of ADHD (MTA). In that study (Pelham et al., 2000), the effects of the STP alone were so large that only minimal effects of additional medication were obtained during that phase of the study. These results have been replicated in five

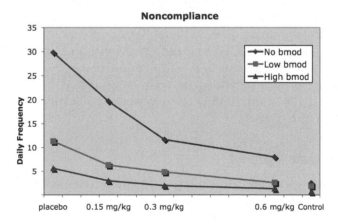

FIGURE 18.2. Daily noncompliance as a function of behavioral treatment and medication (bmod, behavioral medication). From Pelham et al. (2008b).

different STP sites in both university and community settings (Pelham, Fabiano, et al., 2005). Similar positive outcomes have been reported in a Japanese setting (Yamashita et al., in press). Finally, the STP has been included as a component of the psychosocial treatment package in two large National Institute of Health clinical trials (August, Realmuto, Hektner, & Bloomquist, 2001; MTA Cooperative Group, 1999).

A major difference between STP and other treatment programs is that the dropout rate from STP is extremely low, with a completion rate of 98% (Pelham, Fabiano, et al., 2005). Daily attendance is routinely near 100%, as is parent training attendance. Pelham and Hoza (1996) documented that the dropout rate for STP is similarly low across SES, race, and single-parent status, illustrating the utility of the STP across family characteristics that are reliably associated with poor adherence to treatment. A prerequisite to a successful long-term intervention for a chronic disorder such as ADHD is successful completion of the initial stage of treatment, and the STP virtually ensures that outcome.

Perhaps contributing to the high rate of treatment completion, participants in the STP are overwhelmingly satisfied with the intervention. Pelham and Hoza (1996) and Pelham, Fabiano, et al. (2005) report very high parent satisfaction rates at six different STP sites across the United States. Parents routinely rate the STP as superior to other mental health services in which they have been involved. The high rate of consumer satisfaction has also been replicated in the two large studies in which the STP has been utilized as a component of behavioral treatment (August et al., 2001; Pelham et al., 2000).

Finally, additional evidence supporting STP can be found in studies of the behavioral treatment in combination with stimulant medication. Several of the studies reviewed previously have included combined treatment conditions, enabling evaluation of STP as a component of multimodal treatment, including crossover studies comparing the single and combined effects of behavior modification and stimulant medication (e.g., Pelham, Burrows-MacLean, et al., 2005; Fabiano et al., 2007; Pelham et al., 2008a, 2008b). The most recent reports (Fabiano et al., 2007; Pelham, Fabiano, & Massetti, 2005; Pelham et al., 2008a, 2008b) have involved studies of (1) behavioral treatment in the STP with weekly or triweekly crossovers, (2) multiple doses of stimulant medication manipulated in daily repeat crossovers, and (3) medication conditions crossed with the behavioral treatments. These studies have documented findings of major importance: If the STP behavioral treatment—both the lower intensity and the standard conditions—is in place in classroom or recreational settings, then (1) the effect of medication is maximized at a very low methylphenidate dose (0.15 mg/kg/dose) that is insufficient when used alone and that produces no side effects, and (2) the effect of the multimodal intervention is equivalent to a considerably higher dose of medication (0.6 mg/kg/dose) alone. Given the growing concern regarding side effects associated with long-term stimulant use (Swanson et al., 2007), this finding has important implications for chronic intervention with children with ADHD.

Overall Evaluation of the Treatment

In summary, numerous evaluations of the STP have documented program efficacy and effectiveness. Multiple studies utilizing different types of controlled designs, with a variety of measures from multiple settings, domains, and sources, provide detailed documentation of improvements. Notably, these changes are found mainly for behaviors related to functional impairments (e.g., peer relationships, compliance with adult commands, academic work completion). These domains are the putative mediators of long-term outcomes among children with ADHD (Pelham, Fabiano, & Massetti, 2005; Pelham & Fabiano, 2008) and are, therefore, more critical than DSM symptoms as treatment targets and goals. Further, in a large number of these studies, the effects of STP treatment are comparable to the effects of stimulant medication, a well-established intervention for ADHD. Finally, these changes have been obtained by multiple investigators across multiple seasons, samples, and staff members implementing the STP in both university and community settings.

A final benefit of the STP is that it serves as a training site for students who are future mental health, health, and educational professionals. Across years and sites, more than 2,000 undergraduate, graduate, and special education students, teachers, and mental health workers have worked in the STP. Students who receive training in the STP often go on to graduate or medical school and subsequent faculty positions or applied mental health or educational positions. This includes, to our knowledge, more than 100 faculty members in university settings and many times that number in applied settings. All leave the STP trained in state-of-the-art behavior modification strategies for treating ADHD and other childhood problems, and they apply this knowledge across academic, educational, and mental health settings. Many students say that the STP experience was the best of their training careers, and they virtually unanimously recommend it to others.

Evidence Regarding Implementation in Practice

Replications in Clinical Practice

An important issue regarding a comprehensive intervention such as the STP is whether it can be replicated in clinical practice. It is important to understand that the STP was developed as a clinical intervention and has been routinely offered in clinical settings. For example, at the University of Pittsburgh Medical Center, it was conducted through the base service unit of the county mental health system that was operated by the Center's Department of Psychiatry. As such, the procedures utilized (e.g., intakes, treatment plans, progress monitoring and recording, staffing requirements, client reports), fees charged, payment structures (insurance, self-pay, or Medicaid), and regulations governing the STP were those required by the county mental health system with state and Joint Commission on the Accreditation of Healthcare Organizations oversight. Thus, even the STP at Western Psychiatric Institute and Clinic, which has been widely viewed as an academic endeavor, reflected real clinical practice in a psychiatric outpatient setting. In 1994, three community agencies in towns surrounding Pittsburgh received foundation grants to establish STPs. They have conducted STPs since then and now operate 29 STP sites around western Pennsylvania with a predominantly Medicaid client base. Following this model, five community agencies in western New York and New York City have begun STPs in the past several years. Agencies fund their STP programs through the same mechanisms they use to fund other services. Thus, STPs in various states and settings are financed through self-pay, Medicaid, scholarships via private donations, and third-party payers. In Pennsylvania, 29 STP sites are operated by three mental health agencies that focus primarily on Medicaid populations. In the Cleveland Clinic STP, payment is self-pay, third-party insurance, or Medicaid depending on the family's coverage. One STP in New York City is self-pay only, and the other is an exclusively Medicaid population.

In Buffalo, New York Boys' and Girls' Clubs operate STPs using their regular revenue streams.

In addition to community sites, leading medical centers in North America have operated STPs in departments of psychiatry, pediatrics, and psychology (e.g., Cleveland Clinic, New York University, University of Alabama at Birmingham, Vanderbilt University, Emory University, University of Illinois, Chicago, Dalhousie University, Royal Ottawa Hospital, State University of New York at Buffalo). All of these programs have been clinical services, and the majority continue to be offered. In all, the STP has been replicated in clinical practice at more than 25 independent sites in locations ranging from medical centers to community mental health agencies and private practices. A translation of the program has been implemented in Japan for 4 years in a partnership between a department of pediatrics and the local school system (Yamashita et al., in press). Internally, our group has replicated the STP for nearly 30 years with different staff members each time. As the program evaluations reported document, the results across years and sites on a variety of measures have been uniformly positive.

Addressing Barriers to Implementation

The most basic requirement of programmatic replication and implementation in practice is that the procedures are completely documented, and we have done that for the STP, as described previously. The manual and materials necessary to track children's progress are available for purchase from the authors at a very low initial and nonrepeating cost. Materials are provided on a CD-ROM and can be reproduced without limit. We have typically provided consultation and training in the first year of operation for many of these STPs. Each summer, a week-long, intensive centralized training session is provided at low cost at two sites—Buffalo, New York, and Latrobe, Pennsylvania—by experienced STP staff members. Arrangements to purchase materials and attend training or to hire a staff member to conduct training remotely can be made with the authors at *ccf.buffalo.edu*. In subsequent years, sites have typically taken over complete responsibility for their STPs.

The format of the STP removes some of the well-known barriers to treatment associated with poor response and early termination in ADHD and associated disorders (Pelham & Fabiano, 2008; Pelham & Hoza, 1996; Pelham, Fabiano, et al., 2005). For example, parent training sessions are conducted in the evenings and include structured child care activities. The daily contact among counselors, parents, and children maximizes the therapeutic alliance between professionals and parents that is necessary for success in a long-term model of treatment. The fact that almost all children with ADHD very much like attending the STP (Pelham & Hoza, 1996) no doubt contributes to the fact that treatment completion is high. Finally, summer day camps providing activities for children in a manner that allows parents flexibility for their own schedules are ubiquitous in every community in North America. By structuring the STP with the hours and length of a typical summer camp, we have adapted the STP as a mental health service to match what is available for nonhandicapped children. We believe that this approach removes a major barrier to treatment: making services fit with family schedules.

Barriers exist not only for families but also for agencies, and the STP addresses some potential barriers. The STP can be adapted to almost any setting where appropriate facilities (e.g., field space, pool, classrooms) and resources for follow-up are available, including mental health centers, school districts, group private practices, Boys' and Girls' Clubs, and hospitals. The STP treatment package can also be adapted for use in a variety of other treatment settings. For example, several STP community sites have modified and integrated STP components into other services they routinely provide, such as after-school programs, recreation programs, wraparound services, school-based services, and summer school. A major benefit to agencies is that the training in evidence-based behavioral interventions that their staff receive in the STP then carries over to other services that those same staff conduct, improving program implementation agencywide.

A major barrier to implementation of the STP in clinical practice is that the prevailing model of mental health services for children—weekly individual therapy in a clinic for 3–4 months—is incompatible with the approach that is explicit in the STP model. There is an enormous mismatch between the contemporary models of mental health services and the treatments that have an evidence base for ADHD and the other disruptive behavior disorders. These disorders require intensive and ongoing interventions for many if not most children. For example, it has been estimated that a typical child with ADHD has nearly a half million negative interpersonal interactions annually (Pelham & Fabiano, 2008). This means that an 8-year-old child referred for peer problems has a long history of maladaptive learning with regard to peer relationships. It is silly for mental health professionals to assume that a brief intervention (e.g., 12 weekly one-to-one sessions of individual counseling or social skills training) will have an impact on such a strong learning history of maladaptive skills. Instead, intensive summer programs and similar services delivered in schools, after school, and on weekends would appear far more likely to impact this domain positively. Agencies that wish to provide benefit for children with ADHD must adapt their structure, facilities, and staffing patterns to offer these more appropriate and evidence-based services.

DIRECTIONS FOR RESEARCH

There is a very strong evidence base for the short-term effectiveness of the STP. As with all other interventions—both psychosocial and pharmacological—for childhood mental health disorders, there is considerably less evidence for the long-term impact of the STP in children treated for ADHD. Like others, we have argued that systematic plans for maintenance need to be implemented by parents and teachers in order for acute behavioral treatment effects to maintain (Fabiano et al., 2009; Pelham & Fabiano, 2008), and this issue is relevant for the STP (see later discussion). Our group is currently conducting a randomized trial of different "doses" of behavioral treatment for young children with ADHD, and the STP is an integral part of the enhanced behavioral treatment condition. Treatment in this study lasts 3.5 years and will provide controlled information regarding maintenance of STP effects and whether behavioral interventions of varying intensities produce positive outcomes that are sufficient to prevent the need for adjunctive medication.

Elsewhere we have reviewed the evidence for behavioral treatments in ADHD and directions for future research (Pelham & Fabiano, 2008). In our view, a priority for further research is the issue of how to maintain effects over time, or, translated into practice, how to get families and schools to continue the short-term interventions that have proven effective. ADHD is a chronic disorder, and interventions for most children need to be continued in one form or another for very long time periods, perhaps never ended but modified across developmental stages. We have not extensively and systematically investigated the effects of follow-up interventions, but we have used several different types in our clinical practice. One is a 3-hour Saturday treatment program that uses the STP recreational procedures. We also routinely use follow-up school consultations to establish DRCs in the classrooms to which children return after the STP as well as the option for parents to attend booster training group sessions. Our only systematic evaluation of follow-up intervention shows that providing parent boosters and school DRC consultation after an STP results in a substantially lowered probability of the need for stimulant medication during the subsequent school year compared with treatment as usual (Coles et al., 2004). Thus, a key area of future research is how best to incorporate long-term follow-up treatments and to maintain families and teachers in some form of active intervention over the children's lifetime.

One other clear need for future research is intervention for adolescents. It is perhaps unsurprising, given the paucity of treatment research with adolescents with ADHD, that we have not yet evaluated an adolescent version of the STP. Because it is becoming clear that the vast majority of ADHD children continue to have problems with peers, academics, and parents in adolescence, such work is clearly needed.

CONCLUSIONS

We have described the STP, including the intervention, fidelity procedures, outcome measures, and studies supporting its short-term effectiveness. Perhaps reflecting our confidence in its impact on children with ADHD, the STP has received numerous awards. In 1993 it was selected in a national competition as one of 20 Model Programs for Service Delivery for Child and Family Mental Health by the Section on Clinical Child Psychology (Section 1, Division 12) and Division of Child, Youth, and Family Services of the American Psychological Association. In 2003, the STP was named Innovative Program of the Year by Children and Adults with ADHD, a national advocacy organization for people with ADHD. Finally, the STP is included in the Substance Abuse and Mental Health Services Administration National Registry of Effective and Promising Programs (*nrepp. samhsa.gov/programfulldetails.asp?PROGRAM_ID=160*).

Effective treatment for ADHD needs to follow a comprehensive, chronic care model: implemented across domains (peer, family, school); conducted long term; focus on functional impairment rather than DSM symptoms; responsive to family needs; and relatively more intensive than currently common models in the mental health field. As we have outlined previously, STPs add to this model of intervention by offering the potential for unique combinations of treatment components that focus on peer, academic, and home domains and that make treatment especially palatable for families and, therefore, more likely to be continued in a chronic care model than current treatments for ADHD. Competencies such as sports skills that are necessary for children to function well in peer group settings can be intensively taught in STP contexts. Academic intervention can be implemented that adds 80 hours to the 200–250 hours during which children are typically on task in academics during the school year. Parent training can be offered in a setting that doubles the probability of attendance compared with traditional clinic-based training. The STP packs 380 hours of child treatment, sports skills training, academic intervention, and parent training into an 8-week period. We believe that such comprehensive regimens are needed to change the long-term trajectory of most children with ADHD.

REFERENCES

August, G. J., Realmuto, G. M., Hektner, J. M., & Bloomquist, M. L. (2001). An integrated components preventive intervention for aggressive elementary school children: The Early Risers Program. *Journal of Consulting and Clinical Psychology, 69,* 614–626.

Chronis, A. M., Fabiano, G. A., Gnagy, E. M., Onyango, A. N., Pelham, W. E., Williams, A., et al. (2004). An evaluation of the summer treatment program for children with ADHD using a treatment withdrawal design. *Behavior Therapy, 35,* 561–585.

Coles, E. K., Pelham, W. E., Fabiano, G. A., Robb, J., Arnold, F. W., Wymbs, B. T., et al. (2004, November). *Effects of continued interventions following a summer treatment program for children with ADHD.* Poster presented at the annual meeting of the Association for the Advancement of Behavior Therapy, New Orleans, LA.

Cunningham, C. E., Bremner, R., & Secord-Gilbert, M. (1998). *The Community Parent Education (COPE) program: A school based family systems oriented course for parents of children with disruptive behavior disorders.* Unpublished manual, McMaster University and Chedoke-McMaster Hospitals.

Fabiano, G. A., Pelham, W. E., Coles, E. K., Gnagy, E. M., Chronis-Tuscano, A., & O'Connor, B. (2009). A meta-analysis of behavioral treatments for attention-deficit/hyperactivity disorder. *Clinical Psychology Review, 29,* 129–140.

Fabiano, G. A., Pelham, W. E., Gnagy, E. M., Wymbs, B. T., Chacko, A., Coles, E. K., et al. (2007). The single and combined effects of multiple intensities of behavior modification and multiple intensities of methylphenidate in a classroom setting. *School Psychology Review, 36,* 195–216.

Fabiano, G. A., Pelham, W. E., Manos, M. J., Gnagy, E. M., Chronis, A. M., Onyango, A. N., et al. (2004). An evaluation of three time-out procedures for children with attention-deficit/hyperactivity disorder. *Behavior Therapy, 35,* 449–469.

Loe, I. M., & Feldman, H. (2007). Academic and educational outcomes of children with ADHD. *Ambulatory Pediatrics, 7*(Suppl. 1), 82–90.

Lyon, G. R., Fletcher, J. M., Fuchs, L. S., & Chhabra, V. (2006). Learning disabilities. In E. Mash & R. Barkley (Eds.), *Treatment of childhood disorders* (3rd ed., pp. 512–591). New York: Guilford Press.

Molina, B. S. G., Hinshaw, S. P., Swanson, J. M., Arnold, L. E., Vitiello, B., Jensen, P. S., et al. (2009). MTA at 8 years: Prospective follow-up of children treated for combined-type ADHD in a multisite study. *Journal of the American Academy of Child and Adolescent Psychiatry, 48,* 484–500.

MTA Cooperative Group. (1999). 14–month randomized clinical trial of treatment strategies for attention deficit hyperactivity disorder. *Archives of General Psychiatry, 56,* 1073–1086.

Pelham, W. E. (2008). Against the grain: A proposal for a psychosocial-first approach to treating ADHD—The Buffalo treatment algorithm. In K. McBurnett & L. J. Pfiffner (Eds.), *Attention deficit/hyperactivity disorder: Concepts, controversies, new directions* (pp. 301–316). New York: Informa Healthcare.

Pelham, W. E., Burrows-MacLean, L., Gnagy, E. M., Fabiano, G. A., Coles, E. K., Tresco, K. E., et al. (2005). Transdermal methylphenidate, behavioral, and combined treatment for children with ADHD. *Experimental and Clinical Psychopharmacology, 1,* 111–126.

Pelham, W. E., Burrows-MacLean, L., Gnagy, E. M., Fabiano, G. A., Coles, E. K., Wymbs, B. T., et al. (2008a). *A between groups study of behavioral, pharmacological and combined treatment for children with ADHD.* Manuscript in preparation.

Pelham, W. E., Burrows-MacLean, L., Gnagy, E. M., Fabiano, G. A., Coles, E. K., Wymbs, B. T., et al. (2008b). *A dose-ranging crossover study of behavioral, pharmacological, and combined treatment in a recreational setting for children with ADHD.* Manuscript in preparation.

Pelham, W. E., & Fabiano, G. A. (2008). Evidence-based psychosocial treatment for attention deficit/hyperactivity disorder: An update. *Journal of Clinical Child and Adolescent Psychology, 37*(1), 185–214.

Pelham, W. E., Fabiano, G. A., Gnagy, E. M., Greiner, A. R., & Hoza, B. (2005). The role of summer treatment programs in the context of comprehensive treatment for ADHD. In E. Hibbs & P. Jensen (Eds.), *Psychosocial treatments for child and adolescent disorders: Empirically based strategies for clinical practice* (2nd ed., pp. 377–410). Washington DC: American Psychological Association.

Pelham, W. E., Fabiano, G. A., & Massetti, G. M. (2005). Evidence-based assessment of attention-deficit/hyperactivity disorder in children and adolescents. *Journal of Clinical Child and Adolescent Psychology, 34,* 449–476.

Pelham, W. E., Gnagy, E. M., Greiner, A. R., Hoza, B., Hinshaw, S. P., Swanson, J. M., et al. (2000). Behavioral vs. behavioral and pharmacological treatment in ADHD children attending a summer treatment program. *Journal of Abnormal Child Psychology, 28,* 507–526.

Pelham, W. E., Greiner, A. R., & Gnagy, E. M. (1997). *Children's summer treatment program manual.* Buffalo, NY: Comprehensive Treatment for Attention Deficit Disorders.

Pelham, W. E., & Hoza, B. (1996). Intensive treatment: A summer treatment program for children with ADHD. In E. Hibbs & P. Jensen (Eds.), *Psychosocial treatments for child and adolescent disorders: Empirically based strategies for clinical practice* (pp. 311–340). Washington, DC: American Psychological Association.

Swanson, J. M., Elliott, G. R., Greenhill, L. L., Wigal, T., Arnold, L. E., Vitiello, B., et al. (2007). Effects of stimulant medication on growth rates across 3 years in the MTA follow-up. *Journal of the American Academy of Child and Adolescent Psychiatry, 46,* 1015–1027.

Yamashita, Y., Mukasa, A., Muira, N., Honda, Y., Anai, C., Kunisaki, C., et al. (in press). Short-term effects of American summer treatment program for Japanese children with attention deficit hyperactivity disorder. *Brain and Development.*

C

Other Disorders and Special Applications

19

Trauma-Focused Cognitive-Behavioral Therapy for Traumatized Children

JUDITH A. COHEN, ANTHONY P. MANNARINO, and ESTHER DEBLINGER

OVERVIEW

Clinical Problems Addressed

Trauma-focused cognitive behavioral therapy (TF-CBT) addresses problems specifically associated with significantly traumatic events that children experience or witness. Traumatic events are those that are terrifying, shocking, sudden, and potentially threatening to life, safety, or physical integrity. These may include but are not limited to experiences such as sexual or physical abuse or assault, domestic or community violence, bullying, serious accidents, natural or other disasters, fires, traumatic deaths, war, terrorism, and medical traumas. The prototypical disorder associated with trauma exposure is posttraumatic stress disorder (PTSD); TF-CBT targets PTSD symptoms as well as other trauma-related outcomes. After trauma exposure many children develop significant PTSD symptoms without meeting full PTSD diagnostic criteria, and these children are also appropriate candidates for TF-CBT treatment. Other children may develop depressive, anxiety, or behavioral or physical disorders in response to trauma exposure rather than PTSD. Still others may have changed cognitions about themselves, others, and the world (e.g., shame, self-blame, poor self-esteem, diminished sense of safety or trust). Research has demonstrated that traumatized children may experience dysregulation in affective, behavioral, cognitive, and physiological areas of functioning. These problems are addressed in greater detail elsewhere (Cohen, Mannarino, & Deblinger, 2006; Deblinger & Heflin, 1996). TF-CBT includes components that target reregulation in each of these realms, with a goal of optimizing children's adaptive functioning after trauma.

TF-CBT is thus intended for children who have primary trauma symptoms (e.g., PTSD, depressive, anxiety, shame, cognitive distortions) that the core components of this model would be expected to improve. The core target of TF-CBT is to help children

overcome traumatic avoidance, shame, sadness, fear, and other trauma-specific problems. Anger, aggression, oppositional, and other externalized behavior problems are not
typically by themselves core features of traumatized children. Although TF-CBT does
include behavior management components and behavioral dysregulation does improve
for many children who receive this treatment, addressing externalized behaviors is not
the core focus of this model. Thus, TF-CBT would likely not be the first line of treatment
for previously abused children who have no or few symptoms of PTSD or depression
and whose primary presenting problems are conduct symptoms. Such children would be
expected to benefit much more from an evidence-based treatment (EBT) such as parent management training that addresses their core symptoms (i.e., conduct problems)
regardless of the historical fact that abuse had occurred. This is why assessment is so
crucial. Regardless of trauma history, if children's clinical presentation suggests that
their core problems ("what is driving the train" in terms of psychological and functional
problems) are not directly related to the traumatic experiences but rather are due to
another psychopathological process, TF-CBT typically would not be the first treatment
of choice. However, if such children responded to PMT with improved behavioral regulation and then were discovered to have remaining PTSD or depressive symptoms or to
have more significant trauma symptoms than was initially apparent, it would certainly be
appropriate to provide TF-CBT at that point.

Conceptual Model/Underlying Assumptions

TF-CBT is a hybrid model incorporating cognitive-behavioral, attachment, family,
humanistic, and psychodynamic therapy principles as well as research findings about the
psychophysiology of childhood trauma. Traumatic childhood experiences affect children on many different levels and have the potential to disrupt their physical, emotional,
cognitive, behavioral, and social adjustment and development. Cognitive-behavioral
models of treatment assume that overall levels of adjustment in all these areas of functioning impact one another and influence overall well-being. Thus, dysfunction in one
area of well-being likely will lead to difficulties in another. Similarly, improved well-being
in one area (e.g., emotional) will likely enhance well-being in another realm (e.g., physical). TF-CBT is designed to address the impact of childhood trauma across these areas of
functioning, thereby reducing the likelihood of disrupted development and maladaptive
functioning.

Several psychological theories have been proposed to explain the development of
posttraumatic difficulties. Classical conditioning may produce behavioral and emotional
reactions that are natural and, in many cases, productive responses to trauma (e.g.,
arousal, fear). Later these distressing reactions may generalize to innocuous trauma
reminders (e.g., memories, darkness, loud noise, men with beards) that may not warrant,
but automatically elicit, arousal, fear, and other distressing responses. Avoidant behaviors may then develop and may be reinforced (via operant conditioning) in an effort to
minimize the experiencing of trauma-related symptoms and emotions. Unfortunately,
although this avoidance may be adaptive in the short term, it will increasingly limit the
children's capacity to engage in interactions with others as well as the world, which are
critical to healthy emotional and social development. Emotional processing theory (Foa
& Rothbaum, 1998) similarly suggests that posttraumatic symptoms reflect the development of a problematic fear structure comprising many stimuli, responses, and meaning

representations that, when triggered, produce maladaptive reactions. These theories argue for the importance of exposure to trauma memories and reminders by (1) promoting habituation and reducing reinforcement of avoidance and (2) simultaneously allowing the feared memories and emotions to be paired with therapeutic, corrective experiences that may produce new adaptive associations between trauma memories and feelings of safety and mastery. Social-cognitive theory focuses on the impact of trauma on preexisting or developing beliefs about one's self, others, and the world. These theorists highlight the value of reviewing trauma-related feelings and thoughts not for purposes of habituation but rather to fully process the experience, thereby correcting dysfunctional beliefs and addressing secondary emotional reactions such as shame and self-blame. These theories underscore the psychoeducation, skill building, trauma narrative/processing, and *in vivo* components of TF-CBT in that these components are all designed to provide opportunities for corrective experiences and information, enhanced feelings of competence, and the processing of trauma-related thoughts and feelings. Through the use of gradual exposure (GE), included in each of the TF-CBT treatment components, children are able to master and appropriately process trauma reminders rather than be overwhelmed by and feel a need to avoid them.

Attachment, humanistic, family, and psychodynamic theories, with their emphases on the healing potential of relationships, support the central role of the therapist–client relationship as well as the value of parental/family involvement in optimizing outcomes. The TF-CBT model also recognizes the critical contribution of the therapeutic relationship and the importance of parental/family involvement in treatment whenever possible. The therapist serves not only as an educator but also as a role model and coach with respect to skill building and nonavoidance of trauma-related material. Perhaps most importantly, the therapist provides a safe, therapeutic environment for children, adolescents, and parents to share their innermost thoughts and feelings and to overcome the stigma, shame, and self-blame associated with many types of traumatic experiences.

TF-CBT was originally designed to help parents cope with their own distress in the aftermath of trauma while enhancing their skills in responding to their children's trauma-related difficulties. In so doing, TF-CBT reduces parental distress and simultaneously enhances their support for the child, both factors that contribute in important ways to children's enhanced recovery. Although the TF-CBT model was largely developed based on cognitive-behavioral principles, it is perhaps best described as an evolving model that is designed to reflect our most up-to-date scientific understanding of psychosocial theories and research that explain maladaptive and adaptive responses to trauma and recovery in children and adolescents.

GOALS AND THEMES OF TF-CBT

Goals and themes of TF-CBT include (1) mastering skills to manage stress and improve affective, behavioral, and cognitive regulation early in treatment; (2) inclusion of parents or other caretaking adults in treatment whenever feasible; (3) mastering trauma reminders and traumatic avoidance through the use of GE throughout the TF-CBT model; (4) making meaning and contextualizing traumatic experiences through affective and cognitive processing—moving beyond victimization; and (5) enhancing safety and optimizing future development.

CHARACTERISTICS OF TF-CBT

Who Is Seen and in What Format: Special Settings

TF-CBT addresses trauma-related symptoms for children ages 3–18. The treatment model is adapted for children of different developmental levels. Children and their parents or primary caretakers receive TF-CBT in parallel individual sessions as well as joint child–parent or family sessions; children can receive TF-CBT alone if parents or caretakers are not available to participate in treatment. Children in foster care, group homes, residential treatment facilities, day hospitals, and inpatient programs can receive TF-CBT. Cultural adaptations of TF-CBT are available for Latino and Native American children and for HIV-affected Zambian children. TF-CBT treatment materials are available in Spanish, German, Chinese, and Dutch, and cultural adaptations of assessment instruments and TF-CBT treatment for HIV-affected Zambian children using established mixed methods has also been developed.

Content of TF-CBT, Sequence of Sessions

TF-CBT is a components-based model. The TF-CBT components are summarized by the acronym PRACTICE: **P**sychoeducation, **P**arenting skills, **R**elaxation skills, **A**ffective expression and modulation skills, **C**ognitive coping skills, **T**rauma narration and cognitive processing of traumatic experiences, *In vivo* mastery of trauma reminders, **C**onjoint child–parent sessions, and **E**nhancing safety and future developmental trajectory. The sequence of TF-CBT components generally follows the PRACTICE order, with early PRAC skills-based components preceding the more trauma-specific TICE components as described later. The model is progressive, with each component building on previously mastered skills. TF-CBT fidelity checklists are available to monitor therapists' adherence to the treatment model. Fidelity requires the following: (1) All TF-CBT components are provided during treatment unless justification exists to not provide a component (e.g., if no parent is available to participate, parenting skills would not be provided; if no generalization of trauma reminders existed, *in vivo* mastery would not be provided); (2) PRACTICE components are generally provided in sequence unless compelling clinical justification exists to provide a component out of sequence; (3) progression from one component to the next is achieved at a pace that is appropriate for the clinical circumstances (treatment is usually completed within 8–20 sessions; children in foster care or residential settings typically require more sessions than those living in other settings as a result of having experienced multiple placements with inconsistent behavioral expectations, which frequently result in more behavioral dysregulation; (4) GE is included in all treatment components. GE involves incrementally increasing the intensity or duration with which exposure to trauma reminders is included in each sequential TF-CBT component. GE may be achieved through talking, writing, creating arts, or other activities that directly engage the children and parents in mastering avoidance of thoughts, feelings, reminders, and memories of the traumatic experiences. Specific examples of how GE is included in each PRACTICE component are included in the following description.

Skills and Accomplishments Emphasized in TF-CBT: PRACTICE Components

The PRACTICE components are the core of the TF-CBT model. As noted, TF-CBT is optimally provided in parallel individual child and parent sessions, with additional conjoint child–parent sessions. Each component (other than parenting skills) includes interventions provided to both child and parent.

Psychoeducation

Exposure to traumatic events is common, but most families feel alone in their experiences and are afraid of what will become of the children. Psychoeducation provides information to children and parents about the nature of the traumatic experiences, such as the number of other children who experience this type of trauma, its causes, and common reactions of children and parents. Psychoeducation also includes providing information about mental health treatment for many families who have never sought such treatment before, who may believe that therapy suggests serious mental or emotional problems ("My child is crazy"; "I am a terrible parent"; "Someone will take my child away from me") or have misconceptions about what treatment entails. Normalizing children's and parents experience can reassure them that they are not alone or abnormal; providing information that treatment such as TF-CBT is "talk therapy" and is usually time limited and successful brings hope for recovery. Psychoeducation may occur throughout TF-CBT. During initial psychoeducation sessions, GE is implemented by referring to children's traumatic experiences by name (e.g., "sexual abuse"; "domestic violence"; "car accident"; "your father's death") rather than euphemism (e.g., "the bad thing that happened"). This models nonavoidance for the children and parents early in treatment. In a similar manner, children who experience sexual abuse are taught "the doctor's names" for private body parts instead of vaguely referring to them by, for example, nicknames. Domestic violence, physical abuse, bullying, and other traumas are described factually, children who witnessed traumatic death are educated about the cause of death in an age-appropriate manner without the use of euphemisms, and these words are used even with young children to help diminish avoidance and to decrease any shame that might have come to be associated with the experiences. This occurs during psychoeducation, and this information is repeated during other PRAC components. Whenever therapists refer to the children's experiences, they use the words of the children's traumatic experiences with the children and parents. Nonverbal behavior similarly conveys the importance of directly addressing the children's traumatic experiences. TF-CBT therapists are specifically trained to directly look at and face children and parents when using the words that describe the traumatic experiences, not to lower their voice tone in a way that might inadvertently convey secrecy, shame, or discomfort or to say things that suggest that talking about the traumatic experience is something that should be avoided (e.g., "This is going to be really hard to talk about. You can stop whenever you want"). Therapists are also trained to recognize their own avoidance reactions, which are often well-intentioned attempts to avoid retraumatizing the children but may instead encourage the very avoidance that the children are seeking help to address.

Parenting Skills

In the TF-CBT model, parents or other primary caretakers (hereafter referred to as "parents") are viewed as primary agents of change for children. The hour per week that most therapists spend with children is dwarfed by the amount of time parents spend with children during the course of their lives. When parents address their personal traumatic reactions and become sources of strength, support, and belief in the children's recovery, this can strongly contribute to positive child outcomes. As noted, traumatized children experience dysregulation of affect, behavior, and cognitions as well as physical dysregulation. To assist parents in recognizing and optimally addressing these symptoms, the TF-CBT parenting component addresses the children's symptoms, provides parents with interventions that parallel those the children are receiving in sessions, reinforces and practices what the children are learning in treatment, and addresses parents' emotional response to the children's trauma. Depending on whether parents experienced their children's trauma themselves (e.g., a disaster or domestic violence), they may have personal trauma symptoms. Alternatively, parents may develop vicarious trauma symptoms related to hearing about their children's experiences. The parenting skills component focuses on optimizing parents' ability to provide positive parenting to their children (e.g., enhancing the use of praise, positive attention, use of appropriate behavioral interventions for behavioral problems), decreasing parental distress related to the children's trauma, and enhancing parental support of the children and optimizing the overall child–parent relationship. Although TF-CBT is child focused, and the goal is not to address parents' personal past trauma issues, these sometimes arise when children have experienced traumas such as sexual abuse or domestic violence. In these situations, parents may require additional referrals to individual therapy for themselves. GE in the parenting component typically includes making connections between parenting or child behaviors and the children's trauma experiences. For example, a mother brought her child for treatment after the child discovered her brother's dead body on the family's front porch (he had been shot and killed the night before). During treatment, the mother complained that the child had become "a terror," sulking and screaming at her day and night. The mother said, "This is the last thing I need now." She was worried about her daughter developing behavior problems in light of the brother's gang associations, which she believed had led to his death. The mother was so frustrated she admitted that she had started screaming back at the child. The therapist took this opportunity to again talk with the mother about the impact of severe trauma on children's and adults' physiological arousal systems and to explore the symptoms they were both experiencing. The mother described that her daughter was not only screaming, sulking, and irritable but she was also compulsively checking the window and door locks and would jump when she heard loud sounds outside. The therapist suggested that the child's irritability was a symptom of PTSD hyperarousal and her extreme fear of something bad happening to her mother. The therapist also suggested that this was the most terrible experience a mother could go through and that the mother's own alarm system was probably turned up high as well, even if she didn't realize it. The mother started to cry, admitting that both she and her daughter were on edge and they needed help getting their lives back, even if they could never be normal again.

Relaxation Skills

Physiological dysregulation in traumatized children has been documented in several areas of the central and peripheral nervous system. These children also experience increased rates of medical illnesses such as asthma, allergy, headaches and gastrointestinal upset. Relaxation interventions such as focused breathing, progressive muscle relaxation, yoga, and other mind–body techniques have proven effective in reversing some of these adverse impacts in adults. Relaxation skills are also useful as distraction from upsetting and traumatic thoughts: They refocus children and parents on enjoyable activities, they encourage both to learn how to self-soothe, and they are fun. Music, dance, exercise, sports, blowing bubbles, drawing, reading, and praying, among other activities can be included as relaxation or calming techniques. Children and parents develop a relaxation plan; most include different activities for different settings. Teachers or other adults may also be included to assist children in implementing the plan in different settings. Children practice these during the week, and plans are modified each session until the children are able to self-soothe with increasing skill in diverse settings. GE is implemented in this component by helping children and parents develop a variety of relaxation strategies for different scenarios (e.g., at school, bedtime, at friends' houses) when they experience trauma reminders and to practice selecting the best strategy for different specific settings when these reminders occur.

Affective Modulation

Many traumatized children are affectively dysregulated. Some have learned that expressing any feelings is dangerous; for example, some children who have lived with chronic abuse or domestic violence may have correctly learned that protesting against what was being done to them or a parent would further endanger themselves or another family member. Such children may have learned to suppress their feelings. Others may believe that the only "safe" feeling to express is anger. For these children, the first step is to feel safe identifying and expressing feelings in therapy. A variety of techniques are used in TF-CBT to encourage expression of feelings, including the use of games, photographs of faces, drawing, and other creative interventions to encourage affective expression. After affective expression has begun, affective modulation skills are introduced to help children manage disruptive feelings. These include a variety of interpersonal and cognitive techniques, such as problem solving, negotiating, social skills, role-playing, seeking social support, thought interruption, positive imagery, ensuring safety in the moment, and others described elsewhere (Cohen et al., 2006). During their sessions, parents express their own feelings about what has happened to their children and develop personalized optimal ways of coping with them. They also learn to assist children in expressing a variety of feelings; learn to understand, tolerate, and encourage their children's expression of a range of feelings; and are assisted in expressing, their own feelings in therapy. If parents are not able to tolerate affective expression in children, this is addressed in treatment and parents are helped to assist their children with appropriate affective modulation skills. GE is implemented in this component by helping children identify and practice strategies for coping with negative affective states associated with trauma reminders.

Cognitive Coping

Once children start to master affective expression, they are taught the important affective modulation skill of cognitive coping (i.e., understanding the connection among thoughts, feelings, and behaviors). Therapists provide children and parents with examples from daily life (not traumatic experiences) in which their thoughts may not be accurate or helpful. For example, the therapist may present the following scenario, Bobby gets on the school bus, but when his friend Joey doesn't ask Bobby to sit with him, Bobby thinks to himself, "Joey doesn't like me any more." The therapist asks the child, "How would Bobby feel if this were his thought?" The child might respond, "Sad, mad, upset, or rejected." When asked, "If Bobby felt like that, how would he act?, " the child might say, "He would sit by himself, or he might not talk to Joey or he might even hit him." The therapist asks the child, "Can you think of a different thought that Bobby could tell himself, instead of that Joey doesn't like him anymore, that might explain why Joey didn't ask him to sit with him on the bus?" The child might not be able to come up with any explanation, in which case the therapist says, "What if Bobby thinks that maybe Joey's parents had a really bad argument last night and he was upset about that? Or maybe Joey has a big test today that he is worried about? If that was Bobby's thought, how would he feel?" The child says, "He might feel sorry for Joey." The therapist says, "And if he felt sorry for Joey, what would Bobby do?" The child says, "He might ask if he could sit with him, or he might just leave him alone and talk to him later. But he wouldn't be mad at Joey." The therapist then points out to the child that there is no easy way for Bobby to know what Joey was really thinking but that Bobby could change what he himself was thinking. By using examples like this from ordinary life, children and parents learn to examine their own patterns of negative thinking ("Is my thought accurate? Is it helpful? Does it make me feel better?") and to change dysfunctional thoughts both about everyday events and about the traumatic events.

Trauma Narrative and Cognitive Processing

Traumatized children are helped to develop a narrative (often, but not always, in the form of a written book) about their experiences. This occurs over several sessions, during which therapists gradually encourage children to include increasing details about "what happened" during one or more traumatic episodes. Narratives are often organized according to the temporal sequences of the children's life (e.g., Chapter 1: "who I am"; Chapter 2: "before the traumatic event started, including my relationship with the person who perpetrated the trauma; Chapter 3: "the first traumatic event"). The narrative should include "the worst time," "hot spots" (i.e., trauma reminders or triggers), and, for a final chapter, "how I have changed, what I have learned, and what I would tell other children who have gone through this." Some children who have experienced chronic trauma (e.g., those who have lived in multiple foster homes) may prefer to develop a life narrative. This can be accomplished by developing a timeline from birth to the present and filling in important dates (e.g., when the child moved from foster home to foster home, including reasons for these moves). Life narratives should include positive as well as traumatic events, in order to contextualize the children's traumatic experiences (i.e., they have had both good and bad things happen in their lives and are more than the sum of their trauma experiences).

During subsequent sessions, as children read over their trauma narratives, they include more details about what happened as well as how they were feeling, what they were thinking, and their body sensations at the time the traumatic experiences occurred. This allows therapists to identify dysfunctional cognitions that children would not necessarily share during direct questioning. Cognitive processing of the narrative includes addressing these inaccurate and unhelpful cognitions and replacing them with more optimal thoughts, which can be added to the narrative.

While the children develop the narrative, the therapists are typically sharing them with the parents during parallel parent sessions (with child consent). Typically, children are worried about parental reactions to what is being said in the narrative either because of concern about parents' emotional distress or fear that children will be blamed or otherwise get in trouble for what is revealed. It is up to the therapists to intervene in this regard: to assure children that parents are ready and able to tolerate what they are telling in their narratives. If this is not the case, the narratives should not be shared with parents. As noted, if GE has been used properly during the earlier components, developing the narrative should not be a sudden leap in exposure but rather a gradual, incremental increase from previous sessions.

In Vivo Mastery of Trauma Reminders

For children with generalized avoidance of trauma reminders (e.g., those who refuse to go to school after being physically assaulted in the school bathroom), it is first necessary to ascertain whether the feared stimulus (the school) is truly innocuous (i.e., have the perpetrators and other potential assailants been removed from the school?) If not, *in vivo* exposure would not be an appropriate intervention; working with the school, legal interventions, or safety planning would instead be pursued because the stimulus would be an appropriate cue for being vigilant to potential danger. In such a situation, desensitizing a child to danger is not warranted or appropriate. However, if the school were safe, *in vivo* desensitization would be indicated. The therapist, child, parent, and school, in this case, would collaborate to assist the child in tolerating increasingly distressing reminders (e.g., driving to the school without going in; walking into the school building for 5 minutes; staying in the building in the nurse's office for an hour; staying in the building in the nurse's office for an entire day; going to one class; going to two classes; going to class all day for one day; going to class all week). As each milestone is achieved, the child overcomes the maladaptive emotional reactions to trauma reminders and gains additional feelings of mastery, for which he or she is praised. The child uses the PRAC skills learned earlier in treatment to process and tolerate fear and identifies specific trauma cues if these occur in the course of the *in vivo* exposure. The therapist is particularly available during *in vivo* work to provide support and to develop new coping strategies if this occurs. We believe that it is particularly important to help parents and children commit to complete follow-through on the *in vivo* treatment plan: In our experience, abandoning the plan midway can serve to reinforce avoidance even more strongly. GE is of greater intensity during *in vivo* exposure than during the narrative because children are exposed to the feared trauma reminder not only imaginally but in real life.

Conjoint Child–Parent Sessions

Joint sessions can be convened at any time during TF-CBT therapy but are an integral part of treatment after children have completed trauma narrative and processing. At this point in treatment, children are ready to share their narratives with their parents, and parents are prepared to encourage, hear, and praise children for talking openly about their traumatic experiences. This is an important step in transferring remaining agency of change from therapist to parent, as families prepare to move forward together after the end of therapy. In addition to sharing the children's narratives, therapists work to optimize open family communication about the trauma and other issues such as behavior problems and issues that are difficult to talk about (e.g., dating, sex, drugs, appropriate peers). Safety planning is often done during family sessions, as described next. Children in foster care, group homes, or residential settings may ask to share their narratives with another important adult (e.g., an adult sibling, a primary child care worker, previous foster parent) who has not participated in the complete TF-CBT treatment but is still an important figure in their life. This is acceptable as long as the adult is adequately prepared for this component and confidentiality of the contents of the narrative is assured. GE is implemented in this component by sharing the children's narratives as well as through an interchange of questions about the children's traumatic experiences that often occurs between child and parent.

Enhancing Safety and Future Developmental Trajectory

Safety planning is important for children who have experienced trauma, particularly for those who may still encounter dangerous situations, such as those living with ongoing domestic or community violence. Also, because children who have suffered abuse are at high risk for revictimization, personal safety skill training is an important component of treatment. Parents and therapists carefully consider the children's developmental level and actual situation in practicing body safety skills and developing a safety plan. Care is taken to not suggest that the children could or should have done something differently in the past that might have prevented their previous victimization because this is rarely accurate. GE is implemented in this component by discussing prevention of future traumatic events.

Duration and Determining When TF-CBT Is "Finished"

As noted, TF-CBT typically lasts 8–20 sessions. It is completed when all of the components have been provided. However, many children who have experienced trauma have other problems and may need additional interventions or ongoing provision of TF-CBT components to consolidate these skills. Periodic assessment can guide determination of when TF-CBT treatment goals have been met, whether additional treatment goals that go beyond the TF-CBT model need to be established, and when treatment should be terminated. It is important to note, however, that the time-limited nature of TF-CBT may help to enhance clients' commitment to completing the treatment process.

Manuals and Other Supporting Materials

The TF-CBT manual, *Treating Trauma and Traumatic Grief in Children and Adolescents* (Cohen et al., 2006) as well as additional resources are available for implementing TF-CBT, including a free web-based training course, TF-CBT*Web*, which is available at *www.musc.edu/tfcbt*. This web-based course includes many treatment resources such as printable scripts, handouts, streaming video demonstrations, games and books used in the model, and links to other resources. Additional resources include Dutch, German, Chinese, and upcoming Korean, and Japanese translations of the treatment manual, Spanish translations of various treatment resources; year-long TF-CBT Learning Collaboratives sponsored by the National Child Traumatic Stress Network (*www.nctsn.org*); and a TF-CBT Train the Trainer program.

EVIDENCE ON THE EFFECTS OF TF-CBT TREATMENT

Table 19.1 summarizes the completed TF-CBT randomized controlled trials (RCTs). These studies provide significant evidence for the efficacy and effectiveness of TF-CBT in treating PTSD symptoms in children who have experienced sexual abuse and other traumatic events. These studies have also shown that TF-CBT reduces other symptoms, such as depression, behavior problems, shame, and abuse- or trauma-related attributions. Several TF-CBT studies have examined the potential role of mediating factors in symptom reduction. For example, Cohen and Mannarino (1998) documented that for preschool children parental emotional distress and parental support were significant predictors of children's symptoms. Another study (Cohen & Mannarino, 2000) demonstrated that children's abuse-related attributions and perceptions as well as parental support predicted treatment outcome in older sexually abused children. A third study (Deblinger, Mannarino, Cohen, & Steer, 2006) revealed that multiple-trauma history and higher levels of pretreatment depression served as moderator and mediator, respectively, of treatment outcome but only for children receiving child-centered therapy (CCT). This finding, in combination with the overall superiority of TF-CBT documented in the study, suggests that TF-CBT may be particularly preferential to CCT for children with multiple-trauma history and those with higher depressive symptoms at initial intake.

Evidence and Recommendations Regarding Dissemination and Implementation

TF-CBT has been the focus of several dissemination/implementation efforts. Four of these are described here.

TF-CBT for Children of New York Following 9/11

The Child and Adolescent Trauma Treatment and Services (CATS) Consortium was a group of nine community and university-based program funded by the Substance Abuse and Mental Health Services Administration to provide services and treatment to children affected by the terrorist attacks of September 11, 2001 (Hoagwood, 2009). This consortium was also charged with conducting research led by Columbia University. They selected TF-CBT and the University of California, Los Angeles Trauma and Grief Component Therapy (TGCT) models to provide to traumatized children and adolescents, respectively. Training and ongoing consultation calls focused on family engagement strategies, and the respective CBT treatment models were provided to 173 primarily community-based therapists, who were diverse in terms of ethnicity and theoretical orientation. A final sample of 589 youths with mild to severe trauma symptoms was largely Latino and of lower income. Participants with moderate to severe symptoms ($N = 445$) received TF-CBT or TGCT; those with less severe symptoms ($N = 112$) received only the PRAC components without creating personal trauma narratives or *in vivo* exposure components (enhanced services [ES]); and those with the least severe symptoms ($N = 32$) received treatment as usual (TAU). Regression discontinuity analyses were conducted to correct for nonrandom assignment; for these analyses, the ES and TAU groups were combined. All children experienced significant improvement in PTSD symptoms without significant differences between CBT and ES/TAU. This project demonstrated that triaging to different intensities of treatment based on initial symptom severity may work

TABLE 19.1. Summary of Completed TF-CBT Randomized Controlled Trials

Study	Target population (N = Ss starting study or treatment)	Number/length of sessions	Treatment/control (N = Ss in data analyses)	Major findings	Effect sizes between groups	Effect sizes within group
Cohen & Mannarino (1996)	Sexually abused U.S. preschool children, ages 3–6 years; N = 86	12, 1.5 hours	*TF-CBT* 39 TF-CBT 28 NST	TF-CBT superior to NST in improving PTSD, internalizing, and sexual behavior symptoms.	*Weekly Behavior Report* **Completer:** 0.57	*Weekly Behavior Report* 1.18 0.64
Deblinger, Lippmann, & Steer (1996)	Sexually abused U.S. children, 8–14 years; N = 100	12, 1.5 hours	*TF-CBT* 22 TF-CBT parent only 24 TF-CBT child only 22 TF-CBT parent + child 22 community control	TF-CBT provided to child (combined groups) significantly superior to control for improving PTSD symptoms; TF-CBT provided to parents (combined groups) significantly superior to control for improving child depression, behavior problems, and parenting skills.	*K-SADS* Parent vs. control 0.62 Child vs. control 0.85 Parent + child vs. control 0.99 Child vs. parent 0.42 Child vs. Parent + child 0.04 Parent vs. Parent + child 0.33	*K-SADS* 1.56 1.69 2.18 1.08
Cohen & Mannarino (1998)	Sexually abused U.S. children, ages 8–14 years (PTSD symptoms not required for entry); N = 82	12, 1.5 hours	*TF-CBT* 30 TF-CBT 19 NST	TF-CBT superior[a] to NST in improving depression and social competence at posttreatment and in improving PTSD and dissociation at 12-month FU among treatment completers.	*TSCC* **Completer:** 0.22	*TSCC* 0.37 0.16
King et al. (2000)	Sexually abused Australian children, ages 5–17 years; N = 36	20, 100 minutes	*TF-CBT* 12 TF-CBT child 12 TF-CBT family 12 WL	TF-CBT significantly superior to WL in improving PTSD symptoms; inclusion of family only minimally improved child outcomes.	*ADIS* Child vs. WL, 1.09 Family vs. WL, 1.24 Child vs. Family, 0.21	*ADIS* 1.58 1.86 0.63

Study	Sample	Sessions, length	Conditions	Findings	Measures	Effect sizes
Deblinger, Stauffer, & Steer (2001)	Sexually abused children, ages 2–8 years; $N = 44$	11, 1.75 hours	21 TF-CBT group 23 support group	TF-CBT produced larger effect sizes for mothers' symptoms than supportive group and greater gains in children's safety knowledge.	ST, supportive therapy; IES, impact of events scale	*IES (parent)* Intrusion CBT .81 ST .30 *Avoidance* CBT .54 ST .21
Cohen, Deblinger, Mannarino, & Steer (2004)	Sexually abused multiply traumatized U.S. children, ages 8–14 years; $N = 203$	12, 1.5 hours	*TF-CBT* 89 TF-CBT 91 CCT	TF-CBT significantly superior to CCT in improving PTSD, depressive, behavior, and shame symptoms in children, and a number of parenting problems among participating parents.	*K-SADS* 2.13 ITT: 0.61 ADIS, Anxiety Disorder Interview Schedule; TSCC, Trauma Symptom Checklist for Children	*K-SADS* 2.13 1.25
Jaycox et al. (2008)	Children exposed to Hurricane Katrina; $N = 125$	10, 1 hour	CBITS in schools TF-CBT in MH clinic	Access to CBITS superior to TF-CBT. Response to TF-CBT modestly better.	K-SADS, Kiddie Schedule for Affective Disorders and Schizophrenia	

Note. PTSD, posttraumatic stress disorder; TF-CBT, trauma-focused cognitive-behavioral therapy; NST, nonsupportive therapy; CCT, child-centered therapy; WL, wait list; CBITS, Cognitive Behavioral Interventions for Trauma in Schools; MH, mental health; ITT, intention to treat; CBT, cognitive-behavior therapy.
[a]Based on $p < .05$.

for the majority of children, because scores in both groups indicated significant improvement.

Foster Care Children in Illinois

Mental Health Services and Policy Program at Northwestern University (2008) quasi-randomly assigned children in the Illinois foster care Systems of Care (SOC) program to receive either SOC TAU or one of three evidence-based practices (EBPs). Children ages 6–12 years received SOC TAU or TF-CBT. Fidelity to the TF-CBT model was high, as documented by TF-CBT fidelity checklists. Children in all three EBPs experienced significantly less placement disruption than comparable children receiving SOC TAU. Children receiving TF-CBT also experienced significantly greater improvement in PTSD symptoms and in behavioral and emotional symptoms than comparable children receiving SOC TAU.

Web-Based Distance Learning Project

A web-based distance learning course for the TF-CBT model is available to learners who have at least a master's degree. This course, TF-CBT*Web* (*www.musc.edu/tfcbt*) was developed by the Medical University of South Carolina National Crime Victims Research and Treatment Center in collaboration with the TF-CBT developers and several community treatment centers. In its first year of public availability, 12,481 professionals registered—74.6% of master's level (social work or counseling)—and 40% completed the entire course (a very high proportion for free online learning); learners experienced significant knowledge gain in all modules of the course, and virtually all learners who completed the course expressed high levels of satisfaction (National Crime Victims Research and Treatment Center, 2007). After 4 years, the course has had more than 50,000 registrants and 21,000 completers, with the rate of registration and completion slowly increasing over time. Demand for in-person training continues to increase nationally, suggesting that there is ongoing interest in dissemination of EBT for traumatized children and that the availability of free web-based training in this model actually may be contributing to demand for increased training.

Victims of Hurricane Katrina

After Hurricane Katrina, children in three parochial schools in New Orleans participated in a study under the umbrella of Project Fleur-de-Lis (PFDL) in an attempt to develop an algorithm for assigning children to their needed level of intervention postdisaster. Among 197 consenting children in grades 4–8, 125 (63%) met PTSD screening criteria for inclusion in treatment. These children were randomly assigned to receive Cognitive Behavioral Interventions for Trauma in Schools (CBITS; Jaycox, 2003) in school-based groups or TF-CBT individually at Mercy Family Center (MFC), the community clinic overseeing the direction of PFDL. Access to treatment was a significant issue, with school-based CBITS treatment providing significantly superior access to treatment: Of 62 children randomized to receive CBITS, 98% attended the initial treatment session at school, whereas only 37% of children randomized to receive TF-CBT attended an initial TF-CBT assessment session; distance from both home and school to MFC significantly predicted TF-CBT attendance. Improvement in terms of likely PTSD diagnosis was significant among children receiving TF-CBT ($p = .05$) but not those receiving CBITS ($p = .24$). Predictors of ongoing PTSD symptoms among CBITS completers included higher pretreatment PTSD or depressive scores or new trauma exposure during treatment. Thus, both treatments had benefits, with CBITS providing more access to treatment and TF-CBT having greater effectiveness for some children. School-based provision of both treatments may be optimal for future disaster programming.

SUMMARY OF PROGRESS AND DIRECTIONS FOR RESEARCH

TF-CBT has been highly successful in treating diverse samples of traumatized children, with 80–90% remission rates of PTSD diagnosis in some studies. These results compare favorably to outcomes for other child mental health problems. However, many challenges remain. Little work has been done in developing adaptive treatment strategies, that is, adapting TF-CBT for the needs of individual children. Results from the CATS Project suggest that not all children with PTSD symptoms need the entire TF-CBT model; we need better information about which children need which components and how to predict this at the start of treatment. For example, are there factors other than low initial PTSD score that identify children who might recover with less intensive interventions (e.g., only PRAC components, CBITS)? If so, what are they?

Other issues that have not yet been explored pertain to the optimal timing of treatment for traumatized children. Although natural recovery occurs, many children continue to suffer without intervention. For these children, earlier intervention is probably better than waiting for symptoms to become entrenched, but no studies have confirmed this. The issue of optimal timing of interventions is especially critical in the case of large-scale community disasters. No well-designed treatment studies have been conducted in the acute aftermath of disasters because of the many challenges inherent in obtaining institutional review board (IRB) approval and funding to conduct such studies. Data from Hurricane Katrina challenge the presumption that natural recovery is the norm; substantial proportions of children were found to have significant trauma symptoms, many apparently from retriggering of past traumatic experiences. This suggests that there is a pressing need to proactively prepare for, fund, and provide mechanisms for IRB approval before disasters to conduct acute intervention research for children afterward.

Other areas that we need to explore further include how to ensure that TF-CBT fidelity is maintained when dissemination occurs, how organizational readiness is optimally developed before dissemination begins, how to optimally prepare supervisors of therapists delivering TF-CBT when front-line therapists provide more treatment than supervisors and thus gain competency in the model more quickly than supervisors, and whether it is feasible to train students in TF-CBT so that, rather than disseminating it to practitioners who have learned other treatment models, TF-CBT could become a standard model of intervention for a new generation of therapists. All of these are fertile areas for future dissemination research.

The more evidence accumulates about the potentially severe and long-term consequences of childhood trauma, the more crucial it becomes for us to learn what works best for which traumatized child and how to get effective treatments into the hands of the therapists who see these children. In 12 years, we have gone from having no published RCTs to TF-CBT becoming an established EBT for treating traumatized children, with more treatment models (e.g., CBITS, child–parent psychotherapy) accumulating increasing evidence of efficacy. We have come a long way in a short time, but many questions remain.

Our future goals include evaluating comparative models of disseminating TF-CBT. For example, is live training and phone consultation superior to web-based training and web-based consultation? Another goal will be to more thoroughly evaluate stepped-care treatment in collaboration with our CBITS partners and develop and evaluate adaptive treatment strategies for TF-CBT. For example, we have some hypotheses about which children may only need the skills-based components of TF-CBT or may need greater focus on parenting skills and less focus on the trauma narrative. We will design studies to test these hypotheses so that more individualized adaptations of TF-CBT can be applied for specific children. TF-CBT is already being evaluated cross-culturally in Zambia, Germany, the Netherlands, and Norway; pilot work is beginning in Cambodia, and we hope to continue facilitating cross-cultural evaluation of TF-CBT. A new project has just been funded to develop infrastructure for training social work students in TF-CBT during graduate school. We hope to examine the effectiveness of introducing TF-CBT and other evidence-based treatments during graduate training through this and subsequent projects.

We feel very fortunate be in our current position when only several years ago no empirical treatment studies had been published for traumatized children. Our consistent goal is to help children transcend trauma.

REFERENCES

Cohen, J. A., Deblinger, E., Mannarino, A. P., & Steer, R. (2004). A multisite, randomized controlled trial for children with sexual abuse-related PTSD symptoms. *Journal of the American Academy of Child and Adolescent Psychiatry, 43*, 393–402.

Cohen, J. A., & Mannarino, A. P. (1996). A treatment study for sexually abused preschool children: Initial treatment and outcome findings. *Journal of the American Academy of Child and Adolescent Psychiatry, 35*, 42–50.

Cohen, J. A., & Mannarino, A. P. (1998). Factors that mediate treatment outcome of sexually abused preschool children: Six- and 12-month follow-up. *Journal of the American Academy of Child and Adolescent Psychiatry, 37*, 44–51.

Cohen, J. A., & Mannarino, A. P. (2000). Predictors of treatment outcome in sexually abused children. *Child Abuse and Neglect, 24*, 983–994.

Cohen, J. A., Mannarino, A. P., & Deblinger, E. (2006). *Treating trauma and traumatic grief in children and adolescents.* New York: Guilford Press.

Deblinger, E., & Heflin, A. H. (1996). *Treating sexually abused children and their nonoffending parents: A cognitive behavioral approach.* Thousand Oaks, CA: Sage.

Deblinger, E., Lippmann, J., & Steer, R. (1996). Sexually abused children suffering posttraumatic stress symptoms: Initial treatment outcome findings. *Child Maltreatment, 1*, 310–321.

Deblinger, E., Mannarino, A. P., Cohen, J. A., & Steer, R. (2006). A follow-up study of a multi-site, randomized controlled trial for children with sexual abuse-related PTSD symptoms: Examining predictors of treatment response. *Journal of the American Academy of Child and Adolescent Psychiatry, 45*, 1474–1484.

Deblinger, E., Stauffer, L., & Steer, R. (2001). Comparative efficacies of supportive and cognitive behavioral group therapies for children who were sexually abused and their nonoffending mothers. *Child Maltreatment, 6,* 332–343.

Foa, E. B., & Rothbaum, B. O. (1998). *Treating the trauma of rape: Cognitive behavioral therapy for post-traumatic stress disorder.* New York: Guilford Press.

Hoagwood, K. E., & the CATS Consortium. (2009). *Impact of CBT for traumatized children and adolescents affected by the World Trade Center disaster.* Unpublished manuscript, Columbia University.

Jaycox, L. H. (2003). *Cognitive behavioral interventions for trauma in schools.* Longmont, CO: Sopris Press.

Jaycox, L. H., Cohen, J. A., Mannarino, A. P., Walker, D. W., Langley, A. K., Gegenheimer, K. L., et al. (2008). *Children's mental health care following Hurricane Katrina within a randomized field trial of trauma-focused psychotherapies.* Manuscript submitted for publication.

King, N. J., Tonge, B. J., Mullen, P., Myerson, N., Heyne, D., Rollings, S., et al. (2000). Treating sexually abused children with posttraumatic stress symptoms: A randomized clinical trial. *Journal of the American Academy of Child and Adolescent Psychiatry, 39,* 1347–1355.

Mental Health Services and Policy Program, Northwestern University. (2008). *Evaluation of the implementation of three evidence based practices to address trauma for children and youth who are wards of the state of Illinois.* Unpublished manuscript.

National Crime Victims Research and Treatment Center. (2007). *TF-CBTWeb first year report.* Charleston: Medical University of South Carolina. Available from *www.musc.edu/cvc.*

20

Early and Intensive Behavioral Intervention in Autism

TRISTRAM SMITH

OVERVIEW OF THE CLINICAL PROBLEM

Children are diagnosed with autism on the basis of difficulties with reciprocal social interaction, verbal and nonverbal communication, and repetitive or ritualistic behavior. These difficulties usually emerge by 3 years of age and are almost always lifelong without early intervention. The severity of impairments varies greatly among children. Some are so socially isolated that they appear almost completely unaware of others. However, others are clearly attached to caregivers and eager to interact with peers, although they may have poor eye contact and lack appropriate conversational and social skills. Similarly, whereas some children with autism have essentially no verbal or nonverbal language, others speak quite well, although most of what they say may involve reciting scripts from favorite movies, stating requests, or delivering monologues on topics that preoccupy them. They tend to have limited imagination and creative play, instead engaging in repetitive or restricted activities. For some children with autism, these activities involve motor movements such as flapping their hands in front of their eyes or actions with objects such as arranging toys into neat rows or sifting sand. For others, the activities follow an elaborate sequence such as insisting on adhering to an elaborate routine or developing a fascination with an extremely circumscribed area of interest. Many children with autism (but not all) have delays in cognitive development and adaptive skills. Some exhibit challenging behaviors such as tantrums, aggression, self-injury, or overactivity. Many also are either under- or overresponsive to sensory stimuli such as sights or sounds.

The *Diagnostic and Statistical Manual of Mental Disorders* (Fourth edition, text revision [DSM-IV-TR]; American Psychiatric Association, 2000), includes two diagnostic classifications that overlap extensively with autism: (1) Asperger's disorder, which is defined by high rates of autistic behaviors in individuals who do not have a history of delays in cognitive or language development, and (2) pervasive developmental disorder not otherwise specified (PDD-NOS), which is characterized by autistic behaviors that do not meet criteria for autism or Asperger's disorder. In the DSM-IV-TR, autism, Asperger's disorder, and PDD-NOS are all grouped into the category of pervasive developmental disorders. However, a popular alternative term is autism spectrum disorder (ASD), which reflects the view that the three diagnostic classifications may reflect different variants of the same disorder rather than separate conditions. Some studies suggest that, although the intervention model described in this chapter was developed primarily for children with autism, it may also be beneficial for children with PDD-NOS (Smith, Groen, & Wynn, 2000), and some components of the model may be applicable to children with Asperger's disorder (Smith, McAdam, & Napolitano, 2007).

APPLIED BEHAVIOR ANALYSIS AND EARLY INTENSIVE BEHAVIORAL INTERVENTION

Early intensive behavioral intervention (EIBI) begins when children are 4 years or younger, involves 20–40 hours per week of individualized applied behavior analysis (ABA) instruction, and continues for 2 or more years. EIBI is based on ABA, which is a discipline devoted to using principles of learning theory to address socially important problems. Although this chapter focuses on ABA for children with autism, ABA is also used with a variety of other populations in numerous clinical and nonclinical settings (Smith, McAdam, et al., 2007).

The first ABA studies of children with autism took place in the early 1960s, when investigators successfully used operant conditioning to teach simple behaviors such as pulling levers. Although this teaching had no therapeutic benefit, it demonstrated that children with autism could learn in a manner like that of other individuals. Soon investigators discovered that they could also use operant conditioning to teach important skills such as communication and regulation of aggression. Despite many successes in the first generation of ABA interventions, long-term outcomes were disappointing, even heartbreaking (Smith, McAdam, et al., 2007). Intervention gains did not lead to improvements in other skills and failed to transfer to environments outside the treatment setting and to maintain over time. Indeed, many children regressed to pretreatment levels of functioning.

In an effort to improve outcomes, investigators increasingly emphasized implementing interventions in the children's everyday environments instead of in clinical settings, involving parents and peers as change agents in the natural environment, and developing ways to embed instruction into everyday activities rather than in separate therapy sessions. They also focused increasingly on early intervention. From an ABA perspective, it is likely that individuals—children and adults—with autism have the potential to learn from ABA interventions. However, the greatest impact is likely to occur during the toddler and preschool years, because these children have not fallen as far behind or become as set in their ways as older children with autism. Even in young children, however, the intervention may need to be very intensive to match the learning opportunities available to typically developing children. Typically developing children learn from their everyday environment all of their waking hours—7 days a week, 365 days a year—by exploring, playing with peers, modeling, conversing, and so on. Unfortunately, children with autism have little skill or inclination to learn in this manner. Thus, a mismatch arises between these children and environments tailored to typically developing children, with the result that children with autism fail to learn except when their environment is redesigned. These considerations led some behavior analytic investigators, notably O. Ivar Lovaas and his colleagues at the University of California, Los Angeles (UCLA) Young Autism Project, to focus on EIBI.

CHARACTERISTICS OF THE UCLA MODEL OF EIBI

Intervention in the UCLA model is intended to optimize children's functioning in all areas of development. Most studies have enrolled children with autism who are 3 years or younger at intake. In clinical practice, some 4- to 5-year-old children are also enrolled. Most studies also have excluded children with severe global delays such as IQ in the range of severe to profound mental retardation, but clinically such children may be enrolled on a trial basis, with reevaluations every 3–6 months to determine whether they are progressing. Children are unlikely to be offered enrollment if they have medical problems that would preclude full participation in treatment, such as physical disabilities or uncontrolled seizures.

For most children with autism who receive the UCLA intervention, 40 hours per week of one-to-one intervention is recommended. However, fewer hours may be appropriate for (1) children younger than 3, who may start with only 20 hours per week; (2) children near the end of treatment, for whom the number of treatment hours is gradually reduced; and (3) children for whom 40 hours per week is contraindicated for other reasons, such as a history of slow progress with this level of intensity. Treatment usually lasts approximately 3 years, although the precise length is determined on a case-by-case basis.

Intervention in the UCLA model is intended to maximize children's success and prevent failure. Because of their mismatch with the environment, children with autism have already encountered continual frustration in learning situations by the time they begin the intervention. Understandably, many react to such situations with tantrums and other attempts to escape or avoid future failures. During the first year of treatment, intervention takes place mainly in the child's home, and discrete trial training (DTT) is the main intervention procedure. DTT is a highly structured teaching procedure characterized by (1) one-to-one interaction between the practitioner and the child in a distraction-free environment, (2) clear and concise instructions from the practitioner, (3) highly specific procedures for prompting and fading, and (4) immediate reinforcement such as praise or a preferred toy for correct responding.

DTT has the advantage of giving a simplified and predictable structure to the learning situation and creating a large number of learning opportunities (as many as 12 per minute). As children progress, therapists gradually decrease the use of this format and increase their emphasis on naturalistic instruction, similar to those described in the next chapter on pivotal response treatment (PRT). Much of this instruction takes place in group settings outside the home such as classrooms. To maintain children's motivation, sessions include frequent opportunities for successes and a diverse set of instructional programs that focus on skills such as communication, academic skills, self-help, play, and motor activities.

Service Providers

In the UCLA model, there are four levels of service providers: paraprofessionals, team leaders, case supervisors, and project directors. Paraprofessionals implement most of the one-to-one ABA intervention. They are usually either paid staff or undergraduate college students who receive course credit. Before working with children with autism, they complete a college-level course or a 3- to 5-day ABA training workshop. New paraprofessionals work alongside experienced team members for about 25 hours, until observations by senior personnel indicate they are able to conduct sessions themselves. Intervention teams of approximately three to five paraprofessionals are assigned to each child, with every student therapist working a minimum of 5 hours a week. Additionally, each paraprofessional must attend a weekly 1-hour clinic meeting with the child, parents, team leader, and case supervisor.

After a minimum of 6 months, paraprofessionals who excel are eligible to become team leaders. Team leaders continue to provide one-to-one intervention. They also oversee two to four teams and work closely with the case supervisor. Case supervisors are selected from the group of team leaders. Criteria for selection include (1) accumulating a minimum of 1,500 supervised hours of treatment experience, (2) being highly rated by families and student therapists, and (3) passing objective tests of their skill at implementing instructional programs, identifying which skills to teach next, and critiquing others' therapy (Davis, Smith, & Donahoe, 2002). Many case supervisors are board-certified behavior analysts, who have obtained a master's or doctoral degree in ABA or a related profession (e.g., psychology or education with extensive course work in ABA), completed a supervised ABA internship, passed a national written examination, and met requirements for continuing education. Project directors are typically doctoral-level personnel who are licensed in a mental health profession (usually psychology), have postgraduate training in ABA, and have many years of experience implementing the UCLA model. Project directors have daily contact with all case supervisors as well as weekly contact with all other treatment personnel, clients, and families.

Supervisors and project directors meet weekly with each child along with parents, paraprofessionals, and the team leader to review the child's progress. They inspect the child's log book, which contains data on skill acquisition, and ask student therapists to demonstrate programs during the meeting to make sure that all team members are clear on treatment procedures and receive feedback regarding their performance. They also answer questions from parents and the team. On the basis of information obtained during this meeting, they modify the intervention (e.g., introduce new instructional programs when the child has mastered existing ones, alter and assess the format of instructional programs when the child's progress is slow).

Family Participation

Parents are an integral part of their children's intervention teams. Before enrolling their children into the project, they have a 1- to 2-hour intake interview with the project director. In this interview, the project director becomes acquainted with families, confirms information from outside agencies on children's medical and developmental history, and encourages questions from parents. Parents also have the opportunity to receive publications on the UCLA model, view videotapes of intervention, and schedule a time to accompany a case supervisor to observe another child's treatment program, with written permission from that child's parents. The parents then review an informed consent form, which outlines the UCLA model, the parents' role, and the range of outcomes that children achieve after treatment (some making substantial progress but others deriving little or no benefit). In addition to exchanging information, the intake interview affords an opportunity to address the anxiety and stress that parents invariably express about their children's condition. The project director attempts to identify the specific concerns that the parents raise, express empathy and support, and describe how the intervention may help. The director also emphasizes that parents' active participation in treatment is likely to contribute to the children's progress and ease their own stress.

Throughout the intervention, parents attend all team meetings and approve all intervention procedures in advance. Also, for the first 3–4 months of treatment, parents are asked to work alongside an experienced team member for 5 hours per week. During this time, therapists and parents take turns implementing the children's DTT programs and give each other feedback on their work. Thus, parents learn to become effective therapists for their children and make informed decisions about the treatment. Subsequently, many parents reduce their involvement in intervention sessions but continue to generalize and expand skills that children acquire in intervention. For example, they implement incidental teaching procedures to encourage their children to use communication skills in everyday settings, incorporate self-help skills into children's daily routines, and arrange activities that promote further skill development such as outings where children can learn new names for objects or events. Parents also recruit their children's peers to participate in playdates and often oversee the playdates. In addition, they contact school districts about placements for their children, visit the placements that are offered (often accompanied by their case supervisor), and communicate with teachers about children's progress in those and future placements.

Stages of Treatment

Large individual differences exist in children's rate of progress. Nevertheless, the intervention, summarized in Table 20.1, generally follows a predictable sequence. Children who demonstrate mastery of skills that are emphasized in the early stages of the intervention can begin at a more advanced stage.

Stage 1: Establishing a Teaching Relationship

The intervention team aims to schedule the first parent–team meeting as soon as possible after the intake interview. Intervention begins during this meeting. The first hour of intervention tends to be the most upsetting for the child, parents, and team. As noted, many children have already learned to escape or avoid learning situations, often by resorting to intense tantrums that include screaming, crying, hitting team members, and attempting to run away. To address this problem and to optimize the child's success, the team selects one action that the child is likely to perform successfully (e.g., putting a block in a bucket or sitting down in a chair) and request this action. By prompting and reinforcing successful completion while withholding reinforcement for escape or avoid-

TABLE 20.1. Treatment Stages in the UCLA Young Autism Project, with Teaching Formats and Examples of Goals at Each Stage

Stage 1: Establishing a teaching relationship	Stage 2: Teaching foundational skills	Stage 3: Beginning communication	Stage 4: Expanding communication and beginning peer interaction	Stage 5: Advanced communication, adjusting to school
Teaching format: primarily discrete trial training (DTT)	*Teaching format:* primarily DTT	*Teaching formats:* DTT, incidental teaching	*Teaching formats:* DTT, incidental teaching, dyads with typical peers	*Teaching formats:* DTT, incidental teaching, small group, general education preschool
Goals: following one-step directions such as "Sit" or "Come here," reducing interfering behaviors such as tantrums	*Goals:* discriminating between one-step directions, imitating gross motor actions, matching, receptively identifying objects, dressing, beginning play with toys	*Goals:* imitating speech sounds, expressively labeling objects, receptively identifying actions and pictures, expanding self-help and play skills, starting visual communication for children who are slow to acquire speech (picture communication systems or reading and writing)	*Goals:* labeling colors and shapes, beginning language concepts such as big–little and yes–no, recognizing emotions, beginning sentences such as "I want _____" and "I see _____," beginning pretend play and peer interaction, toilet training, entering preschool	*Goals:* using language concepts such as prepositions, pronouns, and past tense; conversing with peers and adults; describing objects and events; comprehending stories; understanding perspective of others; learning from models; participating in groups; working independently; helping with chores

ance behavior, team members increase the child's attentiveness and motivation in the teaching situation while reducing tantrums. The project member explains this process. Then each team member and parent takes a turn requesting the action selected by the team. The project director and case supervisor, who have considerable experience starting treatment, are the first to work with the child. They stay in the meeting throughout the first hour to demonstrate how to implement procedures accurately, point out signs of improvement such as reduced tantrums or increased rates of correct responding, and reassure the team and family that the child is being successful. The first meeting for Shawn, age 2 years 10 months, illustrates how the meeting usually proceeds:

After briefly discussing the plan, the project director went to Shawn and led him by the hand to a set of two toddler-size chairs and a small table. To minimize distractions, the table was bare except for the block and bucket, and Shawn's chair was facing a blank wall. The project director guided Shawn into the chair by nudging him on the shoulders. She then sat facing Shawn and leaned forward so that she was at eye level. The table was placed to Shawn's right (the project director's left). The project director immediately picked up the block, dropped it in the bucket with a clink, handed it to Shawn, and provided hand-over-hand guidance for Shawn to drop the block into the bucket. Shawn screamed, but the block did go in the bucket, whereupon the project director exclaimed,

"Wonderful!," gave him a hug, and placed a small chip in Shawn's hand. This was the end of the first learning trial.

After pausing briefly to let Shawn eat the chip, the project director started a new trial. The trial followed the same format except that the project director changed the reinforcement, saying "Magnificent" and playfully tickling Shawn. Over the next three trials (again following the same format but varying the reinforcement), Shawn successfully put the block in the bucket with guidance from the project director, although he was still screaming. Over the subsequent three trials, Shawn's screaming subsided, and he accurately placed the block in the bucket even when guided only part of the way. The project director announced, "All done," and nudged Shawn on the back of the shoulder to get up. Shawn jumped into his mother's lap and smiled. The whole session lasted about 1 minute.

Shawn was given a break for about 3 minutes, and then the case supervisor ran a session with him, again focusing on teaching Shawn to put the block in the bucket. After another break, the team leader worked with him on "block in the bucket." Already, Shawn was responding correctly without physical guidance, and he often smiled and laughed when his correct responses were reinforced. Each paraprofessional took a turn teaching "block in the bucket," with breaks between each session. Occasionally, Shawn's screaming resumed, and he responded incorrectly on some trials, flipping the block back and forth in his hand instead of releasing it into the bucket. The paraprofessional corrected these responses by saying "No" in a neutral tone of voice, removing the block momentarily, and starting another trial. If he was incorrect on the next trial, the paraprofessional reintroduced hand-over-hand guidance on the following trial and then faded out this assistance on subsequent trials. After the paraprofessionals took their turns, each parent ran a session of "block in the bucket." In the remaining time, the project director and case supervisor worked with Shawn and identified three other requests to teach over the upcoming week: "Come here," "Stand up," and "Do puzzle."

Toward the end of the hour, Shawn, like almost all other children who enter the UCLA program, had made clear progress that was apparent to everyone present and seemed to enjoy the sessions. Team members went to Shawn's home that same day to help transfer his progress by continuing to request the same actions in that setting. Over the next 2–4 weeks, they slowly added other requests that Shawn could also carry out successfully. Each new request was selected in a team meeting, and instruction began in that meeting. At this stage, choosing requests that increased Shawn's skill level was not as important as choosing ones that would help him develop trust in the team members and bolster the parents' confidence that their child can learn.

Stage 2: Teaching Foundational Skills

Once the child has become responsive to the learning situation, the intervention moves to new and more challenging programs that will provide a foundation for learning complex behaviors. At this stage, which usually lasts 1 to 4 months, one focus is on receptive language skills (i.e., responding correctly to what others say) such as sitting down in a chair upon request. Another is on imitation of actions such as putting arms out to the side, touching the head, or stomping feet. Mastery of a dozen or so gross motor actions is followed by imitation of fine motor actions such as facial expressions. An additional focus is on matching and sorting. Although many children with autism already have some matching skills, such as completing inset puzzles, when they enter treatment, extending these skills (e.g., teaching the child to match increasingly complex pictures and three-dimensional objects) helps the child attend to a variety of instructional materials and may facilitate language instruction. Teaching self-care skills such as dressing also begins at this stage. In addition, play skills are introduced such as rolling a car back and forth, rocking a doll, inserting shapes into a shape sorter, rolling a ball, and scribbling with markers. Instructors administer three to eight discrete trials in a sitting, for about 50 minutes of every hour, with the remaining 10 minutes devoted to activities to encourage generalization of skills to everyday settings in the home.

Instruction proceeds in small steps. For example, in teaching early receptive language such as "Come here," the child initially receives a prompt such as a gentle nudge on the back to carry out the instruction and travels only a couple of feet to the adult. As the child progresses, the prompt is gradually reduced so that the child is responding to the verbal request by itself, and the distance to travel increases. To facilitate generalization, the child practices this skill with each team member and parent in multiple settings (e.g., at home, at the clinic). Once the child masters an instruction, team members introduce new instructions one at a time and teach the child to discriminate between them (e.g., coming when the paraprofessional says "Come here" but not when the paraprofessional says "Wave" or selecting the toy named by the paraprofessional out of a group of toys that are on a table). To provide this teaching, team members must be familiar with empirically validated approaches to discriminating training such as procedures for giving instructions, prompting the child to respond correctly, fading prompts, randomizing presentation of instructions, and reinforcing correct behaviors. Learning to discriminate is vital for children because it indicates that they are truly attending to and differentiating among instructions.

Stage 3: Beginning Communication

In this stage, which lasts 6 months or longer, children continue to receive instruction in receptive language, imitation, and matching. They also learn new self-care skills such as toileting, and they expand their play skills. Further, they begin working on expressive language. Team members begin by teaching the child first to imitate speech sounds, then separate words, and finally strings of words. They then use verbal imitation to prompt expressive labeling of objects and events (e.g., the paraprofessional holds up an object such as a ball and says "What is it? Ball").

Although most children complete stages 1 and 2 within the first 5 months of intervention (or sooner), many get stuck at stage 3. Only about half the children in the UCLA program master imitation of speech sounds within the first few months of treatment. This mastery is an important predictor of eventual outcome (Sallows & Graupner, 2005; Smith et al., 2000). Although some children who quickly master verbal imitation encounter difficulties in later stages of the program, many others continue to make rapid progress and achieve favorable outcomes such as IQ in the average range and successful functioning in regular education classes. Those who do not acquire verbal imitation can still learn other skills in treatment but are unlikely to have such favorable outcomes and usually require alternative communication systems such as selecting pictures to indicate what they want.

Stage 4: Expanding Communication and Beginning Peer Interaction

When the child can receptively and expressively identify simple everyday objects and behaviors, the program moves to abstract concepts and grammatically correct sentences (see Table 20.1). Also, children enter a preschool for typically developing children. Although we recognize that many will eventually go into special education classes (as discussed in stage 6), the UCLA model emphasizes general education classes at this stage because research indicates that these classes provide more appropriate peer models and higher academic expectations (Smith, Lovaas, & Lovaas, 2002). Team members help prepare them at home by teaching pretend play skills, age-appropriate games such as "Ring Around the Rosie," songs such as "Wheels on the Bus," and other group activities such as circle time. A paraprofessional accompanies the child to school to facilitate transfer of skills from home to school. Ideally, the paraprofessional is part of the team that is implementing the UCLA model. In practice, however, this individual may be a school employee with little prior experience in ABA, in which case we will seek to collaborate with the school to provide training and ongoing support. At first, classroom time may be as little as 5–10 minutes per day so that the child can be successful and not perceived by the teachers and peers as having a disability. The time is then gradually lengthened to a half-hour and then longer until the child stays for the full preschool session. Regular communication is established among the child's teacher, parents, and ABA team members in order to coordinate efforts across settings. The teacher also may be asked to put the parents in contact with parents of other children to arrange playdates in the child's home and neighborhood.

Stage 5: Advanced Communication, Adjusting to School

At the beginning of this stage, children's time is divided about equally into individual instruction and participation in group settings. Subsequently, time in individual instruction is gradually decreased as time in group settings increases. Team members teach advanced language concepts and preacademic skills, as shown in Table 20.1. Moreover, they provide extensive instruction in social skills such as playing board games, engaging in sociodramatic play with peers, talking about play activities, conversing, making appropriate requests for assistance, and following school rules (e.g., raising hands). They also help children read facial expressions, nonverbal cues, and nonliteral meanings of what people say. They encourage children to problem solve in social situations (e.g., figuring out what to do if they and another child want to play with the same toy). In addition, they aim to teach children to complete academic and self-care tasks independently, without adult prompts. Even at this stage, most children in the UCLA program still learn new skills best by receiving one-to-one instruction and then transferring the skills to other settings. Therefore, a key goal is to increase their ability to learn in everyday situations at home and school. Accordingly, therapists help children respond more to the classroom teacher and peers and less to the aide. They teach observational learning so that the children can learn by modeling peers in group settings. They also prompt and reinforce active engagement in group activities. In addition, they teach children to complete academic assignments, self-care tasks, and activities in the school routine with little direct supervision. As children become less reliant on the paraprofessional, the paraprofessional gradually fades out. For example, the paraprofessional may be assigned partly to the child with autism and partly to classmates or may attend only part time.

Stage 6: Termination of the Intervention

Intervention ends as children enter elementary school. At age 5, children proceed from preschool to a kindergarten class for typically developing children if they display most of the skills that their classmates do and are ready to begin phasing out the paraprofessional. Otherwise, they repeat preschool in order to be with peers closer to their developmental level, have additional time to adjust to the school setting, and continue receiving one-to-one instruction at home. This extra year enables some children to catch up to typically developing children who are entering kindergarten, as evidenced by skills such as engaging in extensive sociodramatic play, cooperating in small groups, and speaking in complex sentences.

If, after repeating preschool and kindergarten, children continue to be delayed relative to their classmates, our research indicates that they will likely need ongoing special services throughout their lives (McEachin, Smith, & Lovaas, 1993). Therefore, the project director and case supervisor evaluate alternative placement options, seeking those in which (1) teachers are willing to collaborate with the EIBI team (most are quite willing, but a few are not), (2) peers model appropriate, adaptive skills for the children with autism, and (3) the class has a clear structure and rules. Potential placements include behavioral classrooms for children with autism, other special education classes, or classes with typically developing children where children with autism receive assistance from an aide. In any of these placements, it is often important to supplement classroom instruction with one-to-one DTT (10 hours/week or more if parents are involved in treatment), because children may still learn most efficiently in this format. Team members from the home program assist in the transition to these placements.

Because of all the complex issues associated with identifying appropriate placements for children who continue to have special needs, such children may be at greater risk for losing skills, developing new maladaptive behaviors, and other difficulties than children who are fully integrated into regular classes. Therefore, project directors discuss this risk with parents and service providers, and they are available for periodic follow-up consultations, as needed. Apart from these consultations, services in the UCLA model for children with special needs usually stop during first grade but sometimes continue for another year in an effort to enhance skill retention and adjustment to school.

EVIDENCE ON THE EFFECTS OF EIBI

In an influential study, Lovaas (1987) compared three groups of children with autism who received 2 or more years of treatment beginning at the age of 2 or 3 years. One group of 19 children received 40 hours of EIBI per week. The other two groups, which included 40 children with autism, either received a less intensive ABA intervention or were served by community agencies independently of Lovaas's project. Assignment was based on whether or not Lovaas's clinic had openings for EIBI services. At follow-up evaluations conducted at ages 7 and 13 years, the EIBI group showed significant improvement relative to the two other groups in educational placement and IQ (McEachin et al.,

1993). Almost half of the children in the intensive group achieved unassisted placements in general education classes and IQs in the average range.

Some investigators hailed the findings of Lovaas's (1987) original EIBI study as a breakthrough and identified a number of strengths in the research design, including groups that appeared well matched on most intake variables, use of an intervention manual, and outcome evaluations conducted by an examiner blind to group assignment. However, others pointed out possible flaws, notably nonrandom assignment to groups, use of different IQ measures at intake and follow-up, failure to measure potentially important outcomes such as changes in behaviors associated with ASD, and impracticality of implementing aspects of the intervention in community settings (e.g., 40 hours of intervention per week). Lovaas and colleagues disputed these critiques but concurred that replications with improved methodological design were required (Smith, McAdam, et al., 2007).

In subsequent studies, investigators have modified Lovaas's original model in some ways. For example, Lovaas (1987) used some intervention procedures that are unacceptable by today's standards, notably contingent aversives such as a slap on the thigh for behavior problems that were severe and unresponsive to other procedures. Shortly thereafter, however, he and his colleagues concluded that a variety of evidence-based alternatives to aversive procedures had become available, and they stopped using such methods (Smith et al., 2000). The intervention manual for the UCLA project was revised (Lovaas, 2003) to include new and more detailed procedures for teaching skills to children with autism. Procedures were also added by Cohen, Amerine-Dickens, and Smith (2006) and Sallows and Graupner (2005) for teaching other advanced social skills, such as taking the perspective of other people. These investigators also adapted the UCLA model for use in community agencies (as opposed to university settings). Although intervention in the UCLA model is usually implemented in the child's home for the first year or more, Eikeseth, Smith, Eldevik, and Jahr (2007) altered the model to administer it entirely in school settings.

Following Lovaas's (1987) study, subsequent studies on the UCLA model have included two randomized clinical trials (RCTs; Sallows & Graupner, 2005; Smith et al., 2000) and three quasi-experimental studies (Cohen et al., 2006; Eikeseth et al., 2007; Smith et al., 1997). Sallows and Graupner's (2005) RCT compared EIBI directed by clinic personnel with EIBI directed by parents. (State funding was available for parents to hire and supervise paraprofessionals.) Children were younger than 42 months at intake and were assessed yearly on a standardized assessment protocol for 4 years. There were few differences between the clinic-directed and the parent-directed groups; both made gains from pre- to postintervention that were comparable to those in the study by Lovaas (1987). For example, 11 of 23 participants (48%) achieved average IQs and unassisted placement in general education at follow-up, similar to the rate of 47% reported by Lovaas (1987). Gains were also reported on measures of adaptive behavior, language, and autism severity. The use of random assignment, a standardized assessment protocol, and multiple outcome measures addressed three of the major criticisms of Lovaas's (1987) study. However, because both groups in the study received EIBI, it did not provide information on outcomes that participants would have attained without EIBI.

The other RCT (Smith et al., 2000) compared 25 hours of EIBI per week with in-home parent training on ABA techniques. Children were younger than 42 months at intake and were followed up at age 7–8 years. At follow-up, the mean IQ for the EIBI group was 16 points higher than that of the control group. The EIBI group also had a higher rate of unassisted placement in general education (four of 15 children vs. none of 13 in the comparison group). These differences were statistically significant but were only about half the size of the effects reported by Lovaas (1987). The EIBI group also obtained higher scores than the control group on measures of nonverbal skills and academic achievement, although the groups did not differ significantly on measures of adaptive behavior, language, and level of behavior problems. Thus, the EIBI group made substantial gains relative to the comparison group on some measures, but the gains were more modest and circumscribed than in the Lovaas (1987) study, possibly because the participants were lower functioning at intake, received fewer treatment hours, and were compared with another group that received ABA intervention. By incorporating random assignment, a standardized assessment protocol, multiple outcome measures, and a comparison group who did not receive EIBI, Smith et al.'s (2000) study may have had the strongest methodology of any published EIBI study thus far.

The three quasi-experiments based on the UCLA model (Cohen et al., 2006; Eikeseth et al., 2007; Smith et al., 1997) also yielded positive results for measures of IQ. Cohen et al. (2006) and Eikeseth et al. (2007) also reported gains in adaptive behavior, but this variable was not assessed in the study by Smith, Eikeseth, Klevstrand, and Lovaas (1997). In addition, Cohen et al. (2006) also found that children in the EIBI group were more likely than control children to have unassisted placements in general education, although Eikeseth et al. (2007) and Smith et al. (1997) did not obtain this result. These studies are noteworthy because they extended the UCLA model in various respects. Cohen et al. (2006) provided intervention in a community agency rather than a university setting. Smith et al. (1997) focused on lower functioning children with ASD and severe developmental delay. Although the children in the Smith et al. (1997) study remained quite delayed following intervention, they made gains on IQ and acquisition of communicative speech. Finally, Eikeseth et al. (2007) studied children who were older than those in Lovaas's (1987) study (4–7 years old at intake), implemented intervention at school instead of in the home, and included a comparison group that received the same number of intervention hours as the EIBI group. Importantly, results were comparable to those obtained with younger children.

All of these replication studies confirm that groups of children who receive the UCLA model of EIBI make substantial gains in IQ and perhaps also in other areas of functioning. Thus, the findings generally support Lovaas's (1987) conclusion that EIBI produces large, beneficial outcomes for many children with autism. However, with the exception of the study by Sallows and Graupner (2005), effect sizes are smaller than in Lovaas's (1987) study.

Given the favorable results, perhaps the next question is whether the replication studies confirm Lovaas's (1987) assertion that some children with autism can be described as normal functioning following intervention. The studies do show that a substantial minority of children (27–48% across studies) perform in the average range on most standardized tests and achieve unassisted placements in general education. However, investigators have replaced the term normal functioning with other descriptors such as best outcome or rapid learners because they have had insufficient data on the extent to which children showed reductions in signs of autism (Cohen et al., 2006).

DIRECTIONS FOR RESEARCH

The findings from replication studies are highly encouraging and have led to widespread acceptance of EIBI as an evidence-based intervention (Smith, McAdam, et al., 2007). However, the studies have limitations. All had small sample sizes. Only two incorporated an RCT design, and only one compared EIBI with an alternate intervention. Outcome measures provide little information on important variables such as effects of EIBI on autistic behaviors and impact on the family. Thus, larger, well-designed studies with more comprehensive assessment protocols are needed.

Additional tests of the effectiveness of EIBI in community settings are also important. Studies suggest that EIBI can be effective in such settings (Cohen et al., 2006; Sallows & Graupner, 2005). However, EIBI is being implemented on a much larger scale than ever before. For example, some EIBI programs cover entire regions such as the province of Ontario, Canada, and serve hundreds of children with autism. Evaluations of such regional programs will be critical.

Lovaas (1987) and subsequent investigators consistently report that some children with autism in EIBI progress to the point where they score in the average range on standardized tests and achieve unassisted placements in general education. However, they also find that other children derive relatively little benefit from EIBI. Unfortunately, reliable predictors of intervention response are not yet available, and other EIBI models (or adaptations of the UCLA model) for children who struggle in the UCLA model have not been developed. Identification of such predictors and models must be a top priority.

For the continued evolution of the UCLA model, several issues may be especially salient. First, given that difficulties in reciprocal social interaction and communication are the defining features of autism, a greater emphasis on these difficulties may be warranted, particularly in the early stages of intervention. For example, problems with joint attention are almost universal among young children who have autism and developmental delays, yet the UCLA model in its present form does not target these problems directly (Lovaas, 2003). Also, DTT may not be the most appropriate instructional format for addressing such difficulties because, in this format, the child is always responding to direction from an adult. More loosely structured formats or child-led interactions such as those used in PRT (see Chapter 21, this volume) may be required. In addition, there are few data on whether 40 hours of intervention per week is optimal or whether another amount (or an amount determined based on assessment of each individual child) would be preferable. Perhaps most importantly, the success of EIBI has spurred efforts to identify children with autism at increasingly younger ages. This, in turn, creates opportunities to increase efficacy by providing very early intervention, beginning when children are 12 or 18 months old instead of 2 or 3 years.

CONCLUSIONS

Although the work of behavior analytic investigators is far from complete, ABA has become the most extensively studied psychoeducational intervention for children with autism. ABA interventions have been implemented successfully for a wide range of difficulties associated with autism, and EIBI may enable some children with autism to make remarkable gains. In a systematic review, Rogers and Vismara (2008) concluded that the

UCLA model met standard criteria for classification as a "well-established" intervention. They further noted that no other psychological, behavioral, or educational intervention for children with autism came close to meeting these criteria, although several other ABA approaches, including PRT, appeared promising and could be classified as "possibly efficacious." Similarly, a meta-analysis based mainly on studies of the UCLA model concluded that EIBI yielded significant and substantial effect sizes (Reichow & Wolery, 2009). Howlin, Magiati, and Charman (2009) were more critical of the quality of the research but still concluded that "there is little question now that early, intensive, behavioural intervention is highly effective for some children." Such conclusions are remarkable because only a generation ago autism was considered to be essentially untreatable (DeMyer, Hingtgen, & Jackson, 1981). The successes of ABA and EIBI provide a strong foundation for ongoing research to improve outcomes.

ACKNOWLEDGMENTS

Preparation of this chapter was supported by Grant Nos. U54 MH066397 (Genotype and Phenotype of Autism) and R01 MH48863-01 (Multi-site Young Autism Project) from the National Institute of Mental Health.

REFERENCES

American Psychiatric Association. (2000). *Diagnostic and statistical manual of mental disorders* (4th ed., text rev.). Washington, DC: Author.

Cohen, H., Amerine-Dickens, M., & Smith, T. (2006). Early intensive behavioral treatment: Replication of the UCLA model in a community setting. *Journal of Developmental and Behavioral Pediatrics, 27,* S145–S155.

Davis, B. J., Smith, T., & Donahoe, P. (2002). Evaluating supervisors in the UCLA treatment model for children with autism: Validation of an assessment procedure. *Behavior Therapy, 31,* 601–614.

DeMyer, M. K., Hingtgen, J. N., & Jackson, R. K. (1981). Infantile autism reviewed: A decade of research. *Schizophrenia Bulletin, 7,* 388–451.

Eikeseth, S., Smith, T., Eldevik, S., & Jahr, E. (2007). Outcome for children with autism who began intensive behavioral treatment between age four and seven: A comparison controlled study. *Behavior Modification, 31,* 264–278.

Howlin, P., Magiati, I., & Charman, T. (2009). Systematic review of early intensive behavioural interventions for children with autism. *American Journal on Intellectual and Developmental Disabilities, 114,* 23–41.

Lovaas, O. I. (1987). Behavioral treatment and normal educational and intellectual functioning in young autistic children. *Journal of Consulting and Clinical Psychology, 55,* 3–9.

Lovaas, O. I. (2003). *Teaching individuals with developmental delays: Basic intervention techniques.* Austin, TX: PRO-ED.

McEachin, J. J., Smith, T., & Lovaas, O. I. (1993). Long-term outcome for children with autism who received early intensive behavioral treatment. *American Journal on Mental Retardation, 97,* 359–372.

Reichow, B., & Wolery, M. (2009). Comprehensive synthesis of early intensive behavioral interventions for young children with autism based on the UCLA Young Autism Project Model. *Journal of Autism Developmental Disorder, 39,* 23–41.

Rogers, S. J., & Vismara, L. A. (2008). Evidence-based comprehensive treatments for early autism. *Journal of Clinical Child and Adolescent Psychology, 37,* 8–38.

Sallows, G., & Graupner, T. (2005). Intensive behavioral treatment for autism: Four-year outcome and predictors. *American Journal on Mental Retardation, 110*, 417–436.

Smith, T., Eikeseth, S., Klevstrand, M., & Lovaas, O. I. (1997). Outcome of early intervention for autistic-like children with severe mental retardation. *American Journal on Mental Retardation, 102*, 228–237.

Smith, T., Groen, A., & Wynn, J. W. (2000). Randomized trial of intensive early intervention for children with pervasive developmental disorder. *American Journal on Mental Retardation, 4*, 269–285.

Smith, T., Lovaas, N. W., & Lovaas, O. I. (2002). Behavior of high-functioning children with autism and their peers when placed with typically developing versus delayed peers: A preliminary study. *Behavioral Interventions, 17*, 1–15.

Smith, T., McAdam, D., & Napolitano, D. (2007). Autism and applied behavior analysis. In P. Sturmey & A. Fitzer (Eds.), *Autism spectrum disorders: Applied behavior analysis evidence and practice* (pp. 1–29). Austin, TX: PRO-ED.

Smith, T., Scahill, L., Dawson, G., Guthrie, D., Lord, C., Odom, S., et al. (2007). Designing research studies on psychosocial interventions in autism. *Journal of Autism and Developmental Disorders, 37*, 354–366.

21

Empirically Supported Pivotal Response Treatment for Children with Autism Spectrum Disorders

ROBERT L. KOEGEL, LYNN KERN KOEGEL, TY W. VERNON, and LAUREN I. BROOKMAN-FRAZEE

OVERVIEW

Autism spectrum disorders have received much attention because of both the steady rise in prevalence and the fact that the etiological basis continues to remain largely unknown. Since Kanner's (1943) recognition of autism as a distinct developmental disorder, the three defining characteristics (impairments in social interaction and communication and restricted and repetitive behaviors) have remained, although the specific diagnostic criteria have changed over the years. Because of difficulties with social communication, individuals with autism spectrum disorders who fail to receive appropriate intervention may also exhibit disruptive behaviors, such as tantrums, aggression, and self-injury. In addition, almost all parents of children with autism experience high levels of stress related to having a child with a disability. Thus, there has been a growing demand for systematically evaluated interventions that address the comprehensive needs of the child and the family as a whole and that result in meaningful outcomes over time and across widespread areas of functioning.

CONCEPTUAL MODEL UNDERLYING TREATMENT

Early interventions, derived from speculative causation theories rather than empirical evidence, were generally ineffective in dealing with the comprehensive needs of children on the spectrum (Koegel, Schreibman, O'Neill, & Burke, 1983). Subsequent scientifically based treatment procedures in the 1960s used operationally defined behavioral principles and resulted in measurable improvements in several target areas of the disorder; however, the interventions proved to be extremely labor and time intensive. In an effort to improve the effectiveness and efficiency of intervention, researchers began to focus on the identification of pivotal responses. The theoretical underpinning of identifying pivotal responses was that if certain core areas were targeted, widespread collateral changes in numerous other untargeted behaviors would occur, resulting in very fluidly integrated behavioral gains. This concept of producing widespread generalized changes is also supported in the research literature in areas such as response covariation (Kazdin, 1982). This chapter focuses on the pivotal area of motivation for children with autism spectrum disorders, which appears to serve a particularly important role in causing widespread collateral behavioral gains in the core areas of the condition of autism as well as increasing the child's learning curve, improving parental and child affect, decreasing parental stress, and decreasing disruptive and interfering behaviors. This core area of motivation underlies other important pivotal areas such as child self-initiations discussed next. Motivation also underlies pivotal areas such as joint attention and responsivity to multiple stimulus input and self-regulation of behavior (not discussed in this chapter). In the next section, we focus on the basic core area of motivation, which appears to be pivotal to almost every area of functioning for children with autism.

Motivation

Motivation to respond to social and environmental stimuli appears to be an essential pivotal area for typical development. The disabilities of children with autism spectrum disorders may cause them to experience repeated failures as well as noncontingent assistance and reinforcement from caregivers. Consequently, they may fail to understand the interconnection between their behavior and the consequences from their environment. This appears to result in lethargy, also seen in conditions of learned helplessness in numerous populations (Koegel, O'Dell, & Dunlap, 1988). Pivotal Response Treatment (PRT) focuses on decreasing the presence of learned helplessness by enhancing the relationship between children's responses and their contingent acquisition of reinforcers. Functionally, this serves to increase the children's subsequent likelihood, rate, and accuracy of responding while decreasing response latency. Such improvements in environmental and social interactions appear to be important for language, social, and cognitive development as well as for creating more positive long-term outcomes. In terms of a transactional model, once children are motivated to respond, a positive feedback loop is created wherein additional learning opportunities are provided, thus generating the social-environmental conditions for the development of more complex behaviors, which are necessary for social, communicative, and cognitive competence.

The PRT paradigm builds on earlier effective techniques described in the applied behavior analysis (ABA) literature but incorporates enhanced motivational strategies. Early ABA interventions focused on using repetitive drill-like practice in a stimulus–response–consequence discrete trial format, teaching one target behavior at a time. Behaviors were followed by edible reinforcers for correct responding and punishment or extinction for incorrect responses. The targeted behaviors were taught within a strict shaping paradigm, and the teaching was repeated in a drill format until criterion was reached on each behavior. PRT differs importantly from traditional discrete trial approaches by focusing on increasing and maintaining the intrinsic motivational qualities within the stimulus–response–consequence interaction.

Several specific motivational strategies used in PRT have been systematically identified through empirical research: child choice, task variation, interspersal of maintenance tasks, reinforcement of response attempts, and the use of natural and direct reinforcement. When provided as a package, these strategies improve children's responsivity to social and environmental learning opportunities. The first empirical study that documented the effectiveness of the treatment package focused on targeting expressive verbal communication with children who were nonverbal and who had undergone lengthy periods of unsuccessful intervention. Data from our center and others suggested that about 50% of nonverbal children would learn functional expressive communication using the traditional ABA procedures. In contrast, when motivational procedures are incorporated, a far greater percentage of children learn to use functional expressive communication. However, age seems to be a variable. If intervention begins before age 3, upward of 95% of the children become verbal; if intervention begins between 3–5 years, more than 85% become verbal; and if intervention begins after age 5, only about 20% of the nonverbal children learn to use expressive verbal communication. Because the communication intervention resembled the way in which typical children learn to communicate, the procedures were called the "Natural Language Paradigm" (NLP). Again, both motivation and age are essential ingredients to better long-term outcomes.

Motivation to Self-Initiate

Self-initiations occur frequently in typically developing children and serve various functions, including information seeking, initiating and maintaining attention, and seeking assistance. Initiations can vary in form, ranging from joint attention bids in prelinguistic children to elaborate question asking in verbal children, and are inherently social in nature because they require a social or verbal response from the communicative partner.

Whereas initiations occur frequently in typically developing children, they occur infrequently or are absent altogether in children with autism. Further, when children with autism do exhibit spontaneous self-initiated communication, it is often exclusively limited to behavior regulation contexts, such as requests or protests. Retrospective research from our center suggests that the presence of self-initiations appears to be a prognostic indicator, associated with more favorable long-term outcomes. Further, the results of a subsequent prospective study showed that children with autism who learn to use self-initiations also have more favorable outcomes than those who do not (Koegel, Koegel, Shoshan, & McNerney, 1999).

This promising research suggests that when children with autism are motivated (through PRT) to self-initiate social interactions, particularly important concomitant changes occur in numerous areas of functioning. Specifically, improvements in social communication and acquisition of linguistic targets as well as reductions in aggression, self-stimulation, self-injury, and tantrums have been documented. Targeting this pivotal area of motivation to self-initiate social interactions results in learning that increases autonomy as children become less reliant on adult-delivered learning opportunities. As well, when children engage in self-initiations, they appear more appropriate on scales of normalcy, sometimes rated as appearing completely appropriate (Koegel et al., 1999). In short, motivating children to engage in initiations provides them with tools that result in learning, thereby decreasing the need for the provision of ongoing learning opportunities created by a parent, teacher, or other adult. Teaching techniques that are not only social in nature but result in learning have the potential to reduce parental stress and have been shown to be pivotal in terms of widespread collateral improvements and related long-term positive outcomes.

Motivation to Socialize

Another successful area of research has focused on using PRT procedures to motivate children with autism to socially interact with their families and typically developing peers. Specifically, the area of child choice has been expanded to the concept of identifying activities that are mutually reinforcing to both the children with autism and their typically developing peers. This results in increased social play, higher levels of positive affect, and increased levels of joint attention. One such technique focuses on incorporating the children's repetitive and restricted areas of interest into age-appropriate social activities (Baker, Koegel, & Koegel, 1998). For example, one child who rarely participated in social play was found to have a ritualistic interest in maps and geography, resulting in a vast accumulation of knowledge on this topic. A playground game of "map tag" was developed as a mutually reinforcing activity (developed from both the typical peer's preference for tag games and the targeted child's preference for map-related themes). In the context of this preferred theme, the child with autism exhibited increases in social play and affect. Furthermore, once the child gained experience with playground games, he was motivated to participate with peers in other playground activities outside of his restricted interests. His increased motivation for nonritualistic play with peers implies that exposure to social play became intrinsically motivating, and that reinforcement hierarchies can be altered if they are carefully created using child choice. Similar successful intervention programs have been developed by creating clubs, playdates, and camp activities around the targeted child's interests (Koegel, Werner, Vismara, & Koegel, 2005).

Recently, research has also begun to explore use of the PRT paradigm to target early joint attention (e.g., Vismara & Lyons, 2007). Using items of perseverative interest as stimuli during PRT intervention for communication resulted in immediate improvements in joint attention without specific intervention for joint attention. Further, over a period of approximately 2 months of PRT intervention, without specifically targeting joint attention, it emerged as a collateral gain (Vismara & Lyons, 2007). This illustrates the important point that PRT is designed to get the child with autism on a typical developmental track through collateral changes in critical early development when motivation is targeted as a core treatment area.

GOALS OF TREATMENT

The goal of PRT is to provide comprehensive intervention in key areas that will increase independence and self-education throughout the day, with rapid widespread improvement in the condition of autism without the need for constant vigilance from an intervention provider, thus resulting in time and cost efficiency (Koegel et al., 2006). In our approach, the teaching of pivotal behaviors is coordinated throughout the children's day with parents, teachers, and other service providers. To maximize the likelihood of a typical developmental trajectory, treatment is provided within natural, inclusive settings (i.e., the same settings and activities in which the individuals would participate if they did not have a disability), with programs developed by individuals with extensive clinical experience in the areas of autism, inclusion, and positive behavior support strategies.

Parent collaboration, education, and empowerment are important features of the program. Of particular importance is the expertise and devotion parents contribute to the intervention process. Parents generally are highly motivated to increase their children's competency and have an intimate knowledge of their children's interests, motivations, and routines. Additionally, they can provide consistency throughout their children's waking hours and over the years as their children move to new teachers and interventionists. Within a parent education model, we use a practice-with-feedback format through a manualized intervention wherein parents work with their children and are given feedback regarding procedures for improving pivotal areas such as motivation and child initiations in the context of social communication, academics, and so on. This type of coordinated model, which emphasizes families' active involvement and building self-initiated interactions, increases the total amount of intervention available for the children. Parent education programs have been effective for addressing a large number of behaviors, including increasing social communication, decreasing disruptive behaviors, and improving the generalization of treatment gains (Laski, Charlop, & Schreibman, 1988). Perhaps most importantly, PRT has been shown to reduce family stress as it is blended into daily routines and developed within individual family values (Koegel, Bimbela, & Schreibman, 1996).

CHARACTERISTICS OF THE TREATMENT PROGRAM: INTERVENTION FORMAT

Families who live geographically near our center are provided with intervention in their homes and local communities. The number of hours provided to each family varies depending on child and family needs. Total intervention time ranges from a few hours per week of parent training to more than 40 hours per week. We have also developed several researched models for families who live in geographically distant areas. Families can participate in either an individual or group intensive workshop that focuses on parent education. Following participation and completion of fidelity of implementation measures, families can also effectively train others who work with their children to implement the PRT procedures that were targeted. Specifically, families participate with their children in a week-long intensive training program, receiving daily 5-hour parent education sessions. Similar multifamily workshops have been implemented wherein families bring in video recordings of themselves using PRT with their children for daily feedback. In addition, we have documented the effectiveness of a trainer-of-trainers format where training was initially implemented by our staff outside of our geographic area, using practice with feedback and videotapes for certification of implementation fidelity (Bryson et al., 2007). Our clients range from infants to adults, may require few or extensive support needs, and represent various cultural backgrounds. Intervention is individualized and dynamic based on each client's presenting symptoms and the family's goals, values, and cultural identity.

PARENT EDUCATION

Intervention is manualized (Koegel, Schreibman, Good, Cerniglia, Murphy, & Koegel, 1989; Koegel, Koegel, Bruinsma, Brookman, & Fredeen, 2003), and each of the motivational procedures (described later) is taught. Teaching examples are provided, and opportunities for parents to apply the procedures to their own children are provided in the context of a curriculum that is based on activities the children would engage in if there were no disability (Koegel et al., 2006). In addition, an integral part of graduate education is teaching the clinicians how to provide feedback to the parents while they work directly with their children. Clinicians are trained to do this through course work and ongoing practicum courses. It is important that the clinicians are able to work together with families to determine target behaviors that will make a difference in their lives and to provide continuous positive feedback while they are learning the PRT procedures.

Throughout the intervention sessions, the clinician provides the parents with immediate *in vivo* feedback on their implementation of the PRT procedures while they work with their children. For most, the initial focus of intervention is on using the motivational strategies to increase their responsivity to learning opportunities. Specifically, parent intervention sessions begin with feedback on the following points:

1. *Use of child-selected stimulus materials.* Procedures that involve child-preferred activities typically increase a child's attention to the task, and the use of natural reinforcers that are integrally related to the target behavior can direct the child's attention to the relevant cues in the activity. Therefore, parents are taught to provide instructional stimuli only when the child is attending and to increase the child's motivation to respond by using child-selected materials, activities, and toys and following the child's lead throughout the teaching interactions. Giving the child input into determining the stimuli to be used during instruction maximizes the child's interest in the learning situation and improves the rate and generalization of learning (e.g. Koegel, Dyer, & Bell, 1987). Child-selected stimuli are not necessarily limited to items and materials; for example, a child may want to choose the topic of conversation or the order of activities.

2. *Direct, natural reinforcers are used whenever possible.* Direct, natural reinforcers are directly and functionally related to the task. In contrast, arbitrary or indirect reinforcers do not fall within the chain of behaviors required to produce the positive consequence. As a simple example, a direct, natural reinforcer for a child saying the word "ball" would be throwing the child a ball as opposed to giving him or her a food item or token reinforcer for the vocalization. Research suggests that the response–reinforcer relationship can be enhanced by providing direct and natural reinforcement, thus improving overall motivation to respond to the interaction (Koegel & Williams, 1980; Williams, Koegel, & Egel, 1981).

3. *Interspersing maintenance trials.* This strategy involves interspersing previously learned tasks with new acquisition tasks. The goal is to increase the success that a child experiences, thereby increasing the likelihood that he or she will attempt the task again.

This phenomenon has also been described as behavioral momentum, such that the child is provided with a target acquisition task following a string of rapid correct responses, thereby increasing the likelihood that the momentum will result in subsequent correct responding. This differs from other techniques that present successive trials of acquisition tasks, which create a more challenging and often frustrating situation for the child and can result in greater levels of avoidance and disruptive behavior.

4. *Reinforcing attempts.* This strategy rewards children's clear, appropriate attempts to respond to instructional materials or natural learning opportunities. Such response attempts are reinforced, even if the response is not a successive approximation to the targeted behavior, as in a strict shaping paradigm. Interestingly, when response attempts are reinforced, the children increase their subsequent correct productions of the target behaviors and do so with a considerable amount of positive affect (Koegel et al., 1988). This component of teaching may be particularly important for children with autism who experience repeated difficulties when they attempt a difficult task and, therefore, may have been extinguished for trying (Koegel & Egel, 1979). Table 21.1 shows a comparison of discrete trial teaching procedures with and without incorporation of these motivational variables.

AMOUNT OF TREATMENT

There appears to be a consensus in the field that children with autism require intensive intervention throughout the day; however, there has also been considerable ambiguity about how to feasibly accomplish this goal. Our approach is that a coordinated effort across all settings and significant individuals can result in large amounts of intervention being delivered on an ongoing basis throughout the child's day without excessive effort on the part of any one individual.

Our research suggests that most individuals can reach our required 80% criterion on fidelity of implementation measures for correct use of the basic motivational procedures within approximately 25 hours. This suggests that it is very feasible to train the significant individuals in the child's environment, thus providing for a comprehensive intervention throughout the child's waking hours.

SELF-INITIATIONS

An additional way to increase the amount of intervention is to teach the children to initiate opportunities for teaching interactions. Typically developing children use a variety of self-initiated queries that result in access to further learning throughout the day. These queries appear within typically developing children's first lexicon and continue throughout the life span. In contrast, most children with autism and other language disabilities use a limited number of such initiations or none at all. Therefore, we specifically target a variety of child-initiated interrogatives, such as "What's that?", "Where is it?", and "Whose is it?" Typically, "what" and "where" questions emerge in about the second year of life, whereas "whose" questions appear in the third year. These queries (and other types of spontaneous initiations such as "Look" and "Help") can serve as a means for the children to obtain additional linguistic information from others throughout the day.

EXAMPLES OF MOTIVATIONAL TREATMENT INTERACTIONS FOR SELF-INITIATED QUERIES

"What's That?"

A rudimentary form of the interrogative "What's that?" appears within typical children's first lexicon and provides them with a self-initiation to access and acquire vocabulary words. To teach children with autism this important strategy, we first identify highly desired items, such as favorite snacks, action figures, and so on. The purpose of starting with highly desired items is to provide a motivational context so that when the children are taught the query, positive consequences will follow. The items are then hidden in an opaque bag, and children are prompted to ask "What's that?" After asking the question, a (highly desired) item is taken out of the bag and labeled "It's a [item name]." Then the children are given the item. The prompt is gradually faded until the children are spontaneously asking the question.

Once children are asking the question and repeating the label, neutral (less desired) items are gradually faded into the bag. Even during the fading of the highly desired items, children are still being provided with a partial schedule of reinforcement that may be helpful in creating a positive context for initiations. This may be partially responsible for the generalized and maintained effects of the intervention. In addition, data show that the procedure is effective for vocabulary acquisition. Thus, a learning situation that parallels typical language development has been created.

"Where Is It?"

Developmentally typical language learners begin using "Where" questions after "What's that?" To teach this interrogative to children with autism, similar motivational strategies are incorporated. Specifically, the children's favorite items are hidden in a variety of different locations. They are prompted to ask "Where is it?", and parents or other adults respond using the targeted preposition (e.g., "*in* the box," "*on* the dresser," or "*next to* the refrigerator"). Access to the favored item serves as a natural reinforcer. Throughout this process, the children are learning both self-initiation and a variety of prepositions.

"Whose Is It?"

Motivating children to self-initiate this later developing interrogative also increasing their opportunities to learn pronouns and possessives. For example, initially, to accomplish this learning task, a parent is instructed to use a variety of items that the child clearly associates with a particular member of the family. The child is prompted to ask, "Whose is it?" The parent then responds and gives the item to the child. Eventually, the child is prompted to repeat the possessive form. The same general teaching format is used to teach "yours" and "mine." Because this reversal of pronouns is typically difficult for children with autism, we use highly desired stimulus items (e.g., a favorite toy or candy). When the parent responds to the child's initiation of "Whose is it?" by saying "It's yours," the child is prompted to say "Mine" and then receives the desired item. With this procedure, children are being naturally reinforced for exhibiting curiosity and for learning pronouns. Because this reinforcement results in a large number of spontaneous learning interactions throughout the day, the procedure not only is an effective teaching technique in its own right but also greatly increases the amount of intervention.

EVIDENCE ON THE EFFECTS OF TREATMENT

Treatment Evaluations

We, along with other researchers in the field, have used a number of different strategies to evaluate the effectiveness of the aforementioned types of PRT. The dependent measures in many of the outcome studies usually fall into one of two categories: (1) child variables and (2) parent and family variables. Although the primary focus is on improving child skills and reducing the symptoms of autism, parent and family variables are also important to assess because of social validity concerns. Our research suggests that parents are not likely to use interventions that are aversive, stressful, or burdensome or strategies that do not fit with their family's particular values. Specific child outcome measures may include child initiations, joint attention, responsivity, reduction of disruptive behavior, spontaneous speech, quality of friendships, academic improvement, and generalization of treatment gains. Parent and family outcome measures include parents' accuracy in using the PRT procedures, parental stress, quality of parent–child interactions, positive affect, positive statements, physical affection, parental empowerment, and reduction of depressive symptoms.

Empirical Evidence for PRT

A number of studies have documented the efficacy of the NLP, or PRT, as a comprehensive intervention for addressing core symptoms characteristic of children with autism. Because the procedures more closely resemble the types of interactions adults have with typically developing children (as contrasted to a more analogue, mass-trial approach that has been traditionally used for children with autism), the PRT language intervention procedures are described as the "natural" language paradigm. Table 21.1 outlines the differences in the procedures for the two models as applied to language intervention. Subsequent research demonstrating the applicability of these NLP procedures to broader areas of nonlanguage behaviors led us to describe the technique as a pivotal response treatment.

Components of PRT

Empirical support for the use of each PRT component has been widely documented in numerous research studies both within our laboratories and in independent laboratories. For example, allowing children to make choices in activities or choose the order of activities was shown to reduce social avoidance behaviors (Koegel, Dyer, & Bell, 1987), increase accuracy and productivity, and decrease disruptive behaviors when embedded within teaching activities. Similarly, interventions in which children respond to a combination of maintenance and acquisition tasks have resulted in increases in correct responding, rate of target behavior acquisition, and positive affect. In addition, a number of studies have also investigated the response–reinforcer relationship in the intervention interactions. For example, when children's attempts at the target behavior are reinforced, as opposed to strictly shaping successive motor approximations, improved speech production occurs as well as increased interest, enthusiasm, and happiness (Koegel et al., 1988). Similarly, reinforcing child responses that are directly or naturally related to the target behavior has been shown to produce more rapid learning (rather than when an

TABLE 21.1. Differences between the Discrete Trial (Individual Target Behavior) and Pivotal Response Treatment (PRT) Paradigms

	Traditional Discrete Trial (individual target behavior) paradigm without a motivational package	Motivational Pivotal Response Treatment paradigm
Stimulus Items	• Chosen by clinician • Repeated until criterion is met • Phonological sounds, irrespective of functionality in the natural environment, shaped into words	• Chosen by child • Varied every few trials • Labels for age-appropriate items/ activities found in the child's natural environment
Prompts	• Manual (e.g., touch tip of tongue or hold lips together)	• Clinician repeats item/activity label
Interaction	• Clinician presents stimulus item; item not functional within interaction	• Clinician and child play with stimulus item (i.e., stimulus item is functional within interaction)
Response	• Correct responses or successive approximations reinforced	• Looser shaping contingency so that intentful attempts to respond are also reinforced
Consequences	• Edible reinforcers paired with social reinforcers (praise)	• Natural reinforcer (e.g., opportunity to play with the stimulus item) paired with social reinforcers

arbitrary reinforcer is provided). That is, it is important that the response is a direct part of the chain leading to the reinforcer (Koegel & Williams, 1980; Williams et al., 1981). Finally, studies show that the presence of child initiations is related to highly favorable outcomes, and that these initiations can be taught to young children who do not demonstrate them (Koegel et al., 1999). In sum, these studies provide strong empirical support for the use of each of the individual motivation components of PRT as well as for the importance of motivating children to exhibit child-initiated interactions.

PRT as an Intervention Package

In addition to the research providing empirical support for individual components of pivotal response interventions, other studies have compared the use of a package combining the components described previously with a package of teaching procedures that does not incorporate the motivational variables. Table 21.2 provides a summary of the empirically based evidence supporting PRT. This body of literature reflects the increased efficacy of the motivational PRT procedures over an approach that targets individual target behaviors in a drill format, without focusing on core motivational variables. Further, improved treatment gains were also observed when parents, rather than clinicians, implemented the treatment. In addition to the positive child outcomes of PRT, the collateral positive effects on family functioning are documented in multiple studies. Finally, more recent empirical research in this area has investigated both the importance of self-initiations as a prognostic indicator and the efficacy of teaching such self-initiations to children who lack them.

(text resumes on p. 340)

TABLE 21.2. Studies Documenting Empirical Evidence for Pivotal Response Treatment (PRT) Interventions

Study	Design	Treatment/ independent variable	Dependent variables	Treatment outcome
Original PRT studies				
Koegel, O'Dell, & Koegel (1987)	Within-subject design: multiple baseline across participants	Traditional discrete trial vs. PRT (called analogue treatment[a] vs. NLP[a])	• Imitative child utterances • Spontaneous child utterances • Generalization	Children produced more imitative and spontaneous utterances in PRT condition. Generalization of treatment gains occurred only in PRT condition.
Koegel, Koegel, & Surratt (1992)	Within-subject design: repeated reversal design with counterbalancing	Traditional discrete trial vs. PRT (called analogue treatment[a] vs. PRT) for teaching of target sounds and words	• Disruptive behavior • Target language responses	Increased responding and less disruptive behaviors occurred during PRT condition compared with analogue condition.
Koegel, Koegel, Shoshan, & McNerney (1999), Phase 1	Retrospective analysis of archival data	High vs. low child-initiated social interactions in PRT treatment	• Language age • Number of initiations • Pragmatic ratings • Social/ community functioning • Adaptive behavior scale scores	Children with poor and favorable outcomes had comparable language ages and adaptive behavior scale scores at preintervention. Children who exhibited high levels of spontaneous initiations at preintervention had more favorable outcomes.
Koegel, Koegel, Shoshan, & McNerney (1999), Phase 2	Clinical replication	PRT teaching of child initiated spontaneous interactions	• Language ages • Number of initiations • Pragmatics ratings • Social/ community functioning • Adaptive behavior scale scores	Following initiation training, children's adaptive and pragmatic scores increased to near chronological age level. They did not retain diagnosis of autism or special education placements. Social/ academic functioning was comparable to typically developing peers.
Koegel, Carter, & Koegel (2003)	Within-subject design: multiple baseline across participants	PRT to teach self-initiated queries as method to access verbs together with temporal morpheme	• Number of verb productions • Number of queries • Use of correct tense • Mean length of utterance (MLU) • Number/diversity of verbs • Generalization	Children were successfully taught to use the queries "What happened?" or "What's happening?" during intervention. Both children generalized the use of "-ing" and "-ed" to other verbs and increased MLU and verb diversity.

(cont.)

TABLE 21.2. *(cont.)*

Study	Design	Treatment/ independent variable	Dependent variables	Treatment outcome
Independent replications of PRT effectiveness with original lab collaboration				
Schreibman, Kaneko, & Koegel (1991)	Group design with random assignment	Traditional Discrete Trial vs. PRT (called individual target behaviors[a] vs. PRT)	• Parental affect (scored by naïve observers)	Parents in PRT condition displayed significantly more positive affect than parents trained in Discrete Trial.
Koegel, Bimbela, & Schreibman (1996)	Group design with random assignment	Discrete Trial vs. PRT (called individual target behaviors[a] vs. PRT)	• Ratings of happiness, interest, stress, communication style during dinnertime probes	Discrete Trial condition resulted in no significant influence on interactions, whereas PRT resulted in positive parent–child interactions.
Koegel, Camarata, Koegel, Ben-Tall, & Smith (1998)	Within-subject design: ABA with counterbalancing to control for order effects	Traditional discrete trial vs. PRT (called analogue Treatment[a] vs. PRT) for teaching target sounds	• Correct production of target sounds in language samples • Intelligibility ratings	Significant gains in correct production of target sounds and speech intelligibility during PRT intervention.
Koegel, Camarata, Valdez-Menchaca, & Koegel (1998)	Within-subject design: multiple baseline across participants	Self-initiated question ("What's that?") using PRT framework	• Spontaneous use of target question • Number of stimulus items labeled correctly	Children consistently and spontaneously initiated "What's that?" across treatment and generalization settings. Significant increase in vocabulary because of item label acquisition.
Bryson et al. (2007)	Clinical replication	Large-scale community training in PRT for interventionists, clinical supervisors, clinical leaders, parents	• Fidelity of implementation • Intervals with functional verbal utterances	Preliminary data show that treatment providers maintained fidelity of implementation across time and increased functional verbal utterances of the participant children
Independent replications of effectiveness of PRT				
Laski, Charlop, & Schreibman (1988)	Within-subject design: multiple baseline across participants	Parent training in PRT (called NLP[a]) at home and in a clinic setting	• Parent verbalizations • Child vocalizations • Frequency of echolalia	Posttreatment increases in parent requests for vocalizations. Increases in children's verbal responsiveness during intervention and generalization.

(cont.)

TABLE 21.2. *(cont.)*

Study	Design	Treatment/ independent variable	Dependent variables	Treatment outcome
Independent replications of effectiveness of PRT (cont.)				
Pierce & Schreibman (1995)	Within-subject design: multiple baseline across participants	Peer-implemented PRT to increase social skills	• Intervals with peer interaction • Conversation initiations • Play initiations • Attention behaviors	Following peer-implemented PRT, children increased interactions to high level of intervals and increased play and conversation initiations. Both children exhibited increases in coordinated and supported joint attention behaviors after treatment.
Thorp, Stahmer, & Schreibman (1995)	Within-subject design: multiple baseline across participants	PRT teaching of sociodramatic play	• Language assessments • Play behaviors (role-playing, make-believe, persistence, social behavior, verbal communication)	All three children increased in all play behavior measures. Play behavior gains maintained during generalization.
Stahmer (1995)	Within-subject design: multiple baseline across participants	Modified PRT using symbolic play as a target behavior	• Symbolic play • Complexity of play • Creativity of play • Generalization across toys, settings, play partners	Increase in symbolic play and play complexity after PRT play training. Maintenance of treatment gains during generalizations.
Pierce & Schreibman (1997)	Within-subject design: multiple baseline across participants	Peer-implemented PRT to increase social skills	• Intervals with peer interaction • Conversation initiations • Play initiations • Generalization to untrained peers	Peer-implemented PRT was successful in producing positive social behavior change across multiple peer implementers. Social behavior change was maintained during generalization with untrained peers.
Sherer & Schreibman (2005)	Clinical replication	PRT administered to groups with two distinct profiles (predicted responders vs. nonresponders)	• Language (echolalia, cued speech, spontaneous speech) • Play (functional, symbolic, and varied play measures) • Social measures (interaction, social initiations)	Children in the responder profile exhibited increases in language, play, and social behavior after PRT intervention.

(cont.)

TABLE 21.2. *(cont.)*

Study	Design	Treatment/ independent variable	Dependent variables	Treatment outcome
Independent replications of effectiveness of PRT *(cont.)*				
Baker-Ericzen, Stahmer, & Burns (2007)	Clinical replication	12-week PRT parent education program	• Vineland Adaptive Behavior Scales domain scores	After parent education in PRT, all children showed significant improvement in adaptive behavior scale scores regardless of gender, age, child/family race/ethnicity.
Vismara & Lyons (2007)	Within-subject design: applied behavior analysis with counterbalancing and alternating treatments in final phase	PRT with child's perseverative interests vs. nonperseverative interests	• Number of joint attention initiations • Contingencies to joint attention initiations • Child affect ratings	Using child's perseverative interests in PRT model increased joint attention initiations.
Gillett & LeBlanc (2007)	Within-subject design: multiple baseline across participants	Parent-implemented PRT (called NLP[a]) to target language and play skills	Frequency of vocalizations Spontaneous vocalizations Appropriate play Social validity questionnaire	Increases in overall rate and spontaneity of utterances for all three children. Children also showed an increase in appropriate play. Parents rated intervention as simple to implement and endorsed continued use of PRT.
Harper, Symon, & Frea (2008)	Within-subject design: multiple baseline across participants	Peer-implemented PRT to increase social play	Attempts at gaining peer's attention Turn-taking interactions Play initiations	After peer implementation of PRT, both children increased initiations and turn-taking initiations. Results were maintained during generalization.

[a]Historically, various terms have been used synonymously in these empirical articles. For example, PRT has been called the natural language paradigm (NLP) when intervention focuses on language. Similarly, Discrete Trial Training has been labeled the individual target behavior condition or the analogue treatment condition in some publications.

SUMMARY OF EMPIRICAL STUDIES

The characteristics of the studies summarized in Table 21.2 on PRT reflect the criteria for an empirically supported treatment for children with autism. The experimental literature on PRT included group design studies that used random assignment to intervention condition; single-subject studies that used multiple baseline designs or ABA experimental designs, or a combination; and clinical replication designs both within and outside of our own laboratories. The procedures in these studies have been manualized, and adherence measures (fidelity of implementation) were used in all studies. The participants in each of the studies were diagnosed with autism by outside agencies based on nationally accepted diagnostic standards. This body of literature also includes studies from multiple independent laboratories using the same manualized treatment proce-dures. The preponderance of evidence shows that PRT leads to greater treatment gains in both targeted behaviors and untargeted, collateral behaviors than the comparison treatments commonly used with children with autism. Thus, from a clinical perspective, empirical evidence shows that PRT is far more effective in producing gains in social com-munication, with concomitant decreases in repetitive and disruptive behaviors. Further, when one examines the data as a whole, the evidence shows massive increases in verbal communication, movement out of special education classes into regular education, and even many children shedding the autism diagnosis.

DIRECTIONS FOR RESEARCH

Autism still continues to be diagnosed in epidemic proportions, and the cause and cure are yet to be found. As such, procedures designed to improve the symptoms of the disabil-ity continue to warrant research so that improved interventions evolve over time. More standardized definitions that are consistent across researchers and practitioners would be helpful. For example, a more careful definition of communication, such as levels of spontaneity, generalization and maintenance of treatment results, and the impact of intervention on an individual's everyday life are all important directions for research.

The training and implementation to increase the availability of empirically vali-dated interventions is also an area in need of research. For example, methods for train-ing interventionists effectively and efficiently, so that individuals on the spectrum can have access to and benefit from the most recent and valuable treatments, are essential. Further, the sustainability and durability of the training is also critical. Although prac-tice with feedback can improve the skills of teachers, paraprofessionals, parents, and other interventionists, research on whether a minimum level of competence is main-tained over time and whether trainees are able to generalize skills to new behaviors and to new children is of great importance. Additionally, questions related to whether or not trainees actually use the procedures in either the immediate or distant future may be as relevant as whether or not they acquired the skills to begin with.

Another area greatly lacking research relates to the age of study participants. That is, most research in the area of autism involves preschool or school-age populations. Given the more positive outcomes of children who receive early intervention services, assessment and intervention procedures that are effective in infancy and the toddler years may significantly improve outcomes. Relatedly, intervention studies for adults are sorely lacking. Even with the interventions currently available, most adults on the spec-trum have difficulty with social relationships, even though research suggests that most have a desire for both friendships and romantic relationships. They also have increased loneliness and depression, rarely live independently or gain meaningful employment, and are unlikely to marry (Howlin, 2000).

Research on social communication and socialization—the foundation for healthy relationships in adulthood—for individuals on the spectrum is scant and research on more personal issues such as intimacy and sexuality almost nonexistent. Comprehen-sive programs addressing social communication, socialization, peer relationships, and pragmatic behavior in everyday settings are of vital importance for long-term positive outcomes and mental health of individuals on the spectrum (Koegel & LaZebnik, 2009). With the geometric in autism spectrum disorder diagnoses that began in the 1980s, and as this population comes of age, all of these areas will undoubtedly be addressed.

CONCLUSIONS

To achieve widespread, long-term, generalized improvements across children's behavioral repertoire, a number of researchers have focused on investigating pivotal responses that might have a broad impact on symptoms of autism and overall development. By treating pivotal areas that have widespread collateral effects, the intervention is less time consuming, more cost efficient, and less labor intensive than those focused on teaching individual target behaviors using mass trial and repetition. For example, data indicate that teaching approaches that specifically incorporate pivotal response motivational techniques result in greatly improved short- and long-term outcomes; however, there is still a very small subpopulation of children who do not seem to learn functional expressive language with the techniques available today. More research regarding these children and specialized procedures for teaching an initial lexicon is warranted. In addition, studies assessing the interrelationship between communication and other variables such as chronological age, disruptive behavior, and repetitive behaviors might enhance our research knowledge. Further information relating to implementation regarding the best settings, times, types, and amount of intervention may also provide valuable advances.

In summary, evidence suggests that intervention programs emphasizing motivation, such as PRT appear to be effective, efficient models of treatment and result in improved generalization of treatment gains as well as improved long-term outcomes. In addition, PRT tends to decrease parental stress in comparison to more traditional interventions, in part because interventions are blended into natural family routines and are individually designed to match family values. Parental stress has been shown to moderate child progress, making parent education procedures that decrease this stress essential.

Finally, we have shown that once children are motivated to respond to and initiate social communication and learning opportunities, there is concomitant achievement of developmental milestones. That is, when parents become proficient in PRT techniques, they are able to engage in naturally occurring teaching interactions, similar to the type of interactions that generally occur with typically developing children. Further research in this area may help us to fully understand the social-communicative trajectories of children with autism and the interventions needed to guide them a typical developmental trajectory at the earliest possible age. We are highly optimistic about the effects that such data-based approaches will have on the condition of autism and the quality of life for affected families.

ACKNOWLEDGMENTS

The research desribed and preparation of this manuscript were supported in part by NIMH Research Grant MH28210 and NIDCD Research Grant DC010924 from the National Institutes of Health (NIH). The content is solely the responsibility of the authors and does not necessarily represent the official views of NIH.

In addition to their employment at the University of California, Santa Barbara, Robert L. Koegel and Lynn Kern Koegel are partners in the private firm, Koegel Autism Consultants, LLC.

REFERENCES

Baker, M. J., Koegel, R. L., & Koegel, L. K. (1998). Increasing the social behavior of young children with autism using their obsessive behaviors. *Journal of the Association for Persons with Severe Handicaps, 23,* 300–308.

Baker-Ericzen, M. J., Stahmer, A. C., & Burns, A. (2007). Child demographics associated with outcomes in a community-based pivotal response training program. *Journal of Positive Behavior Interventions, 9*(1), 52–60.

Bryson, S. E., Koegel, L. K., Koegel, R. L., Openden, D., Smith, I. M., & Nefdt, N. (2007). Large scale dissemination and community implementation of pivotal response treatment: Program description and preliminary data. *Research and Practice for Persons with Severe Disabilities, 32*(2), 142–153.

Gillett, J. N., & LeBlanc, L. A. (2007). Parent-implemented natural language paradigm to increase language and play in children with autism. *Research in Autism Spectrum Disorders, 1,* 247–255.

Harper, C. B., Symon, J. B., & Frea, W. D. (2008). Recess is time-in: Using peers to improve social skills of children with autism. *Journal of Autism and Developmental Disorders, 38,* 815–826.

Howlin, P. (2000). Outcome in adult life for more able individuals with autism or Asperger syndrome. *Autism, 4*(1), 63–83.

Kanner, L. (1943). Autism disturbances of affective contact. *Nervous Child, 2,* 217–250.

Kazdin, A. E. (1982). Symptom substitution, generalization, and response covariation: Implications for psychotherapy outcome. *Psychological Bulletin, 91,* 349–365.

Koegel, L. K., Camarata, S. M., Valdez-Menchaca, M., & Koegel, R. L. (1998). Setting generalization of question-asking by children with autism. *American Journal on Mental Retardation, 102,* 346–357.

Koegel, L. K., Carter, C. M., & Koegel, R. L. (2003). Teaching children with autism self-initiations as a pivotal response. *Topics in Language Disorders, 23,* 134–145.

Koegel, L. K., Koegel, R. L., Bruinsma, Y., Brookman, L., & Fredeen, R. M. (2003). *Teaching first words to children with autism and communication delays using pivotal response training.* Santa Barbara: University of California.

Koegel, L. K., Koegel, R. L., Nefdt, N., Fredeen, R. M., Klein, E., & Bruinsma, Y. (2006). First S.T.E.P.: A model for the early identification of children with autism spectrum disorders. *Journal of Positive Behavior Interventions, 7,* 247–252.

Koegel, L. K., Koegel, R. L., Shoshan, Y., & McNerney, E. (1999). Pivotal response intervention: II. Preliminary long-term outcomes data. *Journal of the Association for Persons with Severe Handicaps, 24,* 186–198.

Koegel, L. K., & LaZebnik, C. (2009). *Growing up on the spectrum: A guide to life, love, and learning for teens and young adults with autism and Asperger's.* New York: Viking/Penguin.

Koegel, R. L., Bimbela, A., & Schreibman, L. (1996). Collateral effects of parent training on family interactions. *Journal of Autism and Developmental Disorders, 26,* 347–359.

Koegel, R. L., Camarata, S., Koegel, L. K., Ben-Tall, A., & Smith, A. E. (1998). Increasing speech intelligibility in children with autism. *Journal of Autism and Developmental Disorders, 28*(3), 241–251.

Koegel, R. L., Camarata, S., Koegel, L. K., & Smith, A. (2008). Increasing speech intelligibility in children with autism. *Journal of Autism and Developmental Disorders, 28*(3), 241–251.

Koegel, R. L., Dyer, K., & Bell, L. K. (1987). The influence of child-preferred activities on autistic children's social behavior. *Journal of Applied Behavior Analysis, 20,* 243–252.

Koegel, R. L., & Egel, A. L. (1979). Motivating autistic children. *Journal of Abnormal Psychology, 88,* 418–426.

Koegel, R. L., Koegel, L. K., & Surratt, A. (1992). Language intervention and disruptive behavior in preschool children with autism. *Journal of Autism and Developmental Disorders, 22,* 141–153.

Koegel, R. L., O'Dell, M. C., & Dunlap, G. (1988). Producing speech use in nonverbal autistic children by reinforcing attempts. *Journal of Autism and Developmental Disorders, 18,* 525–538.

Koegel, R. L., O'Dell, M. C., & Koegel, L. K. (1987) A natural language teaching paradigm for nonverbal autistic children. *Journal of Autism and Developmental Disorders, 2,* 187–200.

Koegel, R. L., Schreibman, L., Good, A., Cerniglia, L., Murphy, C., & Koegel, L. K. (1989). *How to teach pivotal behaviors to children with autism: A training manual.* Santa Barbara, CA: University of California.

Koegel, R. L., Schreibman, L., O'Neill, R. E., & Burke, J. C. (1983). Personality and family interaction characteristics of parents of autistic children. *Journal of Consulting and Clinical Psychology, 16,* 683–692.

Koegel, R. L., Werner, G. A., Vismara, L. A., & Koegel, L. K. (2005). The effectiveness of contextually supported play date interactions between children with autism and typically developing peers. *Research and Practice for Persons with Severe Disabilities, 30,* 93–102.

Koegel, R. L., & Williams, J. A. (1980). Direct versus indirect response-reinforcer relationships in teaching autistic children. *Journal of Abnormal Child Psychology, 8,* 537–547.

Laski, K. E., Charlop, M. H., & Schreibman, L. (1988). Training parents to use the natural language paradigm to increase their autistic children's speech. *Journal of Applied Behavior Analysis, 21,* 391–400.

Pierce, K., & Schreibman, L. (1995). Increasing complex social behaviors in children with autism: Effects of peer-implemented pivotal response training. *Journal of Applied Behavior Analysis, 28,* 285–295.

Pierce, K., & Schreibman, L. (1997). Multiple peer use of pivotal response training to increase social behaviors of classmates with autism: Results from trained and untrained peers. *Journal of Applied Behavior Analysis, 30,* 157–160.

Schreibman, L., Kaneko, W. M., & Koegel, R. L. (1991). Positive affect of parents of autistic children: A comparison across two teaching techniques. *Behavior Therapy, 22,* 479–490.

Sherer, M. R., & Schreibman, L. (2005). Individual behavioral profiles and predictors of treatment effectiveness for children with autism. *Journal of Consulting and Clinical Psychology, 73,* 525–538.

Stahmer, A. C. (1995). Teaching symbolic play skills to children with autism using pivotal response training. *Journal of Autism and Developmental Disorders, 25,* 123–141.

Thorp, D. M., Stahmer, A. C., & Schreibman, L. (1995). Effects of sociodramatic play training on children with autism. *Journal of Autism and Developmental Disorders, 25,* 265–282.

Vismara, L. A., & Lyons, G. L. (2007). Using perseverative interests to elicit joint attention behaviors in young children with autism: Theoretical and clinical implications to understanding motivation. *Journal of Positive Behavior Interventions, 9,* 214–228.

Williams, J. A., Koegel, R. L., & Egel, A. L. (1981). Response-reinforcer relationships and improved learning in autistic children. *Journal of Applied Behavior Analysis, 14,* 53–60.

22

Family Therapy for Adolescents with Anorexia Nervosa

ARTHUR L. ROBIN and DANIEL Le GRANGE

OVERVIEW

Anorexia nervosa (AN) is a life-threatening eating disorder characterized by (1) a refusal to maintain body weight at or above a minimally normal weight for age and height; (2) intense fear of gaining weight or becoming fat, even though the individual is underweight; (3) body weight/shape disturbance or denial of the seriousness of low body weight; and (4) absence of three consecutive menstrual cycles in postmenarchal females (American Psychiatric Association, 2000). The prevalence of AN in 15- to 19-year-old girls has been reported to be about five in 1,000 (Fisher et al., 1995), but the prevalence of eating disorders is lower and not clearly known among younger children. Over 90% of the postpubertal adolescents with AN are female, although the ratio of girls to boys with AN is lower in prepubertal children.

A variety of interventions have been used to treat eating disorders in children and adolescents: inpatient hospitalization, partial hospitalization, individual dynamic therapy, individual cognitive-behavioral therapy, and family therapy. Le Grange and Lock (2005) cited five random-assignment controlled outcome studies that have evaluated the effectiveness of these various treatments for adolescents. All of these studies included some form of family therapy. Although families do not cause AN, they can be essential to treating it. Teenagers with AN are in a deep state of physiological starvation and obsessed with dire fears of weight gain. As a result, their thinking is confused and they often fail to benefit from insight-oriented individual therapy. Someone external to the adolescents must take charge and help them get out of starvation. Parents and siblings are the natural resource to help restore weight in adolescents with AN.

Family therapy proved to be the most effective intervention for adolescents with eating disorders in the five random assignment studies, helping approximately two-thirds of the patients return to health. Key elements of the successful family therapy approaches included (1) refraining from blaming the adolescents or their parents for AN; (2) placing the parents in charge of restoring their adolescents' weight; (3) requiring parents and adolescents to attend therapy sessions together; (4) directly discussing weight restoration and coaching parents *in vivo* to become successful at encouraging the adolescents to eat more than they had intended to; (5) gradually returning control over eating to the adolescents when sufficient weight gain has been achieved; and (6) emphasizing adolescent developmental issues, cognitive distortions, and family relations after weight restoration had been successfully accomplished.

This chapter describes, compares, and reviews the research for two similar but independently developed family therapies for treating adolescents with AN that incorporate these six key features: behavioral family systems therapy (BFST), developed by Arthur L. Robin, and the Maudsley family-based treatment (FBT), which Le Grange has helped to develop and has extensively researched.

BFST: CHARACTERISTICS OF THE TREATMENT PROGRAM

BFST combines behavioral, cognitive, and family systems perspectives and interventions to help adolescents and their parents overcome AN. Strategic interventions are used to place parents in charge of refeeding their adolescents. Parents are taught to develop and implement a behavioral weight gain program at home akin to those used in inpatient facilities. Later, cognitive restructuring is used to overcome cognitive distortions associated with the eating disorder. When the adolescents reach target weight, control over eating is returned to them, and therapy focuses on the normal developmental task of individuation from the family.

The treatment program can roughly be divided into three phases: (1) assessment, (2) weight gain, and (3) weight maintenance. In the first two phases, typically lasting 6–12 months, the adolescents and the parents are seen together weekly for 55 minutes per session. In the third phase, which typically lasts 3–4 months, sessions are scheduled twice per month. Siblings are invited to attend family sessions when an issue arises that involves them. The therapist works as a team together with a physician and a dietician. The physician sets target weights and rates of weight gain, makes decisions about hospitalization, and conducts regular medical follow-ups; and the dietician provides information about the types and amounts of food to be eaten. Adolescents are weighed before each session by either the physician or the therapist. An unpublished treatment manual describing the four phases of the intervention is available from Arthur L. Robin.

Phase 1: Assessment

During the first of two assessment sessions, the therapist meets separately with the patient and the parents. The therapist establishes rapport with the adolescent and then encourages him or her to relate the story of dieting and weight loss, fears and body dissatisfaction, family relationships, school, peers, and anything else he or she considers important. Listening empathetically, the therapist separates the person from the disorder by explaining how AN has taken over the patient's body and mind, but AN is not who the adolescent is.

With the parents, the therapist takes a history of the onset and course of dieting, weight loss, eating habits and attitudes, previous treatment attempts, general medical and developmental histories, school and peer functioning, and family relations. The team approach is described, and parents are instructed to schedule a physical with the physician and an initial consultation for the family with the dietician and to keep a written log of everything that the patient eats over the next week.

Meeting jointly with the parents and the patient for the second session, the therapist examines the food records. This serves as a springboard to learn about family interactions during mealtime. The therapist picks a representative meal and asks for a "blow-by-blow" description of what happened. Their description provides a further opportunity to assess parental teamwork, parent–child coalitions, and triangulated behavior. The adolescent patient's reactions to the meal open up a host of issues regarding distorted cognitions about food, weight, shape, and family life. From this discussion, the therapist builds a picture of family interactions, coalitions, and family structure. Next, the dire medical situation is reviewed, and the therapist asks the family to make a commitment to participate regularly in family therapy.

Phase 2: Weight Gain

During this phase of intervention, the therapist teaches the parents the skills necessary to take charge of refeeding the patient. This begins with the control rationale:

> "AN is a life-threatening disease. When a child is sick, we consult the doctor, who usually prescribes medicine. You have consulted the doctors, and food has been prescribed as the only medicine that can cure AN. But your child's disease causes a fear of taking the medicine that is so desperately needed. When a child is unable to take the medicine on his or her own for any other disease, the parents, who love the child, give the medicine. Similarly, in this case you are going to need to give your child the medicine, that is, the food, that is needed to recover. Temporarily, you will take over complete control of everything related to eating. You will plan the menu based on the dietician's recommendations. You will do the shopping. You will select and prepare her food. You will present the food and sit with your daughter to make sure it is eaten. You will record everything that she eats on the sheets I give you. You will praise and reward her for eating all of her food, and you will arrange for energy to be preserved by not allowing her to engage in any activities if it proves too difficult to eat all of her food. I understand that this is a very big responsibility. I will help you work as a team to divide this responsibility between the two of you. When she approaches the target weight and demonstrates readiness to take back responsibility for food and eating, I will help you gradually return it to her. I know that I am asking you to do something that is very difficult, but I also know how much you love your child and I feel completely confident that you can help her take the food, which is the only medicine."

Afterward, the therapist assesses each family member's reactions. The patient's objections are empathetically acknowledged, but the therapist reiterates that through no fault of her own starvation has clouded her mind and prevented healthy eating. The parents' resistance is empathetically reframed as the natural apprehension and fear of a loving couple who want to heal their child but don't know how to go about it. Strategically, the therapist "goes with the resistance," creatively finding a graceful path to navigate around it.

When the parents do make the commitment to take charge of their adolescent's eating, the therapist coaches them to develop a behavioral weight gain program. The therapist further prompts them to designate positive incentives for eating meals as well as longer term incentives for achieving 25%, 50%, and 75% of the required weight. Powerful incentives have included money, access to video games, and favorite hobbies or recreational pursuits. For example, one patient who loved to ride horses and who took care of her own horse daily had to eat all of her meals before she could go to the barn to see her horse. An athlete on the school swimming team had to achieve 75% of his target weight before he could participate in swim practice and swim meets on a limited basis. Another patient had to eat all of her meals before she could use her cell phone and computer. During the remaining sessions of the weight gain phase, the therapist teaches the family the skills necessary to fine-tune the behavioral weight gain program, closing off any loopholes and continuing the program as the patient gradually gains weight and moves toward the target weight.

When the patient eats most of the required foods and gains weight regularly, the therapist shifts the focus to non-*food*-related issues. Cognitive restructuring is introduced to correct distorted thinking about certain foods, body parts, and body size. Cognitive restructuring involves (1) identifying a distorted cognition, (2) challenging it logically, (3) suggesting a more appropriate cognition, (4) proposing an experiment to determine which cognition makes more sense based on the evidence collected by the teen, and (5) reviewing the results of the experiment. For example, as 15-year-old Nicole slowly approached her target weight range, she became increasingly distraught about the change in her appearance. "My stomach sticks out and I look gross" was her distorted cognition. The therapist gently challenged this distortion by suggesting that perhaps there were other ways to interpret the changes in her body that accompanied weight gain; Nicole was skeptical. The therapist proposed an experiment to test the validity of Nicole's belief. Asked to identify four people whom she trusted, Nicole named her grandmother, aunt, a close friend, and her English teacher. The therapist asked Nicole to bring in photos of herself before she began to lose weight, at various points afterward, and during weight gain. The four trusted people reviewed the photos and selected the one that represented the "healthiest" image. Three of the four raters selected the photo in which Nicole was closest to her target weight as "healthiest," and none thought her stomach stuck out. Nicole was taken aback and found cause to reevaluate her self-perceptions.

Phase 3: Weight Maintenance

As the patient approaches the target weight, the weight maintenance phase of BFST begins. The therapist teaches the parents the skills necessary to gradually return the responsibility for eating to the patient. The parents consult the dietician to reduce caloric intake to facilitate weight-maintenance rather than weight gain. The therapist helps the family delineate the steps for giving the patient more decision-making control over eating. At first, the teenager might plan one of the meals, measure and prepare some of the food, eat a meal without supervision, or write down the foods for the meal.

Later, the teenager might eat a meal without supervision, plan the menus for an entire day, eat several meals without supervision, and so on. Eventually, the patient may eat all of the meals for a day without any parental intervention or monitoring.

The therapist also focuses on adolescent development and encourages (1) the patient to seek age-appropriate individuation and autonomy from the parents and (2) the parents to refocus their energies on their strengthening their marital bonds. The patient is assigned tasks to engage in more autonomous behaviors such as spending more time with peers and less time with parents. Parents are assigned tasks to spend more time with each other; this makes it easier for the adolescent to individuate and spend more time with peers. If parents are experiencing marital problems, they may focus too much energy on the eating-disordered adolescent, which may interfere with the adolescent's individuation and increased involvement in peer relationships.

When the patient has maintained the target weight for at least 3 months, the therapist plans for termination. The interval between sessions is increased to 1 month. The therapist discusses methods of coping with possible relapses with the family. The changes that have occurred are reviewed, and the family is left with the framework that coping with AN may be a lifelong process, and that they can return for more therapy at any time.

FBT: CHARACTERISTICS OF THE TREATMENT PROGRAM

The theoretical underpinning of FBT is that the adolescent patient is embedded in the family and that the parent's involvement in therapy is vital for the ultimate success of treatment. From a developmental perspective, in the area of food and eating, the adolescent is functioning like a much younger child (e.g., normal adolescent development has been arrested by the presence of the eating disorder). The parents are temporarily put in charge of the adolescent's eating to help reduce the hold that this disorder has over the teenager's life. When the eating disorder is no longer controlling the adolescent's life, the parents will return control over eating to the adolescent and return to the usual role of helping him or her achieve the developmental tasks of adolescence.

FBT progresses through three clearly defined phases: (1) temporary parental control over weight restoration; (2) negotiation for a new pattern of relationships in which control over eating is returned to the adolescent; and (3) adolescent developmental issues and termination. Treatment is provided by a primary mental health clinician (psychologist, psychiatrist, social worker) along with a consulting team comprising a pediatrician for medical monitoring and a child/adolescent psychiatrist to manage any psychiatric comorbidity. The primary clinician sees the patient and family regularly and maintains regular contact with the other team members so everyone is "on the same page." The patient is weighed at the beginning of each session by the therapist. Sessions last 60 minutes, except for the 90-minute family meal session. A published therapy manual is available (Lock, Le Grange, Agras, & Dare, 2001).

Phase 1: Refeeding the Patient

Weekly therapy sessions are focused primarily on restoring the patient's weight and include a family meal session, which gives the therapist an opportunity for direct observation of family interaction patterns at mealtime and direct intervention to change these patterns. The parents are placed in charge of restoring the patient's weight, supported and encouraged to work as a team, and absolved from any responsibility for causing AN. The adolescent patient is helped to align with his or her siblings for support. In the first session of this phase, the therapist engages the family in therapy, obtains each member's perspective on how AN is affecting the family, and obtains preliminary information about how the family functions (e.g., coalitions, authority structure, conflicts). After greeting each family member in a courteous and serious manner and listening to all perspectives on the problems, the therapist separates the illness from the patient, emphasizing how AN has taken over the adolescent's life but does not identify the patient (e.g., the adolescent has an identity apart from AN). Then, in a nonblameful manner, the therapist raises the parents' anxiety about the dire consequences of this serious disorder, culminating in charging the parents with the task of weight restoration. Specific advice about calories and food and the details of restoring the patient's weight are not given; the therapist appeals instead to the parents' intuitive knowledge about good nutrition and supports their explorations and attempts at weight restoration. At the end of the session, the parents are instructed to bring food for everyone to the next session, including a portion for the patient that meets the nutritional requirements to begin the process of reversing weight loss.

The second session involves a family meal. The parents are asked to convince their teenager to eat at least one mouthful more than she is prepared to. To support the parents in this difficult task and help them succeed when they believe they cannot, the therapist will emphasize a persistent effort on their part, one that sends a clear message to the adolescent that her parents will persevere in their insistence that she eat adequate amounts of nutritious food. For instance, the therapist can suggest that the parents sit on either side of the patient, put on her plate exactly what they think she should eat, and then kindly yet firmly encourage her to eat. The therapist coaches the parents by urging them to make repetitive and insistent suggestions as to how to act uniformly so that the teenager will eat. The therapist also notes that there are few alternatives available, and the parents must be prepared to persevere until their child eats and to repeat this effort frequently. The siblings have a very specific role to play that does not involve mealtimes. They are asked to align with the adolescent and provide support by spending time with him or her in age-appropriate endeavors, which can include activities such as surfing the Internet, watching a favorite television program, or merely sharing a joke.

The remaining three to 10 sessions of phase 1 continue to focus on helping the parents refeed the patient. After an initial weigh-in, the therapist reviews with the parents their attempts at refeeding to systematically advise them how to proceed in controlling the influence of the eating disorder on the patient. Parental teamwork is strongly reinforced, and siblings are urged to continue providing support to the patient outside mealtimes.

Phase 2: Negotiating for a New Pattern of Relationships

The patient's surrender to her parents' demands to increase food intake, accompanied by steady weight gain, as well as the parents' relief after having taken charge of the eating disorder signal readiness to start phase 2 of treatment. More specifically, the patient is ready for phase 2 when weight is at a minimum of 87% of ideal body weight, the patient is able to eat without undue cajoling by parents, and the parents report they feel empowered in the refeeding process. As was the case in phase 1, the main task of phase 2 is to return the adolescent to physical health. To accomplish this goal, the therapist continues to support and assist the parents in managing weight restoration and the eating-disordered symptoms but changes from direct coaching to a more supportive role in helping them continue with weight restoration.

When the patient is approaching an ideal body weight and the therapist judges that this improvement will likely continue with less parental supervision, the therapist assists the parents and adolescent in bringing about a careful, mutually agreed-upon return of age-appropriate responsibility over eating to the adolescent. This process is tailored to each family's unique rituals or habits of regular eating activities before the eating disorder changed the family's mealtimes.

When eating is no longer the primary focus of discussion, it is time for the therapist and family to begin examining adolescent development issues. The patient is strongly encouraged to engage in age-appropriate socialization with same- and opposite-sex peers. The therapist coaches the adolescent to plan peer activities and become involved in dating and prompts the family to problem solve how eating will be handled during peer activities (e.g., how the adolescent will make wise food choices at restaurants and at friends' homes). Phase 2 usually lasts two to six sessions, which are scheduled at 2- to 3-week intervals.

Phase 3: Adolescent Issues and Termination

During this final, brief phase of FBT, the therapist continues the focus on adolescent developmental issues, actively prompts the family to problem solve these issues, continues to refocus the parents on their own relationship, and gradually terminates treatment. Phase 3 typically lasts two to four sessions, with intervals stretched to 4–6 weeks. The family is ready for phase 3 when the patient's weight is under control (95–100% of ideal body weight) and the responsibility for eating has been successfully transferred. The therapist begins by giving the parents a primer of adolescent development. Then specific issues pertinent to the patient are identified (e.g., choice of friends, dating, curfew, chores, college planning, sex, parent–teen relationships issues), and the family is helped to problem solve them. All of these issues are directly discussed without reference to the eating disorder. At the same time, the parents are pushed into more activities as a couple so that they can defocus on caring for their now-recovering adolescent. In the last session, the therapist anticipates and plans for future problems, listens carefully to each family member's feedback regarding the therapy experience, and thanks them for their participation.

COMPARISON OF BFST AND FBT

Table 22.1 compares BFST and FBT. These two interventions are similar in that they both adhere to the six key elements of effective family therapy outlined earlier in this chapter. However, they differ in certain respects:

TABLE 22.1. A Comparison of Behavioral Family System Therapy and Family-Based Treatment

Variable	BFST	FBT
Place parents in charge of restoring weight	X	X
Refrain from blaming	X	X
Parents and adolescent attend sessions together	X	X
Entire family (e.g., siblings too) attend sessions together		X
Eating, weight restoration direct focus of discussion	X	X
Gradually return control over eating to adolescent during maintenance	X	X
Emphasize adolescent development issues after weight restoration	X	X
Dietician is regularly involved	X	
Give parents detailed instructions for behavioral weight gain program	X	
Use cognitive restructuring for body image concerns, distorted thinking	X	
Includes a family meal session		X

1. BFST always involves a dietician, who outlines the foods to be eaten and adjusts them as the adolescent gains weight. In contrast, FBT involves a dietician only as consultant to the treatment team.
2. In BFST the therapist provides parents with a detailed structure of a behavioral weight gain program, including stimulus control over the eating setting and positive incentives for eating the required foods. In FBT the therapist appeals to parents' intuitive knowledge of good nutrition, does not delineate a structured eating regimen, and does not systematically program positive incentives contingent on appropriate eating.
3. BFST includes cognitive restructuring surrounding extreme cognitions and body image distortions; FBT does not.
4. In FBT the entire family is encouraged to attend all sessions, whereas in BFST patient and the parents attend all BFST sessions, with only occasional sibling involvement.
5. On average, BFST takes longer than FBT.
6. FBT includes a family meal session. BFST does not; instead, the therapist systematically assesses home-based family meals.

These differences arose because the two therapies heralded from different traditions, FBT from a strategic/structural adolescent developmental framework and BFST from a cognitive-behavioral framework with a strategic/structural component added. To date, no research has examined whether these differences impact the outcomes of family intervention for adolescents with AN. Future researchers are urged to evaluate whether such differences matter and, if so, for what subgroups of eating disordered patients.

EVIDENCE ON THE EFFECTS OF TREATMENT

Since our own earlier review (Le Grange & Lock, 2005), five randomized controlled trials (RCTs) of family therapy for AN have been published and most have been relatively small (Table 22.2). In the first and perhaps most influential of these, Russell, Szmukler, Dare, and Eisler (1987) at the Maudsley Hospital in London tested the relative efficacy of family therapy and individual supportive therapy in maintaining weight gain as a follow-up treatment posthospitalization. A total sample of 80 patients of all ages was prospectively subdivided into four subgroups based on patient diagnosis or age or both. All patients were first admitted for weight restoration to the inpatient program for a mean of 10 weeks. After discharge, patients were randomly allocated to either outpatient family therapy or individual control treatment. For the purposes of this discussion, we focus on the first of the four subgroups, which comprised 21 adolescents with AN. For all, age of onset was 18 years or younger and duration of illness was less than 3 years. Although the findings were inconclusive for adolescents with AN who had been ill for more than 3 years (subgroup 2), adults with AN (subgroup 3), or patients with a diagnosis of bulimia nervosa (BN; subgroup 4), findings for patients in the first subgroup favored family therapy. Outcome was defined by a composite score that took both biological (weight and menses) and psychological (psychosocial and psychosexual development) markers into account. At 5-year follow-up, adolescents in this subgroup, who received family therapy, continued to do well, with 90% having a good outcome (Eisler et al., 1997). Although adolescents who had received the individual control treatment also continued to improve, almost half of this group still had significant eating disorder symptoms at follow-up. This follow-up study was the first to demonstrate that the benefits of family therapy were maintained 5 years posttreatment.

Building on this seminal work from Russell and his group, three subsequent studies compared different forms of family interventions. In the first of these, and also from the Maudsley group, Le Grange, Eisler, Dare, and Russell (1992) in a pilot study (*N* = 18) and Eisler et al. (2000) in a larger RCT (*N* = 40) compared conjoint family therapy (CFT) and separated family therapy (SFT) among a total of 58 patients. The treatment goals for

TABLE 22.2. Completed Randomized Controlled Trials using Family Treatments for Adolescent Anorexia Nervosa

Study	N	Mean age	Treatment	Duration	Mean sessions	End treatment outcome (Morgan–Russell: good + intermediate)
Russell et al. (1987)	21	15.3	Conj FBT vs. IT	10.3 weeks	13	Conj FBT, 90%; IT, 18% $p < .02$
Le Grange et al. (1992)	18	15.3	Conj FBT vs. Sep FBT	6 months	9	Overall 68% NS
Robin et al. (1999)	37	13.9	BFST vs. EOIT	1–1.5 yrs	47	BFST, 94%; EOIT, 65% $p < .05$
Eisler et al. (2000)	40	15.5	Conj FBT vs. Sep FBT	1 year	16	Overall 63% NS
Lock et al. (2005)	86	15.1	Low-dose FBT vs. high-dose FBT	6 months vs. 12 months	10 vs. 20	Overall 90% NS

Note. Conj BFT, conjoint family-based treatment; IT, individual therapy; Sep FBT, separated family-based treatment; BFST, behavioral family systems therapy; EOIT, ego-oriented individual therapy.

CFT and SFT were the same. However, in SFT the same therapist first met separately with the adolescent before meeting with the parents separately in another session. In contrast to the Russell et al. (1987) study, patients were not hospitalized; both treatments were provided on an outpatient basis. Overall, results were similar for both the Le Grange and Eisler studies, with significant improvements in the primary outcome measure reported for patients in both CFT and SFT. Utilizing the Morgan and Russell outcome criteria to assess weight, menses, and individual psychological functioning, more than 60% of patients were classified as having a good or intermediate outcome posttreatment irrespective of type of family therapy. However, families with high levels of parental criticism (as defined by expressed emotion) did worse in CFT. On the other hand, significantly more change was demonstrated for CFT in terms of both individual psychological and family functioning (Eisler et al., 2000). As was the case in the first RCT (i.e., Russell et al., 1987), patients continued to improve after the treatment ended and at 5-year follow-up, the majority had a good (75%) or intermediate (15%) outcome, with only 10% failing to respond to treatment (Eisler, Simic, Russell, & Dare, 2007).

In a design that shares some similarities with these Maudsley studies, Robin and colleagues (1999) in Detroit compared CFT (BFST) with ego-oriented individual therapy (EOIT) in 38 adolescents with AN. BFST has been discussed in some detail earlier in this chapter. The comparison treatment in this RCT (i.e., EOIT) comprised weekly individual sessions for the adolescent and bimonthly collateral sessions with the parents. We have carefully highlighted the similarities and differences between BFST and FBT in the prior discussion. EOIT is superficially similar to SFT, although the aims are quite different whereas SFT emphasizes helping parents take a strong role in the management of the symptoms, EOIT aims to help parents relinquish control over their child's eating and prepares them to accept a more assertive adolescent. The similarities between EOIT and SFT are equally important. Both treatments provide the adolescent with regular individual therapy in which he or she has the opportunity to address personal and relationship issues as well as matters directly related to eating difficulties. Although the parallel sessions with the parents differ in frequency and content, both treatments encourage parents to take an active and supportive role in their child's recovery and to reflect on some of the family dynamics that might have gotten caught up with the eating disorder.

Posttreatment results demonstrated significant improvements for both BFST and EOIT, with 67% of patients reaching target weight and 80% regaining menstruation. Patients continued to improve during the follow-up period, and at 1-year follow-up approximately 75% had reached their target weight and 85% were menstruating (Robin et al., 1999). In terms of physiological improvements, changes in weight and menses were superior for patients in BFST at posttreatment and follow-up. As for psychological measures (i.e., eating attitudes, mood, self-reported eating-related family conflict), improvements were comparable for the two groups. In an offshoot of their study, Robin, Siegel, and Moye (1995) also reported results of observational ratings of family interaction. These researchers demonstrated a significant decrease in maternal negative communication as well as a corresponding increase in positive communication in BFST but not in EOIT.

Some of the differences between Robin et al.'s Detroit (BFST) study and Le Grange et al.'s Maudsley (FBT) study, already alluded to, could also have had an impact on outcome. First, in Robin et al., patients at less than 75% of ideal body weight (IBW) were hospitalized at the outset of treatment (almost half the sample) and remained in the inpatient setting until they have achieved 80% IBW. In contrast, the second-generation Maudsley studies were conducted on an outpatient basis, and patients were admitted to the inpatient unit only if outpatient therapy failed to arrest weight loss (four of 58 were admitted during the study). Second, the duration and dose intensity of treatment were lower in the Maudsley studies (6–12 months of treatment with a mean of ~10 sessions) than in the Detroit study (12–18 months of treatment with a mean of ~30 sessions). Finally, compared with the Detroit group, patients from the Maudsley studies appeared to have been ill for a longer period, the majority had had previous treatment, and a higher percentage were suffering from depression.

Improvements in the design of treatment studies to follow this early work were made possible by a manualized form of the family therapy originally developed by Dare and Eisler and their group in London. This treatment is called Family-Based Treatment for AN (FBT-AN) in its manualized format and was discussed in more detail earlier in this chapter. The process of manualizing this treatment was outlined by Lock and Le Grange (2001), and more extensive details about the goals and techniques of this therapy are provided in the clinician's manual, also authored by the same team (Lock et al., 2001). The first study to utilize FBT-AN was conducted by Lock, Agras, Bryson, and Helena (2005). These authors examined the treatment dose among 86 adolescents and found that a brief 6-month 10-session version of FBT-AN was as effective as a year-long 20-session version. However, the longer version was superior for two groups of patients: (1) those who came from nonintact families and (2) those who presented with higher levels of obsessions and compulsions about eating. Findings at 4-year follow-up were encouraging in that FBT-AN was equally effective regardless of treatment dose. Moreover, at follow-up about two-thirds of patients achieved healthy body weights and had Eating Disorder Examination scores within the normal range (Lock, Couturier, Agras, & Bryson, 2006).

As a result of the development of this clinician's manual, three groups in the United States utilized case series data to demonstrate that manualized FBT-AN (1) is feasible and effective for consecutive patients referred to a specialist eating disorder clinic (Le Grange, Binford, & Loeb, 2005), (2) can be disseminated and administered by investigators other than its developers (Loeb et al., 2007), and (3) appears to be as effective for children as it is for adolescents (Lock et al., 2006). FBT-AN has also been adapted to treat adolescent BN (FBT-BN) in the form of a clinical manual and has been evaluated in an RCT (Le Grange, Crosby, Rathouz, & Leventhal, 2007). This RCT compared FBT-BN with supportive psychotherapy (SPT) and found the family treatment to have both a statistical and a clinical advantage over SPT in terms of the primary outcome measure (i.e., binge and purge abstinence).

DIRECTIONS FOR RESEARCH

The evidence to date supports family therapy for this patient population. However, enthusiasm for this approach to treatment should be tempered because the positive findings may, at least in part, be due to the lack of research on other treatments. Ego-oriented, cognitive, and psychodynamic treatments have all been described in the literature. With the exception of the former, however, these treatments have not been systematically evaluated with adolescent AN. Consequently, their relative merits in comparison with a family-based approach are not known. Likewise, little systematic evidence is available that can guide us in deciding the suitability of a family-based approach for one family as opposed to another. Until more information is available regarding mediators and moderators of treatment, our clinical experience leads us to proceed with caution before engaging in therapy when there is (1) significant parental psychopathology, such as an active eating disorder or a severe mood disorder; (2) serious discord between parents, enough to precipitate discussions about divorce because differences between the spouses are seen as irreconcilable; and (3) significant challenges in terms of the typical logistical resources that can aid parents in engaging in treatment and fulfill the rather high expectations in terms of time and energy requirements.

Efforts are now underway to overcome some of the shortcomings in the evidence base. Researchers at Maudsley Hospital in London are about to complete a systematic evaluation of the effectiveness of a multiple-family day treatment program, a promising new treatment development described in some detail elsewhere (see Le Grange & Eisler, 2009). Additional projects also in progress are an adaptation of FBT for early intervention in subsyndromal AN (Katharine Loeb, PhD, Mount Sinai Medical Center New York), a parent group format of FBT for adolescent AN (Nancy Zucker, PhD, Duke University, Raleigh-Durham, NC), an adaptation of FBT for young adults with AN (Daniel le Grange, PhD, and Eunice Chen, PhD, University of Chicago), and FBT for pediatric overweight (Katharine Loeb, PhD, Mount Sinai Medical Center and Daniel le Grange, PhD, University of Chicago).

CONCLUSIONS

The studies discussed in this chapter consistently show that adolescents with AN respond well to treatment when their parents are included in these efforts. If family therapy is implemented, inpatient treatment can usually be avoided, with between 50–75% of weight restored by the end of treatment. However, most patients will not have started or resumed menses. Three follow-up studies have now been published and consistently show that 4–5 years after family therapy the majority of patients (80–90%) will have fully recovered and only 10–15% will still be seriously ill (Eisler et al., 1997, 2007; Lock et al., 2006).

Any comparison between different kinds of family interventions ought to be interpreted with caution given the small number of such studies as well as the relatively small sample size included. Notwithstanding, treatments that promote parents' active role in challenging their child's AN seem most effective and may have benefits over treatments in which parents are involved in a supportive role but are nevertheless encouraged to step back from the eating problem. For instance, the initial RCT for AN has shown that excluding parents from treatment (i.e., the individual supportive psychotherapy) leads to a deleterious outcome and may even delay recovery to a considerable degree (Russell et al., 1987; Eisler et al., 1997). Another advantage of seeing families in conjoint format appears to be that both family and individual psychological issues are addressed. However, this form of family intervention may be disadvantageous for families with high levels of parental hostility or criticism directed at the adolescent with AN (Le Grange et al., 1992). Although such families may perhaps be more difficult to engage in family treatment, this challenge is exacerbated when the family is seen as a whole. One reason for this scenario might be that feelings of guilt and blame are increased as a consequence of criticisms or confrontations occurring during family sessions. Our clinical experience suggests that conjoint sessions may be more useful for these families at a stage in treatment when the concerns about eating disorder symptoms have dissipated. In the meantime, clinicians may be well advised to utilize the separated format of this treatment for such families (Eisler et al., 2000; Le Grange et al., 1992). It is important to note, however, that the differences between the various forms of family therapy that have been studied are relatively small, especially when compared with improvements on the whole.

Notwithstanding, reviewers recently concluded that there is convincing evidence for the effectiveness of family interventions for adolescents with AN (e.g., Le Grange & Lock, 2005). Given the status of the current available evidence, although limited, a family-based approach is probably the treatment of choice for most adolescents with AN who have been ill for a relative brief period (i.e., less than 3 years) and who are medically stable for outpatient treatment.

REFERENCES

American Psychiatric Association (2000). *Diagnostic and statistical manual of mental disorders* (4th ed., text rev.). Washington, DC: Author.

Eisler, I., Dare, C., Hodes, M., Russell, G. F. M., Dodge, E., & Le Grange, D. (2000). Family therapy for adolescent anorexia nervosa: The results of a controlled comparison of two family interventions. *Journal of Child Psychology and Psychiatry, 41,* 727–736.

Eisler, I., Dare, C., Russell, G. F. M., Szmukler, G.I., Le Grange, D., & Dodge, E. (1997). Family and individual therapy in anorexia nervosa: A five-year follow-up. *Archives of General Psychiatry, 54,* 1025–1030.

Eisler, I., Simic, M., Russell, G., & Dare, C. (2007). A randomized controlled treatment trial of two forms of family therapy in adolescent anorexia nervosa: A five-year follow-up. *Journal of Child Psychology and Psychiatry, 48,* 552–560.

Fisher, M., Golden, N. H., Katzman, D. K., Kreipe, R. E., Rees, J., Schebendach, J., et al. (1995). Eating disorders in adolescents: A background paper. *Journal of Adolescent Health, 16,* 420–437.

Le Grange, D., Binford, R., & Loeb, K. (2005). Manualized family-based treatment for anorexia nervosa: A case series. *Journal of the American Academy of Child and Adolescent Psychiatry, 44,* 41–46.

Le Grange, D., Crosby, R. D., Rathouz, P. J., & Leventhal, B. L. (2007). A randomized controlled comparison of family-based treatment and supportive psychotherapy for adolescent bulimia nervosa. *Archives of General Psychiatry, 64,* 1049–1056.

Le Grange, D., & Eisler, I. (2009). Family interventions in adolescent anorexia nervosa. *Child and Adolescent Psychiatric Clinics of North America, 18,* 159–173.

Le Grange, D., Eisler, I., Dare, C., & Russell, G. F. M. (1992). Evaluation of family treatments in adolescent anorexia nervosa: A pilot study. *International Journal of Eating Disorders, 12,* 347–357.

Le Grange, D., & Lock, J. (2005). The dearth of psychological treatment studies for anorexia nervosa. *International Journal of Eating Disorders, 37,* 79–91.

Lock, J., Agras, W. S., Bryson, S., & Helena, K. (2005). A comparison of short- and long-term family therapy for adolescent anorexia nervosa. *Journal of the American Academy of Child and Adolescent Psychiatry, 44,* 632–639.

Lock, J., Couturier, J., Agras, W. S., & Bryson, S. (2006). Comparison of long-term outcomes in adolescents with anorexia nervosa treated with family therapy. *Journal of the American Academy of Child and Adolescent Psychiatry, 45,* 666–672.

Lock, J., & Le Grange, D. (2001). Can family-based treatment of anorexia nervosa be manualized? *Journal of Psychotherapy Practice and Research, 10,* 253–261.

Lock, J., Le Grange, D., Agras, W. S., & Dare, C. (2001). *Treatment manual for anorexia nervosa: A family-based approach.* New York: Guilford Press.

Loeb, K. L., Walsh, B. T., Lock, J., Le Grange, D., Jones, J., Marcus, S., et al. (2007). Open trial of family-based treatment for adolescent anorexia nervosa: Evidence of successful dissemination. *Journal of the American Academy of Child and Adolescent Psychiatry, 46,* 792–800.

Robin, A. L., Siegel, P. T., & Moye, A. (1995). Family versus individual therapy for anorexia: Impact on family conflict. *International Journal of Eating Disorders, 17,* 313–322.

Robin, A. L., Siegel, P. T., Moye, A. W., Gilroy, M., Dennis, A. B., & Sikand, A. (1999). A controlled comparison of family versus individual therapy for adolescents with anorexia nervosa. *Journal of the American Academy of Child and Adolescent Psychiatry, 38,* 1428–1429.

Russell, G. F. M., Szmukler, G. I., Dare, C., & Eisler, I. (1987). An evaluation of family therapy in anorexia nervosa and bulimia nervosa. *Archives of General Psychiatry, 44,* 1047–1056.

23

Behavioral Treatment for Enuresis

ARTHUR C. HOUTS

OVERVIEW

Bedwetting is a problem for 1 of every 10 secondary school-age children. The prevalence at 6 years of age is about 15% and declines to about 1% among 18-year-olds. Only 15 of every 100 will outgrow the problem in a year. Continued bedwetting leads to restricted social activities, embarrassment about a family secret, and diminished confidence. Given that a 4-month course of treatment can permanently fix the problem in about 75% of children, this treatment should be pursued once a child is 6 years old. I have never met or heard of a child who preferred to keep wetting. Unfortunately, most parents do not know what to do, and many get bad advice from professionals.

Of the 7 to 10 million bedwetting children in the United States, about 85% are monosymptomatic primary enuretics (MPEs). They have no medical problems, they wet only at night, and they have never been dry for at least 6 consecutive months. MPEs are ideal candidates for behavioral treatment. Children who have daytime wetting need more medical attention and may enter behavioral treatment when the daytime wetting is resolved. Children with this secondary bedwetting also need more careful evaluation for distress associated with the return of bedwetting.

All children should receive a basic physical examination and urinalysis. Consultation with a pediatric urologist can be useful to obtain a bladder and renal sonogram. Again, 90% of children will have no medical complications, but no one wants children to fail behavioral treatment because an easily curable infection was overlooked.

Active Avoidance Learning and the Urine Alarm

All children start out wetting the bed, and most stop without special help. On average, children attain daytime control of urination at 2½ years of age, and nighttime control generally follows within 1 year. Regular bedwetting beyond age 4 may indicate that the developmental window for acquiring the responses needed to be dry at night was missed. For practical reasons, behavioral treatment is generally not instituted until a child is at least 5 years old. Children get control either by waking up to go to the toilet or by physically inhibiting urination while asleep. Learning either response is facilitated by the natural discomfort of a wet bed. If for any number of reasons (e.g., failure to arouse, not feeling the discomfort from prolonged use of disposable underpants or diapers) a child repeatedly fails to respond to the aversive conditions of nature, he or she will fail to learn the physical responses needed to be dry. Continued wetting, then, is a failure to learn how to be dry from natural conditions. From a biobehavioral perspective, MPE is caused by an interaction between delays in physical development that are genetically transmitted and behavioral histories that delay active avoidance responses (e.g., waking or pelvic floor contraction in sleep; Houts, 1991; Lovibond, 1963).

Urine alarm treatment re-creates conditions to perform an active avoidance response to inhibit urination (details of the procedure are shown in Figure 23.1 and discussed later). Urination starts with contraction of the bladder detrussor muscle, and this contraction can be stopped by actively contracting the muscles of the pelvic floor. The alarm is an aversive stimulus that produces a conditioned avoidance response of contracting the pelvic floor along with the external sphincter of the bladder neck. This avoidance response is maintained by negative reinforcement. So long as the response is made, the child avoids having to wake and avoids wetting the bed. This model is consistent with findings from nighttime recording of pelvic floor activity. Norgaard observed that when wetting was avoided, children interrupted detrussor contractions by spontaneously contracting pelvic floor muscles (Norgaard, 1989). In contrast, wetting without arousal was preceded by relaxation of the pelvic floor. When wetting was avoided, children were inhibiting bladder contractions by spontaneously contracting the pelvic floor.

With alarm treatment, pelvic floor activity that occurs when a child either arouses to or sleeps through the sensation of a full bladder is a conditioned response produced by startling the child with the alarm. The sound of the alarm startles the child and causes contraction of the pelvic floor. Over time, this physiological response gets conditioned to detrussor contractions associated with a full bladder. The conditioned pelvic floor contraction is maintained to avoid being startled and having to awaken. We obtained indirect evidence for this formulation in a study of children who completed daytime pelvic floor electromyography (EMG) assessments over the course of urine alarm treatment. Compared with those who failed to become completely dry, those who did become dry showed a steady increase in average peak voltage over the 16-week course of treatment even though their initial muscular response was weaker. The EMG assessments confirmed that muscle conditioning did, in fact, occur in those children who became dry. Responders compared with nonresponders appeared to acquire more pelvic floor reactivity and responsiveness (Scott, 1993). These findings support the view that the urine alarm works by training the child to make an inhibitory pelvic floor response during sleep. More direct confirmation can be obtained by future investigations assessing pelvic floor reactivity during sleep as urine alarm treatment progresses.

Bladder Capacity and Maintenance of Dry Nights

Some bedwetting may be due to developmental delays in bladder capacity. In our original formulation of full-spectrum home training (FSHT), we regarded this problem as a complicating factor rather than a primary cause. Subsequent evidence has suggested that there may be a small proportion of children whose bedwetting is due primarily to the fact that their bladders cannot accommodate the volume of urine produced at night. These are likely children who wet multiple times each night, and they are likely to be that small proportion who actually do fail to produce normal amounts of antidiuretic hormone at night. Whether one approaches this from the standpoint of increasing capacity or reducing the volume produced, such techniques alone are not sufficient (Houts, Berman, & Abramson, 1994); the alarm is essential.

If nothing is done to prevent relapse, relapse after successful urine alarm treatment may be as high as 40% within a year. In FSHT we address the problem by incorporating overlearning. In early studies, we followed standard procedure of having the child consume 16 ounces of water immediately before bedtime. This started after the child attained 14 consecutive dry nights and continued until the child attained another 14 in a row. We replicated previous findings of cutting the relapse rate in half, from 40% to 20% (Young & Morgan, 1972). Most recently, we modified overlearning to gradually increase the amount of water consumed. This gradual overlearning has reduced the relapse rate in half once again, from 20% down to just less than 10%.

Family Involvement

As with any child problem, behavioral treatment for bedwetting requires concerted and cooperative effort from the family. The most demanding part of FSHT is training children to wake to the alarm within the first 4 weeks. Many children require parental assistance. Parents have to wake the children and require them to get out of bed before turning off the alarm. Cooperation and firm resolve are essential. Children, too, have to be ready to do the hard work.

Fortunately, most MPEs come from families with resources and skills. Enuresis is not an epidemiological marker for family dysfunction. Obviously, where there is significant marital discord, extreme distress, chaotic family structure, parental neglect or abuse, or significant child conduct disorder, such problems must be resolved before implementing treatment. Routine use of screening instruments for marital distress and child conduct disorder can identify such problematic cases.

CHARACTERISTICS OF TREATMENT

FSHT includes four components: (1) basic urine alarm treatment, (2) cleanliness training, (3) retention control training, and (4) overlearning. Components are presented in a manual for parents to follow, and a contract between parents and children forms the basis for implementing the treatment.[1]

The Family Support Agreement

The parents and child complete the family support agreement as a trainer illustrates each step (see Figure 23.1). The children follows the rule to get out of bed and stand up before turning off the alarm. Parents are told never to turn off the alarm for the child. The steps involved in cleanliness training are displayed on a wall chart (Daily Steps to a Dry Bed) placed in the child's bedroom. The chart also displays a record of progress

1. John and Mom and Dad agree to do the training just like it is described in order to reach the goal of a dry bed.
2. Everyone agrees to follow the program for at least 84 days (12 weeks). Children who wet more than once a night will probably take longer to be completely dry.
3. The whole family agrees not to punish, scold, ridicule, or say anything negative about "bedwetting" during the training.
4. Both parents and child understand that training is most effective when the child is not overtired or stressed. Therefore, John and Mom and Dad agree that 8:30 P.M. is a reasonable bedtime, and John agrees to go to bed at that time every night.
5. NO RESTRICTIONS ON LIQUIDS. John will be allowed to drink as much liquid as desired at all times.
6. Parents and family agree to provide support, help, and understanding to John. They will praise him when dry and provide encouragement that progress will be made. However, they understand that the training itself includes sufficient pressure and agree they will not urge him to try harder or do better.
7. Parents and family agree not to complain about the effects of the training on them or about the urine alarm but to support and help instead. John also agrees not to complain about the training and to cooperate fully.
8. The family will provide a relatively stress-free environment at home during training. During the training, parents will not ask the child to do extra jobs around the house.
9. John and Mom and Dad agree to participate in self-control training once a day during the hours of 4:30 and 6:30 P.M. as explained in the Parent Guide. Parents will give John money for each success according to the Reward Schedule for Self-Control Training.
10. John agrees to follow the procedure of cleanliness training as outlined on the wall chart and to put wet sheets and underwear in the clothes hamper in his room. Parents agree to keep clean sheets and clean underwear in the dresser in John's room for him to use when remaking the bed.
11. Parents agree to wake John immediately if the buzzer rings and he does not wake up. IT IS ESSENTIAL THAT THE PERSON RESPONSIBLE FOR WAKING THE CHILD WILL BE ABLE TO HEAR AND BE AWAKENED BY THE ALARM. NOTHING ELSE SHOULD BE DONE TO WAKE THE CHILD DURING THE NIGHT. The alarm must do this.
12. Parents agree to check the batteries regularly and to have replacement batteries ready when needed.
13. John and Mom and Dad agree that ONLY John WILL TOUCH THE ALARM, except for alarm testing as described previously.
14. Parents agree to assume all responsibilities associated with training for a dry bed as spelled out in the Parent Guide. John agrees to follow the Daily Steps to a Dry Bed outlined on the wall chart.
15. OVERLEARNING. When John has been dry for 14 consecutive nights, the overlearning procedures will be followed until the child is dry for 14 more nights in a row. Overlearning will be explained when the child attains 14 dry nights in a row.
16. It is understood that every child has an occasional wet bed, especially when sick or under stress. DO NOT WORRY ABOUT THIS. TELL YOUR CHILD NOT TO WORRY.

FIGURE 23.1. Completed example of the family support agreement of full-spectrum home training.

and is colored in as either wet or dry for each day. Parents are instructed to have the child go through with the full procedure of remaking the bed even if the sheets are not wet, something that typically happens in the latter part of training. A child may be very difficult to arouse in the first 4 weeks. It is imperative that the child be awakened so that he or she turns off the alarm. Even if this means that a parent must share the room with the child early on, training the child to awaken to the alarm is crucial. It is important to give parents an easy way to determine whether their child is truly awake. Short-term memory tasks such as choosing a password each night before bedtime or asking the child to spell a familiar word backward are simple ways to determine whether the child is fully awake.

Retention control training is done once a day, and the child is given money for postponing urination for increasing amounts of time in a step-by-step fashion up to a 45-minute holding time. The total amount of money the child receives for reaching all 15 3-minute incremented goals is $12.00. The child is encouraged to save the money in a prominent place as a reminder of the accomplishments. Retention control training ends when the child attains the 45-minute goal, typically within 3 weeks.

The first goal of treatment is to attain 14 consecutive dry nights. This takes an average of 8–12 weeks. For children who wet more than once a night, the average time is 16–20 weeks. Overlearning begins immediately and is an essential ingredient for preventing relapse.

Our gradual overlearning begins by determining a maximum amount of water. The maximum is 1 ounce for each year of age plus 2 ounces. For example, the maximum amount for an 8-year-old child is 10 ounces. Children begin by drinking 4 ounces of water 15 minutes before bedtime. If they remain dry for two nights while drinking 4 ounces, the amount increases to 6 ounces. If they remain dry for two nights at 6 ounces, the amount is increased to 8 ounces. The water increases continue in this fashion—2 ounces more for every 2 consecutive dry nights—until the children's maximum reached. The children continue to drink this maximum until 14 consecutive dry nights are attained. In the event children wet, and most do at least once, a simple rule is followed: They go back to whatever amount was consumed on the immediate last dry night and continue with that amount until there are 5 nights in a row dry. If the children are not already at the maximum, the procedure continues as before increasing by 2 ounces for every 2 dry nights. The goal remains 14 consecutive dry nights during overlearning. Some children end up having all 14 at the maximum amount, but this is not required for the relapse prevention effect.

Optional Waking Schedule

Occasionally, it may be necessary to disrupt the child's sleep routine with a waking schedule to achieve 14 consecutive dry nights. Parents are told to wake their child hourly using a minimal amount of prompting throughout the first night. Each time the child is awakened, he or she is praised for a dry bed and encouraged to void in the toilet. Any time the child wets the bed and consequently activates the alarm, the cleanliness training program is followed. The second night the child is awakened only once, 3 hours after falling asleep. From the second night forward, the waking schedule continues, with the child being awakened only once each night. Following a dry night, the parents wake the child 30 minutes earlier than the previous night. If the child wets during the night, then the time of waking remains the same as the previous night. The nightly waking schedule ends when the scheduled time for awakening the child is 30 minutes immediately following bedtime. The waking schedule resumes only if the child has two or more wet nights in 7 days. When resumption is necessary, the waking schedule begins at 3 hours after bedtime and decreases in the same manner (Azrin, Sneed, & Foxx, 1973; Bollard & Nettelbeck, 1982). The waking schedule is not a routine part of FSHT and is indicated only when there are extreme difficulties training a child to awaken to the alarm.

Minimal-Visit and Multiple-Visit Protocols

We have implemented this treatment in single-visit and dual-visit protocols with comparable results. In the single-visit protocol, the entire program is covered in one 90-minute session where the parents and child complete the family support agreement and observe a demonstration for each component. In the dual-visit protocol, the first nine items of the family support agreement are covered. This takes about 30 minutes. The remaining 30 minutes are devoted to building rapport and presenting information about bedwetting. This information emphasizes the learning basis of the therapy and the fact that learning the new skills will take time and patience on the part of everyone. In the second 60-minute visit, the preceding week's records for retention control training are reviewed, and the alarm is demonstrated. The family then continues retention control training and begins the urine alarm procedures.

Regardless of how the treatment is introduced, follow-up contact is important. We have achieved good results with minimal contact such as having biweekly phone contact. Somewhat better results can be expected with more therapist contact. This can take the schedule of two initial visits followed by a 30-minute visit within the first 2 weeks of starting the alarm. Thereafter, half-hour visits can be scheduled about every 3 weeks to provide encouragement and to solve minor problems. We have also implemented the protocol where the start of overlearning triggers a return visit. FSHT can be implemented with as few as one or two visits. Rarely have I ever conducted the treatment with more than six visits over the course of 16–20 weeks.

Group and Individual Session Formats

FSHT has been successfully delivered in both group and individual formats. As summarized next, we have replicated the effectiveness of group-administered FSHT in a series of five studies. With the exception of differing relapse rates as a result of different forms of overlearning, outcomes were comparable. In these studies, families attended group training sessions held in university classrooms large enough to accommodate up to 10 families at a single demonstration. Presentations to adolescents differ in terms of how much control the child is given. In most cases, these young people are highly motivated and want to train themselves with minimal assistance from adults.

Individual administration of FSHT has been conducted by numerous practitioners who requested and used the treatment materials over the past 20 years.[2] In that same period, I collected effectiveness data on individual administration using both single-visit and dual-visit initial sessions. Those outcome data are presented later and suggest results comparable to group administration.

Reinforcing Accomplishments and Reducing Frustrations

Although we have shown that effective behavioral treatment can be delivered in a cost-efficient manner using minimal contact groups, it is important to note that our study protocols always included regular contact with the child and family, even if that contact was confined to phone consultations. Again, the major weakness of any behavioral treatment is lack of compliance. General therapeutic skills and practical problem solving are needed to forestall noncompliance and dropout.

A focus on reinforcing accomplishments during treatment is very helpful. Children who wet multiple times each night are easily discouraged. These families need to understand that it will take 12–16 weeks as opposed to the average of 8–12 weeks for the child to get the first 14 consecutive dry nights. Informing such children that their first goal is to get from multiple wettings to a single wetting episode each night adjusts their expectations and prevents some of the frustration.

Pointing out that progress can be measured by monitoring the size of wet spots helps to focus on the process and recognize that even though every night has been a "wet night," the child is responding more readily to the alarm. As the size of the wet spot gets smaller and smaller, the child is learning to make the active avoidance response sooner and sooner. Dry nights are sure to follow. In focusing on the goal of 14 consecutive dry nights, the parents and child often need to be reminded of the overall picture. Even though a child may not have reached the 14-night goal, he or she may have been 90% dry for the past 6 weeks. This can give the family a positive perspective and encouragement to proceed.

Many children enjoy the challenge of overcoming bedwetting, and it is easy to engage their competitive spirit. Some bring their wall charts to follow-up visits to show off their work. Others set goals of beating the 42-day record for completing FSHT. So long as their goals are not outlandish and beyond reach, this energetic approach to eliminating the problem is welcomed because the energy can be directed to accomplishing the daily tasks of treatment.

Parents often want to add other incentives, and this is not typically a good idea. What can be helpful is to redirect parents to use contingent praise for completion of the various tasks. Praising children for their hard work of waking to the alarm, remaking the bed, and taking the soiled linens to the laundry is directly beneficial. Outcome-related rewards such as a new mattress or new bed upon completion of the program can be helpful. We place the emphasis on the inherent attraction of no longer wetting the bed, and children understand instantly that this is a very big reward.

Relapse Prevention and Follow-Up

Carrying out overlearning can be especially challenging for children who have struggled and finally attained the first 14 dry nights in a row. Children and their parents often fear the prospect of overlearning: Once a child wets again, they worry the child will never recover. We typically tell such families that overlearning is designed precisely to show them that their fear is unwarranted. In this regard, it is important to emphasize that almost all children wet at least once during overlearning. The process of having a programmed relapse can build confidence in all.

Overlearning is introduced by citing the data. The chance of a relapse without overlearning is four in 10 (Morgan, 1978). The chance of relapse is less than one in 10 if the child does gradual overlearning. The benefit far outweighs the time and effort. Occasionally, a child simply cannot complete overlearning (i.e., cannot attain 14 consecutive dry nights during the drinking procedure). Although our outcome trials have been conducted under rigorous procedures that required completion of overlearning to be counted a treatment success, in the effectiveness work based on clinical flexibility I have followed the procedure of suspending overlearning if a child has not completed this within 8 weeks. In such cases, the child stops nighttime drinking and simply continues with the alarm until 14 consecutive dry nights without the drinking are attained. The child then proceeds to follow-up. This does not seem to lead to any worse outcome and makes me suspect that the benefit of overlearning as a relapse prevention procedure may be as much psychological as it is physiological. The added water load before bedtime forces almost all children to wet at least one night. When they overcome this set back, they gain new confidence in their ability to stay dry. This may also contribute to their confidence to accept invitations for sleepovers away from home, a practice strongly encouraged once treatment is completed.

Follow-up in FSHT has been for 1 year or more. In both the efficacy and the effectiveness data, we have monitored children for 3 months, 6 months, and 1 year. In the outcome studies, we did not offer retreatment in the event of relapse because we were interested in estimating the relapse rates. In data collection efforts, our focus has been on relapse prevention rather than retreatment of relapsers, a procedure that is strongly recommended for clinical practice.

In clinical applications, we have offered retreatment in the event a child wets four or more times in 14 days. The parents and child were instructed to contact the clinic in the event of a relapse and to reinstate the alarm until the child was dry for 14 consecutive nights. Such retreatment permanently stops the recurrence in more than 95% of cases.

One other note about follow-up bears mentioning. Over the past 25 years, I have received numerous postcards, letters, and greetings from parents and former adolescent clients who have themselves become parents. Helping a family overcome a child's bedwetting problem is rewarding work, and the children and families are typically very grateful.

EVIDENCE ON THE EFFECTS OF TREATMENT

We have collected both efficacy and effectiveness data on FSHT. Compared with urine alarm procedures without any ancillary procedures such as retention control training and overlearning, FSHT is an improvement over the urine alarm alone. In fact, it is not good practice to use the urine alarm without some relapse prevention. Our components breakdown analysis of FSHT suggested that the addition of retention control training was helpful to get children to the first 14 dry nights in a row. Children who did the retention training attained the 14-night goal faster (Houts, Peterson, & Whelan, 1986). This is important to motivate the family and speed progress toward the ultimate goal.

Controlled Outcome Trials in Group Format

Figure 23.2 summarizes 1-year follow-up from six observations of FSHT. Four are from published studies indicated by their respective dates (Houts, Liebert, & Padawer, 1983; Houts et al., 1986; Houts, Whelan, & Peterson, 1987; Whelan & Houts, 1990). The 1991 sample shows outcomes from an unpublished randomized clinical trial comparing FSHT with imipramine and oxybutynin treatment. The 137 cases identified by the year 2000 were accumulated in our private enuresis clinic over a period of 14 years.

On the basis of five efficacy trials, about three of every four children can be expected to stop wetting at the end of a mean of 12 weeks. It is important to remember that these

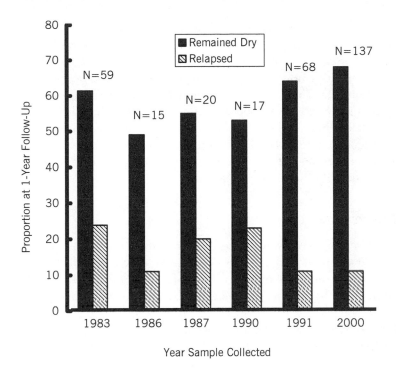

FIGURE 23.2. Mean percentage of children who remained dry or relapsed at 1-year follow-up with full-spectrum treatment for five samples. Relapse was defined as two or more wet nights in 1 week.

data were obtained under research protocol conditions in which flexibility was highly constrained. Further, these samples did not include secondary enuretics and children with clinically significant behavioral problems such as conduct disorder and attention-deficit/hyperactivity disorder (ADHD). Single-parent households were represented, as were low-income families. However, the samples did not include families with marked marital discord or clinically significant family dysfunction. Although these demographic limitations constrain the applicability of findings, it also should be remembered that these samples are quite representative of bedwetting children, most of whom do not have these additional problems.

At 1-year follow-up, six of every 10 children are permanently dry. The lower relapse rates observed in the 1991 and 2000 samples were for children who did our gradual over-learning. In the other samples, overlearning was done in the original fashion of having children consume 16 ounces of water regardless of age. We now consistently find that slightly less than 10% of children relapse using the gradual overlearning.

Effectiveness Outcomes in Individual Format

For FSHT, effectiveness data mirror efficacy data. The 137 cases from our private clinic (last bar in Figure 23.1) were referred by pediatricians and pediatric urologists. More so than in the research trials, this sample included children with additional problems, most often ADHD. The issues in dealing with such children are the same as those for children with other behavioral problems. Parents who use coercive parenting and engage in repeated struggles with a noncompliant child cannot expect to be successful with FSHT. In fact, I tell them that I will not provide the treatment until they first solve the other problems so that the child has a good chance for success with bedwetting treatment.

In this context, I have also treated a number of secondary enuretics, or children who resumed wetting after a period of 6 months or more of continuous continence. The issue with secondary enuresis is not the history of bedwetting but rather the family environment and ancillary child behavior problems.

Important Research Directions

In FSHT, we have not completely solved the problem of relapse. A quantitative study of the effects of retreatment of relapses is needed. We may very well be able to claim that behavioral treatment permanently cures more than 90% of MPEs who follow through with the full treatment program. As it now stands, we can safely make this claim for about 70–75%.

There are true nonresponders. Excluding those cases where the child defeats the alarm and where the parents fail to provide support, there are still some 10–15% of patients who do not respond despite the fact that they carry out the treatment to the fullest. An intensive study of true treatment failures is necessary. This would be beneficial for improving treatment and screening. It would also be useful from an etiological point of view. Like many other problems in the field of behavior, bedwetting is most likely the outcome of multiple causal pathways. Classifying failures to respond could shed some light on the types of causal pathways not adequately addressed by urine alarm treatment. For example, some children never learn to awaken to the alarm. Such may require a different type of alarm that is louder and provides tactile vibration. Oddly enough, a precursor to today's urine alarm was not an alarm at all but a spring-loaded metal bed that catapulted the child across the room when urine closed the pad contacts and activated a solenoid that released the bed frame (Mowrer, 1980). Waking the child at the correct time is both practically and theoretically important. Surely some of the nonresponses to behavioral treatment are due to failure to arouse to the alarm, and methods for improving arousability are important to pursue. Technological innovations, behavioral additions such as the waking schedule, and pharmacological methods are all worth pursuing.

Another important type of failure involves children who continue multiple wetting and never move to single-episode wetting. These children most likely have a deficit in the natural production of anti-diuretic hormone. They are also good candidates for combining behavioral treatment with synthetic antidiuretic hormone (Bradbury & Meadow, 1995; Sukhai, Mol, & Harris, 1989).

The role of airborne and food allergies also merits further investigation. There are occasional references to the co-occurrence of these problems with bedwetting, but systematic investigations are lacking. With all of the aforementioned problems, the difficulty is the very low base rate. It is difficult to accumulate a sufficient sample for study of the mechanisms relating such problems to bedwetting.

HISTORY AND THE FUTURE

Current behavioral treatment of childhood enuresis with the urine alarm is one of the best examples of a highly effective intervention for a widespread problem where the intervention has been based on laboratory-derived principles of learning and conditioning. As one of the oldest forms of 20th century behavior therapy, the object lesson offered by the history of this treatment is important for the 21st century. This history reflects the larger issues for empirically supported psychological treatments more generally. Will children of the 21st century be medicated for their difficulties to the exclusion of alternative and adjunctive behavioral interventions? What is it about our culture in the United States that makes pharmacotherapy so attractive and so easily sold? What does it take to make a treatment available once it has been shown to be effective?

History of Urine Alarm Treatment

At the time that Mowrer faced the challenge of designing a solution to bedwetting, he was part of a group of Yale University psychologists who were attempting to translate Hullian learning theory into clinically relevant terms. In the height of the Great Depression, even a Yale professor could not earn enough to make ends meet, so Mowrer and his wife took up residence in a home for misfit boys, many of whom wet the bed. As house parents, the burden of 12 or so wet beds every night was apparently enough adversity to give birth to invention. From the impracticality, not to mention the danger, of the spring-loaded bed, Mowrer reasoned his way to the urine alarm. Interestingly, there were some earlier independent applications of alarm devices (Kazdin, 1978) that were unknown to Mowrer at the time. Some version of the urine alarm that uses moisture pads has been in use since the first publication by the two Mowrers in 1938 (Mowrer, 1980; Mowrer & Mowrer, 1938). The Mowrers did not patent the device, nor did they copyright the procedures. In fact, they did not pursue the subject beyond their seminal 1938 publication.

In the early 1950s, several companies were formed in the United States to sell treatment for bedwetting, and these companies featured their own alarm devices, which were typically "leased" to the family for an exorbitant price. The business model for these companies is to place sales personnel in certain regions and then blanket it with advertisements. A salesperson then comes to the home in response to returned postcards and attempts to sell the family a treatment program. Today the contract costs about $2,000. The point is, these companies are still in business some 50 years later.

Where are the psychologists? Throughout the 1940s, theoretical interest in bedwetting took hold not in the United States but in the United Kingdom. Among the first clinical psychologists trained at the Maudsley program by Eysenck were a number of investigators who did empirical studies of conditioning treatment. The net effect has been that within the National Health Service of the United Kingdom and throughout much of Australia, urine alarm treatment is widely available. Intellectual interest in principles of classical conditioning and avoidance learning spawned a keener awareness of conditioning treatment and provided a solution that medical professionals did not have.

By way of contrast, developments in the United States followed a different course. Interest in the problem of enuresis as a laboratory for testing various conditioning formulations did not take hold. Compared with the British and Australian empirical publications, relatively little work was conducted in the United States until the mid-1970s, when Azrin and his colleagues challenged the idea that the urine alarm worked via classical conditioning (Azrin et al., 1973; Azrin, Thienes-Hontos, & Besalel-Azrin, 1979; Azrin & Thienes, 1978). When others failed to replicate the Azrin results and showed instead that the urine alarm was an essential component to successful treatment, the theoretical dispute about classical conditioning was largely settled (Bollard & Nettelbeck, 1982; Nettelbeck & Langeluddecke, 1979).

As graduate students at Stony Brook University in the late 1970s, we enjoyed debates about classical versus operant conditioning explanations for urine alarm treatment. We followed the experiments (we did not call them clinical trials) with theoretical interest to see how the issues would be resolved by data. In retrospect, this intellectual interest in models of conditioning was probably atypical and was certainly short lived in the broader scheme of U.S. training programs. Within a decade, everything and everyone went "cognitive," so much so that a fellow graduate student who was interested in the theoretical implications of enuresis treatment and who had since gone on to teach at the University of Illinois remarked to me that he had to give this up because graduate students responded to the subject matter like a "wet blanket." In the United States there has never really been sustained intellectual interest in enuresis.

Recent History of Pharmaceutical Treatment

Another important part of the historical picture concerns the role of medical professionals and the pharmaceutical industry. Before the introduction of DDAVP in the United States in 1989, the modal treatment for bedwetting recommended by medical doctors was to wait for the child to outgrow it. If treatment was offered, it was the antidepressant imipramine, which carried risks of poisoning and adverse cardiovascular events. Moreover, it was not effective. The medical community was generally not educated about behavioral treatment, and among those few who were, there were no providers readily available to deliver it. Behavioral treatment was never integrated into primary care as it had been in the United Kingdom and Australia.

Bringing DDAVP to American medicine offered primary care physicians an option to that was safer and possibly effective. As it turns out, the evidence clearly favors urine alarm over DDAVP, but this has been practically negated by the powerful advertising campaigns of drug companies. The selling of DDAVP as a treatment for bedwetting is very instructive, and to the extent that pharmaceutical companies can successfully sell medications for other problem behaviors, this does not bode well for the future of psychological treatments more generally. What is so fascinating about the case of enuresis is that an inferior and more expensive treatment has become the de facto standard of care even in a scientific climate that features evidence-based medicine and an economic climate that features cost containment. How did this happen?

Pharmaceutical advertising has become very sophisticated. The obvious influences are easily recognized. Medical doctors in training receive gifts of all types. Physicians in practice are routinely visited by representatives, who provide free samples, coffee mugs, pens, and even dinners and cruises called seminars. What is less obvious is the advertising that takes place in the form of studies and publications. When you examine the literature on enuresis over the past 15 years, there is an elephant in the library. The manufacturer of DDAVP has sponsored numerous publications and special issues of journals and has spent millions of dollars to conduct and publish research, much of which was designed to provide a rationale for the use of its product. Their message is subtle but clear: Use their product instead of the urine alarm. What is left out of their messages is more telling than what is in them. Their materials refer to the inconvenience of urine alarm treatment and emphasize the safety of long-term use of DDAVP. They even question the durability of urine alarm treatment as if we do not know full well that urine alarm treatment is far more durable than DDAVP. Promoters of DDAVP routinely visit pediatricians. There is no comparable promotion for urine alarm treatment.

Promotion alone, however, does not account for the business success of DDAVP. Having the right cultural niche is also important, and this has been provided in the United States by popular culture and by the rise of managed health care.

Popular Culture Disinformation and Managed Care

Another influence on misconceptions about treatment for bedwetting comes through popular culture in television advertisements for special underpants, a euphemism for diapers. Diaper manufacturers remind parents to discuss the problem with the child's doctor and point out that the doctor will tell them there are no guarantees with any treatment. The idea that wearing diapers might further habituate a child to the sensations of a wet bed that might otherwise prompt waking and learning to be dry is never mentioned. In fact, waiting until the child is 11–15 years old is the main message of the diaper purveyors. After all, the sooner a child stops bedwetting, the sooner their product is no longer needed. No wonder parents are confused. Television advertisements convey the message that wearing diapers is normal for an adolescent who wets the bed.

In addition to such confusing messages within popular culture, there is the influence of managed care on what treatments for bedwetting are supported. Managed care companies routinely pay for prescription medicines, and they often question nonmedical services. Most insurance plans have different reimbursement rates for care provided under mental health as opposed to physical health. Hence, psychologists who provide treatment for bedwetting receive a lower rate of reimbursement and parents pay a larger portion of the fee out of pocket. Thus, even when behavioral treatment for bedwetting is covered by third-party payers, the immediate contingencies for parents are such that it is cheaper for them to get the more expensive and less effective medication treatment. These market forces have led to greater ignorance about behavioral treatment.

Where Can We Go from Here?

Twenty-five years ago, I imagined that we might have an efficient delivery system for successful behavioral treatment (Houts et al., 1983). We are far from that, but I remain hopeful. Several things are needed to bring about change.

First, behavioral treatment needs a sponsor that can compete with the pharmaceutical and diaper companies. The obvious organization is the American Psychological Association (APA). Psychologists developed urine alarm treatment, and they remain the most likely providers who have the background to implement it successfully.

Second, through its accredited training programs, the APA should provide incentives for teaching of behavioral treatment to new psychologists. Providing programs with the training materials and publishing those materials on the Internet would make them widely available. Accreditation reviews can require evidence that students are instructed in empirically based therapies. Some of this has already started to happen.

Third, advertising is clearly important. Organizations such as the APA can work with manufacturers of urine alarms to promote behavioral treatment. This can be done through print and media advertising.

Finally, primary providers, mostly primary care physicians and pediatricians, must be adequately educated. Psychologists and medical educators need to collaborate to find ways to convey to medical students the importance of research methodology in the assessment of claims for treatment efficacy. This includes the publication in medical journals of primary studies of behavioral treatment, something that has been sadly rare.

CONCLUSIONS

Bedwetting is a problem for some 5–7 million secondary school-age children in the United States. This problem can be solved in most cases. FSHT is a behavioral treatment that has been tested in several clinical trials and has been shown to be efficacious. This treatment has also been used in clinical settings with demonstrated effectiveness. A key feature of FSHT is that it contains a modified overlearning procedure to prevent relapse, and this gradual overlearning is both effective and practical.

Although it is of considerable theoretical interest to document how the urine alarm works, this type of investigation involving all-night sleep studies is very expensive and unlikely to be pursued. Hypotheses regarding the role of antidiuretic hormone in bedwetting have been investigated extensively because the pharmaceutical companies have a vested interest in such studies. Despite such extensive study, there is little reason to believe that the cause of bedwetting is some defect in production of antidiuretic hormone. At best, such an etiological hypothesis might be true for about 10% of children who wet multiple times each night.

In the larger scheme of health care, the problem with behavioral treatment is that it is not being delivered. There are economic and social structural barriers. Unlike medication and stop-gap approaches such as diapers, behavioral treatment has no corporate backing. Ironically, the APA has engaged in a massive campaign to obtain prescribing privileges for psychologists. The history of treatment for bedwetting has some interesting lessons to teach regarding the relative role of medications as contrasted with conditioning-based behavior therapies. Alarm-based treatment is by far the most effective current treatment and costs considerably less than alternative medication treatments (Glazener, Evans, & Peto, 2003; Houts, 2000; Houts et al., 1994). At least in the case of bedwetting, behavior therapy is the treatment of choice. Whether this will hold for other child problems remains to be seen. What is abundantly clear from the example of bedwetting is that establishing the superiority of one treatment over all others is no guarantee that the best treatment will be delivered in a market-driven health care economy that is steered by sophisticated advertising and clever infiltration of the scientific literature.

ACKNOWLEDGMENTS

Partial support was provided by a Centers of Excellence grant from the state of Tennessee to the Department of Psychology, University of Memphis, and by National Institutes of Health Grant No. R01 HD21736 to Arthur C. Houts.

NOTES

1. The manual and wall chart are available for free as pdf downloads at the following website: *www.drhouts.com*. An affordable and durable body-worn urine alarm, Malem Ultimate with Sound and Vibration, is available from *www.bedwettingstore.com/index.htm* or *www.malem.co.uk*.
2. I have maintained a list of professionals who requested the manual, and over the past 25 years have accumulated about 150 names.

REFERENCES

Azrin, N. H., Sneed, T. J., & Foxx, R. M. (1973). Dry bed: A rapid method of eliminating bedwetting (enuresis) of the retarded. *Behaviour Research and Therapy, 11*, 427–434.

Azrin, N. H., & Thienes, P. M. (1978). Rapid elimination of enuresis by intensive learning without a conditioning apparatus. *Behavior Therapy, 9*, 342–354.

Azrin, N. H., Thienes-Hontos, P., & Besalel-Azrin, V. (1979). Elimination of enuresis without a conditioning apparatus: An extension by office instruction of the child and parents. *Behavior Therapy, 10*, 14–19.

Bollard, J., & Nettelbeck, T. (1982). A component analysis of dry-bed training for treatment for bedwetting. *Behaviour Research and Therapy, 20*, 383–390.

Bradbury, M. G., & Meadow, S. R. (1995). Combined treatment with enuresis alarm and desmopressin for nocturnal enuresis. *Acta Pediatrica, 84*(9), 1014–1018.

Glazener, C. M., Evans, J. H., & Peto, R. E. (2003). Alarm interventions for nocturnal enuresis in children. *Cochrane Database System Review*(2), CD002911.

Houts, A. C. (1991). Nocturnal enuresis as a biobehavioral problem. *Behavior Therapy, 22*, 133–151.

Houts, A. C. (2000). Commentary: Treatments for enuresis: criteria, mechanisms, and health care policy. *Journal of Pediatric Psychology, 25*(1), 219–224.

Houts, A. C., Berman, J. S., & Abramson, H. A. (1994). The effectiveness of psychological and pharmacological treatments for nocturnal enuresis. *Journal of Consulting and Clinical Psychology, 62*, 737–745.

Houts, A. C., Liebert, R. M., & Padawer, W. (1983). A delivery system for the treatment of primary enuresis. *Journal of Abnormal Child Psychology, 11*, 513–519.

Houts, A. C., Peterson, J. K., & Whelan, J. P. (1986). Prevention of relapse in full-spectrum home training for primary enuresis: A components analysis. *Behavior Therapy, 17*, 462–469.

Houts, A. C., Whelan, J. P., & Peterson, J. K. (1987). Filmed vs. live delivery of full-spectrum home training for primary enuresis: Presenting the information is not enough. *Journal of Consulting and Clinical Psychology, 55*, 902–906.

Kazdin, A. E. (1978). *History of behavior modification: Experimental foundations of contemporary research.* Baltimore: University Park Press.

Lovibond, S. H. (1963). The mechanism of conditioning treatment of enuresis. *Behaviour Research and Therapy, 1*, 17–21.

Morgan, R. T. T. (1978). Relapse and therapeutic response in the conditioning treatment of enuresis: A review of recent findings on intermittent reinforcement, overlearning and stimulus intensity. *Behaviour Research and Therapy, 16*, 273–279.

Mowrer, O. H. (1980). Enuresis: The beginning work—What really happened. *Journal of the History of the Behavioral Sciences, 16,* 25–30.

Mowrer, O. H., & Mowrer, W. M. (1938). Enuresis: A method for its study and treatment. *American Journal of Orthopsychiatry, 8,* 436–459.

Nettelbeck, T., & Langeluddecke, P. (1979). Dry-bed training without an enuresis machine. *Behaviour Research and Therapy, 17,* 403–404.

Norgaard, J. P. (1989). Urodynamics in enuretics: I. Reservoir function. *Neurourology and Urodynamics, 8,* 199–211.

Scott, M. A. (1993). *Facilitating pelvic floor conditioning in primary nocturnal enuresis.* Unpublished doctoral dissertation, University of Memphis.

Sukhai, R. N., Mol, J., & Harris, A. S. (1989). Combined therapy of enuresis alarm and desmopressin in the treatment of nocturnal enuresis. *European Journal of Pediatrics, 148*(5), 465–467.

Whelan, J. P., & Houts, A. C. (1990). Effects of a waking schedule on the outcome of primary enuretic children treated with full-spectrum home training. *Health Psychology, 9,* 164–176.

Young, G. C., & Morgan, R. T. T. (1972). Overlearning in the conditioning treatment of enuresis: A long-term follow-up study. *Behaviour Research and Therapy, 10,* 419–420.

24

Treating Hispanic Youths Using Brief Strategic Family Therapy

MICHAEL S. ROBBINS, VIVIANA HORIGIAN, JOSÉ SZAPOCZNIK, and JESSICA UCHA

OVERVIEW OF BRIEF STRATEGIC FAMILY THERAPY

Overview of the Clinical Problem

Brief strategic family therapy (BSFT), an empirically based family intervention for the treatment of adolescent drug use and co-occuring problem behaviors, has evolved within the context of a rigorous program of clinical research over the past three decades. Co-occurring problem behaviors that have been targeted in BSFT include conduct problems at home and at school, oppositional behavior, delinquency, associating with antisocial peers, aggressive and violent behavior, and risky sexual behavior.

The intervention began as a direct response to identifying the treatment needs of Hispanic adolescents with behavior problems in Miami in the early 1970s. The importance of research and practice in clinical model development has been an essential ingredient in the emergence of BSFT as a viable intervention for Hispanic adolescents with drug use, delinquency, and other behavior problems. As such, BSFT is intended to address the constellation of behavior problems presented by youths. In fact, the model was developed and refined with clinical samples who presented with high rates of co-occurring behavior problems.

Adolescent drug abuse continues to represent one of the most pressing public health issues in the United States. Although trends over the prior years indicate that individual drug use may vary slightly from year to year, our nation's teenagers continue to use illicit drugs at a stable rate. In 2007, the lifetime prevalence rates for any illicit substance use were 19%, 36%, and 47% in grades 8, 10, and 12, respectively (Johnston, O'Malley, Bachman, & Schulenberg, 2008b). In particular, Hispanics have the highest reported rates of use for nearly all classes of drugs, with the exception of amphetamines,

375

in grades eight and twelve and highest reported rates of use for some drugs such as heroin, methamphetamine, and crystal methamphetamine (Johnston et al., 2008b). In 2007, the annual prevalence rates for any illicit substance use for Hispanics were 17%, 27%, and 32% in grades 8, 10, and 12, respectively (Johnston, O'Malley, Bachman, & Schulenberg, 2008a).

Drug use is just one the many behavior problems in adolescence that can interfere with youths' ability to master normal developmental skills and to function effectively in their environment. The term behavior problems is often used to characterize acting-out and externalizing-type behaviors manifested by youths during adolescence: conduct problems at home and at school, oppositional behavior, delinquency, associating with antisocial peers, aggressive and violent behavior, and risky sexual behavior. Given the prevalence of these behavior problems and consequences for the adolescent as well as the family, the need for effective treatment is imperative. Even more alarming, the Youth Risk Behavior Surveillance reports that adolescents are continuing to engage in behaviors that place them at risk for death (Eaton et al., 2008). Students in grades 9–12 were assessed on their participation in problem as well as risky behavior. In 2007, 36% of adolescents were in a physical fight in the last 12 months; 22% were offered, sold, or given illegal drugs at school; 18% carried a weapon (gun, knife, club) at least one day in the past 30 days; and 39% of currently sexually active high school students had not used a condom during their last sexual intercourse (Eaton et al., 2008).

Conceptual Model and Assumptions of BSFT

The primary goal of BSFT is to improve family relationships and relationships between the family and other important systems that influence youths (e.g., school, peers). By strategically targeting maladaptive family interactions, BSFT is intended to reduce adolescent behavior problems by improving maladaptive family interactions. BSFT is best articulated around three central constructs: *system, structure/patterns of interactions, and strategy.*

A system is made up of component parts that are interdependent and interrelated. Families are systems that are made up of individuals (parts) who are responsive to each other's behaviors (interrelated). Family members become accustomed to the behavior of other family members, because such behaviors have occurred thousands of times over many years. These behaviors synergistically work together to organize a family's system.

Whereas the concept of systems tells us that family members are interdependent, structure explains the set of repetitive patterns of interactions that are idiosyncratic to a family system. A maladaptive family structure is characterized by repetitive family interactions that persist despite the fact that these interactions fail to meet the needs of the family or its individual members. BSFT specifically targets those patterns of interaction that have been shown in the research literature to be predictors of drug abuse and related antisocial behaviors (Szapocznik & Coatsworth, 1999).

The third fundamental concept of BSFT, strategy, is defined by interventions that are practical, problem focused, and planned. Practical interventions are selected for their likelihood to work quickly and effectively. The problem-focused aspect of BSFT targets family interaction patterns that are the most directly related to the presenting problem as a way of limiting the scope of treatment. As such, intervention strategies are very well planned and are specifically intended to help the family shift from one set of interactions that maintain symptomatic behaviors in youths to another set that will reduce symptomatic behaviors.

Goals and Main Themes of BSFT

BSFT is predicated on several key assumptions: (1) changing family interaction patterns is the most effective way of changing individual behavior, (2) changing an individual and then returning her or him to a detrimental or negative environment increases risk for the reemergence of behavior problems, and (3) changes in one central or powerful individual can result in changes in the rest of the family. However, to achieve these changes in individuals and family interaction patterns, interventions must be strategic and directive. For both individual and family change to be successful and maintained over time, BSFT proposes a treatment model that simultaneously addresses both domains. Goals targeted include eliminating or reducing the use of drugs and associated problem behaviors and changing family members' behaviors that are linked with each other and related to the adolescent's drug abuse. Table 24.1 lists the specific change goals targeted in BSFT.

CHARACTERISTICS OF BSFT

Who Is Seen and in What Format

BSFT targets children and adolescents ages 8–17 years who present with behavior problems such as drug use, conduct problems at home and at school, oppositional behavior, delinquency, associating with antisocial peers, aggressive and violent behavior, and risky

TABLE 24.1. Change Goals of Brief Strategic Family Therapy

Structural level	Specific goals
Family	Increased parental figure involvement with one another and improved balance of involvement of the parent figures with the child
	Improved effective parenting, including successful management of children's behavior
	Improved family cohesiveness, collaboration, and affect and reduced family negativity
	Improved "appropriate" bonding between children and parents
	Improved family communication, conflict resolution, and problem-solving skills
	Correct assignment and effective performance of the roles and responsibilities of the family
Individual child/adolescent	Reduced behavior problems
	Improved self-control
	Reduced associations with antisocial peers
	Reduced substance use
	Development of prosocial behaviors
	Bonding to family
	Good school attendance, conduct, and achievement

sexual behavior. Treatment involves the entire family, which typically includes everyone who lives in the adolescent's household as well as other individuals with whom the adolescent has regular contact. Foster families have been excluded from prior research and clinical work because in many circumstances these families are less stable than traditional families and the adolescent transitions to different households during the 6-month period after referral.

BSFT consists of 12–16 sessions (range, 8–24) delivered once a week for 1–1½ hours over a 4-month period either in the office or at the family's home. However, the actual number of sessions and length of service are based on the therapist's ability to achieve necessary improvements in specific behavioral criteria and the severity of family problems. Sessions may occur more frequently around crises times because these are opportune moments for change. BSFT can be implemented in a variety of settings, including community social services agencies, mental health clinics, health agencies, and family clinics. Location of services is flexible and should not become an obstacle to the delivery of BSFT. BSFT family therapy sessions are taped and supervised to ensure therapist adherence and competent delivery of the model.

Content of BSFT: Sequence of Therapy Sessions

BSFT follows a prescribed process format that is flexible and adapted to the content of each family's central concerns. There are three intervention components in BSFT: joining, diagnosis, and restructuring.

The first pillar, joining, involves establishing a therapeutic alliance with each family member and with the family as a whole. A number of specific techniques can be used in establishing a therapeutic alliance, including maintenance, tracking, and mimesis. Maintenance involves the therapist supporting the family's structure and entering the system by accepting its rules. This entails supporting areas of family strength, rewarding or affiliating with a family member, and supporting an individual member who feels threatened by therapy. A creative therapist may be able to establish an alliance around the common goal of ridding the family of its undesirable problem and of the stress that it is experiencing. By offering each family member something she or he would like to achieve, the therapist is able to establish a therapeutic alliance with the family in which they are all committed to working together to improve things. Tracking involves utilizing the nature of family interactions to join with the family. Tracking does not involve direct confrontation, but uses the content and process of the session to move the family's process from what it is to what is desired. The counselor encourages the family to interact in front of her or him so as to observe patterns of interactions, because these are the primary targets of interest in the counselor's work. This is called enactment. Finally, mimesis is directed at the family's style and affect and involves therapist attempts to match the tempo, mood, and style of family member interactions as a way of blending in with the family.

The second pillar, diagnosis, involves identifying family strengths and problematic interactions and developing a treatment plan. Effective diagnosis is facilitated by encouraging family members to behave as they normally would if the counselor were not present. When family members speak with each other, they are more likely to interact in their usual way of behaving and relating. From the observations of family interactions, the therapist is able to proceed with the diagnosis of both family strengths and problematic interactions. Emphasis is given to those problematic interactions that are linked to the youth's problem behaviors or that interfere with parent figures' ability to correct the youth's problem behaviors. To derive a diagnosis of the family, family interactions are assessed along five dimensions: organization, resonance, developmental stage, identified patienthood, and conflict resolution.

Organization refers to repetitive patterns of interactions that give the family a specific form. Therapists evaluate whether parents are in charge of maintaining behavior control by observing who keeps the order in the family, who disciplines, and whether these attempts to discipline are successful or are ignored. Leadership should be with the parental figures, although some leadership can be delegated to older children as long as such delegation is not overly burdensome, is age appropriate, and is delegated and not usurped. Therapists should also learn who provides advice in the family, who are the family "teachers," and whether the advice has an impact on family interaction. In general, parent figures should be responsible for providing guidance, although some of this responsibility can be delegated to other family members. In working with Hispanic families, a common organization pattern involves an adolescent who, because of his or her increased English fluency, is inadvertently placed in an authority role, having to communicate and serve as translator. The centralization of adolescents in this communication process does not necessarily indicate that there is a serious dysfunction in family processes; however, there are times when parents become disempowered and the adolescent empowered, giving rise to an inverted hierarchy.

Resonance is the sensitivity and connection of family members to one another. When assessing family resonance, therapists evaluate interpersonal boundaries, which is a way of denoting where one person or group ends and the next ones begins. Family boundaries reflect how connected or disconnected family members are with each other. Both enmeshment, which occurs when members of the family overreact to one another and emotional and psychological boundaries are weak, and disengagement, when family members are emotionally distant from each other and emotional and psychological boundaries are excessively strong, may signal a problem in the family. Many families and relationships may have some features of one or the other and sometimes both; however, problems emerge when the patterns become rigid and extreme. It should be noted that some cultures have a tendency toward more or less interpersonal connection. Irrespective of these tendencies, however, if over- or underinvolvement creates problems within the family, it must be targeted in therapy.

The third dimension of family functioning involves developmental stages. Families are composed of multiple individuals who are often at different stages of development. It is not always understood, however, that families also go through a series of developmental stages; and in order for its members to continue to function in a healthy way, family members need to behave in ways that are appropriate at each developmental level. When a family's developmental stage is assessed, four major sets of tasks and roles are assessed: parenting tasks and roles, marital tasks and roles, sibling tasks and roles, and extended family's tasks and roles. How each of these family subgroups is functioning is evaluated in reference to what is normative or expected at that stage of individual and familial development. A maladaptive pattern may include a child who is overwhelmed with adult tasks (e.g., a Hispanic family in which a child is asked by a parent not only to translate but then to make a family decision "because the child understands better how things work in this country"). When a child is placed in such a powerful family role, the child acquires considerable power in the family. Consequently, if the child were to choose to disobey his parents, the parents would be unable to set limits.

Identified patienthood refers to adolescents with behavioral problems who often are viewed by the family as the sole cause of all family problems. Identified patients are easy to distinguish because family interactions tend to revolve around them. The more family members blame and centralize the adolescent, the more difficult it will be to change the family's repetitive maladaptive interactions.

The last dimension in family functioning is conflict resolution. A family can approach and attempt to manage conflicts in five ways: denial, avoidance, diffusion, conflict emergence without resolution, and conflict emergence with resolution. For a family to function well, it must use the full range of styles in solving conflicts.

The next step is to develop a treatment plan that systematically addresses the problems that are directly linked to the youth's problem behaviors. The treatment plan is strategic in that the most relevant problems that are identified as problematic relations are the primary targets of intervention. All interventions are planned to capitalize on each family's and individual family member's unique strengths.

The third pillar of BSFT, restructuring, involves the implementation of those change strategies needed to transform family relations from problematic to effective and mutually supportive. In this work, the therapist is planful, problem focused, directive, and practical. BSFT therapists use a range of techniques that fall within three broad categories: working in the present, reframing, and working with boundaries and alliances.

Working in the present refers to focusing on the present interactions that occur between family members and that are observable to the therapist. For this reason, enactments are a critical feature of BSFT. Enactments refer to the therapeutic focus of encouraging, helping, or allowing family members to behave and interact in their characteristic manner (i.e., as they would naturally if the therapist were not present). To facilitate enactments, the therapist systematically redirects communications to encourage interactions between session participants rather than interactions between session participants and the therapist. It is important to remember that in BSFT therapists are interested in having the family behave differently within and following the intervention sessions and not simply talk about behaving differently. This will require that the therapist remain decentralized or, in other words, have the interactions occur among family members and not between the family members and the therapist. If the enactment breaks down, the therapist either comments on what went wrong or urges family members to continue. As the reader will note, enactments permit a seamless transition from joining to restructuring. The therapist tracks and elicits responses by systematically redirecting communications to encourage interactions between session participants. Tracking then transitions to restructuring the process of transforming characteristic patterns of interaction by the therapist directing and orchestrating interactions as they occur in the session.

The second category of restructuring interventions is reframing. Reframing interventions are intended to create a different sense of reality, to give the family the opportunity to perceive their interactions or their situation from a different perspective. That is, when the family is stuck, when it is behaving in a rigidly, repetitive fashion, when it is unable to break out of its maladaptive interactions, the therapist's job is to create the opportunity for the family to behave/interact in a new way. Reframing serves two extremely important functions: to change negativity and apparent uncaring into positivity and caring and shift the focus from blaming and castigating the identified patient to a nonblaming, relational focus (e.g., a family pain or loss).

The last category of restructuring interventions is working with boundaries and alliances. The life context of a drug-using youth is likely to be composed of a complex set of alliances. Boundaries are the social walls that exist around groups of people who are allied with each other and that stand between individuals not allied with each other. A common pattern with drug-using youths involves one-parent-to-youth alliances that cross generational lines and work against the effective functioning of the executive parental hierarchy. Shifting boundaries thus involves creating a more solid boundary around the parental subsystem so the parental figures make executive parental decisions together, removing the inappropriate parent–child alliance to decrease the child's influence on the executive parental subsystem, and replacing it with an appropriate alliance between both parents or the parent figure and the youth that meets the youth's needs for support and nurturance.

Skills and Accomplishments Emphasized in BSFT

Two main goals are emphasized in BSFT: to eliminate or reduce the adolescent's use of drugs and associated problem behaviors, known as symptom focus, and to change the family interactions that are associated with the adolescent's drug abuse and behavior problems, known as system focus. An example of family system focus is when the counselor intervenes to change the way family members act toward each other (i.e., patterns of interaction). This will prompt family members to speak and act in ways that promote more positive family interaction. These new family interactions are then used to effectively address the adolescent's drug use and problematic behavior.

Duration and How to Determine When Treatment Is "Finished"

Termination occurs when it is clear that the family has met the goals of the treatment plan; that is, family functioning has improved and adolescent behavior problems have been reduced or eliminated. Thus, termination is not determined by the number of sessions provided but by the improvement in identified behavioral criteria. A good prognostic sign of readiness for termination is the family's ability to effectively manage a crisis without therapist intervention. The family is empowered by the knowledge that even when behavior problems recur, they are equipped to rein in their adolescent's behavior. After successful termination, families may come across some of the old or even some new problems for which they may receive booster sessions. At this point, even a troubled situation for the family is different from previous occasions because each member has already enjoyed the benefits of a better functioning family.

BSFT Manual and Other Supporting Materials

BSFT is extremely adaptable to a broad range of family and youth situations and problems. BSFT, however, is not a simple recipe. Rather, it is an advanced clinical model that establishes a set of principles and guidelines that requires considerable clinical skill on the part of the counselor. Training and certification on the BSFT manualized intervention are available through the BSFT Training Institute. The National Institute on Drug

Abuse (NIDA) included BSFT in its *Treatment Manual Series*. Treatment Manual 5: *Brief Strategic Family Therapy for Adolescent Drug Abuse* can be found on NIDA's website: *www. drugabuse.gov/pdf/Manual5.pdf*.

EVIDENCE ON THE EFFECTS OF BSFT

How BSFT Is Evaluated

BSFT has been evaluated for children and adolescent with behavior problems. Efficacy research has established the benefits of BSFT compared with alternative interventions. In these studies, measures of behavior problems have included the Child Behavior Checklist and the Revised Behavior Problem Checklist. More recently, in our effectiveness research, we have included the Youth Self Report and Timeline Followback to assess behavior problems and drug use, respectively. One of the most important aspects of our research has been the development of the Structural Family Systems Ratings (SFSR) to measure theoretically relevant aspects of family functioning that are addressed in BSFT. The SFSR has been critical in examining the impact of BSFT and alternative interventions on family functioning along the five dimensions targeted by BSFT.

Status of Evidence

As noted, BSFT has emerged from more than three decades of clinical research. In some respects, the research focus can be described as occurring within three "eras of research," which roughly correspond to each decade of research. The first era focused extensively on treatment development and feasibility of family therapy and the second on outcome research within controlled efficacy trials; the third era has expanded to include dissemination (effectiveness) research and the widespread training of therapists in community agencies.

During the first era of research, our initial focus was to identify a viable treatment alternative for Hispanic (at the time predominately Cuban) immigrant adolescents and their families in Miami, Florida. This was a particularly important issue because there was a dearth of programs in the area available to serve Spanish-speaking populations, and Hispanics were also not using existing services. To address this problem, the Spanish Family Guidance Center (now the Center for Family Studies) was established to identify and develop a culturally appropriate treatment intervention for Cuban youths with behavior problems. After conducting a series of studies examining the values of the Cuban population, structural family therapy (cf. Minuchin, 1974; Minuchin & Fishman, 1981) was adopted as the center's core approach, and structural theory and therapy have provided the foundation for every clinical development and innovation of the center's work in culturally diverse contexts (Szapocznik, Scopetta, & King, 1978; Szapocznik & Williams, 2000).

Our initial clinical work with adolescents in Miami revealed that failure to include families in treatment led to failure to retain the youths in treatment, and that therapists who adopted an active, directive, present-oriented leadership role that attended to family hierarchy matched the values and expectations of the population (Szapocznik et al., 1978). Based on our clinical work with Cuban and Central and South American families, it became evident that the youths and parents had become adversaries around a struggle that was culturally flavored: Americanism versus Hispanicism. To adequately address youths' problem behaviors, it was necessary to examine the context of immigrant Hispanic families that had been immersed in mainstream culture (Szapocznik et al., 1978). Only within this larger social and cultural context was it possible to understand the profound impact of immigration on family functioning, and, in turn, on adolescent behavior problems. Our clinical focus was expanded to include not only the family as the immediate social context of the youths but also the larger cultural streams, which were differentially affecting the youths and their parents (Szapocznik & Kurtines, 1993).

Although the majority of immigrant families successfully manage in host contexts, many experience conflict as normal developmental family processes. This is especially true for those families with intergenerational differences in the acculturation process. For example, in immigrant Hispanic families, two interdependent processes converged to create acculturative conflict: adolescents' normal striving for independence combined with their powerful acculturation to the American cultural value of individualism (Szapocznik, Santisteban, Rio, Perez-Vidal, Kurtines, & Hervis, 1986) on the one hand and parents' normal tendency to preserve family integrity and adherence to the Hispanic traditional cultural value of strong family cohesion and parental control on the other. The additive effects of intergenerational (adolescent seeks autonomy; parents seek family integrity) and cultural differences (American individualism; Hispanic parental control) produce an exacerbated and intensified intrafamilial conflict in which parents and adolescents feel alienated from each other.

The latter part of our first era of research also focused on addressing challenges that were encountered in our clinical work with Hispanic families. For example, many therapists reported that they preferred to work with the entire family to address adolescent drug use; however, they reported that it was very difficult to bring whole families into treatment. In response to this challenge, we developed an adaptation of BSFT called one-person BSFT, which achieved the goals of BSFT without requiring the presence of the whole family in treatment sessions (Szapocznik, Kurtines, Perez-Vidal, Hervis, & Foote, 1990).

Randomized clinical trials were conducted to compare the efficacy of one-person BSFT with conjoint BSFT. The samples consisted of 35 (Szapocznik, Kurtines, Foote, Perez-Vidal, & Hervis, 1986) and 37 (Szapocznik, Kurtines, Foote, Perez-Vidal, & Hervis, 1983) Hispanic families with a drug-abusing adolescent. These 72 adolescents and their families were randomly assigned to the one-person (involving only the drug-abusing adolescent) or conjoint (involving the whole family) BSFT modalities (Szapocznik, et al., 1983; Szapocznik, Kurtines, Foote, Perez-Vidal, & Hervis, 1986). Both conditions were designed to use exactly the same BSFT theory, so that only one variable (one person vs. conjoint) would differ between the conditions. The families in both treatment conditions were assessed at three time points: pretreatment, posttreatment, and follow-up. The results showed that one-person BSFT was as efficacious as conjoint BSFT in significantly reducing youth drug use and behavior problems as well as improving family functioning (Szapocznik et al., 1983; Szapocznik, Kurtines, Foote, Perez-Vidal, & Hervis, 1986). It appears that an individual modality, conceptualized in family terms (Szapocznik, et al., 1983; Szapocznik, Kurtines, Foote, Perez-Vidal, & Hervis, 1986), such as one-person BSFT can bring about improvements in family functioning.

Nonetheless, our clinical experience implementing one-person BSFT suggested that it was very difficult to change family functioning and adolescent behavior problems through one family member. Therapists had to maintain a consistent focus on family interactions and not fall into the trap of becoming individual focused. In many ways, the one-person techniques can be thought of as the most sophisticated and difficult-to-implement strategies in BSFT.

Building on the success of these early studies, we developed a more effective tool for engaging and retaining adolescents and family members in treatment that was heavily influenced by the theoretical principles of our one-person approach. The BSFT engagement module conceptualized resistance to participation in systemic terms, both in terms of the family systemic process that prevented whole families from entering treatment as well as from therapist–family systemic process that suggested that therapist's behaviors could be changed to overcome family systemic processes that prevented families from coming into treatment. The efficacy of BSFT engagement has been tested in three studies with Hispanic youths.

The first study (Szapocznik et al., 1988) included mostly Cuban families with adolescents who had behavior problems and who were suspected of or observed using drugs by their parents or school counselors. Families were randomly assigned to one of two therapies: BSFT engagement or engagement as usual (the control therapy). Successful engagement was defined as the conjoint family (minimally the identified patient and his or her parents and siblings living in the same household) attending the first BSFT session. Treatment integrity analyses revealed that interventions in the BSFT engagement modality adhered to prescribed guidelines, and that BSFT engagement and engagement as usual were clearly distinguishable by both level of engagement effort applied and the techniques used.

The efficacy of the two methods of engagement (BSFT vs. usual) was measured by the percentage of families who entered treatment and the percentage who completed treatment. The results were statistically significant: For the families in engagement as usual, 42% were successfully engaged and 25% of the engaged cases successfully completed treatment, whereas for the families in BSFT engagement, 93% were successfully engaged and 77% of engaged cases successfully completed treatment. Improvements in adolescent symptoms occurred but were not significantly different between the two methods of engagement. Thus, the critical distinction between the treatments was in their different rates of engagement and retention. Therefore, BSFT engagement had a wider impact on more families than did engagement as usual.

In addition to replicating the previous engagement study, the second study (Santisteban et al. 1996) also explored factors that might moderate the efficacy of the engagement interventions and more stringently defined the success of engagement as a minimum of two office visits: the intake session and the first therapy session. The researchers randomly assigned 193 Hispanic families to one experimental (BSFT plus BSFT engagement) and two control (BSFT plus engagement as usual; group counseling plus engagement as usual) treatments.

The statistically significant results indicated that 81% of families were successfully engaged in the BSFT plus BSFT engagement experimental treatment, whereas 60% of families in the two control therapies were successfully engaged. However, the efficacy of the experimental therapy procedures was moderated by the cultural/ethnic identity of the Hispanic families in the study, supporting the widely held belief that therapeutic interactions must be responsive to contextual changes in the treatment population. Among families assigned to BSFT engagement, 93% of the non-Cuban Hispanics and

64% of the Cuban Hispanics were engaged. These findings have led to further study of the mechanism by which culture/ethnicity and other contextual factors may influence clinical processes related to engagement (Santisteban et al., 1996, 2003).

A third study (Coatsworth, Santisteban, McBride, & Szapocznik, 2001) compared BSFT with a community control intervention, administered by an outside treatment agency, in terms of its ability to engage and retain adolescents and their families in treatment. As in previous studies, findings showed that BSFT was significantly more successful at engaging adolescents and their families in treatment (81% vs. 61%), retaining those engaged in treatment (71% vs. 42%), and having clients complete treatment (58% vs. 25%) than the community control treatment. In addition, in BSFT, families of adolescents with more severe conduct problem symptoms were more likely to remain in treatment than those of adolescents whose conduct problem symptoms were less severe. The opposite pattern was evident in the community control intervention. These findings are particularly important because they suggest that adolescents who are most in need of services are more likely to stay in BSFT than in the community treatment control.

The second era of research focused on empirically comparing BSFT with other modalities. The first compares structural family therapy/BSFT with individual psychodynamic child therapy for emotionally and behaviorally troubled children. The second compares BSFT and group counseling for adolescents with behavior problems.

The first study (Szapocznik, Rio, Murray, Cohen, Scopetta, Rivas-Vasquez, et al., 1989) tested the relative efficacy, and investigated the mechanisms of, therapeutic change of structural family therapy/BSFT compared with individual psychodynamic child-centered psychotherapy and a recreational control condition. Sixty-nine moderately emotionally or behaviorally troubled Hispanic boys were randomly assigned to one of the three intervention conditions. The results revealed that, first, the recreational control condition was significantly less effective in retaining cases than the two treatment conditions. Second, both BSFT and individual psychodynamic child therapy were more effective than the recreational control group in reducing behavior problems and improving child psychodynamic functioning, and no significant differences between the two intervention groups were observed on these variables. Third, BSFT was significantly more effective than individual child psychodynamic therapy in protecting family functioning at 1-year follow-up.

The second study examined the efficacy of BSFT versus a group therapy control condition (Santisteban et al., 2003) in Hispanic adolescents with externalizing problems. Results indicated that adolescents in the BSFT condition showed significantly greater reductions in measures of conduct disorder, delinquency in the company of peers, and marijuana use than youths in the group control condition. In addition, a substantially and significantly larger proportion of BSFT than control cases demonstrated clinically significant improvement. With respect to family functioning, families were partitioned into two groups: better baseline family functioning at intake and worse baseline family functioning at intake based on a median split. Examination of the patterns of change showed that for families classified as worse baseline family functioning, BSFT cases showed significant improvements in family functioning, whereas group cases showed no improvement. A different picture emerged for the better family functioning group. Analyses demonstrated that BSFT cases showed no significant change in family functioning (good functioning was maintained), whereas group therapy cases showed a statistically significant deterioration in family functioning. Together, these two studies provide some empirical support for the efficacy of BSFT with troubled Hispanic children and adolescents.

The final era of BSFT research involves efforts to establish the effectiveness of the model and its dissemination, in addition to generalizing to other populations. From 2002 to 2008, within NIDA's Clinical Trials Network, BSFT was compared with treatment as usual (TAU) in a multisite, prospective randomized clinical trial for drug-using adolescents and their families in outpatient settings. The effectiveness of BSFT was compared with TAU in reducing adolescent drug use, conduct problems, and sexually risky behaviors as well as in improving family functioning and adolescent prosocial behaviors. Four hundred eighty adolescents and family members from eight community treatment providers in Arizona, California, Colorado, Florida ($n = 2$), North Carolina, Ohio, and Puerto Rico participated. The BSFT study enrolled more than 2,000 individuals, including pilot participants, adolescent-identified participants, family members, and therapist participants (the latter were also randomized). At present, analyses are being conducted to examine the impact of BSFT on adolescent and family outcomes and to examine rates of engagement and retention in treatment. In addition, the BSFT Training Institute has been established to disseminate BSFT to community agencies and practitioners. The institute provides a broad range of training programs and has trained hundreds of therapists nationally and internationally. Training is tailored to agency needs and clinical populations and is offered in Spanish and English. The overall BSFT training program includes 140 hours over approximately 5–6 months. Didactic material, live consultation, and supervision are completed during four 3-day workshops. Group supervision is conducted via telephone and involves the review of counselor trainee's DVD recordings of family sessions with training cases. Therapists are trained to achieve competency in the key elements of BSFT. A major goal of the training program is to develop an on-site leader/supervisor of the clinical team to enhance adherence sustainability beyond the training period. Ongoing adherence checks and booster training sessions are also conducted to maintain fidelity and to address staff turnover.

Training has been conducted in numerous settings with diverse clinical and racial/ethnic groups. Therapist trainees have varied academic backgrounds and levels of clinical experience. Before training at any agency, on-site visits with agency leadership are conducted to ensure that the site has the capacity for training in BSFT, including number of qualified therapists, number of appropriate adolescent referrals, and procedures for working with families (e.g., billing for family services, space for family sessions, home-based service options, flexibility for participation in training and supervision activities). In addition, the site visit is necessary to adapt the training program to the special needs of the agency. A recent development in our training program is the utilization of video teleconference for supervision sessions. This has substantially improved the quality of communication and relationship between the trainer/supervisor and the trainees. BSFT training, certification, and technical assistance are available through the BSFT Training Institute.

Overall Evaluation of BSFT

BSFT, like many other treatment approaches, has its strengths and limitations. As evident by its name, BSFT is a brief intervention that targets self-sustaining changes in the family context that are expected to persist after the treatment is completed. As such, the changes made during treatment continue to provide a context for preventing future problems in the target adolescent as well as siblings. Another strength of BSFT appeals to cultural groups that emphasize family and interpersonal relationships. Perhaps its primary strength is that BSFT is a flexible approach that can be adapted to a broad range of family situations in a variety of service settings and treatment modalities.

BSFT is an advanced clinical modality that requires therapeutic skill and sophistication. In the past 5 years, our experience has been that, when therapists are screened both by the agency seeking treatment and the BSFT Training Institute, one in every four therapists has difficulty mastering the implementation of BSFT. Another potential limitation is that research on BSFT has been conducted primarily with Hispanic adolescents and their families. Although we have recently completed a large multisite effectiveness study with a diverse sample, the effectiveness of BSFT (compared with TAU) in reducing adolescent drug use and conduct problems with racially/ethnically diverse youths has not yet been established.

EVIDENCE, RECOMMENDATIONS, AND QUESTIONS REGARDING IMPLEMENTATION IN PRACTICE

Despite our ability to publish manuals to disseminate BSFT, we recognize the considerable challenges in transporting BSFT. Indeed, psychotherapy researchers fall short in their ability to communicate the findings of their research to stakeholders such as consumers, policymakers, and society at large (Newman & Tejeda, 1996). To address this challenge, we need to examine the costs and cost-effectiveness of BSFT to more effectively address the concerns raised by managed care companies and other stakeholders in systems of care to evaluate the utility of BSFT and its various applications.

Fidelity to the intervention model may be critical to achieving expected outcomes in practice settings. Our intensive training model, which includes the review of DVD recordings, provides a unique opportunity for evaluating therapist fidelity and linking level of fidelity to clinical outcomes as well as to examine in-session mechanisms of action that may account for some of the variation in clinical outcomes that is observed across sites.

Additional future research challenges include the following: (1) conducting trials comparing BSFT with other empirically validated family-based and non-family-based interventions for adolescent drug abuse and problem behavior; (2) linking specific therapists behaviors to proximal and distal family and individual outcomes (currently underway) to refine and improve the intervention; (3) conducting research on applications to non-Hispanic populations and Hispanic populations in different parts of the country; and (4) conducting research on methods for transporting BSFT to practice settings. Although transportability to practice settings is challenging, fortunately during the last 15 years we have always applied BSFT with populations obtained from the usual referral sources to community agencies. Our current studies obtain most of their referrals from the justice system, and therapy is conducted in homes and other settings in the life context of the participating families. Overall, our work appears to meet guidelines for an adequate program of research that will be informative to consumers, practitioners, policymakers, and the public at large.

DIRECTIONS FOR RESEARCH

At present, research on BSFT is focused on three areas: effectiveness research, process research, and expansion of the intervention to target adolescents' social ecology. As is the case throughout the mental health and drug abuse field, there is a substantial gap between the interventions validated in research studies and the interventions implemented in community settings. Thus, our most recent activities have involved a multisite effectiveness study in community treatment sites. The results are expected to be available for dissemination in 2009.

A second area of ongoing and future research studies involves examining the clinical interior of BSFT to identify processes that are related to successful and unsuccessful outcomes. Process studies are fundamental in model development and therapist training, and the results of these studies are immediately applicable to practicing clinicians. The rich theoretical base about the change process as well as the detailed definitions and examples contained in the treatment manual about joining, diagnosing, and restructuring family interactions provide a solid foundation for the design and implementation of process studies. The Center for Family Studies has maintained a DVD/videotape library that contains thousands of BSFT session recordings collected as part of several clinical research studies, which provides a unique opportunity for linking in-session processes to treatment outcomes. Currently, a process study is underway that is focused on identifying aspects of BSFT that may be related to retention in treatment. Specifically, this study examines the therapist role as a change agent in family therapy by examining interventions that impact family members' behaviors presumed to be directly related to retention in treatment. To date, we have published one study demonstrating the critical importance of maintaining balanced alliances in BSFT (Robbins et al., 2008). In this study alliance was defined as each family member's working relationship with the therapist. Balanced alliance was conceptualized as differences in the parent's alliance with therapist and the adolescent's alliance with therapist (parent minus adolescent). Greater imbalances in alliance were observed among clients who dropped out of treatment than among those who completed treatment. Current analyses are being conducted to examine the relationship between therapist supportive interventions, family member–therapist alliance, and family conflict and dropout from treatment.

Finally, as briefly noted in prior sections, we plan to examine aspects of the transportation process that contribute to the successful implementation of BSFT in real-world settings. This includes conducting studies on aspects of training and site characteristics that promote or interfere with the successful adoption of BSFT by front-line providers at community agencies as well as studies examining the impact of BSFT on clinical outcomes for adolescents and family members who are seen in these agencies.

CONCLUSIONS

The primary goal of the Center for Family Studies has been to identify and develop a culturally appropriate intervention for Hispanic youths with behavior problems. BSFT continues to be adapted through a program of research that involves the rigorous and continuous interplay among theory, research, and application.

As a family intervention, the focus of BSFT is not the child or adolescent but rather the entire family system. A central tenet of BSFT is that problematic family interactions play a key role in the evolution and maintenance of behavior problems. The strategic, problem-focused aspect of BSFT refers to targeting those maladaptive family interaction patterns that are most directly relevant to the symptomatic behavior.

BSFT was developed from within a Hispanic perspective and recognizes the influence of cultural factors in the development and maintenance of behavior problems. BSFT was first used to target specific problematic interactions that developed as a result of differential rates of acculturation between parents and youths as well as generic maladaptive patterns of family interactions. Our training of clinicians pays specific attention to Hispanic-specific family processes.

Research on the efficacy of BSFT has documented the positive impact of BSFT children and adolescents with behavior problem including reductions in conduct problems, delinquency, and drug use and improvements in family functioning. In addition to the immediate impact on behavior problems, BSFT has also been found to have a wider impact than alternative adolescent therapies by engaging and retaining more adolescents and their families in treatment. Present and future research is focused on the effectiveness of BSFT in real-world settings and on the identification of in-session mechanisms of action (process research) that may account for the success of BSFT. Future studies examining characteristics of transporting BSFT into community agencies are being planned.

ACKNOWLEDGMENTS

This work was supported by the National Institute on Drug Abuse Grant No. U10-DA13720 (José Szapocznik, Principal Investigator).

REFERENCES

Coatsworth, J. D., Santisteban, D. A., McBride, C. K., & Szapocznik, J. (2001). Brief strategic family therapy versus community control: Engagement, retention, and an exploration of the moderating role of adolescent symptom severity. *Family Process, 40*(3), 313–332.

Eaton, D. K., Kann, L., Kinchen, S., Shanklin, S., Ross, J., Hawkins, J., et al. (2008). Youth risk behavior surveillance—United States, 2007. *Morbidity and Mortality Weekly Report Surveillance Summaries, 57*, 1–131.

Johnston, L. D., O'Malley, P. M., Bachman, J. G., & Schulenberg, J. E. (2008a). *Demographic subgroup trends for various licit and illicit drugs, 1975–2007* (Monitoring the Future Occasional Paper No. 69). Ann Arbor, MI: Institute for Social Research.

Johnston, L. D., O'Malley, P. M., Bachman, J. G., & Schulenberg, J. E. (2008b). *Monitoring the future national results on adolescent drug use: Overview of key findings, 2007* (NIH Publication No. 08-6418). Bethesda, MD: National Institute on Drug Abuse.

Minuchin, S. N. (1974). *Families and family therapy.* Cambridge, MA: Harvard University Press.

Minuchin, S. N., & Fishman, C. H. (1981). *Family therapy techniques.* Cambridge, MA: Harvard University Press.

Newman, F. L., & Tejeda, M. J. (1996) The need for research that is designed to support decisions in the delivery of mental health services. *The American Psychologist, 51*(10), 1040–1049.

Robbins, M. S., Turner, C. W., Mayorga, C. C., Alexander, J. F., Mitrani, V. B., & Szapocznik, J.

(2008). Adolescent and parent alliances with therapists in brief strategic family therapy with drug using Hispanic adolescents. *Journal of Marital and Family Therapy, 34*(3), 316–328.

Santisteban, D., Coatsworth, J. D., Perez-Vidal, A., Kurtines, W. M., Schwartz, S. J., LaPerriere, A., et al. (2003). The efficacy of brief strategic family therapy in modifying Hispanic adolescent behavior problems and substance use. *Journal of Family Psychology, 17*(1), 121–133.

Santisteban, D. A., Szapocznik, J., Perez-Vidal, A., Kurtines, W. M., Murray, E. J., & Laperriere, A. (1996). Efficacy of intervention for engaging youth and families into treatment and some variables that may contribute to differential effectiveness. *Journal of Family Psychology, 10*(1), 35–44.

Szapocznik, J., & Coatsworth, J. D. (1999). An ecodevelopmental framework for organizing the influences on drug abuse: A developmental model of risk and protection. In M. D. Glantz & C. R. Hartel (Eds.), *Drug abuse: Origins and interventions* (pp. 331–366). Washington, DC: American Psychological Association.

Szapocznik, J., & Kurtines, W. M. (1993). Family psychology and cultural diversity: Opportunities for theory, research, and application. *American Psychologist, 48*(4), 400–407.

Szapocznik, J., Kurtines, W. M., Foote, F., Perez-Vidal, A., & Hervis, O. E. (1983). Conjoint versus one-person family therapy: Some evidence for effectiveness of conducting family therapy through one person. *Journal of Consulting and Clinical Psychology, 51*, 889–899.

Szapocznik, J., Kurtines, W. M., Foote, F., Perez-Vidal, A., & Hervis, O. E. (1986). Conjoint versus one-person family therapy: Further evidence for the effectiveness of conducting family therapy through one person with drug-abusing adolescents. *Journal of Consulting and Clinical Psychology, 54*(3), 395–397.

Szapocznik, J., Kurtines, W. M., Perez-Vidal, A., Hervis, O., & Foote, F. H. (1990). Interplay of advances between theory, research, and application in treatment interventions aimed at behavior problem children and adolescents. *Journal of Consultation and Clinical Psychology, 58*(6), 696–703.

Szapocznik, J., Perez-Vidal, A., Brickman, A., Foote, F. H., Santisteban, D. A., Hervis, O., et al. (1988). Engaging adolescent drug abusers and their families into treatment: A strategic structural systems approach. *Journal of Consulting and Clinical Psychology, 56*(4), 552–557.

Szapocznik, J., Rio, A. T., Murray, E., Cohen, R., Scopetta, M. A., Rivas-Vasquez, A., et al. (1989). Structural family versus psychodynamic child therapy for problematic Hispanic boys. *Journal of Consulting and Clinical Psychology, 57*, 571–578.

Szapocznik, J., Santisteban, D., Rio, A., Perez-Vidal, A., Kurtines, W., & Hervis, O. (1986). Bicultural effectiveness training (BET): An intervention modality for families experiencing inter-generational/intercultural conflict. *Hispanic Journal of Behavioral Sciences, 8*(4), 303–330.

Szapocznik, J., Scopetta, M. A., & King, O. E. (1978). Theory and practice in matching treatment to the special characteristics and problems of Cuban immigrants. *Journal of Community Psychology, 6*, 112–122.

Szapocznik, J., & Williams, R. A. (2000). Brief Strategic Family Therapy: Twenty-five years of interplay among theory, research and practice in adolescent behavior problems and drug abuse. *Clinical Child and Family Psychology Review, 3*(2), 117–135.

25

Treating Hispanic Children and Adolescents Using Narrative Therapy

ROBERT G. MALGADY

OVERVIEW

This chapter describes a program of psychotherapeutic treatment–outcome research addressing behavioral conduct disorders and anxiety disorders common to young Puerto Rican children and adolescents in New York City public schools. The clinical problem has been associated with this population's low socioeconomic status, the ubiquity of single parent (usually female-headed) households, marginal levels of acculturation, and a reluctance to seek traditional mental health services (Rogler, Malgady, & Rodriguez, 1989). The treatment model is based on narrative techniques to instantiate adaptive behavior by reinforcing modeling of culturally similar characters drawn from Puerto Rican literature and history. Three treatment models were investigated within this context, varying the modality according to children's and adolescents' age cohorts.

Treatment Models: Three Forms of Narrative Therapy

The first intervention, cuento/folktale therapy, involved the presentation of Puerto Rican folktales (Costantino, Malgady, & Rogler, 1986) of a well-known fictional character in Puerto Rican folklore, Juan Bobo for John the Fool. Juan, a hapless character, falls into a variety of precarious situations, much to his chagrin. After trying several maladaptive escape mechanisms, ultimately Juan resolves his situations in a socially acceptable manner exhibiting appropriate adaptive behavior. Children were encouraged to discuss the fables, describe how they would have resolved such dilemmas, and finally engage in role-playing sessions. Behaviorally adaptive solutions were verbally reinforced by the therapist, while maladaptive solutions were not, and children and their peers were prompted to explore more appropriate resolutions of the conflicts at hand.

In the second intervention, biographies of nonfictional characters were presented to Puerto Rican adolescents. Following a historical literary search of prominent Puerto Ricans, beginning with the native Taino Indians through modern-day times, a team composed of psychologists, anthropologists, and historians selected male and female figures from a variety of walks of life who would serve as heroes and heroines to the behaviorally troubled Hispanic youths. This treatment was termed hero/heroine modeling therapy (Malgady, Rogler, & Costantino, 1990).

The third intervention was storytelling therapy, also with young adolescents, in which the youths were exposed to pictures from a culturally sensitive projective test (TEMAS, or Tell Me a Story; see Malgady, 1996; Costantino, Dana, & Malgady, 2008; Costantino, Malgady, & Primavera, in press). The pictures depicted bipolar solutions, one adaptive and the other maladaptive, to scenarios such as helping with or stealing groceries from an elderly woman or saving money to await a larger reward versus immediate gratification by impulsive spending. Similar to the folktale and hero/heroine versions of narrative therapy, behaviorally adaptive resolutions of the conflicts presented in the pictures were reinforced by the therapist, while maladaptive solutions were discussed and more socially acceptable outcomes were invoked, followed once again by role-playing of the adaptive ending to the adolescents' stories.

Assumptions Underlying the Model

The assumptions underlying this psychotherapeutic approach were that culturally marginalized children and adolescents exhibiting behavioral conduct problems and associated anxiety symptomatology would be more amenable to engagement in treatment and acquire more remedial treatment outcomes when exposed to stimuli that were culturally relevant to their lives as opposed to the content of mainstream treatments with which they have difficulty identifying. These children and adolescents, by assumption and based on circumstantial empirical evidence, experience emotional distress growing up in a cultural environment from which they are alienated, leading to weakened cultural values (not valued or reinforced in mainstream society), a feeling of distance from society, a lack of pride in their cultural roots, and the inability of the poverty-stricken, single-parent household structure to serve as an agent for their socialization. The narrative approach was taken because of the Hispanic oral tradition of passing down cultural and familial values within the family and because, as Howard (1991) has argued, psychopathology is a life story gone awry while the goal of treatment is to reconstruct a healthy story within behaviorally disordered youths.

CHARACTERISTICS OF THE TREATMENT PROGRAM

The three treatment interventions involved similar procedures for participant selection. Superintendents in three inner-city public school districts in Brooklyn and the Bronx, New York, serving large, primarily Puerto Rican communities were approached for their district's participation. The purpose of the research and scope of preliminary screening, testing, and therapeutic activities proposed were explained to both parents and the prospective participants, and all signed informed consent forms. At the first level of screening, children were identified by classroom teacher referrals for problems of acting out and disruptive behavior and apparent evidence of possible anxious or depressive moods. Subsequently, teachers and parents were administered standardized behavioral rating scales (Conner's Behavior Rating Scale [CBRS]) to identify the most problematic students. About 300–500 students were screened per study, and those with the most pathological scores were selected for participation. Approximately 80% of those screened and invited to participate ultimately volunteered. The target sample size was at least 200 per study in order to achieve sufficient statistical power to detect moderate treatment effects at the standard .05 level of significance. The practicality of sample size was another consideration, given project resources and the capacity of schools and a local mental health clinic to manage the groups.

The therapy was administered by trained psychotherapists (graduate doctoral interns in clinical and school psychology), who followed a standardized treatment manual outline. Initial training sessions were videotaped with clients at the local clinical treatment center, and feedback was provided by supervising licensed psychologists. All three versions of narrative therapy were conducted with the children and adolescents in a small-group format of six to eight participants per session. Sessions were conducted weekly. In the case of cuento/folktale therapy, children's mothers also participated in the group sessions. Cuento and storytelling therapies were conducted within the participating clinic, and the hero/heroine therapy was presented as an after-school program in lieu of alternative school activities.

Cuento and Hero/Heroine Therapy

Two versions of cuento therapy were conducted, one based on the original folktales about the Juan Bobo character from Puerto Rican folklore and a second based on an adaptation of the cuentos to a modern-day Hispanic community setting. For instance, in the adapted cuentos, apple trees in a rural Puerto Rican farm were transformed to an apple stand in a local community bodega; a farmer became a local storekeeper; and horses became taxi cabs. It was predicted that this manipulation would promote greater identification with the main character as a vehicle for therapeutic change while retaining the essential cultural elements of the cuentos.

Cuento and hero/heroine therapies were conducted in twenty 90-minute sessions, while the storytelling therapy was conducted as a brief intervention with eight 90-minute sessions. The decision to terminate experimental treatments was based on protocol design (i.e., the number of cuentos, hero/heroine, and TEMAS stimulus pictures preselected for the research). Participants who were considered by therapists as needing continuing mental health care were referred to the local community mental health center following completion of the study.

In the hero/heroine intervention, which was conducted with 12- to 15-year-olds, 10 male and 10 female biographies were selected from Puerto Rican history. The selection criteria targeted persons who had confronted adversities in their lives and had managed to overcome them through adaptive behavioral resolution of their dilemmas. In particular, the biographies exemplified themes such as confronting racial/ethnic prejudice, poverty, educational and athletic achievement, and maintenance of a positive self-image and cultural pride. Biographies ranged from the time of Columbus and Ponce de León to modern figures such as athletes Roberto Clemente (professional baseball star) and Angelita Lind (track and field star) as well as those fighting political causes on the island such as Carlos Albizu Campos, a black, Harvard University-educated lawyer who was jailed, persecuted, and exiled for his efforts to achieve Puerto Rico's independence from the United States.

Storytelling Intervention

In the storytelling intervention, older children (preadolescents), ages 9–11 (grades 4–6), were randomly assigned to discuss TEMAS pictures or read nontherapeutic stories (attention control). Eight pictures were selected for their intended "pull" of various themes, such as complying with a parental request for a child to purchase something at a local bodega versus running off to play with friends; a character sitting at a desk doing homework, with mental images of scoring an F from a scolding teacher versus an A from a smiling teacher; a group of girls or boys molesting a peer versus helping him or her repair a broken bicycle. Similar to the previous intervention, verbal reinforcement accompanied stories emphasizing positive themes and socially adaptive behavior, while maladaptive stories were not reinforced and children were prompted to seek more socially acceptable alternatives.

Study Designs

In each study, outcomes of the experimental treatment intervention were compared with those of a control group. Half of the participants, stratified by gender, were randomly assigned to an experimental narrative treatment or a control group who received play therapy in the case of the cuento and hero/heroine studies and an equal-attention control group who read nontherapeutic stories (e.g., *Tom Sawyer*) in the storytelling study.

Intervention Procedures

The 90-minute group sessions were structured according to four stages. First, the therapist read aloud the cuentos and biographies in the first two studies along with the participants. In the third study, therapists represented scenarios of TEMAS pictures for approximately 15 minutes, describing the pictures overall with prompts: "What is happening in this picture?" What happened before?" "How does the story end"? "How does the main character in the story feel at the end?"

Second, participants were asked to relate the content of the narratives to events and emotional feelings in their own lives for about 30 minutes of a session. Goals of the initial sessions (up to three) were primarily to establish therapeutic rapport, therapeutic alliance, and confidence in sharing openly among a peer group. The remaining sessions were expected to have greater therapeutic impact on participants' distress, culminating in reduced maladaptive behavior and anxiety and increased self-esteem and instilling a sense of ethnic identity and pride in their Puerto Rican cultural roots.

Third, possible adaptive resolutions of conflicts and distress that were articulated were the subject of group discussion (30 minutes). For instance, in one cuento, Juan Bobo is stealing apples from a local farmer. His dilemma, upon being caught by his mother, is whether to return the apples, admit his misbehavior, and face the attendant consequences of his actions or abscond with the apples, eat them for immediate gratification, and attempt to cover up his misbehavior. Some interesting qualitative observations reported by the therapists were that during early sessions the children—in grades K–3—tended toward the latter option. They were accustomed to this manner of behavior to satisfy their immediate needs. Although the intention of the intervention was not to necessarily instill a sense of morality in the children, their themes changed in this direction as sessions progressed. They enjoyed the "comical" Juan Bobo figure and could readily identify with his behavior. As Juan's plight took on negative consequence, also a factor in their personal experience, remorse and suggestions for more socially appropriate behavior began to emerge in the sessions. Finally, the group engaged in role-playing of a single cuento, biographical character, or TEMAS narrative selected by the group for the remaining 15 minutes. The role-playing exercises were videotaped and played back to the group for further discussion and reinforcement.

Throughout stages 2–4, verbal reinforcement was provided by the therapist and solicited from peer participants. To reinforce behavior more tangibly and promote continuation in therapy, inasmuch as research by Sue and Zane (1987) has reported up to 50% dropout rates after a single session among ethnic minorities, token rewards such as t-shirts and school supplies were awarded after every two consecutive sessions attended.

Treatment materials were developed as standardized protocols to be followed by the therapists; cuentos and hero/heroine biographies are available from the author. TEMAS pictures used in the storytelling intervention are copyrighted by Western Psychological Services (Los Angeles, CA) and are available from the publisher.

EVIDENCE ON THE EFFECTS OF TREATMENT

Cuento Therapy

In the initial study of cuento therapy (Costantino et al., 1986), 210 boys and girls (ages 5–8) were randomly assigned to four groups: original cuentos, adapted cuentos, art/play therapy, or no-treatment control. Participants were tested before treatment, after treatment, and again at 1-year follow-up ($n = 178$). Anxiety symptoms were measured by the 10-item Trait subtest of the Spielberger State-Trait Anxiety Inventory. Social judgment was measured by the Comprehension subtest of the Wechsler Intelligence Scale for Children–Revised. Observational rating measures were developed by the authors to measure aggression (in response to an experimenter-induced provocation), disruptiveness (compliance with instruction to remain silent during a 10-minute task), and delay of gratification (number of days awaiting an increasingly larger monetary award).

With respect to anxiety, first graders differed between groups on the immediate posttest, with the adapted cuento group evidencing more favorable effects than the other three groups. The original cuento group evidenced less anxiety than the no-treatment controls but did not differ from the art/play therapy group. After 1 year, the adapted cuento group evidenced less anxiety than the art/play and no-treatment groups but not the original cuento group, who, in turn, differed only from the no-treatment group. After 1 year, treatment effects were direct and not moderated by either age/grade level or gender. Adapted cuentos remained the most effective treatment but did not differ significantly from the original cuentos treatment.

Social judgment differences between treatment groups were evident on the immediate posttest but not as the 1-year follow-up. Both cuento treatments enhanced social judgment relative to art/play and no treatment. This suggests that the culturally based treatments facilitated children's ability to understand, verbalize, and evaluate socially acquired knowledge in an adaptive manner.

There were no effects on disruptive behavior, which may be due to a measurement problem. The observation rating scale was devised by the authors and not standardized or tested for reliability or validity in traditional ways; on the other hand, when interrater reliability was assessed, it was high, at .80. Unexpectedly, adapted and original cuento therapy reduced children's aggressiveness relative to art/play therapy but not to no treatment. One explanation is that the art/play therapy enabled children to express their feelings by acting out, which promoted aggressive behavior in comparison to the more benign themes in the cuentos. However, aggressive themes appearing in the cuentos may have induced aggression relative to no treatment (nonexposure to aggression). Thus, the children may indeed have modeled the behaviors presented in cuentos but may not have internalized the consequences of aggression in the stories; if this was the case, it would suggest that change of aggressive behavior may require more powerful reinforcement techniques than those provided via the cuentos.

Hero/Heroine Therapy

Interviews with older children (third graders) participating in the cuento study, conducted in debriefing sessions, revealed an interesting qualitative finding. Many reportedly found the cuentos to be too juvenile and cartoon-like. They expressed feelings of being treated as children younger than their age, which may partially explain some of the nonsignificant findings. This suggests that they were reluctant to identify with the Juan Bobo character and, therefore did not engage in imitative role modeling. This inspired greater consideration of the age appropriateness of the treatment modality, leading to the development of the hero/heroine therapy.

This study was conducted with 90 male and female Puerto Rican adolescents in grades 8–9 (ages 13–15), who were randomly assigned to either the hero/heroine treatment or an equal-attention control group. Treatment outcomes were measured using the Piers–Harris Self Concept Scale, the Trait scale of the Spielberger State–Trait Anxiety Inventory, the Symptom Checklist-90 (SCL-90), Distress (scored for global severity), and a Puerto Rican identity scale (Rogler, Cortes, & Malgady, 1991).

The analysis of anxiety outcomes revealed a significant treatment x grade level interaction, with differences between treatment groups, in favor of the hero/heroine treatment but only among eighth graders. Once again, qualitative interview data shed some light on these findings. The ninth graders in particular reportedly found the treatment sessions too repetitive in content; the themes of facing and overcoming poverty and prejudice, successful achievement, and the like were instilled after about four sessions. Thus, their interest in and attentiveness to the biographies may have waned as the sessions drew on, again despite verbal reinforcement by the therapist and peers and tangible rewards.

Although there was no effect on the measure of self-concept, there was a moderate effect of hero/heroine therapy in promoting ethnic identity relative to the equal-attention control group. There were, however, interaction effects with respect to both self-concept and ethnic identity as a function of gender and household structure (father presence in the household). Treatments did not differ among girls in father-absent households nor among boys in father-present households. Boys from father-absent households showed much greater ethnic identity in the hero/heroine treatment compared with controls.

Girls, on the other hand, showed greater ethnic identity when they came from father-present households.

One supposition about these findings is that the female adolescents may have already strongly identified with their mothers, so the culturally sensitive treatment did not impact their identities. Lacking a father in the household may be more stressful for boys during adolescence; consequently, the male biographical figures in hero/heroine therapy may have provided role models with whom boys could readily identify.

On self-concept, the interaction effects were also curious. The therapeutic role models promoted self-concept more for girls than boys in father-absent families. Perhaps most interesting, despite the intention of the intervention and research logic to enhance self-esteem, there was a strong negative treatment effect among female adolescents from intact (two-parent) families. Although the girls from intact families felt "more Puerto Rican" as a result of treatment, their self-image paradoxically diminished in the process. Two reasons come to mind for this discrepant finding. The role models presented in therapy may have aroused conflict about the girls' own parents as role models, and as a result of own-parent identification the idealized role models may have invoked feelings of parental inadequacy. Their own fallible parents were being judged against the most heroic figures in Puerto Rican history. In addition, many of the female biographies were stories that may have provoked sex-role conflicts inasmuch as many were in non-traditional female roles (particularly for Puerto Ricans), such as professional athletes, lawyers, and politicians.

Turning to debriefing information, qualitative interviews exposed a consensus among females about one of the particular heroes selected by the panel of research experts. This concerned the biography of Carlos Albizu Campos, which the researchers found most compelling and heroic of all. The female adolescents viewed this biography rather unheroically. The fact that he had to leave his family and spent years in jail and political exile fighting for Puerto Rico's independence was quite dismaying to the young girls. His abandonment of family overrode whatever significance his contributions to the culture and political climate of Puerto Rico may have had. In this case, it seems clear that the adult researchers' culture differed dramatically from that of the young female adolescents, who were most concerned with maintaining an intact family system.

Storytelling Therapy

In the third study (Costantino, Malgady, & Rogler, 1994), 90 Puerto Rican male and female preadolescents (ages 9–11) were randomly assigned to either the TEMAS storytelling treatment or an equal-attention control group. Evidence indicated that there were no differences between treatments or interactions involving gender or grade level with respect to adolescents' depression, as measured by the Center for Epidemiological Studies Depression Scale. There were, however, interactions on teacher ratings of student conduct, as measured by the CBRS. Specifically, there was a treatment x grade level interaction on CBRS ratings such that treatment groups differed in favor of the storytelling intervention among sixth graders but not among youths in lower grades. Further analysis revealed that this was due to effects on the Conduct Problem and Hyperactivity subscales.

There was also a main effect of treatment on the SCL-90 Anxiety subscale but no interaction effects. Thus, the effect of culturally based storytelling therapy reduced anxiety regardless of adolescents' gender or age within the range studied. More complex findings emerged from an analysis of phobic symptomatology on the SCL-90. A three-way interaction (treatment x gender x grade level) emerged, such that for boys story-telling therapy reduced phobic symptoms relative to controls at the sixth-grade level, whereas for girls this pattern occurred at both the fifth- and sixth-grade levels. Thus, this study was consistent with earlier studies showing that narrative therapies are effective treatment models for Puerto Rican children and adolescents, but treatment effects are moderated by factors such as household structure, gender, and age.

DIRECTIONS FOR RESEARCH

One important consideration emerging from this program of research on narrative therapy, and perhaps the most interesting, is the serendipitous finding of myriad interaction effects involving children's and adolescents' gender, age/grade level, and household structure. What works for one does not necessarily work for all. Clearly, such findings call for further systematic research to explore other possible moderator effects in relation to culturally oriented therapies. The question of potential mediator effects, to my knowledge, has not been investigated in this realm. Studies conducted with more substantial sample sizes are needed to permit more sophisticated statistical analyses of how treatments and their moderators and mediators influence outcomes; with adequate sample size and appropriate measurement models, these analyses might use such techniques as structural equation modeling.

Another issue concerns the generalizability of findings from this particular program of treatment–outcome research. The studies were conducted in the northeast United States (New York City), where the Hispanic population largely consists of persons of descent or immigrants from Puerto Rico and, lately, the Dominican Republic. Generalizability to the highly diverse Hispanic population in this country is questionable (Malgady, 1994), given the vast socioeconomic, educational, linguistic, and even subcultural differences between such groups as Cubans (predominantly in the southeast) and Mexican Americans (primarily in the southwest).

Despite the encouraging findings about narrative therapy and the establishment of at least a foundation for an evidence base, further research is needed to explore the underlying processes related to the treatment effects and to build a theoretical understanding of the issues raises by the findings. A recent PsychINFO literature search revealed only two studies in the past 2 years that attempted to apply culturally oriented psychotherapy to ethnic minorities. Despite the attention given to cultural competence in the American Psychological Association (APA; 1993) guidelines as well as to diagnostic considerations in the *Diagnostic and Statistical Manual of Mental Disorders* (fourth edition; American Psychiatry Association, 1994), during the past decade little new light has been shed on the fundamental problem of how best to provide effective mental health services to the high-risk, high-need, underserved Hispanic population in this country.

This chapter has described a program of treatment–outcome research based on the use of narrative techniques in psychotherapy with Puerto Rican children and adolescents. The evidence-based conclusion is that such culturally oriented treatment leads to more favorable treatment outcomes compared with traditional therapy and equal-attention and no-treatment control conditions. However, this conclusion is qualified by important interactions indicating that treatment effects may differ widely across subsets of our study samples.

The latest study in this programmatic research effort introduces a new concept into the literature, namely cultural congruence, which refers to the fit of the cultural competence of mental health service providers with the cultural needs of the consumers of such services. A standardized index has been developed to quantify the degree of fit between provider and consumer, and preliminary data suggest that it is predictive of outcomes as a moderator of treatment.

CONCLUSIONS

More than two decades ago, a comprehensive review of the relatively sparse research addressing the special needs of ethnic minority clients receiving mental health services uncovered three fundamental approaches to treatment, or what was then called "cultural sensitivity" (Rogler, Malgady, Costantino, & Blumenthal, 1987). These approaches included matching the ethnicity/race of treatment providers with that of their clients, at the most fundamental level, while providing services in a culturally appropriate ambiance and adapting to any language issues in the case of nonnative English-speaking clients. The second level was to select a treatment from our menu of mainstream treatments that best fit the minority group's cultural character. The third level of culturally sensitive treatment was to develop new modalities or adapt mainstream treatments to clients' culture, as in the case of cuento therapy for young Puerto Rican children.

Since then, there has been growing recognition of the importance of bridging cultural gaps between the mental health service system and the needs of typically low-socioeconomic, unacculturated, minority clients who are increasingly underrepresented in the mental health service population. More recently, the most commonly used terminology is "cultural competence," which has been extensively defined in the Guidelines for Providers of Mental Health Services by the APA (2003) to address disparities in mental health care among underserved minority populations.

Despite the presence of clearly articulated guidelines, supported by the APA, there has been no research designed to systematically measure the construct of cultural competence across a variety of mental health care settings in relation to treatment outcomes. Moreover, the focus of service providers on cultural characteristics has taken place largely in the absence of refined assessments of individual clients' cultural needs in treatment. For example, a second- or third-generation Latino, who is racially white and middle class and speaks little or no Spanish might not require the same degree of consideration of Latino culture in mental health treatment as, for example, a racially black, immigrant Latino speaking little or no English and living at the poverty level. Cultural congruence (Costantino et al., in press) refers to the distance between the cultural competence of the mental health service provider and the cultural neediness of the individual client seeking treatment. As the distance increases, there is a culture gap, disparity, or incongruence between the culture of services delivered and the culture being served. As the gap narrows, clients' cultural needs are able to be accommodated by the mental health service system at hand. Our preliminary findings have indicated that cultural congruence does not predict treatment outcomes directly, but it moderates the effects of other factors (i.e., integrated primary care vs. direct referral to psychiatrists) influencing treatment outcomes, such as anxiety, depression, and substance abuse.

The program of research described in this chapter provides an evidence base in support of a narrative approach to psychotherapeutic intervention with Hispanic children and adolescents, who characteristically exhibit higher prevalence of mental health disorders and less favorable treatment outcomes compared with their nonminority counterparts. This research supports the view that minority youths can be effectively treated by increasing the relevance of therapeutic stimuli, such as cuentos, heroic biographies, and TEMAS pictures, to children's and adolescents' cultural roots, but the research also reveals numerous interactions, tempering conclusions about overall treatment effects and suggesting many useful directions for future research. In the years ahead, there is much to be learned about the potential benefits of interventions relying on identification with culturally relevant characters and modeling of their adaptive behavior to resolve everyday dilemmas as a treatment vehicle for behaviorally troubled Hispanic youths.

REFERENCES

American Psychiatric Association. (1994). *Diagnostic and statistical manual of mental disorders* (4th ed.). Washington, DC: Author.

American Psychological Association. (1993). Guidelines for providers of psychological services to ethnic, linguistic, and culturally diverse populations. *American Psychologist, 48*, 44–48.

Costantino, G., Dana, R., & Malgady, R. G. (2008). *The TEMAS test: Research and applications.* Hillsdale, NJ: Erlbaum.

Costantino, G., Malgady, R. G., & Primavera, L. P. (in press). *Journal of Consulting and Clinical Psychology.*

Costantino, G., Malgady, R. G., & Rogler, L. (1986). Cuento therapy: A culturally sensitive treatment modality for Puerto Rican children. *Journal of Consulting and Clinical Psychology, 54,* 739–746.

Costantino, G., Malgady, R. G., & Rogler, L. H. (1994). Storytelling through pictures: Culturally sensitive psychotherapy for Hispanic children and adolescents. *Journal of Clinical Child Psychology, 23,* 13–20.

Howard, G. S. (1991). Culture tales: A narrative approach to thinking, cross-cultural psychology, and psychotherapy. *American Psychologist, 48,* 127–141.

Malgady, R. G. (1994). Hispanic diversity and the need for culturally sensitive mental health services. In R. G. Malgady & O. Rodriguez (Eds.), *Theoretical and conceptual issues in Hispanic mental health* (pp. 27–54). Melbourne, FL: Krieger.

Malgady, R. G. (1996). The question of cultural bias in assessment and diagnosis of ethnic minority clients: Let's reject the null hypothesis anyway. *Professional Psychology: Research and Practice, 27,* 73–77.

Malgady, R. G., Rogler, L. H., & Costantino, G. (1990). Hero/heroine modeling for Puerto Rican adolescents. *Journal of Consulting and Clinical Psychology, 58,* 469–474.

Rogler, L. H., Cortes, D. H., & Malgady, R. G. (1991). Acculturation and mental health status among Hispanics: Convergence and directions for new research. *American Psychologist, 46,* 585–597.

Rogler, L. H., Malgady, R. G., Costantino, G., & Blumenthal, R. (1987). What do culturally sensitive mental health services mean?: The case of Hispanics. *American Psychologist, 47,* 565–570.

Rogler, L. H., Malgady, R. G., & Rodriguez, O. (1989). *Hispanics and mental health: A framework for research.* Melbourne, FL: Krieger.

Sue, S., & Zane, N. (1987). The role of culture and cultural techniques in psychotherapy: A critique and reformulation. *American Psychologist, 42,* 37–45.

26

Functional Family Therapy for Adolescent Substance Use Disorders

HOLLY BARRETT WALDRON and JANET L. BRODY

OVERVIEW OF THE CLINICAL PROBLEM

Adolescent substance use disorders (SUDs) encompass a broad spectrum of phenomena involving distinct substances used, a range in quantity and frequency of use, an array of associated problem behaviors, and multiple ecological influences (Winters, Stinchfield, & Bukstein, 2008). SUDs are often viewed as just another manifestation of adolescent disruptive behavior. However, the pharmacological effects and physiologically addictive properties of alcohol and illicit drugs have important and unique implications for treatment relative to those for other adolescent disorders. In addition, unlike other clinical problems, the development and maintenance of SUDs may be influenced by the immediate social environment, including the extent of peer or parent substance abuse, the availability of substances, and the prevailing societal influences (e.g., tobacco and alcohol taxes, stringent law enforcement, bans on nonprescription medications). Another unique feature of adolescent SUDs is that substance use is a covert behavior not always readily apparent to parents, teachers, and health professionals. The majority of teens with SUDs are characterized by lack of motivation to change and resistance to treatment, entering treatment only under a court mandate or in lieu of school suspension.

The consequences associated with SUDs can be severe. Potential adverse consequences include school failure and dropout, substance-related injuries, and increased risk for sexually transmitted infections, HIV/AIDS, teen pregnancy, violent exchanges, overdose, and death. Substance use can also interfere with crucial developmental tasks, such as prosocial identity formation, interpersonal and educational skill acquisition, and meeting family and work responsibilities (Bentler, 1992). Youths with SUDs often have co-occurring conduct, depressive, bipolar, posttraumatic stress, and anxiety disorders, bulimia, and other problem behaviors (Kaminer & Bukstein, 2008). Evidence indicates that dual diagnosis increases the likelihood of continued problem behaviors and is associated with poorer treatment outcomes. The negative consequences associated with SUDs, the co-occurrence of other psychiatric disorders, and the associated problems facing these youths and their families underscore the need for evidence-based practice.

The influence of the family on the development and maintenance of substance use problems is widely recognized. Parental and sibling use, family members' attitudes toward use, poor family management practices, disturbed marital and family relationship functioning, and a host of other family factors have been linked to adolescent substance abuse and have been conceptualized as interdependent and bidirectional influences. Moreover, treatment–outcome research has shown that family-based interventions are associated with higher rates of treatment engagement and retention, significant reductions in substance use, and improved functioning in other behavioral domains (Stanton & Shadish, 1997; Waldron & Turner, 2008).

FUNCTIONAL FAMILY THERAPY: CHARACTERISTICS OF THE TREATMENT PROGRAM

The focus of this chapter is the functional family therapy (FFT) approach for adolescents with SUDs and their families. FFT is a widely disseminated evidence-based treatment developed for youths with conduct disorder, delinquency, and other disruptive behaviors (Alexander et al., 1998). FFT has also been implemented with families of adolescents with SUDs (Friedman, 1989; Waldron, Slesnick, Brody, Turner, & Peterson, 2001) and has emerged as a well-established treatment for youths with alcohol, marijuana, and other illicit substance use disorders (Waldron & Turner, 2008). The purpose of this chapter is to provide an introduction to FFT for clinicians in diverse settings who treat adolescents with SUDs and related problem behaviors and to serve as a guide for clinicians already familiar with FFT with respect to integrating strategies for drug-abusing youths into their FFT practice.

Conceptual Overview

The FFT model is an ecological approach that, like other systemic family models, conceptualizes alcohol and drug abuse as problem behaviors that develop and are maintained in the context of maladaptive family relationships (Alexander et al., 1998). Thus, changing family interactions and improving relationship functioning are key to reducing adolescents' involvement with alcohol and other drugs. The essential core and distinguishing feature of family systems models, relative to other treatment models, is that the locus of problem behavior is relational, transcending the individual; therefore, the focus of treatment should also be relational. The FFT model goes beyond systems theory, integrating and conceptually linking behavioral and cognitive intervention strategies to the ecological formulation of the family disturbance.

The treatment goals for families of adolescents with substance abuse are to reduce adolescent substance use and other problem behaviors, improve family relationships, and increase adolescents' productive use of time. Underlying these goals is the emphasis on changing interaction patterns in the family such that the functions served by substance use are met through other, more adaptive behaviors. The specific methods used to achieve treatment goals are accomplished in three distinct phases: engagement/motivation, behavior change, and generalization/termination. Each of the phases has associated goals, intervention strategies and techniques, and therapist skills. The phases occur in sequence such that the tasks of one phase are completed before the therapist proceeds to the next phase.

Contents of the Treatment

FFT usually involves 12–16 sessions lasting 60–75 minutes, with sessions scheduled twice weekly at the beginning of treatment to potentiate the initial change process. This is followed by a period of weekly sessions to space learning and allow time between sessions for practice, concluding with sessions that occur several weeks apart as families are able to maintain new behaviors independently. Homework is an integral part of treatment and is tailored to the unique tasks of each phase. FFT is designed to include all family members who are living together and any other extended family members or significant others who are central to family functioning. With such an inclusive focus, getting the whole family to become involved in therapy may be the therapist's first great challenge and initial target of intervention.

Phase 1: Engagement/Motivation

The engagement/motivation phase focuses on readiness to change and involves creating the context in which behavior change can occur. The aims are to (1) engage the family in therapy and begin to develop a therapeutic relationship, (2) enhance the family's motivation for change, and (3) assess the relevant aspects of individual and family functioning to be addressed in treatment.

Engaging Families

The process of engaging families relies primarily on creating positive expectations for therapy. A host of variables can influence treatment expectancies, including characteristics of the service delivery system (e.g., reputation, location, friendliness of staff), family attitudes and beliefs, and therapist characteristics (e.g., age, gender, ethnicity, cultural sensitivity, education, experience, humor, interpersonal warmth). Adopting the language system used by the family, normalizing problems, and expressing confidence are only a few of the many ways therapists can influence family expectations for change.

Families with substance use problems frequently enter treatment with an established pattern of interaction involving intense negative affect and malevolent attributions (Waldron & Slesnick, 1998). These patterns and behaviors represent a major impediment to change at the onset of treatment. However, because confrontation is associated with family resistance, maintaining a nonblaming, nonjudgmental tone lowers family defensiveness and hostility and allows change to occur without forcing family members to admit fault for previous failures. The therapist's aim is to create a cognitive framework compatible with systemic change by offering families a relational perspective on their problems. The primary strategies for motivating families include (1) emphasizing the connections in thoughts, feelings, and behaviors of family members by focusing on the relational aspects of behaviors rather than on the individual-oriented complaints presented, (2) reframing, and (3) actively managing aversive interactions, all while maintaining a nonblaming stance. FFT therapists also strive for a balanced alliance with family members, taking care to avoid forming a coalition with one family member at the expense of another. Each family member should experience the therapist support while also coming to accept that all family members share in the responsibility for the family's problems.

Relationship Focus. In disturbed families, individuals rarely view their own behavior as contributing to their current difficulties in a contingent or interdependent fashion. Rather, their behavior is often seen as a necessary reaction to the misbehavior of other members. The therapist highlights the interactions between family members to increase their awareness of how they affect each other and how the relationship affects their own behavior. The therapist can facilitate a relationship focus by asking questions and identifying sequences of behavior that focus on the relational impact of family behaviors, thoughts, and feelings and guide the family away from discussions of the adolescent's problem behavior. For example, if a mother complains about having to constantly remind her daughter about chores and responsibilities, the therapist could turn to another sibling and ask, "Do you need Mom to keep after you like your sister? Or is your job to be the 'good' child?" Given the context of the mother's blaming, asking such a question redirects the exchange, focuses on family relationships, "takes the heat off" the referred family member, and increases the likelihood that the family will begin to experience the sense that they are "all in this together."

Reframing. Reframing problem behavior is a core technique of FFT aimed at changing the meaning and value of negative emotions and behaviors in the family. If family members can be helped to consider that their own and others' behaviors are motivated and maintained by variables other than individual malevolence (e.g., anger reflects underlying hurt or worry), they are more likely to see change as possible and become more motivated.

Some reframes may focus on motives (e.g., "So letting Brett live at home, even though he takes money from your purse, is one way you feel you can make sure he's safe and, at the same time, keep you from experiencing the loss of having him move out"). Other reframes emphasize a common experience shared by all family members and evolve into overarching themes that can be returned to throughout therapy to help redirect the family focus toward change (e.g., "A lot of times it sounds like important things don't get said in this family because you want to protect one another from pain and hurt"). The therapist can use knowledge, inferences, and guesswork about the family in relabeling. This strategy can continue for as many sessions as needed until the negativity is reduced and family members have adopted the shift in perspective.

Managing Aversive Interactions. Actively interrupting families during hostile exchanges is critical to avoid an escalation of the kind of interactions families typically experience at home and allows the family to experience a change, albeit brief, in the usual outcome. The therapist can redirect a hostile exchange using reframing or relational comments, making comments on the process just observed, or may interrupt the process specifically to slow down the pace of therapy, using summary statements to moderate the rate of exchange. Process comments, like summary statements or relational comments, slow the pace of therapy and help disrupt a negative cycle before it escalates. Process comments can also focus on the meaning family members ascribe to others' behaviors, can be used to dissect or analyze the points at which interactions become negative, and can be used to interconnect the affect, behavior, and cognitions of family members. One caution in managing aversive interactions, however, is that the traditional counseling technique of reflective listening and expressing empathy in response to a family member's blaming statement can be countertherapeutic. Empathy and reflection may verbally reinforce hostile expressions and escalate aversive exchanges.

SUD Engagement/Motivation Strategies

The FFT therapist will encounter many different types of family dynamics related to substance use, and there is no single approach that will be effective for all families. This section identifies some of the common therapeutic challenges encountered when working with these families and provides examples of specific strategies that may be effective in addressing the issues when they arise. These challenges often require creative use of the standard techniques prescribed in FFT treatment.

Establish the Meaning of Substance Use in the Family

Therapists should attempt to identify current or prior experiences that may be exacerbating certain views about substance use. Perhaps substance use means different things to different members of the family, and the differences in meaning create difficulty in communication or understanding individual behavior within the family. For example, suppose Mom had a brother who died of a drug overdose. She sees her son using drugs and is very frightened that he will escalate his drug use like her brother did and will die, too. For Mom, the son's drug use means he's engaging in behavior that is potentially life threatening. Dad, on the other hand, was a drug user in high school, just like his son, and stopped using over time. For Dad, drug use is a "normal" teenage activity that elicits little concern. In a family dynamic like this, Mom will tend to address the drug use as zealously as Dad minimizes it, leaving her feeling increasingly unsupported and frustrated. The son will receive a mixed message from his parents, hearing tacit approval from Dad while engaging in heated exchanges with Mom as she exerts pressure on him to stop using drugs. By examining differences in meaning, the therapist can focus the intervention on providing reframes that highlight the relational nature of the problem: "Mom's reaction is intense because her life experience leads her to worry more than Dad about what might happen to you with the drug use. Dad didn't suffer the same loss as your Mom. For her, this is about making sure nothing bad happens to the son she loves so much. That's why she tries so hard to control what you're doing. When Mom yells, that's her way of saying 'I'm really frightened.'"

When parents disagree about the importance of drug use as a problem, the therapist should not directly challenge positive drug use attitudes. Instead, the therapist points out how the difference of opinion limits the ability of the parents to work together as a team, creating bad feelings with the more concerned parent, who ends up feeling less supported. It also sends the message to the adolescent that the more the parents disagree, the more he or she will probably be able to get away with continuing the problem behavior.

Punitive Stance toward Drug Use

Some families adopt a rigid, punitive parenting approach in response to drug use, focusing much attention on the drug use behavior. The adolescents are viewed primarily in terms of their problem with drugs (e.g., they are addicts). There is often limited attention to other aspects of the relationship and few positive family interactions. Many times these families tend to get stuck in a cycle of escalating negative consequences. Rules are set for the adolescents, the rules are broken, and then increasing punishments are applied. Privileges are lost (e.g., grounding, no access to car keys, door removed from room, possessions taken away). The adolescents often become defiant under these punitive conditions and conflict escalates. A common trajectory is that parents repeatedly threaten to kick the adolescents out of the house. Although this pattern is also common in families facing other adolescent disruptive behaviors, a unique substance-related issue is that a substance use lapse is a normative aspect of recovery that can provide a useful opportunity to evaluate the antecedents of the lapse and problem solve how to avoid a recurrence. Thus, parents who define any evidence of substance use as a rule violation and an indicant of treatment failure will likely set the stage for crises that disrupt treatment and interfere with the expected process of recovery. One particularly effective reframe is to offer a longer term perspective for the families: "One of the goals of the family is to help Michael launch into adulthood. It might be time for Michael to move toward independence and living on his own, but we want that to happen as constructively as possible, with your support, so he's not moving out in anger."

A second strategy for these families is to expand the focus of the relationship beyond the negative emphasis on rules and behaviors to reestablishing a strong positive bond. Strengthening the bond can also serve to increase motivation to change. Homework assignments involving previously enjoyed family activities or new activities that have a high likelihood for success (e.g., send a positive text message) are good ways to begin the process.

Parental Substance Abuse

A particularly challenging situation is a family in which one parent is a chronic alcoholic or drug user, and the family enters therapy with the united belief that the parent's use is responsible for the adolescent's drug problem. The parent's acceptance of blame and regular apology for both his or her own drinking or drug use as well as for the adolescent's drug use serve to perpetuate the drug use. Rather than accepting the family's interpretation of the problem, the therapist must reframe the parent's substance use behavior to provide an alternative relational focus for the problem. "It sounds like it's been really important to the family to have someone who takes responsibility for all the problems, and that's clearly your role. I'm wondering whether the family has communicated how important it is to have you available for the other aspects of family life. I'm talking about the fun parts of being a member of this family, like sharing at dinner or coming home early and watching a movie together. And, I'm curious, are you responsible for Sally's talent in art too, or is Mom the one who gets credit for the good stuff?" The intent of this type of reframe is to help the family think about the roles in a different way. In this scenario, we have a good parent–bad parent dynamic that actually reinforces the current behavioral patterns and allows the dysfunctional behavior patterns to continue.

By challenging the rigid roles, the therapist helps everyone take responsibility for the dysfunctional behavior, expanding the ways family members can interact.

Talking about Drug Use in Sessions

In FFT, the presenting problem is de-emphasized as a topic of discussion because the individual problem behavior is viewed as a symptom of a dysfunctional relational pattern and the focus of the intervention is on the relational interactions. However, in families where the substance use is a direct component of the relationship (e.g., family members using together), it is important to highlight the connection between use and relationship contact. Yet the therapist also needs to avoid allowing the family to focus on drug use content alone and to maintain an emphasis on clarifying the meaning of drug use for the relationship. Moreover, the therapist will have to negotiate situations in which the parent views his or her own drug use as acceptable but views the adolescent's use as a problem behavior. One effective technique in this situation is to use reframing in conjunction with questions about the circumstances and behavioral sequences associated with conjoint substance-using behavior. This is followed by a reframe that emphasizes the positive or negative role the drug use is playing in the relationship and points to a relational motivation for reducing the use. For example, in response to a mother saying, "When we're using together we're just able to relax," the therapist could say, "It's really important for both of you to share downtime and the drugs have helped you do that. It sounds like what we need to do is figure out other ways you two can enjoy each other's company, because that's important to you, but we want to do that without the drug use, since the drugs are getting in the way of your son's success in school." This approach avoids directly focusing on the parent's substance use as a cause of the adolescent's drug problem. Therapists should avoid confronting or blaming the parent, because that will result in defensiveness. Instead, the therapist focuses on the relational impact of the drug use, framing the problem as a need to find ways of enhancing the relationship in a manner that does not involve drug use.

Assessment

Assessment takes place at two levels to identify what change is needed (e.g., drug use, other problem behavior) and how the behavior change needs to occur in order to maintain the functions served by the behavior. Specific recommendations for substance use assessment are reviewed elsewhere (e.g., Winters et al., 2008). The concept of the interpersonal function of behavior is unique to the FFT model and is an essential element in determining how behavior change techniques should be implemented in the family. By integrating drug use and relationship function information, the therapist can devise a unique plan for each family that takes into account the characteristics and needs of each individual as well as the fit between these individual characteristics at the relationship level.

Relational functions are defined in terms of the interpersonal relatedness or interdependency they allow each family member to achieve with each other. Each family member has a relational function, closeness, distance, or midpointing, with each other member of the family (e.g., mother with son, son with mother, mother with father,

father with son). The essence of understanding the interpersonal function of behaviors between members of each dyad is to look at the outcome of the behavior. If a behavior is associated with repeated interaction patterns in families that result in family members experiencing significant physical or psychological separation from one another, then the function of the behavior is distance. If the outcome of behavior is that family members experience greater connection or interdependency, the function is closeness. Some relationships involve a blending of distance and closeness, or midpointing.

Although certain behaviors more commonly produce certain functions (e.g., intoxication is distancing), a particular behavior is never assumed to create a specific function. Adolescent drug use could create considerable distance in that the youth spends the majority of free time with other drug-abusing peers. Alternatively, drug use may cue a repeated behavioral sequence in the family that routinely results in increased closeness when mother and father rally around the adolescent in a renewed effort to support him or her.

Although closeness and intimacy are generally viewed as socially desirable and distance as undesirable, FFT functions are not conceptualized as inherently good or bad. In addition to healthy forms of closeness, "smothering" or enmeshed relationships represent maladaptive forms. Although some forms of distance are unhealthy (e.g., isolating oneself from other family members, being nonresponsive), maintaining distance from other people may facilitate the development of independent thinking and a sense of autonomy and competence. Midpointing can also be expressed in either adaptive or maladaptive ways. For example, a young adult with a drug problem may at times use the addiction as a way of escaping from the family and at other times as a way of connecting with them: "I lost my license, so you need to drive me to work." The identification of the functions for each dyad in the family allows the therapist to develop a change plan that will address maladaptive behaviors while ensuring that each family member's functions with others are maintained, thereby increasing the likelihood that behavioral changes will be successful.

Phase 2: Behavior Change

Behavior change focuses on establishing and maintaining behavior change both at the individual level and for the family as a whole. In this phase, the motivational framework created and the assessment data obtained in engagement/motivation are used to guide the selection and implementation of specific behavioral techniques. The primary goal of this phase is to establish new behaviors and patterns of interaction that will replace old ones, preventing maladaptive patterns from reappearing and producing long-term change in the family. During behavior change, techniques are used to change the meaning of behavior, the attributions family members have about one another, and family members' motivations. Although such changes are important prerequisites to long-term change, they will not be maintained unless interaction patterns follow a specific plan.

During this phase, therapists draw from a menu of treatment strategies and techniques in order to achieve the objectives for change for each target behavior in the treatment plan. In addition, therapists can implement other specialized evidence-based strategies as needed (e.g., trauma intervention, anxiety management) to tailor treatment to the individual needs of adolescents or families. Strategies are implemented to be consistent with each family member's interpersonal function with each other family member.

An early goal in the behavior change phase is to enhance the family's experience of positive change by increasing positive activities and interactions. Throughout the behavior change phase, interactions are highly structured and the therapist is active and directive. By maximizing the success experiences of families, the positive momentum and family motivation established in the treatment readiness phase will continue.

The specific techniques introduced by the therapist in the behavior change phase can include any strategies or devices capable of changing behavior and accomplishing these goals. The FFT model has not created a new set of techniques for changing behavior. Rather, clinicians are directed to the broader literature on evidence-based cognitive and behavioral treatments to integrate other behavior-change strategies into FFT as needed. The most commonly used behavior change session topics are presented in Table 26.1. Communication and problem-solving skills training are considered core behavior change strategies and are implemented in some form with virtually all families. Other topics may or may not be used and are presented as a menu of options. In addition, a host of technical aids can be integrated into behavior change sessions to support families' change efforts (Alexander et al., 1998).

The unique emphasis of the FFT model is on the application of techniques in the context of the assessment of functional payoffs in the family and tailored to each set of family relationships. For example, the manner in which the therapist incorporates communication or problem-solving skills into family interactions may range from instituting nightly, formal family meetings (high contact, low distance) to occasional, informal, as-needed checkups between family members or even written notes used to convey messages and solve problems (low contact, high distance). Similarly, community-based approaches such as Alcoholics Anonymous could be incorporated into treatment, for example, with a father and son with drinking problems attending meetings together or attending different meetings on alternating nights of the week, again depending on their assessed relationship functions.

TABLE 26.1. Menu of Behavior Change Session Topics

Increasing pleasant family activities

Communication training ("feeling heard")

Problem-solving skills

Anger management

Depression and negative mood management

Assertiveness training

Contingency management

Functional analysis of substance use behavior

Coping with drug and alcohol urges and cravings

Substance refusal skills

Decision making for drug avoidance ("seemingly irrelevant decisions")

Enhancing behaviors that compete with drugs

Relapse prevention

Job skills

SUD Behavior Change Strategies

There are a variety of behavior change techniques for the unique problems associated with substance abuse. However, the behavior change program selected for families will be based on the specific problems associated with each family and on the family functions identified during the engagement/motivation phase. When both the adolescent and the parent are involved in substance use, conducting a functional analysis of their use behavior (i.e., identifying antecedents and consequences of use as well as the quantity, frequency, and circumstances surrounding use) can help reinforce the relational nature of the substance use problems and identify specific ways in which the adolescent and parent can support each other in reducing use. This technique can be effective in motivating parents to address their own use and can be introduced as an informational exercise for parents who resist changing their own behavior.

Despite improvements in family relationships, actual drug use reduction can be hampered by difficulties coping with the urges and cravings associated with the addictive properties of drugs. Several techniques exist for identifying and coping with urges and cravings. One strategy that can be implemented in the behavior change when the adolescent has a contact or midpointing function with one or both parents parent is to have the adolescent seek support from the parents to help monitor and cope with urges to use. Similarly, relapse prevention techniques can be discussed with the entire family, and specific responsibilities can be assigned to family members to help support the adolescent's sobriety. For example, when the adolescent is invited to a party, if the mother has a distancing function, she can help her daughter figure out what triggers for drug use might come up and be available by phone to pick the daughter up as part of a safety plan.

Communication between the adolescent and the parent is often compromised because of escalated reactions to the adolescent's drug use. A common FFT behavior change strategy to help individuals regulate negative moods and emotions (e.g., anger management, coping with negative thoughts) can be effective in this situation. The process involves examining and challenging automatic and irrational thoughts associated with a particular situation and then demonstrating the link between these thoughts, negative moods, and poor family communication. ("When I see Adam getting high, it makes me think about my brother, who did the same thing and ended up homeless, spending all his money on drugs. I get so worried that I just yell at him to stop, then he gets mad and we get into a fight"). By challenging the belief that Adam will turn out like her brother, the parent is then able to substitute more useful thoughts (e.g., "Adam isn't my brother and it probably is frustrating to him that I keep comparing them. I'm just going to thank him for bringing his dishes down from his room"). This process will deescalate emotional responses and help the family implement more effective communication strategies.

Phase 3: Generalization and Termination

The final phase of FFT is designed to facilitate maintenance of behavior change and the generalization of treatment gains to the natural environment. As behavioral changes are established in the family, the focus of therapy shifts toward maintenance of change and establishing the family's independence from the therapy, with the therapist gradually taking a less active role and the interval between sessions extended. A key goal of the generalization phase is for families to apply their newly acquired behavioral skills to novel situations outside the therapy room. Families are continually faced with new challenges that can quickly send them back into prior behavior patterns. While still in therapy, it is helpful to review the families' attempts during the week to use their newly acquired behavior change skills. Even one successful experience using the behavior change strategies outside of the therapy room can be very powerful for motivating families to continue their efforts.

Another area of emphasis related to generalizing behavior change is the focus on multiple system issues. Many extrafamilial factors cannot be changed, such as neighborhood crime or availability of specific drugs. However, other factors may be modifiable for a family, such as responsiveness of school personnel. The therapist may interact directly with legal and educational systems on behalf of the family, particularly during the later stages of therapy when a family is about to complete therapy. In addition, the therapist should help families interact more effectively with extrafamilial influences on their own. For example, an adolescent could be encouraged to use his or her new communication skills to assertively refuse the offer of drugs in the neighborhood or to ask for help from a teacher at school. A mother may identify ways to support her adolescent by helping him to communicate effectively with a probation officer or to practice for a job interview.

The therapist may also help the family anticipate future problems and potential solutions (e.g., how the family will handle a lapse if the adolescent ends up using at a party, steps Mom can take to calm herself when she angry, how parents resolve disagreements about punishment when their son comes home high). By helping families anticipate appropriate solutions, the therapist will increase the possibility that the families will respond effectively when situations arise, further solidifying their use of behavior change techniques. Therapy moves toward termination when (1) drug and alcohol use and other problem behaviors are reduced or eliminated, (2) adaptive interaction patterns and problem-solving styles have been developed and occur independent of the therapist, and (3) the family appears to have the necessary motivation, skills, and resources to maintain a positive clinical trajectory without the support of ongoing services.

EVIDENCE ON THE EFFECTS OF TREATMENT

FFT has received considerable research attention during the past 25 years. Initially developed and evaluated for crisis intervention with juvenile offenders and their families, the effectiveness of FFT has been replicated across sites and settings for substance use problems and a wide range of other problem behaviors (Alexander et al., 1998; Barton, Alexander, Waldron, Turner, & Warburton, 1985; Gordon, Graves, & Arbuthnot, 1995; Klein, Alexander, & Parsons, 1976).

The FFT was evaluated by Friedman (1989) in a randomized trial involving 135 families of youths ages 14–21 years presenting with heavy alcohol and drug use (e.g., daily cannabis use). Friedman compared FFT with a parenting skills group intervention. Both the FFT and parent training groups showed significant reductions in substance use of more than 50% at follow-up, with improvements in other areas of functioning as well. Although no differences were found between the two treatment groups for treated families, engagement rates differed dramatically (93% in FFT vs. 67% in the parenting condition). In a reanalysis of the entire intention-to-treat sample (i.e., including treatment dropouts as failures), Stanton and Shadish (1997) found significantly greater substance use reductions for FFT than the comparison condition.

Tentative support for FFT was also found in a study by Lewis, Piercy, Sprenkle, and Trepper (1990) with 136 youths described as regular substance users. They compared an integrative family therapy model, described as a combination of elements drawn from FFT and structural strategic systems therapy, with a didactic, family-oriented parenting skills intervention similar to Friedman's parent group and an educational intervention that included all family members. The integrated treatment and a parenting skills intervention both showed significant pre- to posttreatment reductions in drug use, with a greater percentage of youths in family therapy decreasing their use. Although the family intervention involved an adapted form of FFT, the findings provide additional indirect support for the model with SUD youths.

More recently, we conducted a series of three randomized trials comparing FFT with group and individual cognitive-behavioral therapy (CBT). The total sample included 129 adolescents (30 girls, 99 boys) ranging in age from 13–17 ($M = 15.54$). Families identified their race/ethnicity as follows: Hispanic, 35%; Anglo, 41%; Native American, 6%; mixed, 15%; and other, 3%. In the first study, referred adolescents ($N = 120$) were randomly assigned to FFT, individual CBT, a combined FFT and individual CBT intervention, or a group skills-based intervention (Waldron et al., 2001). Adolescents received 12 hours of FFT, CBT, or group intervention or 24 hours of therapy in the combined condition (Waldron et al., 2001). Substance use, including self-report and urine toxicology screening, was measured at baseline and 4, 7, and 19 months after treatment initiation. Adolescents in both of the FFT conditions showed significant reductions in the percentage of days using marijuana from baseline to the 4-month follow-up. Significant reductions also occurred at the 7-month and 19-month assessments. Adolescent marijuana use in the group condition was not significantly lower than at baseline at the 4-month assessment, but it was significantly lower at the 7-month and 19-month assessments. The CBT condition was not significantly different from baseline at any of the three follow-up measurement conditions. The findings supported the short-term benefit of FFT for substance-abusing youths.

The second study focused on alcohol and extended the work of the marijuana study (cf. Waldron & Turner, 2008). In this trial, drinking teens ($N = 146$) were randomly assigned the same four intervention conditions, although in this study the combined FFT and CBT treatment was integrated so that treatment dose was equated with the other conditions (14 sessions). In this integrated condition, families were scheduled to receive approximately eight FFT sessions. In all other respects, the two studies were virtually identical. Because drinking teens also used marijuana and other illicit drugs, the primary dependent variables included percentage of days of alcohol use and marijuana use in the past 3 months..All four conditions were associated with significant reductions in the percentage of days of alcohol use from pre- to posttreatment. Significant reductions in marijuana use were also shown in the FFT only and individual CBT conditions. Thus, FFT and CBT were the only conditions associated with improvement for both alcohol and marijuana.

The third randomized trial evaluated the efficacy of our integrated FFT + CBT intervention relative to CBT alone for Anglo and Hispanic drug-abusing adolescents across two project sites, one in New Mexico and the other in Oregon (cf. Waldron

& Turner, 2008). Each site included 60 Anglo and 60 Mexican American youths. In addition, the New Mexico site included 60 New Mexican Hispanic youths, a primarily English-speaking, highly acculturated Hispanic group with a 500-year presence in the state. Both interventions involved 14 sessions, with approximately eight FFT sessions in the integrated condition. Assessments occurred at baseline and at 5, 8, and 18 months after treatment initiation.

Results of the analysis for Hispanic participants revealed a statistically significant treatment condition × time interaction. To further evaluate the interaction effect, we compared the difference between treatments at each assessment. We found significant reductions from baseline to 5-month follow-up for both conditions, with significantly greater reductions for the FFT + CBT condition. No differences were found between the two groups at later follow-ups. A similar analysis was performed for the Anglo sample. The analysis revealed a statistically significant main effect for time, with no differences between the two treatments. Anglo youths in FFT and in CBT showed significant reductions in drug use at each posttreatment assessment point.

Outcomes for our three FFT studies were included in a recent meta-analytic study (Waldron & Turner, 2008). In this meta-analysis, we examined 46 different treatment conditions that included 2,307 adolescents treated for SUDs. The combined sample evaluated several family therapy models, including FFT, group CBT, individual CBT, and a minimal treatment condition. The effect size for the pre- to posttreatment change in the minimal treatment condition was 0.21, which reflected a significant reduction in drug use. For families who received FFT, the effect size for the change from pre- to posttreatment was 0.65, a significantly larger effect than for the minimal treatment condition. For families who received a lighter dose of FFT (eight sessions) when FFT was offered in combination with CBT, the effect size for the pre- to posttreatment change was 0.36. Although this effect size reflects a significant reduction in drug use, it is not significantly different from the minimal treatment condition. Thus, the strongest support for FFT for the three clinical trials included in the meta-analysis was for the higher dose of FFT.

DIRECTIONS FOR RESEARCH

Individual adolescent outcomes in SUD treatment research have varied widely across randomized clinical trials. Because no single treatment approach appears to be equally efficacious for all youths, research focusing on understanding who might benefit from particular treatments, including FFT, is a high priority. Moreover, given relapse trajectories for a substantial subgroup of treated youths, FFT strategies designed to enhance the maintenance of treatment gains among youths at risk for relapse are urgently needed. One approach that has potential for addressing problems associated with variability in treatment response is adaptive, progressive treatments (Collins, Murphy, & Bierman, 2004). Although FFT allows tremendous flexibility in implementation, the basic model does not take into account the breadth of individual differences in the presentation of adolescent SUDs that might make aspects of the approach less relevant or inefficient for certain individuals. In adaptive research designs, treatment algorithms that vary treatment components and dosages in response to the needs of the individuals are used to guide clinical decision making. In FFT, early treatment responders could step out of treatment, with follow-up or booster sessions offered as needed, while nonresponders could progress to FFT with a contingency management component involving incentives earned for family therapy compliance and achievement of drug abstinence.

Another major research direction involves understanding the parameters surrounding the efficient transfer of FFT into community settings. Through a formal dissemination organization, FFT has been established in more than 250 clinical settings worldwide. Yet research examining the transfer process has been rare. Poor adherence of therapists to treatment models has been cited as one of the major limitations to successfully establishing evidence-based practices outside of research settings. Research linking specific training and supervision approaches to treatment adherence and outcome could inform administrators and treatment providers in clinical service delivery systems regarding sustainable implementation practices. Improved implementation could have a substantial impact on increased FFT services for SUD youths. Such research could also examine the organizational and system-level variables related to treatment utilization and outcomes.

Future research should also include an emphasis on mechanisms associated with FFT effectiveness. In particular, process–outcome research is essential within all phases of FFT to increase our understanding of how manual-guided interventions should be implemented or could be enhanced. Such research could also examine how therapist behavior is linked to changes in adolescent and family functioning.

CONCLUSIONS

FFT is an integrated systems and behavioral family-based intervention in which SUDs are conceptualized as problem behaviors that develop and are maintained in the context of maladaptive family relationships. The intervention is designed to change family interactions as a means for reducing adolescents' involvement with alcohol and illicit drugs. Taken together, FFT outcome studies have demonstrated consistent decreases in substance use from baseline to follow-up. Moreover, a recent meta-analysis showed that FFT was superior to treatment as usual. Research is needed to identify SUD youths most likely to benefit from FFT and to enhance the FFT intervention to improve outcomes for youths at risk for relapse. Future research should also begin to evaluate individually tailored adaptive, progressive approaches for integrating FFT into a continuum of SUD treatments, to examine the process of dissemination of FFT into community settings, and to identify mechanisms associated with treatment effectiveness.

ACKNOWLEDGMENTS

This research was supported in part by grants from the National Institute on Drug Abuse (Nos. R01 DA11955, R01DA13350, R01DA13354) and the National Institute on Alcohol Abuse and Alcoholism (No. R01 AA12183). We are also grateful to Hyman Hops for his ongoing support of our efforts and his editorial feedback on drafts of the chapter.

REFERENCES

Alexander, J. F., Barton, C., Gordon, D., Grotpeter, J., Hansson, K., Harrison, R., et al. (1998). *Blueprints for violence prevention.* Boulder, CO: Venture.

Barton, C., Alexander, J. F., Waldron, H., Turner, C. W., & Warburton, J. (1985). Generalizing treatment effects of functional family therapy: Three replications. *Journal of Marriage and Family Therapy, 13*, 16–26.

Bentler, P. M. (1992). Etiologies and consequences of adolescent drug use: Implications for prevention. *Journal of Addictive Diseases, 11*, 47–61.

Collins, L. M., Murphy, S. A., & Bierman, K. L. (2004). A conceptual framework for adaptive preventive interventions. *Prevention Science, 5*, 185–196.

Friedman, A. S. (1989). Family therapy vs. parent groups: Effects on adolescent drug abusers. *American Journal of Family Therapy, 17*, 335–347.

Gordon, D. A., Graves, K., & Arbuthnot, J. (1995). The effect of functional family therapy for delinquents on adult criminal behavior. *Criminal Justice and Behavior, 22*, 60–73.

Kaminer, Y., & Bukstein, O. G. (Eds.). (2008). *Adolescent substance abuse: Psychiatric cormorbidity and high-risk behaviors.* New York: Routledge.

Klein, N. C., Alexander, J. F., & Parsons, B. V. (1976). Impact of family systems intervention on recidivism and sibling delinquency: A model of primary prevention and program evaluation. *Journal of Consulting and Clinical Psychology, 45*, 469–474.

Lewis, R. A., Piercy, F. P., Sprenkle, D. H., & Trepper, T. S. (1990). Family-based interventions for helping drug-abusing adolescents. *Journal of Adolescent Research, 5*, 82–95.

Stanton, M. D., & Shadish, W. R. (1997). Outcome, attrition, and family/couples treatment for drug abuse: A review of the controlled, comparative studies. *Psychological Bulletin, 122*, 170–191.

Waldron, H. B., & Slesnick, N. (1998). Treating the family. In W. R. Miller & N. Heather (Eds.), *Treating addictive behaviors: Processes of change* (2nd ed., pp. 271–285). New York: Plenum.

Waldron, H. B., Slesnick, N., Brody, J. L., Turner, C. W., & Peterson, T. R. (2001). Treatment outcomes for adolescent substance abuse at 4- and 7-month assessments. *Journal of Consulting and Clinical Psychology, 69*, 802–813.

Waldron, H. B., & Turner, C. W. (2008). Evidence-based psychosocial treatments for adolescent substance abuse. *Journal of Clinical Child and Adolescent Psychology, 37*, 238–261.

Winters, K. C., Stinchfield, R., & Bukstein, O. G. (2008). Assessing adolescent substance use and abuse. In Y. Kaminer & O. G. Bukstein (Eds.), *Adolescent substance abuse: Psychiatric cormorbidity and high-risk behaviors* (pp. 53–85). New York: Routledge.

27

Treating Adolescent Substance Abuse Using Multidimensional Family Therapy

HOWARD A. LIDDLE

OVERVIEW OF THE CLINICAL PROBLEM

The nature of a clinically referred adolescent's presenting problems makes treating teen drug abuse challenging. These problems are multivariate, such as the often secretive aspects of drug use; involvement in illegal and criminal activities with antisocial or drug-using peers; despairing, stressed, and poorly functioning families; involvement in multiple social agencies; disengagement from school and other prosocial contexts of development; and lack of intrinsic motivation to change. Many new developments in the drug abuse and delinquency specialties provide guidance and hope. We have witnessed an unprecedented volume of basic and treatment research, increased funding for specialized youth services, and a burgeoning interest in the problems of youths from basic research and applied prevention and treatment scientists, policymakers, clinicians and prevention programmers, professional and scientific societies, mass media and the arts, and the public at large. Developmental psychology and developmental psychopathology research has revealed the forces and factors that combine and contribute to the genesis of teen drug experimentation and abuse. Perhaps a consensus about a preferred conceptualization and intervention strategy has been reached. Leading figures in the field now conclude that drug abuse results from both intraindividual and environmental factors. For this reason, unidimensional models of drug abuse are inadequate and multidimensional research and intervention approaches are necessary.

This chapter summarizes multidimensional family therapy (MDFT), a family-based therapy with considerable empirical support for its effectiveness with teen drug abuse and delinquency (Liddle, 2004). Three frameworks help therapists use the research knowledge base on teen drug use. The *risk and protective factor* framework informs clinicians about the known antecedents of dysfunction and resilience. It identifies factors from different domains of functioning (psychological, social, biological, neighborhood/community) relevant to positive adaptation and threats to development. It also helps therapists to think in interactional or process terms about the many clinically germane dimensions of a teen's and family's current life circumstances.

The *developmental perspective* (developmental psychology and developmental psychopathology research) is another useful framework. This knowledge base informs therapists about the course of individual adaptation and dysfunction through the lens of normative development. Developmental psychopathology moves beyond considerations of symptoms only to understand a youth's ability to cope with the developmental milestones at hand, and considers the implications of stressful experiences and developmental failures in one developmental period for (mal)adaptation in future periods. Because multiple pathways of adjustment and deviation may unfold from any given point, emphasis is placed equally on understanding competence and resilience in the face of risk. Adolescent substance abuse is conceptualized as a problem of development, a deviation from the normal developmental pathway. Substance abuse is a failure to meet developmental challenges and a set of behaviors that compromises hope to achieve future developmental milestones.

The third framework, the *ecological perspective,* articulates the intersecting web of social influences that form the context of human development. Ecological theory regards the family as a principal developmental arena, and it takes a keen interest in how both intrapersonal and intrafamilial processes are affected by and affect extrafamilial systems (i.e., significant others involved with the youth and family, such as school, job, or juvenile justice personnel). This theory coincides with contemporary ideas about reciprocal effects in human relationships, and it underscores how problems nest at different levels and how circumstances in one domain can affect other domains.

Assumptions Underlying Treatment: Ten Principles of MDFT

1. *Adolescent drug abuse is a multidimensional phenomenon.* Individual biological, social, cognitive, personality, interpersonal, familial, developmental, and social ecological aspects can all contribute to the development, continuation, worsening, and chronicity of drug problems.

2. *Family functioning is instrumental in creating new, developmentally adaptive lifestyle alternatives for adolescents.* The teen's relationships with parents, siblings, and other family members are fundamental areas of assessment and change. The adolescent's day-to-day family environment offers numerous and essential opportunities to retrack developmental functioning.

3. *Problem situations provide information and opportunity.* Symptoms and problem situations provide assessment information as well as essential intervention opportunities.

4. *Change is multifaceted, multidetermined, and stage oriented.* Behavioral change emerges from interaction among systems and levels of systems, people, domains of functioning, and intrapersonal and interpersonal processes. A multivariate conception of change commits the clinician to a coordinated, sequential use of multiple change methods and to working multiple change pathways.

5. *Motivation is malleable but it is not assumed.* Motivation to enter treatment or to change will not always be present with adolescents or their parents. Treatment receptiv-

ity and motivation vary in individual family members and relevant extrafamilial others. Treatment reluctance is not pathologized. Motivating teens and family members about treatment participation and change is a fundamental therapeutic task.

6. *Multiple therapeutic alliances are required and they create a foundation for change.* Therapists create individual working relationships with the adolescent, individual parents or caregivers, and individuals outside of the family who are or should be involved with the youth.

7. *Individualized interventions foster developmental competencies.* Interventions have generic or universal aspects. For instance, one always wants to create opportunities to build adolescent and parental competence during and between sessions, but all interventions must be personalized, tailored or individualized to each person and situation. Interventions are customized according to the family's background, history, interactional style, culture, and experiences. Structure and flexibility are two sides of the same therapeutic coin.

8. *Treatment occurs in stages; continuity is stressed.* Core operations (e.g., adolescent or parent treatment engagement and theme formation), parts of a session, whole sessions, stages of therapy, and therapy overall are conceived and organized in stages. Continuity— linking pieces of therapeutic work together—is critical. A session's components and the parts of treatment overall are woven together; continuity across sessions creates change-enabling circumstances.

9. *Therapist responsibility is emphasized.* Therapists promote participation and enhance motivation of all relevant persons; create a workable agenda and clinical focus; provide thematic focus and consistency throughout treatment; prompt behavior change; evaluate, with the family and extrafamilial others, the ongoing success of interventions; and, per this feedback, collaboratively revise interventions as needed.

10. *Therapist attitude is fundamental to success.* Clinicians are neither "child savers" nor unidimensional "tough love" proponents; they advocate for adolescents *and* parents. Therapists are optimistic but not naïve or Pollyannaish about change. Their sensitivity to contextual or societal influences stimulates intervention possibilities rather than reasons for how problems began or excuses for why change is not occurring. As instruments of change, a clinician's personal functioning enhances or handicaps one's work.

CHARACTERISTICS OF THE TREATMENT PROGRAM

Multidimensional Assessment

Assessment yields a therapeutic blueprint, an indication about where and how to intervene across multiple domains and settings of the teen's life. A comprehensive, multidimensional assessment process identifies risk and protective factors in relevant areas and prioritizes and targets specific areas for change. Information about functioning in each target area comes from referral source information and dynamics, individual and family interviews, observations of spontaneous and instigated family interactions, and interchanges with influential others outside of the family. MDFT's four overall targets are (1) adolescent, (2) parent, (3) family interaction, and (4) extrafamilial social systems. Attending to deficits and hidden areas of strength, we obtain a clinical picture of the unique combination of weaknesses and assets in the adolescent, family, and social system. A contextualized portrait includes a multisystems formulation of how the current situation and behaviors are understandable, given the youth's and family's developmental history and current risk and resilience profile. Interventions decrease risk processes known to be related to dysfunction development or progression (e.g., parenting problems, affiliation with drug-using peers, disengagement from and poor outcomes in school) and enhance protection, first within what the therapist finds to be the most accessible and malleable domains. An ongoing process rather than a single event, assessment continues throughout treatment as new information emerges and experience accumulates. Assessments and therapeutic planning overall are revised according to feedback from our interventions.

A home-based or clinic-based family session generally starts treatment. Telephone conversations with a parent, and sometimes the teen, typically precede the first session. These calls may be important in beginning motivation enhancement and the assessment process. Therapists stimulate family interaction on important topics, noting to themselves how individuals contribute to the adolescent's life and current circumstances. We also meet alone with the youth, the parents, and other family members within the first session or two. These meetings reveal the unique perspective of each family member, how events have transpired (e.g., legal and drug problems, neighborhood and negative peer influences, school and family relationship difficulties), what family members have done to address the problems, what they believe needs to change with the youth and family, as well as their own concerns and problems, perhaps unrelated to the adolescent.

Therapists elicit the adolescent's life story during early individual sessions. Sharing one's life experiences facilitates teen engagement. It provides a detailed picture of the nature and severity of the youth's circumstances and drug use, individual beliefs and attitude about drugs, trajectory of drug use over time, family history, peer relationships, school and legal problems, any other social context factors, and important life events. Adolescents sketch out an eco-map, representing one's current life space. This includes the neighborhood, indicating where the teen hangs or buys and uses drugs, where friends live, and school or work locales. Per protocols (Marvel, Rowe, Colon, DiClemente, & Liddle, 2009), clinicians inquire about health and lifestyle issues, including sexual behavior. Comorbid mental health problems are assessed by reviewing records and reports, the clinical interview process, and psychiatric evaluations. Adolescent substance abuse screening devices, including urine drug screens (used extensively in therapy), are invaluable in obtaining a comprehensive picture of the teen's and family's circumstances.

Parents assessment includes their functioning both as parents and as adults, with individual, unique histories, and concerns. We assess strengths and weaknesses in terms of parenting knowledge, skills and parenting style, parenting beliefs, and emotional connection to one's child. Inquiring in detail about parenting practices, clinicians promote parent–teen discussions and in this process watch for relationship indicators such as supportiveness and attachment. Parents discuss their experiences of family life when they were growing up, because these may be used to motivate or shape needed changes in current parenting style and beliefs. Nothing is more vital to ascertain and facilitate than parents' emotional connection to and investment in their child. Parent mental health and substance use are also appraised and addressed directly as potential challenges to improved parenting. On occasion we make referrals for a parent's adjunctive treatment of drug or alcohol abuse or serious mental health problems.

Information on extrafamilial influences is integrated with the adolescent's and family's reports to yield a comprehensive picture of individual and family functioning relative to external systems. A new component of our approach provides on-site educational academic tutoring that meshes with core MDFT work. We assess school- and job-related issues thoroughly, and well-planned parent–teen meetings with school personnel are frequent. Therapists cultivate relationships and work closely with juvenile court personnel, particularly probation officers, who sort out the youth's charges and legal requirements. Facing juvenile justice and legal issues can become emotional. Clinicians help parents understand the potential harm of continued negative or deepening legal outcomes. Using a nonpunitive tone, we help teens face and take needed action regarding their legal situation. Friendship network assessment encourages teens to talk forthrightly and in detail about peers, school, and neighborhoods. Friends may be asked to be part of sessions. They can be met during sessions in the family's home. A driving force in MDFT is the creation of concrete alternatives that use family, community, or other resources to provide prosocial, development-enhancing day-to-day activities.

Adolescent Focus

Clinicians build a firm therapeutic foundation by establishing a working alliance with the teenager, a relationship that is distinct from but related to identical efforts with the parent. We present therapy as a collaborative process, following through on this proposition by collaboratively establishing therapeutic goals that are practical and personally meaningful to the adolescent. Goals become apparent as teens express their experience and evaluation of their life so far. Treatment attends to these "big picture" dimensions. Problem solving, creating practical, attainable alternatives to a drug-using and delinquent lifestyle—these remediation efforts exist within an approach that addresses an adolescent's conception of his or her own life, values, life's direction, and meaning. Success in one's alliance with the teenager is noticed by parents. Parents expect and appreciate how clinicians reach out to and form a distinct relationship and therapeutic focus with their child. Individual sessions are indispensable; their purpose is defined in "both/and" terms. These sessions access and focus on individual and parent–teen and other relationship issues through methods that might be construed as belonging within an individual therapy (vs. multiple systems) approach. Individual parent and teen meetings also prepare (i.e., motivate, coach, rehearse) for joint sessions.

Parent Focus

We focus on reaching the caregivers as adults with individual issues and needs and as parents who may have declining motivation or faith in their ability to influence the child. Objectives include enhancing feelings of parental love and emotional connection, underscoring parents' past efforts, acknowledging difficult past and present circumstances, generating hope, and improving parenting. When parents enter into, think, talk about, and experience these processes, their emotional and behavioral investment in their adolescent deepens. This process, the expansion of parents' commitment to their child's welfare, is fundamental to the MDFT change model. Achieving these therapeutic tasks sets the stage for later changes. Taking the first step toward change with the parents, these interventions grow parents' motivation and, gradually, parents' capacity to address relationship improvement and parenting strategies. Increasing parental involvement with one's adolescent (e.g., showing an interest, initiating conversations, creating a new interpersonal environment in day-to-day transactions) creates a new foundation for attitudinal shifts, enhanced repertoire, and changes in parenting. We foster parental competence by teaching and behavioral coaching about normative characteristics of parent–adolescent relationships, consistent and age-appropriate limit setting, monitoring, and emotional support, all research-established parental behaviors that enhance relationships, individual, and family development.

Cooperation is achieved and motivation enhanced by underscoring the serious, often life-threatening circumstances of the youth's life and establishing an overt, discussable connection (i.e., a logic model) between that caregiver's involvement and creating behavioral and relational alternatives for the adolescent. This follows the general procedure used with parents, promoting caring and connection through several means: First through an intense focusing and detailing of the youth's difficult and sometimes dire circumstances, making sure that these realities are experienced deeply by the parent (although there is description of the youth's circumstances, the presumed mechanism of action here is experiential and not didactic or psychoeducational), which then flows into the need for the parents to reengage and work hard to help the youth change.

Parent–Adolescent Interaction Focus

MDFT interventions also change development-detouring transactions directly. Shaping changes in the parent–adolescent relationship are made in sessions through the structural family therapy technique of enactment. A clinical method and a set of ideas about how change occurs, enactment involves elicitation and frank discussion in family sessions of important topics or relationship themes. These discussions reveal relationship strengths and problems. Expanding their repertoire of experience, perceptions, and behavioral alternatives, therapists assist family members to discuss and solve problems in new ways. This method creates behavioral alternatives as clinicians actively guide, coach, and shape increasingly positive and constructive family interactions. For discussions to involve problem solving and relationship healing, family members must be able to communicate without excessive blame, defensiveness, or recrimination. Therapists guide retreats from extreme stances, because these actions undermine problem solving, instigate hurt feelings, and discourage motivation and hope for change. Individual sessions sharpen and process these important issues and prepare family members for family sessions where the issues are discussed and new ways of relating are attempted. The content focus of any given session is important. Skilled therapists focus in-session conversations on personal and meaningful topics in a patient, sensitive way.

Focus on Social Systems External to the Family

Clinicians help the family and adolescent interact more effectively with extrafamilial systems. Families may be involved with multiple community agencies. Success or failure in interacting with these systems affects short term, and in some cases longer term, outcomes. A give-and-take collaboration with school, legal, employment, mental health, and health systems influencing the youth's life is critical for engagement and durable change. An overwhelmed parent appreciates a therapist who can understand and negotiate with complex and intimidating bureaucracies and obtain adjunctive services. Achieving these practical outcomes lessens parental stress and burden, enhances engagement, and bolsters parental efficacy. Therapists team with parents to organize meetings with school personnel or probation officers. Because successful compliance with the legal supervision requirements is an instrumental therapeutic focus, therapists prepare the family for and attend the youth's disposition hearings. School or job placement outcomes are additional core aspects: They represent real-world settings where the teen can develop competence and build escape routes from deviant peers and drugs. In some cases, medical or immigration matters or financial problems may be urgent areas of stress and need. We understand the interconnection and synergy of these life circumstances in improving family life, parenting, and a teen's reclaiming of his or her life from the perils of the street. Not all multisystem problems are solvable. Nonetheless, in every case, our rule of thumb is to assess comprehensively, declare priorities, and, as much as possible, work actively and directively to help the family achieve better day-to-day outcomes relative to the most consequential and malleable areas in the four target domains.

Decision Rules about Individual, Family, or Extrafamilial Sessions

MDFT works from "parts" (subsystems) to larger "wholes" (systems) as well as from these larger units (families/family relationships) back down to smaller units (individuals). Session composition is not random or at the discretion of the family or extrafamilial others, although sometimes this is unavoidable. Session goals drive decisions about session participants. Goals may exist in one or more categories. At any given point there may be session-specific goals suggesting who should be present for all or part of an interview. For instance, a significant part of the first sessions, from strategic (i.e., relationship formation, giving a message about family involvement) and information-gathering (i.e., family interaction is a key part of what therapists access, assess and ultimately attempt to change) perspectives, include all family members.

MDFT works in four interdependent and mutually influencing subsystems with each case. The rationale for this multiperson focus is theory based and practical. Some family-based interventions might address parenting practices by working alone with the parent for most or all of treatment. Others might only conduct whole-family sessions throughout (i.e., family interaction as the single pathway of youth change). MDFT is unique in how it works with the parents alone and with the teen alone as well, apart from the parent and family sessions, in addition to targeting family-level change *in vivo* and multisystems change efforts (i.e., multiple pathways of change). Individual sessions have communicational, relationship-building, strategic, and substantive (change focused) value. They provide "point of view" information and reveal feeling states and historical events not always forthcoming in family sessions. We establish multiple therapeutic relationships rather than a single alliance, as is the case in individual treatment. Success in those relationships connects to clinical success. A therapist's relationship with different people in the mosaic comprising the teen's and family's lives is the starting place for inviting and instigating change attempts. The strategic aspects of these actions are probably obvious by now. There is a leveraging, a shuttle diplomacy, that occurs in the individual sessions as they work to determine content and grow motivation, readiness, and capability to address other family members in joint sessions.

Manuals and Other Supporting Materials

A new version of the MDFT manual containing all core sessions and clinical and supervision protocols is forthcoming (Liddle, in press). MDFT has an online training program, which includes a curriculum, worksheets, and therapy video segments for clinical sites training in the approach. A multistep certification procedure includes site readiness preparation; clinical and supervision training procedures, including supervisor/trainer preparation protocols; and adherence and quality assurance procedures. Independent MDFT training institutes have been established in the United States and Europe. Many clinical articles have been written over the years, and two MDFT DVDs are available (Liddle, 1994, 2008, 2009; Rodriguez, Dakof, Kanzki, & Marvel, 2005).

EVIDENCE ON THE EFFECTS OF TREATMENT

MDFT has been developed and tested since 1985. In 2010, we will complete our 10th MDFT randomized controlled trial (RCT). This research program has produced considerable evidence supporting the intervention's effectiveness for adolescent substance abuse and antisocial behavior. Four types of studies have been conducted: efficacy/effectiveness RCTs, process studies, cost studies, and implementation/dissemination studies. The projects have been conducted at sites across the United States with diverse samples of adolescents (African American, Hispanic, and Caucasian youths ages 11–18) of varying socioeconomic backgrounds. Internationally, a multinational MDFT controlled trial in Germany, France, Switzerland, Belgium, and the Netherlands is complete and publications are forthcoming. Study participants across studies met diagnostic criteria for adolescent substance abuse disorder and included teens with serious drug abuse and delinquency. MDFT has demonstrated efficacy in comparison to several other state-of-the-art active treatments, including a psychoeducational multifamily group intervention, peer group treatment, individual cognitive-behavioral therapy (CBT), and residential treatment. Table 27.1 summarizes key outcomes and studies contributing to the MDFT evidence base.

Substance Abuse

MDFT participants' substance use is reduced significantly. Using an example from one study, MDFT youths reduced drug use by 41–66% from baseline to treatment completion. These outcomes remained consistent at 1-year follow-up (Liddle et al., 2001; Liddle, Dakof, Turner, Henderson, & Greenbaum, 2008; Liddle, Rowe, Dakof, Henderson, & Greenbaum, 2009; Liddle, Rowe, Ungaro, Dakof, & Henderson, 2004). MDFT youths also have demonstrated abstinence from illicit drugs after treatment significantly more than teens in comparison treatments (Liddle & Dakof, 2002; Liddle et al., 2001, 2008,

(text resumes on p. 427)

TABLE 27.1. Multidimensional Family Therapy (MDFT) Representative Controlled Trials: Summary of Primary Outcomes

Study	Population	Treatment conditions	Assessments	Findings
Liddle et al. (2001)	$N = 182$; mean age, 16 (range: 13–18); 80% male; 51% white, non-Hispanic; 18% African American; 15% Hispanic; 6% Asian; 10% other; 61% juvenile justice involved	Adolescent group therapy (AGT); multifamily educational intervention (MEI); vs. MDFT, once weekly for 4 months, clinic based	Baseline, treatment termination, 6 and 12 months	MDFT youths showed greater reduction in substance use ($\eta^2 = .12$). MDFT reduced substance use 54%; group therapy, 18%; multifamily therapy, 24%. MDFT substance use reduction retained at 12 months, MDFT youths showed greater increase in school grades ($\eta^2 = .09$) and improved family functioning ($\eta^2 = .16$) (videotape ratings).
Liddle & Dakof (2002)	$N = 113$; mean age, 15; 67% male; 79% Hispanic; 81% juvenile justice involved	Residential treatment (RT) vs. MDFT, 1–3 sessions weekly for 4–6 months, clinic and home based	4, 12, 18, 24, 36, and 48 months	MDFT retained 95% for 90 days or more. Compared with RT, MDFT youths more rapidly decreased drug use problem severity, self- and parent-reported aggressive behavior and delinquent activity, and substance use frequency. RT youths spent an average of 60 more days in controlled environments (jail, RT) during the 18-month follow-up (FU) period than MDFT youths. Treatment differences between intake and 18-month FU favor MDFT in parent-reported aggressive behavior and delinquent activity maintained at 4-year FU. RT: Drug use problems increased from 18 month to 4-year FU; MDFT maintained treatment gains. Substance use increased over the 4-year FU period for RT youths and treatment gains remained level for MDFT teens. At 4-year FU, RT youths increased their HIV risk more than MDFT youths.
Dennis et al. (2004)	$N = 300$; mean age, 15; 18% female, 82% male; 49% Caucasian, 49% African American; 82% juvenile justice involved	Adolescent community reinforcement approach (ACRA), motivational enhancement treatment/cognitive-behavior therapy (MET/CBT5) vs. MDFT, once weekly for 12 weeks, clinic based	Baseline, 6, 12, and 30 months	All Cannabis Youth Treatment (CYT) treatments are more effective clinically and cost less than current practice (treatment administrators' report). MDFT assessment by an independent investigator (Dennis, 2000; Dennis, personal communication, February 23, 2001) found that MDFT delivered at two sites (per study design) replicates results from earlier RCTs. At 6-month FU, MDFT youths reported 49% and 36% reductions (two sites). MDFT and other treatment costs were significantly less than both the mean and median costs of adolescent outpatient treatment. Benefit–cost analysis indicated that MDFT had a statistically significant baseline to

Study	Sample	Design	Assessment points	Findings
				12-month reduction in drug use consequences. MDFT had approximately equivalent net benefits associated with reduced drug use consequences as MET/CBT5, and both had relatively greater net benefits than ACRA.
Liddle et al. (2006)	N = 104; mean age, 15; 77% males, 23% females; 79% Hispanic (38% of Cuban descent), 13% African American, 1% white, non-Hispanic, 7% other (Haitian, Jamaican)	Quasi-experimental; interrupted-time series design; MDFT, 1–3 sessions per week, clinic based	1 month after intake, discharge from treatment, and 9 months after intake	Following training, therapists successfully delivered MDFT, with 36% increase in number of weekly individual therapy sessions, 150% increase in number of weekly family sessions, 390% increase in contact with probation officers, and 1,400% increase in school contacts compared with baseline (before training). Following withdrawal of all MDFT clinical staff, therapists continued to deliver MDFT according to protocol. Program factors (organization, clarity in expectations) improved after introduction of MDFT. Client outcomes significantly improved after staff MDFT training (substance use, internalizing and externalizing symptoms, fewer out-of-home placements). Improvements were sustained in durability phase, 1 year after withdrawal of MDFT trainers.
Liddle et al. (2008)	N = 224; mean age, 15 (range: 12–17.5); 81% male; 72% African American, 18% white, non-Hispanic, 10% Hispanic	Individual CBT vs. MDFT, once weekly for 4–6 months, clinic based	Baseline, 12 months	MDFT showed greater reductions in substance use problem severity, drug use, abstinence; impact was strongest after treatment completion. MDFT youths had 77% decrease in hard drug use; CBT teens increased drug use over the same time period. One year after intake 64% of MDFT youths showed minimal use compared with 44% for CBT youths. MDFT was more effective than CBT with more impaired cases.
Liddle et al. (2004, 2009)	N = 83; mean age, 14 (range: 11–15); 74% male; 42% Hispanic, 38% African American	Manualized peer group therapy vs. MDFT, 1–3 sessions per week for 3–4 months; clinic based	6 weeks from intake; treatment discharge; 6 and 12 months from intake	MDFT youths: more improvement than group treatment on all outcomes, demonstrated more improvement in substance use, delinquency, affiliation with delinquent peers, internalized distress, family and school functioning. MDFT youths were 2.3 times more likely to progress from having substance use problems at intake to not having problems at 12 months. At 12-month FU, MDFT teens were less likely to be arrested (23% vs. 44%), placed on probation (10% vs. 30%), and report delinquent behavior than group therapy participants.

(cont.)

TABLE 27.1. (cont.)

Study	Population	Treatment conditions	Assessments	Findings
Liddle et al. (in press)	$N = 154$; mean age, 15; 82% male; 60% African American; 22% Hispanic, 17% white, non-Hispanic	Enhanced services as usual (ESAU) vs. MDFT, 1–3 sessions per week, clinic based	Discharge from detention and at 3, 6, 9, and 24 months after detention release	MDFT-HIV intervention engaged 99% of youths successfully in detention and 97% in outpatient phase. Across treatments, drug use between intake and the 9-month FU decreased. Baseline: average of 46 days of drug use in the previous 90 days (measured by a timeline follow-back procedure) and decreased it over 60% over the 9-month FU. Between-treatment effects favored MDFT, especially those who received MDFT at the site characterized by greater therapist–JPO collaboration and more severely impaired youth (d = .75). MDFT reduced delinquency and days confined in detention (following the initial release from detention). MDFT youth showed superior outcomes for comorbid internalizing and externalizing problems—these youths continued to improve between 6 and 9 months, whereas comparison youths' symptoms increased. HIV prevention and reduction of high-risk sexual behavior outcomes: 76% of participants at intake engaged in moderate- to high-risk behaviors over the previous 90 days, and 11% of the sample tested positive for an STD. FU: MDFT youth were less likely to engage in unprotected sex acts over the 9-month FU than ESAU youth.

2009). For instance, in a recent study (at posttreatment and at 1-year follow-up) MDFT participants had 64% drug abstinence rates compared with 44% for CBT (Liddle et al., 2008); in another study, MDFT achieved a 93% abstinence outcome compared with 67% for group treatment (Liddle et al., 2009). MDFT has been effective as a community-based drug prevention program as well. And using a brief 12-session (over 3 months), in-clinic (community treatment setting) weekly protocol, MDFT has successfully treated clinically referred younger adolescents who recently initiated drug use (Liddle et al., 2009).

Substance abuse-related problems (e.g., antisocial, delinquent, externalizing behaviors) were reduced significantly in MDFT versus comparison interventions, including manual-guided active treatments. Ninety-three percent of MDFT youths report no substance-related problems at 1-year follow-up (Liddle et al., 2009).

School Functioning

School functioning improves more dramatically in MDFT versus comparison treatments. MDFT clients have been shown to return to school and receive passing grades at higher rates (Liddle et al., 2001, 2009) and also show significantly greater increases in conduct grades than a comparison peer group treatment (Liddle et al., 2009).

Psychiatric Symptoms

Psychiatric symptoms show greater reductions during treatment in MDFT than comparison treatments (30–85% within-treatment reductions in behavior problems, including delinquent acts and mental health problems such as anxiety and depression, Liddle et al., 2006, 2009). Compared with individual CBT, MDFT had better drug abuse outcomes for teens with co-occurring problems and decreased externalizing and internalizing symptoms, thus demonstrating superior and stable outcomes (1 year) with the more severely impaired adolescents (Liddle et al., 2008).

Delinquent Behavior and Association with Delinquent Peers

MDFT-treated youths have shown decreased delinquent behavior and associations with delinquent peers, whereas peer group treatment comparisons reported increases in delinquency and affiliation with delinquent peers. These outcomes maintain at 1-year follow-up (Liddle et al., 2004, 2009; Liddle, Dakof, Henderson, & Rowe, in press). Department of Juvenile Justice records indicate that, compared with teens in usual services, MDFT participants are less likely to be arrested or placed on probation and have fewer findings of wrongdoing during the study period. MDFT-treated youths also require fewer out-of-home placements than comparison teens (Liddle et al., 2006). Importantly, parents, teens, and collaborating professionals have found the approach acceptable and feasible to administer and participate in (Liddle et al., in press).

Theory-Related Changes: Family Functioning

MDFT youths report improvements in relationships with their parents (Liddle et al., 2009). On behavioral ratings, family functioning improves (e.g., reductions in family conflict, increases in family cohesion) to a greater extent in MDFT than family group therapy or peer group therapy (observational measures), and these gains are seen at 1-year follow-up (Liddle et al., 2001). In another example, MDFT-treated youths report gains in individual, developmental functioning on self-esteem and social skill measures.

Studies on the Therapeutic Process and Change Mechanisms

MDFT studies show improvements in family functioning by targeting in-session family interaction (Diamond & Liddle, 1996) and how therapists build productive therapeutic alliances with teens and parents (Diamond, Liddle, Hogue, & Dakof, 1999). Adolescents are more likely to complete treatment and decrease their drug taking when therapists have effective therapeutic relationships with their parents (Hogue, Liddle, Singer, & Leckrone, 2005) and with the teens as well (Robbins et al., 2006). Strong therapeutic alliances with adolescents predict greater decreases in their drug use (Shelef, Diamond, Diamond, & Liddle, 2005). Another process study found a linear adherence–outcome relation for drug use and externalizing symptoms (Hogue et al., 2005). MDFT process studies found that parents' skills improve during therapy and, critically, these changes predict teen symptom reduction (Henderson, Rowe, Dakof, Hawes, & Liddle, 2009; Schmidt, Liddle, & Dakof, 1996). Culturally responsive protocols have demonstrated increases in adolescent treatment participation (Jackson-Gilfort, Liddle, Tejeda, & Dakof, 2001). We are beginning to understand the relationship of particular kinds of interventions to key target outcomes. In one example, interventions focusing on in-session family change produced differences in drug use and emotional and behavioral problems (Hogue, Liddle, Dauber, & Samuolis, 2004).

Economic Analyses

The average weekly costs of treatment are significantly less for MDFT ($164) than for standard treatment ($365). An intensive version of MDFT has been designed as an alternative to residential treatment and provides superior clinical outcomes at significantly less cost (average weekly costs of $384 vs. $1,068 [French et al., 2003; Zavala et al., 2005]).

Implementation Research

MDFT integrated successfully into a representative day treatment program for adolescent drug abusers (Liddle et al., 2006). There were several noteworthy findings. First, after training, therapists delivered MDFT with superb fidelity (e.g., broadened treatment focus posttraining, addressed more approach-specific content themes, focused more on adolescents' thoughts and feelings about themselves and extrafamilial systems), with model adherence at 1-year follow-up. Second, client outcomes were significantly better, and these outcomes maintained at follow-up as well. Third, association with delinquent peers decreased more rapidly after therapists received MDFT training (Liddle et al., 2006) and drug use decreased by 25% before and 50% after a MDFT training and organizational intervention (and the probability of out-of-home placements for non-MDFT youths was significantly greater before MDFT was used in the program). Fourth, program or system-level factors improved dramatically as well, according to, for example, adolescents' perceptions of a program's increased organization and clarity of expectations (Liddle et al., 2004).

DIRECTIONS FOR RESEARCH

Our newest projects all address the model's capacity to retain efficacy while expanding the range of settings in which the approach can be used. A juvenile drug court study and a new juvenile justice diversion study are testing in controlled trials the additive value of MDFT when integrated into juvenile justice programs. This work is in accord with other juvenile-justice focused projects that demonstrated success with a version of MDFT that began with the youth in a juvenile detention facility (and conducted parent sessions in the home) and then continued upon the youth's release (Liddle et al., in press). Another adaptation of the approach is being tested in a controlled study that integrates evidence-based trauma and loss focused methods with the core MDFT approach for adolescents and families who suffered in the disaster of Hurricane Katrina.

Additional work focuses on new avenues of model refinement in the area of HIV prevention. We developed a standardized protocol that included parents in targeting the high-risk sexual behavior of their adolescents (Marvel et al., 2009). We tested this approach with a juvenile offender sample and found the intervention to be feasible and acceptable; interim findings show it to be effective as well, as evidenced by biological markers of sexually transmitted disease (STD) acquisition. This new protocol, in conjunction with the standard MDFT approach, reduced youths' high-risk sexual behavior, HIV, and STD risk (laboratory-confirmed STDs; Liddle et al., in press). Another area of current and future work concerns additional moderator and mediator analyses. Using formal meditational analyses, for instance, we have established a causal link between MDFT changes in parenting practices and posttreatment youth outcomes (Henderson et al., 2009). This work complements earlier therapy process studies, research that used intensive videotape analysis to articulate facilitative in-session therapeutic processes and assess the connection of therapists' technique to desired changes in sessions and beyond. Future work will include more independent national and international evaluations and dissemination, additional moderator and mediator analyses to understand how MDFT achieves its effects, and continued implementation research investigating the most effective ways to teach and supervise clinicians as well as, relatedly, the kind of systemic and organizational systems issues that enable or constrain the implementation of evidence-based programs.

CONCLUSIONS

MDFT is one of the most extensively studied therapies for teen substance abuse and delinquency. Several aspects of the approach can be highlighted at this stage of its 25-year history. MDFT is a flexible treatment system. Different versions of the model have been implemented successfully in diverse community settings by agency clinicians with both male and female adolescents from varied ethnic, minority, and racial groups. Study participants were not narrowly defined, rarefied research samples: Participants were drug users and generally showed psychiatric comorbidity and delinquency, with juvenile justice involvement. Assessments included state-of-the-science measures, theory-related dimensions, and measures of clinical and practical knowledge, important to the everyday functioning of target youth and families. MDFT has been tested against active, empirically validated treatments, including individual CBT and high-quality peer group and multifamily approaches as well as treatment as usual. It has been varied on dimensions such as treatment intensity and has demonstrated favorable outcomes in its different forms. An intensive version of MDFT was found to be a clinically effective alternative to residential treatment. On the other end of the spectrum, MDFT has been effective as a prevention program with at-risk, nonclinically referred youths and as an effective intervention for clinically referred young adolescents in the early stages of drug and criminal justice involvement. The research program has used the most rigorous designs in conducting efficacy/effectiveness trials, followed Consolidated Standards of Reporting Trials guidelines, used intent-to-treat analyses, and has been tested in multisite RCTs. We developed psychometrically sound adherence measures (Hogue et al., 1998) and successfully trained therapists, supervisors, and trainers in drug abuse and criminal justice settings nationally and internationally. MDFT process studies have illuminated the model's internal workings and confirmed hypotheses about the model's mechanisms of action. Cost analyses indicate that MDFT is an affordable alternative compared with standard outpatient or inpatient treatment costs. Although often thought of as a drug abuse treatment only, MDFT also has generated evidence in multiple trials of favorable outcomes far beyond drug taking and drug abuse. Delinquency and externalizing, and internalizing symptoms have improved significantly in MDFT trials. HIV and STD risks have decreased in our newest work (developing a family-based HIV prevention module). We have also demonstrated the capacity to target and change key components of the outcome equation (e.g., affiliation with drug-using peers, family and school functioning). Our RCTs routinely track outcomes with 1-year follow-ups, and the outcomes are maintained at this assessment. Newer studies include 4-year postintake assessments.

MDFT offers a unique clinical focus in how it establishes individual relationships with parents and teens, works with each alone in individual sessions, targets family interactional changes, and also works with individuals and parents vis-à-vis teens' and their family's social context. MDFT's treatment development tradition is strong, given its process studies and use of behavioral ratings of videotapes. The approach's revisions and extensions now include manual-guided modules that begin MDFT with youths in juvenile detention and continue after release as part of the regular MDFT outpatient phase (3–4 months) and an integrated parent-involved youth HIV/STD prevention intervention. Training, supervision, and quality assurance protocols are well developed, and our online training course includes the model's core sessions and clinician microskills via streaming video segments.

Impressive advances have been made in the development and testing of evidence-based treatments for adolescents, as this current volume testifies. At the same time, the pace of implementing these interventions into, for example, regular community settings of mental health and addictions clinics, schools, and juvenile justice remains painfully and unacceptably slow. Clearly, although treatment developers and researchers have responded admirably in many ways to previous developmental eras that questioned the relevance of their treatments and research, much more needs to be done to create effective therapies for nonresearch contexts.

ACKNOWLEDGMENTS

MDFT research has been supported since 1985 by the National Institute on Drug Abuse (NIDA). The support of former and current NIDA staff Liz Rahdert, Redonna Chandler, Bennett Fletcher, Akiva Liberman, Melissa Racioppo Riddle, and Jerry Flanzer has been instrumental to this work's development. Over the years, other research support has come from Substance Abuse and Mental Health Administration's Center for Substance Abuse Treatment and Center for Substance Abuse Prevention and recently from entities such as the Children's Trust of Miami, the Miami Dade Youth Crime Task Force, and the Health Foundation of South Florida. I acknowledge with deep gratitude these many forms of research support. Finally, I thank the adolescents and their families and the supervisors and clinicians who have participated in our studies.

REFERENCES

Dennis, M., Godley, S. H., Diamond, G., Tims, F. M., Babor, T., Donaldson, J., et al. (2004). Main findings of the Cannabis Youth Treatment (CYT) randomized field experiment. *Journal of Substance Abuse Treatment, 27*, 197–213.

Diamond, G. M., Liddle, H. A., Hogue, A., & Dakof, G. A. (1999). Alliance-building interventions with adolescents in family therapy: A process study. *Psychotherapy: Theory, Research, Practice, and Training, 36*, 355–368.

Diamond, G. S., & Liddle, H. (1996). Resolving a therapeutic impasse between parents and adolescents in multidimensional family therapy. *Journal of Consulting and Clinical Psychology, 64*, 481–488.

French, M. T., Roebuck, M. C., Dennis, M., Godley, S., Liddle, H. A., & Tims, F. (2003). Outpatient marijuana treatment for adolescents: Economic evaluation of a multisite field experiment. *Evaluation Review, 27*, 421–459.

Henderson, C. E., Rowe, C. L., Dakof, G. A., Hawes, S. W., & Liddle, H. A. (2009). Parenting practices as mediators of treatment effects in an early-intervention trial of multidimensional family therapy. *American Journal of Drug and Alcohol Abuse, 56*, 220–226.

Hogue, A., Liddle, H. A., Dauber, S., & Samuolis, J. (2004). Linking session focus to treatment outcome in evidence-based treatments for adolescent substance abuse. *Psychotherapy: Theory, Research, Practice, and Training, 41*, 83–96.

Hogue, A., Liddle, H. A., Rowe, C., Turner, R. M., Dakof, G. A., & LaPann, K. (1998). Treatment adherence and differentiation in individual versus family therapy for adolescent substance abuse. *Journal of Counseling Psychology, 45*, 104–114.

Hogue, A., Liddle, H. A., Singer, A., & Leckrone, J. (2005). Intervention fidelity in family-based prevention counseling for adolescent problem behaviors. *Journal of Community Psychology, 33*, 191–211.

Jackson-Gilfort, A., Liddle, H. A., Tejeda, M. J., & Dakof, G. A., (2001). Facilitating engagement of African American male adolescents in family therapy: A cultural theme process study. *Journal of Black Psychology, 27*, 321–340.

Liddle, H. A. (1994). The anatomy of emotions in family therapy with adolescents. *Journal of Adolescent Research, 9*(1), 120–157.

Liddle, H. A. (2004). Family-based therapies for adolescent alcohol and drug use: Research contributions and future research needs. *Addiction, 99*(Suppl. 2), 76–92.

Liddle, H. A. (2008). *Multidimensional family therapy* [DVD and Instructional Booklet]. Washington, DC: American Psychological Association.

Liddle, H. A. (2009). *Multidimensional family therapy for adolescent drug abuse* [Clinician's manual and DVD]. Center City, MN: Hazelden.

Liddle, H. A. (in press). *Multidimensional family therapy for adolescent drug abuse and delinquency*. New York: Guilford Press.

Liddle, H. A., & Dakof, G. A. (2002). A randomized controlled trial of intensive outpatient, family based therapy vs. residential drug treatment for co-morbid adolescent drug abusers. *Drug and Alcohol Dependence, 66,* S103.

Liddle, H. A., Dakof, G. A., Henderson, C. E., & Rowe, C. L. (in press). Implementation outcomes of Multidimensional Family Therapy—Detention to Community (DTC)—A reintegration program for drug-using juvenile detainees. *International Journal of Offender Therapy and Comparative Criminology.*

Liddle, H. A., Dakof, G. A., Parker, K., Diamond, G. S., Barrett, K., & Tejeda, M. (2001). Multidimensional family therapy for adolescent drug abuse: Results of a randomized clinical trial. *American Journal of Drug and Alcohol Abuse, 27,* 651–688.

Liddle, H. A., Dakof, G. A., Turner, R. M., Henderson, C. E., & Greenbaum, P. E. (2008). Treating adolescent drug abuse: A randomized trial comparing multidimensional family therapy and cognitive behavior therapy. *Addiction, 103,* 1660–1670.

Liddle, H. A., Rodriguez, R. A., Dakof, G. A., Kanzki, E., & March, F. A. (2005). Multidimensional Family Therapy: A science-based treatment for adolescent drug abuse. In J. Lebow (Ed.), *Handbook of clinical family therapy* (pp. 128–163). New York: Wiley.

Liddle, H. A., Rowe, C. L., Dakof, G. A., Henderson, C. E., & Greenbaum, P. E. (2009). Multidimensional family therapy for early adolescent substance abusers: Twelve month outcomes of a randomized controlled trial. *Journal of Consulting and Clinical Psychology, 77,* 12–25.

Liddle, H. A., Rowe, C. L., Gonzalez, A., Henderson, C. E., Dakof, G. A., & Greenbaum, P. E. (2006). Changing provider practices, program environment, and improving outcomes by transporting multidimensional family therapy to an adolescent drug treatment setting. *American Journal on Addictions, 15,* 102–112.

Liddle, H. A., Rowe, C. L., Quille, T. J., Dakof, G. A., Mills, D. S., Sakran, E., & Biaggi, H. (2002). Transporting a research-based adolescent drug treatment into practice. *Journal of Substance Abuse Treatment, 22,* 231–243.

Liddle, H. A., Rowe, C. L., Ungaro, R. A., Dakof, G. A., & Henderson, C. (2004). Early intervention for adolescent substance abuse: Pretreatment to posttreatment outcomes of a randomized controlled trial comparing multidimensional family therapy and peer group treatment. *Journal of Psychoactive Drugs, 36,* 2–37.

Marvel, F. A., Rowe, C. R., Colon, L., DiClemente, R., & Liddle, H. A. (2009). Multidimensional family therapy HIV/STD risk-reduction intervention: An integrative family-based model for drug-involved juvenile offenders. *Family Process, 48,* 69–83.

Robbins, M. S., Liddle, H. A., Turner, C. W., Dakof, G. A., Alexander, J. F., & Kogan, S. M. (2006). Adolescent and parent therapeutic alliances as predictors of dropout in multidimensional family therapy. *Journal of Family Psychology, 20,* 108–116.

Schmidt, S. E., Liddle, H. A., & Dakof, G. A. (1996). Changes in parenting practices and adolescent drug abuse during multidimensional family therapy. *Journal of Family Psychology, 10,* 12–27.

Shelef, K., Diamond, G. M., Diamond, G. S., & Liddle, H. A. (2005). Adolescent and parent alliance and treatment outcome in multidimensional family therapy. *Journal of Consulting and Clinical Psychology, 73,* 689–698.

Zavala, S. K., French, M. T., Henderson, C. E., Alberga, L., Rowe, C. L., & Liddle, H. A. (2005). Guidelines and challenges for estimating the economic costs and benefits of adolescent substance abuse treatments. *Journal of Substance Abuse Treatment, 29,* 191–205.

IMPLEMENTATION AND DISSEMINATION
Extending Treatments to New Populations and New Settings

28

Implementation of Evidence-Based Treatments for Children and Adolescents

Research Findings and Their Implications for the Future

DEAN L. FIXSEN, KAREN A. BLASE, MICHELLE A. DUDA, SANDRA F. NAOOM, and MELISSA VAN DYKE

OVERVIEW

A growing number of evidence-based psychotherapies hold the promise of substantial benefits for children, families, and society. These therapies are the product of a tremendous investment in research on interventions over the past few decades. For the benefits of evidence-based programs to be realized on a scale sufficient to be useful to individuals and society, evidence-based psychotherapies need to be put into practice outside of controlled clinical trials. Efforts to make use of evidence-based programs in typical service settings have not gone well. As the evidence-based program movement has unfolded, national reviews across service sectors have documented:

- The "science-to-service gap."
- The variability and lack of effectiveness commonly found in typical human services.
- The lack of sustainability of various pilot and demonstration programs.
- The lack of progress toward achieving socially important outcomes.

These deficiencies have occurred despite dramatic improvements in the number and quality of evidence-based practices and programs (e.g., Clancy, 2006; Institute of Medicine, 2001; U.S. Department of Health and Human Services, 1999).

As indicated in these reviews, the process of putting evidence-based programs into practice is where some of the best therapies fail. Fortunately, we are coming to understand more fully that the "to" in "science to service" represents implementation: that is, "science implemented in practice." As it turns out, implementation is an active process. Our goal for this chapter is to outline the progress that has been made toward creating the science and practice of implementation, a field that is quite separate and distinct from the science related to developing new prevention or intervention practices. In this chapter we provide a brief overview of our experiences with implementation to set a context for the practice of implementation. Next, we present an overview of the development of the science and practice of implementation and summarize the key components that seem to be associated with successful endeavors across a number of fields. We conclude with an appeal for greater investment in implementation research and practice.

The brevity of this chapter permits only a few references to the key science and best practice literature related to implementation components. Interested readers can find relevant citations and more detailed information in Fixsen, Naoom, Blase, Friedman, and Wallace (2005); Blase, Fixsen, Naoom, and Wallace (2005); Greenhalgh, Robert, MacFarlane, Bate, and Kyriakidou (2004); and Schoenwald, Kelleher, and Weisz (2008); and on websites for the National Implementation Research Network (*nirn.fpg.unc.edu/*) and State Implementation & Scaling-up of Evidence-based Practices (*www.scalingup. org*).

IMPLEMENTATION FAILURES: TRIAL AND LEARNING

Our early experiences with implementation began in the context of developing an evidence-based program, although that was not the language we used in those days. In 1967 the opening of Achievement Place, a family-style group home for six teenagers referred by the juvenile court, marked the beginning of several decades of research on effective treatment practices (e.g., relationship development, teaching appropriate alternative behavior, self-government and rational problem solving, motivation systems) to help adolescents be more successful at home, in school, and in the community. This research led to the establishment of the Teaching-Family Model (a bibliography and related information are available at *www.teaching-family.org*). It was cited as a model program by the American Psychological Association in its initial review of evidence-based programs in the early 1990s and as one of three evidence-based residential programs in the U.S. Surgeon General's report (U.S. Department of Health and Human Services, 1999). The Teaching-Family Model serves as an early example of an evidence-based program and currently (more than 40 years later) is in use in a variety of group home treatment, home-based treatment, treatment foster care, supported independent living, and school-based intervention settings.

Based on evidence-based treatment practices, exemplary results were obtained with the teaching parents (the married couple who staffed the family-style home) in the prototype program. Starting in 1971, our initial attempts to replicate the group home treatment program did not go well, but we soon learned the rudiments of how to teach, coach, and evaluate new teaching parents (our introduction to implementation; Wolf, Kirigin, Fixsen, Blase, & Braukmann, 1995). Our replication strategy in the early days was to focus on preparing and supporting practitioners. However, in the next few years, we found that the group home treatment programs we had established were closing about as fast as we were creating new ones. For example, only 15% of the first 84 group homes lasted 6 years or more (Fixsen, Blase, Timbers, & Wolf, 2001), even though the practitioners routinely met treatment performance criteria (fidelity). This led us to begin working with whole organizations instead of just practitioners in single group homes.

IMPLEMENTATION SUCCESS

We soon developed a purveyor organization that specialized in implementation and learned how to change organizations to support the cost-effective use of the Teaching-Family Model in community-based and campus-based group homes (Blase, Fixsen, & Phillips, 1984; Kingsley, 2006). We finally had learned how to implement the treatment program purposefully and successfully in typical service environments! By the mid-1980s organizations of effective Teaching-Family group home treatment programs were being developed in about 3 years, with 80% of the attempted implementation sites meeting the site certification standards established and independently monitored by the Teaching-Family Association (Fixsen et al., 2001). In retrospect, we can see how our experiences from 1967 to 1987 and the implementation-related data we were collecting led us down the path of greater understanding of implementation, although at the time it was not so clear.

IMPLEMENTATION SCIENCE AND PRACTICE

Our initial implementation failures prompted a quest to learn more about the mysteries of effective implementation practices. Through our associations with other early purveyor organizations (e.g., Fairweather, Sanders, & Tornatzky, 1974; Watkins, 1995), we knew our experiences were not unique. However, it was not until we completed thorough reviews of the implementation evaluation literature (Fixsen et al., 2005) and implementation best practices (Blase et al., 2005) that we more clearly understood, in retrospect, our own implementation experiences and those of others. The components associated with successful implementation endeavors are the subject of this chapter.

Greenhalgh et al. (2004) outlined a classification system that is very useful for understanding implementation practices. These authors noted that over the past several decades putting science into service has moved from "letting it happen" or "helping it happen" to "making it happen" styles of implementation. We have used the Greenhalgh et al. classifications to assess implementation attempts. In the "letting it happen" style, researchers and innovators publish their findings regarding interventions, and it is up to practitioners and managers to find the information, assess its usefulness, and apply it to their situation. In the "helping it happen" style, summaries of new findings are provided directly to practitioners and others via handbooks, tool kits, and websites as well as through training or other technical assistance. Both of these approaches hold practitioners accountable. Practitioners are responsible for (1) learning about the intervention so they know what it is and how to do it in the context of their daily practice and (2) learning about implementation so they know what it is and how to do it in the context of organization functioning and system demands. Over the years, the "letting it happen" and "helping it happen" (do-it-yourself) approaches to implementation have resulted in only modest outcomes for consumers across a variety of fields (e.g., Institute of Medicine, 2001).

As we note later, in the "making it happen" approach, purveyor organizations take responsibility for helping practitioners and others learn how to use evidence-based practices with fidelity and for creating hospitable environments in which those practitioners can work to produce good outcomes for consumers. Thus, "making it happen" is not some heavy-handed approach to implementation; rather, it makes full use of implementation knowledge, with accountability for results resting fully with the purveyor organization. The frameworks outlined in this chapter help to define many of the key features of the "making it happen" approach to implementation.

IMPLEMENTATION: MAKING IT HAPPEN

To focus implementation practice and research activities, we offer a framework for implementation. The components of the theoretical framework are based on findings from more than 40 years of program development and national implementation experience (e.g., Blase et al., 1984; Fairweather et al., 1974; Fixsen et al., 2001; Watkins, 1995; Wolf et al., 1995), thorough reviews of the implementation and dissemination evaluation literature (e.g., Fixsen et al., 2005; Greenhalgh et al., 2004), and intensive reviews of current implementation best practices across several successful purveyor organizations (e.g., Blase et al., 2005). The key components of successful implementation are shown in Table 28.1.

Across a wide range of business, education, engineering, human services, and manufacturing fields, reliably producing predictable science-based outcomes for consumers seems to be related to a common set of components:

1. Purveyor organizations to do the work of helping others use science in practice.
2. Methods for operationalizing interventions.
3. Methods for developing a competent workforce.
4. Establishing organizational supports for practitioners.
5. Locating and developing facilitative leadership.

When all components are working harmoniously, large-scale and long-lasting benefits can be realized (e.g., Khatri & Frieden, 2002; Ogden, Forgatch, Askeland, Patterson, & Bullock, 2005). When the components are not working harmoniously, substantial benefits and sustainability are not realized (e.g., Goldman et al., 2002). Currently, successful, large-scale, systematic efforts to move science to service appear to make good use of these fundamental implementation components (e.g., Khatri & Frieden, 2002: implementation of the directly observed treatment system for tuberculosis treatment with more than 1 million patients across many regions of India; Ogden et al., 2005: nationwide implementation of the parent management training—Oregon model in Norway; Henggeler, Schoenwald, Borduin, Rowland, & Cunningham, 2009: implementation of multisystemic treatment across hundreds of delinquency treatment teams nationally and internationally; Sugai, Sprague, Horner, & Walker, 2000: implementation of positive behavior support whole-school interventions in more than 8,000 schools nationally).

TABLE 28.1. A Summary of the Key Components of Successful Implementation

Components	Critical features and functions	Rationale
Purveyor organization	Purveyor organizations are composed of individuals who (1) know interventions from a practice point of view, (2) are skillful users of implementation methods, and (3) are thoroughly engaged in continuous quality improvement cycles in all aspects of their activities.	Some of the most successful examples of well-implemented evidence-based programs (e.g. Behavior Tech, MST Services, PBIS Technical Assistance Center) have developed strong purveyor organizations that take responsibility for ensuring full and effective uses of dialectical behavior therapy, multisystemic therapy, and school-wide positive behavior support in typical service settings nationally and internationally.
Operational definition	The implementation process begins with a clear understanding and description of the intervention. It is difficult to implement anything unless you know what "it" is you are trying to do.	This is an important issue when it comes to implementing evidence-based programs on a scale sufficient to solve social problems. To be useful across thousands of practitioners and organizations operating in hundreds of social service systems, purveyor organizations need to know what to train, what to coach, and what performance to assess to make full and effective use of a well-researched evidence-based program. Purveyor organizations need to know what "it" is so they can efficiently and effectively ensure proper use of the intervention now and improve "it" over time.
Creating competency	A fundamental goal of implementation is to have practitioners (e.g., caseworkers, foster parents, physicians, teachers, therapists) use innovations fully and effectively in their interactions with consumers. Reducing variability and increasing effectiveness of human services is a high priority and a driving force behind the evidence-based program movement internationally.	Four factors appear to be important to developing competent users of evidence-based practices: staff selection, training, ongoing coaching, and performance evaluation. Purveyor organizations need to be proficient in best practices in these areas in order to ensure implementation of evidence-based programs on a useful scale.
Organization supports	Practitioners cannot make effective use of evidence-based practices without the support of the organizations in which they work. Selection, training, coaching, and performance assessments must be initiated and continue to be supported and improved if generations of practitioners are going to be available and able to make effective use of evidence-based practices.	Successful implementation ensures the effective and continuing use of organized decision support data systems, facilitative administrative supports, and systems interventions to create and sustain benefits to consumers.
Leadership	Leadership is not one person but multiple individuals engaging in different kinds of leadership behavior as needed to establish and sustain effective programs as circumstances change over time.	Leadership needs change as implementation progresses, from adaptive leadership styles to "champion change" in the beginning to more technical leadership styles to manage the continuing implementation supports for evidence-based programs over the long run.

The key components of successful implementation are outlined in Table 28.1 and their associated factors are described next.

PURVEYOR ORGANIZATIONS

Purveyor organizations have emerged as a critical component of "science implemented in practice" (Fixsen et al., 2005). A purveyor organization consists of individuals who (1) know interventions from a practice point of view, (2) are skillful users of implementation methods, and (3) are thoroughly engaged in continuous quality improvement cycles in all aspects of their activities. Some purveyor organizations such as Behavior Tech, MST Services, and the PBIS Technical Assistance Center are focused on one intervention (dialectical behavior therapy, multisystemic therapy, and school-wide positive behavior support, respectively). Other purveyor organizations, such as those supported by the California Institute of Mental Health (*www.cimh.org/Home.aspx*) and the Ohio Center for Innovative Practices (*www.cipohio.org*), serve as "intermediary organizations" that help communities and organizations make use of multiple evidence-based programs. Many purveyor organization members have been practitioners themselves so they know the intervention and associated craft knowledge from a practice point of view (often learned from the original program developers). Members also acquire the knowledge and skills related to implementation practice and science, either through the "school of hard knocks" or through organized professional development experiences. Finally, members understand and apply the PDSA (**P**lan, **D**o, **S**tudy, **A**ct) improvement cycles (described later) as an embedded part of all of their activities. For example, each time training or coaching is provided to practitioners (or staff in other positions), purveyor organization members are examining their own behavior (e.g., a new approach to behavior rehears-als; a new way to present sensitive information about performance) and results (e.g., pre–post training tests of knowledge and skills; feedback from the practitioner) and are purposefully making changes to try to improve outcomes next time.

Currently, purveyor organizations are not commonly available, and only a few states are in the beginning stages of developing an infrastructure for implementation by form-ing sufficient numbers of purveyor groups to make full and effective use of evidence-based programs statewide (e.g., Ogden et al., 2005; *www.scalingup.org*). Purveyor organi-zations may be embedded in larger service organizations and in groups of collaborating human service agencies or may be part of transformed human service systems. Nations such as Norway and India and states such as California, Illinois, Michigan, Minnesota, Ohio, and Oregon systematically are creating purveyor organizations to improve the suc-cess of moving science to service to benefit children, families, adults, and communities on a socially important scale.

OPERATIONALIZING INTERVENTIONS

It is difficult to implement anything unless you know what "it" is you are trying to do. Thus, the implementation process begins with a clear understanding and description of the intervention. Although this may seem very basic (and it is), documentation of an intervention (the independent variable) is not common in the research community, ranging from about 5–30% in a series of reviews of nearly 1,000 outcome studies (e.g., Durlak & DuPre, 2008). Even when the intervention was documented (e.g., a detailed manual was available), only a few investigators actually measured the presence or strength of the intervention (the independent variable) and fewer still included the measure of the presence or strength of the intervention in analyses of the results. As a result, the published literature is a poor source of information for the functional components of human service interventions.

Without documentation and measures of an intervention, we are left wondering what "it" is that was done to achieve the marvelous results we admire. Currently, there is little empirical evidence to support assertions that the components named by an evidence-based program developer are, in fact, necessary for producing the effects (e.g., Abraham & Michie, 2008). There may be other unnamed, unmeasured components involved in a treatment that actually produce the effects, and the components identified by the program developer may or may not be important to the outcomes achieved. The mention or lack of mention of these components by a developer should not be confused with function or lack of function in a therapeutic exchange.

This is not a trivial issue when it comes to implementation of evidence-based programs on a scale sufficient to solve social problems. To be useful to consumers and functional across thousands of practitioners and organizations operating in locations across the country, purveyor organizations need to know what to train, what to coach, and what performance to assess to make full and effective use of a well-researched evidence-based program. Purveyor organizations need to know what "it" (intervention components) is so they can efficiently and effectively ensure proper use of the intervention now and improve "it" over time.

In our own experience and those of other developers who have successfully implemented an evidence-based program, we have made unintentional use of the PDSA cycle originally developed by applied researchers in the Bell Labs in the 1920s (e.g., Deming, 1986). The benefits of the PDSA cycle in highly interactive environments have been evaluated across many domains, including manufacturing, health, and substance abuse treatment. Although the PDSA cycle is thought of as an improvement cycle, this trial-and-learning approach also allows developers of complex human service programs to identify the essential components of the intervention itself and can further evaluate or discard nonessential components. The brief history of the development of the Teaching-Family Model that introduced this chapter is one example of the use of a PDSA approach over many years to develop successful intervention and implementation practices.

When applied to human services, the plan can be the intervention as the developer intends it to be used in practice. To carry out the "do" part of the PDSA cycle, the plan needs to be operationalized (what we will do and say to enact the plan). This compels attention to the core intervention components and provides an opportunity to begin to develop a training and coaching process (e.g., here is how to do the plan) and to create a measure of fidelity (e.g., Did we "do" the plan?). As a newly trained practitioner begins working with children and families in an actual service environment, the budding fidelity measure can be used to interpret the outcomes in the "study" part of the PDSA cycle (e.g., Did we do what we intended? Did doing what we intended result in desired outcomes?). In human services, program developers may use the PDSA cycle many times over to arrive at a functional version of an intervention that is effective in practice and can be implemented with fidelity on a national scale (e.g., Fixsen et al., 2001; Wolf et al.,

1995). Once the components of an intervention have been identified, functional analyses can be done to determine empirically the extent to which key components contribute to significant outcomes. For the 70–95% of interventions that have not been operationalized by the developers, purveyor organizations will need to make use of PDSA improvement cycles to uncover the core intervention components before they can proceed with broader scale implementation.

METHODS FOR DEVELOPING A COMPETENT WORKFORCE

Innovations cannot produce benefits for consumers unless the intended beneficiaries experience the innovation (Dobson & Cook, 1980). Thus, a fundamental goal of implementation is to have practitioners (e.g., caseworkers, foster parents, physicians, teachers, therapists) use innovations fully and effectively in their interactions with children and families. The Institute of Medicine (2001) highlighted a common finding that health and human services, as currently practiced, are highly variable, often ineffective, and sometimes harmful to consumers. Thus, reducing variability and increasing effectiveness of human services is a high priority and a driving force behind the evidence-based program movement internationally. In the reviews of implementation evaluation literature and implementation best practices, four factors appeared to be important to developing competent users of evidence-based practices: (1) staff selection; (2) staff training; (3) ongoing, on-the-job coaching of staff; and (4) regular assessments of staff performance. Purveyor organizations need to be proficient in these areas in order to ensure implementation of evidence-based programs on a useful scale. For a new evidence-based program, the foundations for selection, training, coaching, and performance evaluations are developed during the early PDSA testing, as described previously. Functional selection, training, coaching, and performance evaluations are those processes that increase the likelihood that practitioners will appropriately and skillfully use the relevant dimensions of the intervention (i.e., the core components of the intervention that make it effective) in their interactions with children and families.

Staff selection is the beginning point for building a competent workforce that has the knowledge, skills, and abilities to carry out evidence-based practices with benefits to consumers. Beyond academic qualifications or experience factors, what essential skills are required? Certain practitioner characteristics critical to the use of an evidence-based program are difficult to teach in training sessions and so must be part of the selection criteria (e.g., basic professional skills, basic social skills, common sense, empathy, good judgment, knowledge of the field, personal ethics, sense of social justice, willingness to intervene, willingness to learn). Implementation of evidence-based programs on a useful scale requires:

- Specification of required skills and abilities within the pool of candidates.
- Methods for recruiting likely candidates who possess these skills and abilities.
- Protocols for interviewing candidates.
- Criteria for selecting practitioners with those skills and abilities.

Even when implementation is occurring in an organization with a well-established staff group, the new way of work can be described and volunteers recruited and interviewed to select the first practitioners to make use of an evidence-based intervention. The pre–post test scores for training provide an immediate source of selection outcome data, and performance assessment/fidelity scores provide a more important but longer term source of feedback on the usefulness of the selection process. Purveyor organizations make use of these data in PDSA cycles to continue to improve recruitment and selection methods.

Staff training is important because innovations such as evidence-based practices and programs represent new ways of providing treatment and support. Innovation-based training helps practitioners (and others) at an implementation site learn when, where, how, and with whom to use (and not to use) new approaches and new skills. Even though training is an ineffective implementation strategy when used alone (e.g., Joyce & Showers, 2002), staff training is an efficient way to:

- Provide knowledge related to the history, theory, philosophy, and values of the program.
- Introduce the components and rationales of key practices.
- Provide opportunities to practice new skills to criterion and receive feedback in a safe and supportive training environment.

Implementation best practices and science indicate that good training includes ample opportunities for demonstrations of evidence-based practice-related skills, behavior rehearsal to criterion, and pre–post tests of knowledge and skill. The results of posttests of training are provided to the coach for each practitioner so the coach will know the areas of strength and areas of weakness on which to focus early in the coaching relationship.

Staff Coaching is essential because most skills needed by successful practitioners can be assessed during selection and introduced in training but actually are learned on the job with the help of a coach. An effective coach provides craft information along with advice, encouragement, and opportunities to practice and use skills specific to the innovation (e.g., engagement, treatment planning, clinical judgment). The full and effective use of human service innovations requires behavior change at the practitioner, supervisory, and administrative support levels. Training and coaching are the principal implementation methods in which behavior change is brought about for carefully selected staff in the beginning stages of implementation and throughout the life of evidence-based practices and programs (e.g., Schoenwald, Sheidow, & Letourneau, 2004).

Staff performance assessment is designed to assess the use and outcomes of the skills that are reflected in the selection criteria, taught in training, and reinforced and expanded in coaching processes. Assessments of practitioner performance and measures of fidelity also provide feedback useful to key participants (interviewers, trainers, coaches, program managers, and purveyor organizations) regarding the progress of implementation efforts and the usefulness of selection, training, and coaching methods. For example, purveyor organizations consistently monitor current performance assessments in search of common strengths and weaknesses. If performance assessments of, for example, the last 20 practitioners show a common area of subcriterion performance, the purveyor organization uses the PDSA improvement cycle to make adjustments in how selection, training, and coaching are conducted to help strengthen skills related to that area. The purveyor organization remains accountable for ensuring that current and future practitioners will achieve high levels of effective performance when working with children, families, and others. In addition, the results of practitioner performance assessments over time and across a number of practitioners provide an evaluation of the effectiveness of the purveyor organization itself.

ORGANIZATIONAL SUPPORTS FOR PRACTITIONERS

Practitioners cannot make effective and continuing use of evidence-based practices without the support of the organizations in which they work. Selection, training, coaching, and performance assessments must be initiated and must continue to be supported and improved if generations of practitioners are going to be available and able to make effective use of evidence-based practices. Reviews of implementation practices and research point to the importance of decision support data systems, facilitative administrative supports, and systems interventions. These factors help to create and sustain benefits to consumers. The specific organizational supports required for a given evidence-based program can be identified during the initial development of an intervention. For example, for a new evidence-based program, attention to PDSA testing strategies during attempts to implement the intervention in the first 30–40 organizations likely will provide the data and experience purveyor organizations need to learn the nature and content of organization structures and supports that are required to sustain high-fidelity implementation (e.g., Fixsen et al., 2001; Khatri & Frieden, 2002).

Decision support data systems are sources of information used to help make good decisions internal to an organization. Effective organizations make use of a variety of measures to assess key aspects of the overall performance of the organization, provide data to support decision making, and ensure continuing implementation of the evidence-based intervention and benefits to consumers over time. All modern organizations have a financial data collection and reporting system that regularly is monitored internally and externally (e.g., through employment of professional financial managers and clerks in the organization, careful attention from the governing board, and annual audits by external experts). Effective organizations also have data collection and reporting systems for their treatment and management processes and outcomes. Decision support data systems are an important part of continuous quality improvement for interventions, implementation supports, and organization functioning (e.g., used as the "study" part of the never-ending PDSA cycle). Purveyor organizations help organizations establish and evolve their data systems so information is immediately accessible and useful to practitioners, trainers, coaches, and managers for short-term and long-term planning and improvement at clinical and organizational levels. Human service organizations and systems are dynamic, so there is ebb and flow to the relative contribution of each component to the overall outcomes (e.g., Panzano et al., 2004). The decision support data system feedback loops appear to be critical to keeping an evidence-based program on track in the midst of a sea of change. If the feedback loops (staff performance evaluations and decision support data systems) indicate needed changes, then the purveyor organization adjusts the integrated system to improve effectiveness and efficiency.

Facilitative administration provides leadership and makes use of a range of data inputs to inform decision making, support the overall intervention and implementation processes, and keep staff organized and focused on the desired intervention outcomes. In an organization with a facilitative administration, careful attention is given to policies, procedures, structures, culture, and climate to ensure alignment of these aspects of an organization with the needs of practitioners (e.g., Fleuren, Wiefferink, & Paulussen, 2004). Practitioners' interactions with consumers are the keys to any successful intervention. Facilitative administrators and others make full use of available resources to ensure that practitioners have the time, skills, and supports they need to perform at a high level of effectiveness with every consumer even as practitioners, coaches, managers, and others come and go year after year. With training, coaching, and technical assistance from a purveyor organization, administrators continue to find more and better ways to support practitioners. In their surveys of organizations, investigators are beginning to look at the potential interactions among these larger units of analysis and their contributions to implementation and intervention outcomes (e.g., Panzano et al., 2004; Glisson et al., 2008).

Finally, systems interventions are strategies to work with external systems to ensure the availability of the financial, organizational, and human resources required to support the work of the practitioners. Alignment of these external systems to specifically support the work of practitioners is an important aspect of systems interventions (e.g., Mihalic & Irwin, 2003; Panzano et al., 2004). Systems interventions take on issues that impact the ability to provide evidence-based services within organizations. Systems interventions are designed to help create a generally supportive context in which effective services can be provided, maintained, and improved over the years.

LOCATING AND DEVELOPING LEADERSHIP

Over the decades it has been rare to find a description of implementation that does not include some discussion of the critical role of leadership at organizational and system levels. It has been equally rare to find a description of what good leaders do and when they do those things to achieve benefits to consumers. Fortunately, recent advances have shed some light on this important aspect of implementation. As one part of an exemplary study of implementation, Panzano et al. (2004) measured dimensions of leadership across several agencies attempting to make use of a variety of evidence-based programs across time. Panzano and colleagues found that "leadership" is not one person but multiple individuals engaging in different kinds of leadership behavior as needed to establish and sustain effective programs as circumstances change over time. For example, leadership needs change as implementation progresses, from adaptive leadership styles to "champion change" in the beginning to more technical leadership styles to manage the continuing implementation supports (e.g., selection, performance assessments, system interventions) for evidence-based programs over the long run.

INTEGRATED AND COMPENSATORY IMPLEMENTATION COMPONENTS

It seems the implementation components described previously interact with one another in endless combinations. In successful applications, these interactive components are integrated and focused on full use of one or more innovations to make the most of their influence on staff behavior, organization supports, and system functioning in order to maximize benefits to children and families. The interactive components also compensate for one another so that a weakness in one component can be overcome by strengths in other components. The compensatory nature of the implementation components seems to be especially important as members of purveyor organizations come and go (e.g., trainers, coaches). With turnover, the quality of implementation supports will vary over time. For example, the strength of coaching is diminished when an expert coach leaves and is replaced by an inexperienced coach. In this case, a purveyor organization might compensate by strengthening the skill development sections of a practitioner training workshop and increasing the frequency of practitioner performance assessments to give the practitioner and the new coach greater opportunities to more quickly develop their respective competencies.

Data and experience suggest that selection, training, coaching, and performance assessments need to be integrated to increase the likelihood that full benefits for consumers can be achieved (e.g., Blase et al., 1984; Huber et al., 2003). The importance of integration was illustrated in a meta-analysis of research on training and coaching by Joyce and Showers (2002). They found that training that consisted of theory and discussion coupled with demonstration, practice, and feedback resulted in only 5% of the teachers using the new skills in the classroom. When on-the-job coaching was added to training, however, large gains were seen in knowledge and teachers' ability to demonstrate the skills, and most importantly, about 95% of the teachers used the new skills in the classroom with students. Joyce and Showers (2002) also noted that training and coaching only can be done with the full support and participation of school administrators (facilitative administration) and works best with teachers who are willing and able to be fully involved (selection factors). A purveyor organization continually monitors the effectiveness of the methods for developing a competent workforce and makes adjustments as needed to selection processes, training content and procedures, and staff performance evaluations to ensure that consumers are provided with well-implemented interventions over time and across practitioners.

DIRECTIONS FOR RESEARCH

For many years there has been broad agreement that implementation is a complex process simultaneously involving multiple factors at several levels of functioning. In 1975 Van Meter and Van Horn stated:

> The difficulties inherent in implementation have "discouraged detailed study of the process of implementation. The problems of implementation are overwhelmingly complex and scholars have frequently been deterred by methodological considerations. A comprehensive analysis of implementation requires that attention be given to multiple actions over an extended period of time. (pp. 450–451)

Three decades later, essentially the same conclusion was drawn by review teams (e.g., Improved Clinical Effectiveness through Behavioural Research Group, 2006; Wensing, Wollersheim, & Grol, 2006), who noted that the lack of a unifying view of implementation and the wide variation in methodology, measures, and terminology across studies are major impediments to the development of implementation science.

If children, families, and society are to benefit from the growing number of evidence-based psychotherapies, there is much to be done to establish solid foundations for a science of implementation. Significant advances in the science have been made in the past decade as interest and research activities in implementation have increased (e.g., Schoenwald et al., 2008). Thanks to the growing number of research teams, we now know it is possible to study implementation variables under overwhelmingly complex conditions. Research is needed to begin testing and validating a comprehensive theoretical framework to guide the practice and science of implementation. Frameworks such as those outlined in this chapter can be used to organize our approaches to practice and research, establish a common vocabulary to describe what we mean by implementation, and develop methods to consistently measure the multiple levels of complex components apparently important to successful uses of innovations.

With the advent of purveyor organizations and research groups focused on implementation, we expect the science and practice of implementation to advance more rapidly in the next decade than it has in the past five decades. Implementation practices are improving and are becoming better organized and more purposeful. These efforts are creating better laboratories in which more potent implementation components can be studied. The integrated and compensatory nature of the implementation components presents a challenge for implementation researchers, who need to account for multiple variables at multiple levels of functioning in order to understand their individual and collective contributions to successful practice (e.g., Panzano et al., 2004). With purveyor organizations organizing and ensuring practitioner competency (i.e., staff selection, training, coaching, and performance assessments), strong organization components (i.e., decision support data systems, facilitative administration, systems interventions), and human service systems that generally are supportive of the new ways of work (e.g., changes in funding, regulations, and accountability structures designed to facilitate the new ways of work at practice and organizational levels), we can expect evidence-based practices to have sustainable, high-fidelity implementations with benefits to children, families, and society.

CONCLUSIONS

Hollin and McMurran (2001) summarized the tasks of a purveyor organization by stating that the group that "treads in the deep waters of implementation needs a daunting range of attributes spanning policy formulation, developing treatment procedures, tact and diplomacy (lots!), management awareness, training skills, political awareness, practice skills, and committee and consultancy skills" (p. xvii). Perhaps that is why the development of a science of implementation has lagged far behind the science concerned with developing evidence-based interventions (e.g., Weisz, Jensen-Doss, & Hawley, 2006).

Since the early 1990s, researchers and policymakers have focused considerable attention on the development of evidence-based programs and methods to assess the methodological rigor of the evidence concerning those programs. The development of effective interventions is a critical first step toward solving the persistent problems faced by children, families, adults, and communities across the nation. However, the use of effective interventions on a scale sufficient to benefit society requires careful attention to implementation strategies as well. One without the other is like serum without a syringe; the cure is available, but the delivery system is not. For example, even if we had a well-researched school-based prevention program that was 100% effective in solving all behavioral health problems of all children, how could we effectively and efficiently deliver it to all 65 million children being taught by more than 6 million teachers and staff in over 100,000 schools in the United States? Our inability to answer this question exposes a fundamental gap in knowledge facing our society and our science today.

The implementation components outlined here provide a starting point for an organized, multidisciplinary effort to rapidly advance the practice and science of implementation. Based on best practices and the best available research, the framework offers a tool for planning implementation efforts and an outline for creating measures of important implementation variables and implementation outcomes. The framework also postulates the connections among the components to encourage research not only on the components but also (especially) on the interactive relationships among the components. There is much to do if we are to develop the practice and science of reliably and effectively using science in practice.

REFERENCES

Abraham, C., & Michie, S. (2008). A taxonomy of behavior change techniques used in interventions. *Health Psychology, 27,* 379–387.

Blase, K. A., Fixsen, D. L., Naoom, S. F., & Wallace, F. (2005). *Operationalizing implementation: Strategies and methods.* Tampa: University of South Florida, Louis de la Parte Florida Mental Health Institute, National Implementation Research Network.

Blase, K. A., Fixsen, D. L., & Phillips, E. L. (1984). Residential treatment for troubled children: Developing service delivery systems. In S. C. Paine, G. T. Bellamy, & B. Wilcox (Eds.), *Human services that work: From innovation to standard practice* (pp. 149–165). Baltimore: Brookes.

Clancy, C. (2006). The $1.6 trillion question: If we're spending so much on healthcare, why so little improvement in quality? *Medscape General Medicine, 8*(2), 58. Retrieved July 15, 2009, from *www.pubmedcentral.nih.gov/articlevender.fcgi?artid-1785188.*

Deming, W. E. (1986). *Out of the crisis.* Cambridge, MA: MIT Press.

Dobson, L., & Cook, T. (1980). Avoiding type III error in program evaluation: Results from a field experiment. *Evaluation and Program Planning, 3,* 269–276.

Durlak, J. A., & DuPre, E. P. (2008). Implementation matters: A review of research on the influence of implementation on program outcomes and the factors affecting implementation. *American Journal of Community Psychology, 41,* 327–350.

Fairweather, G. W., Sanders, D. H., & Tornatzky, L. G. (1974). The essential conditions for activating adoption. In G. W. Fairweather (Ed.), *Creating change in mental health organizations* (pp. 137–161). Elmsford, NY: Pergamon Press.

Fixsen, D. L., Blase, K. A., Timbers, G. D., & Wolf, M. M. (2001). In search of program implementation: 792 replications of the teaching-family model. In G. A. Bernfeld, D. P. Farrington, & A. W. Leschied (Eds.), *Offender rehabilitation in practice: Implementing and evaluating effective programs* (pp. 149–166). London: Wiley.

Fixsen, D. L., Naoom, S. F., Blase, K. A., Friedman, R. M., & Wallace, F. (2005). *Implementation research: A synthesis of the literature* (FMHI Publication No. 231) . Tampa, FL: University of South Florida, Louis de la Parte Florida Mental Health Institute, National Implementation Research Network.

Fleuren, M., Wiefferink, K., & Paulussen, T. (2004). Determinants of innovation within health care organizations. *International Journal for Quality in Health Care, 16,* 107–123.

Glisson, C., Schoenwald, S. K., Kelleher, K., Landsverk, J., Hoagwood, K. E., Mayberg, S., et al. (2008). Therapist turnover and new program sustainability in mental health clinics as a function of organizational culture, climate, and service structure. *Administration and Policy in Mental Health, 35*, 124–133.

Goldman, H. H., Morrissey, J. P., Rosenheck, R. A., Cocozza, J., Blasinsky, M., Randolph, F., et al. (2002). Lessons from the evaluation of the ACCESS Program. *Psychiatric Services, 53*, 967–969.

Greenhalgh, T., Robert, G., MacFarlane, F., Bate, P., & Kyriakidou, O. (2004). Diffusion of innovations in service organizations: Systematic review and recommendations. *The Milbank Quarterly, 82*, 581–629.

Henggeler, S. W., Schoenwald, S. K., Borduin, C. M., Rowland, M. D., & Cunningham, P. B. (2009). *Multisystemic treatment of antisocial behavior in children and adolescents* (2nd ed.). New York: Guilford Press.

Hollin, C., & McMurran, M. (2001). Series editors' preface. In G. A. Bernfeld, D. P. Farrington, & A. W. Leschied (Eds.), *Offender rehabilitation in practice: Implementing and evaluating effective programs* (pp. xv–xviii). London: Wiley.

Huber, T. P., Godfrey, M. M., Nelson, E. C., Mohr, J. J., Campbell, C., & Batalden, P. B. (2003). Microsystems in health care: Part 8. Developing people and improving work life: What frontline staff told us. *Joint Commission Journal on Quality and Safety, 29*, 512–522.

Improved Clinical Effectiveness through Behavioural Research Group. (2006). Designing theoretically-informed implementation interventions. *Implementation Science, 1*, 4.

Institute of Medicine, Committee on Quality of Health Care in America. (2001). *Crossing the quality chasm: A new health system for the 21st century.* Washington, DC: National Academy Press.

Joyce, B., & Showers, B. (2002). *Student achievement through staff development* (3rd ed.). Alexandria, VA: Association for Supervision and Curriculum Development.

Khatri, G. R., & Frieden, T. R. (2002). Rapid DOTS expansion in India. *Bulletin of the World Health Organization, 80*, 457–463.

Kingsley, D. E. (2006). The Teaching-Family Model and post-treatment recidivism: A critical review of the conventional wisdom. *International Journal of Behavioral and Consultation Therapy, 2*, 481–497.

Mihalic, S. F., & Irwin, K. (2003). Blueprints for violence prevention: From research to real-world settings-factors influencing the successful replication of model programs. *Youth Violence and Juvenile Justice, 1*, 307–329.

Ogden, T., Forgatch, M. S., Askeland, E., Patterson, G. R., & Bullock, B. M. (2005). Large scale implementation of parent management training at the national level: The case of Norway. *Journal of Social Work Practice, 19*, 317–329.

Panzano, P. C., Seffrin, B., Chaney-Jones, S., Roth, D., Crane-Ross, D., Massatti, R., et al. (2004). The Innovation Diffusion and Adoption Research Project (IDARP): Moving from the diffusion of research results to promoting the adoption of evidence-based innovations in the Ohio mental health system. In D. Roth & W. Lutz (Eds.), *New research in mental health* (Vol. 16, pp. 78–89). Columbus: Ohio Department of Mental Health Office of Program Evaluation and Research.

Schoenwald, S. K., Kelleher, K., & Weisz, J. R. (2008). Building bridges to evidence-based practice: The MacArthur Foundation Child System and Treatment Enhancement Projects (Child STEPs). *Administration and Policy in Mental Health, 35*, 66–72.

Schoenwald, S. K., Sheidow, A. J., & Letourneau, E. J. (2004). Toward effective quality assurance in evidence-based practice: Links between expert consultation, therapist fidelity, and child outcomes. *Journal of Clinical Child and Adolescent Psychology, 33*, 94–104.

Sugai, G., Sprague, J., Horner, R., & Walker, H. (2000). Preventing school violence: The use of office discipline referrals to assess and monitor school-wide discipline interventions. *Journal of Emotional and Behavioral Disorders, 8*, 94–101.

U.S. Department of Health and Human Services. (1999). *Mental health: A report of the Surgeon General.* Rockville, MD: U.S. Department of Health and Human Services, Substance Abuse and

Mental Health Services Administration, Center for Mental Health Services, National Institutes of Health, National Institute of Mental Health.

Van Meter, D. S., & Van Horn, C. E. (1975). The policy implementation process: A conceptual framework. *Administration and Society, 6*, 445–488.

Watkins, C. L. (1995). Follow through: Why didn't we? *Effective School Practices, 15*, 57–66.

Weisz, J. R., Jensen-Doss, A., & Hawley, K. M. (2006). Evidence-based youth psychotherapies versus usual clinical care. *American Psychologist, 61*, 671–689.

Wensing, M., Wollersheim, H., & Grol, R. (2006). Organizational interventions to implement improvements in patient care: A structured review of reviews. *Implementation Science, 1*, 2.

Wolf, M. M., Kirigin, K. A., Fixsen, D. L., Blase, K. A., & Braukmann, C. J. (1995). The Teaching-Family Model: A case study in data-based program development and refinement (and dragon wrestling). *Journal of Organizational Behavior Management, 15*, 11–68.

29

Assessing the Effects of Evidence-Based Psychotherapies with Ethnic Minority Youths

STANLEY J. HUEY, JR., and ANTONIO J. POLO

OVERVIEW

Nearly 45% of youth in the United States are ethnic minority or multiracial, and minority youth currently represent a numerical majority or near majority in 25% of U.S. counties (Pollard & Mather, 2009). Not surprisingly, ethnic minority youth also make up a large percentage of those who utilize mental health services in the United States (McCabe et al., 1999), particularly in large metropolitan areas. Yet our understanding of optimal ways to treat ethnic minority youth with behavioral/emotional problems is limited. Although evidence-based treatments (EBTs) exist for youth with diverse mental health problems, many doubt whether standard EBTs can be used effectively to treat ethnic minorities (e.g., Hall, 2001).

In debates over treatment efficacy with ethnic minorities, the *ethnic disparity* and *ethnic invariance* perspectives make different predictions concerning the possibility of ethnic differences in therapy outcomes. The ethnic disparity perspective argues that EBTs are less effective for ethnic minorities than for European Americans. EBTs might shortchange ethnic minorities because conventional treatments are developed by and for European Americans, and thus clinicians and clinical researchers may be more inclined to ignore cultural considerations. In contrast, the ethnic invariance perspective suggests that EBTs affect all cultural groups equally because basic principles of therapeutic change are universal.

The goal of this chapter is to shed some light on this debate by summarizing what we know about EBTs for ethnic minority youth with psychosocial problems. Specifically, we examine several questions regarding psychotherapy efficacy and engagement with minority youth. First, what treatments are efficacious for ethnic minority youth and how

451

robust are treatment effects? Second, are treatments equally efficacious for European American and ethnic minority youth? Third, what adaptations are made to EBTs that incorporate the needs of ethnic minority populations, and do these adaptations enhance treatment effects for ethnic minority youth? Finally, what evidence-based methods exist for successfully engaging ethnic minorities in mental health treatment? We draw primarily from our recent review and meta-analysis of EBTs with ethnic minority youth (Huey & Polo, 2008); however, we also summarize findings from other empirical work addressing treatment outcome issues with ethnic minority youth. The focus is on U.S. youth ages 18 years or younger with preexisting behavioral and emotional problems.

EFFICACIOUS TREATMENTS FOR ETHNIC MINORITY YOUTH

To address the extent to which treatments are efficacious for ethnic minority youth, we reviewed published randomized trials comparing active treatment with no-treatment, placebo, or treatment-as-usual (TAU) control groups (Huey & Polo, 2008). Efficacious treatments had to meet criteria as well-established, probably efficacious, or possibly efficacious based on standards developed by the Task Force on Promotion and Dissemination of Psychological Procedures (Chambless et al., 1998). Well-established treatments require support from at least two randomized trials by independent research teams showing that treatment is superior to placebo or another treatment (or equivalent to an established treatment). Probably efficacious treatments require only one placebo-controlled trial, or two trials comparing treatment and no treatment. Possibly efficacious treatments require only one study showing that a treatment is more efficacious than control but does not meet criteria as well-established or probably efficacious. In addition, studies had to meet one or more of the following conditions: (1) At least 75% of participants were ethnic minorities, (2) separate analyses with ethnic minority youth showed that treatment was superior to control conditions, and (3) analyses showed that ethnicity did not moderate treatment effects or that treatment was effective with ethnic minority youth despite moderator effects (Huey & Polo, 2008). If these criteria were met for a particular treatment, it was classified as an ethnic minority EBT, and supporting studies were included in our meta-analysis.

Overall, 13 treatments were considered as probably efficacious for ethnic minority youth and 17 as possibly efficacious (Huey & Polo, 2008). None met criteria for a well established treatment for ethnic minority youth. Efficacious treatments were found for minority youth with a broad array of psychosocial problems, including attention-deficit/hyperactivity disorder, conduct problems, trauma-related problems (e.g., posttraumatic stress disorder), depression, substance use problems, anxiety-related problems, suicidal behavior, and mixed/comorbid problems (i.e., no one target problem predominated) (Table 29.1).

The overwhelming majority of EBTs were group- or family-based treatments identified either for African American or Latino youth. Also, cognitive-behavioral approaches (e.g., treatments derived from social learning principles and cognitive theories of psychopathology) showed the strongest record of success with minority youth, although interpersonal psychotherapy and family systems interventions (i.e., brief strategic family therapy [BSFT], multidimensional family therapy, and multisystemic therapy [MST]) were also efficacious. Moreover, treatments for conduct problems constituted more than

TABLE 29.1. Probably Efficacious and Possibly Efficacious Treatments for Ethnic Minority Youth with Behavioral/Emotional Problems

Problem domain	Youth ethnicity	Evidence-based treatments
ADHD	African American and Hispanic/Latino	Behavioral treatment + stimulant medication
Anxiety-related problems	African American	AMT, group CBT, modified AMT, study skills training
	Hispanic/Latino	Group CBT
Conduct problems	African American	Anger management group training, assertive training, attribution training, behavioral contracting, cognitive restructuring, Coping Power, MST, response cost, social relations training
	Hispanic/Latino	Brief strategic family therapy, child-centered play therapy
	Mixed/other ethnicity	Rational emotive education, structured problem solving
Depression	Hispanic/Latino	CBT, interpersonal psychotherapy
Substance use problems	African American	MST
	Mixed/other ethnicity	Multidimensional family therapy
Suicidal behavior	African American	MST
Trauma-related problems	African American	Fostering individualized assistance program, resilient peer treatment, trauma focused CBT
	Hispanic/Latino	School-based group CBT
Mixed/comorbid problems	African American	Reaching educators, children, and parents
	Multiracial Hawaiian	MST

Note. ADHD, attention-deficit/hyperactivity disorder; AMT, anxiety management training; CBT, cognitive-behavioral treatment; MST, multisystemic therapy. Data from Huey and Polo (2008).

40% of all EBTs for minority youth. For example, seven treatments were probably efficacious for minority youth with conduct problems (i.e., anger management group training, attribution training, BSFT, child-centered play therapy, coping power, MST, rational emotive education), and six were possibly efficacious (i.e., behavioral contracting, cognitive restructuring, response cost, assertive training, social relations training, structured problem solving).

We also calculated effect size coefficients (Cohen's *d*) to provide a quantitative overview of treatment effects, assess the clinical relevance of treatment, and discern whether certain factors influenced treatment outcomes (Huey & Polo, 2008). Each study that met our ethnic minority criteria and reported appropriate effect size data was included, regardless of whether all participants were ethnic minorities. A coefficient of about 0.2 represents a small effect; 0.5, a medium effect; and 0.8, a large effect. Positive effects indicate that treated youth show more favorable outcomes than comparison youth. Results showed that the mean posttreatment effect size for these EBTs is $d = .44$, which represents a medium effect. This indicates that in the typical ethnic minority clinical trial 67% of treated participants were better off at posttreatment than the average control participant. At various follow-up periods (4–6 months, 1–1.7 years, 4 years, 13.7 years) treatment effects were generally maintained. Also, effects were stronger when treatment was compared with no treatment or placebo versus TAU (see Figure 29.1). However, type of target problem (externalizing vs. internalizing), problem severity (clinically significant vs. not clinically significant), and diagnostic status (*Diagnostic and Statistical Manual of Mental Disorders* diagnosis vs. no diagnosis) did not affect outcomes (Huey & Polo, 2008).

Next, studies were divided into those that compared active treatment with no treatment or placebo control, or compared active treatment with TAU, and effect sizes were recalculated. These results were then contrasted with two conventional treatment meta-analyses that included studies with mostly nonminority youth (or youth with unspecified ethnicity; Weisz, Weiss, Han, Granger, & Morton, 1995; Weisz, Jensen-Doss, & Hawley, 2006). Figure 29.2 shows that our effect sizes for ethnic minorities were roughly equivalent to those found in conventional youth treatment meta-analyses.

Thus, EBTs exist for ethnic minority youth with a broad array of behavioral and emotional problems (particularly conduct problems), although no treatments met the highest level of empirical support (i.e., well-established). Also, similar to findings with nonminority youth (Weisz et al., 1995), treatment effects were generally of medium magnitude and did not vary by problem type or severity. Moreover, although cognitive-behavioral treatments predominated, other forms of treatment were also identified as efficacious for ethnic minority youth.

However, our review revealed that there is still much that we do not know about effective treatments for ethnic minority youth. For example, whereas dozens of EBTs were found for African American and Latino youth, other ethnic minority groups (e.g., Asians, Pacific Islanders, Native Americans) are mostly absent from this literature. Also, despite the availability of effective approaches for autism, eating disorders, and other clinical syndromes with predominantly White youth, we know little about how minority youth might respond to these treatments. Finally, the majority of EBTs summarized

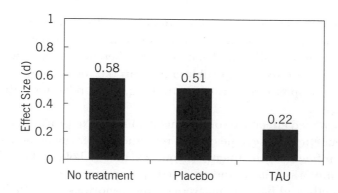

FIGURE 29.1. Type of comparison group as moderator of treatment effects for ethnic minority youth (TAU, treatment-as-usual). Data from Huey and Polo (2008).

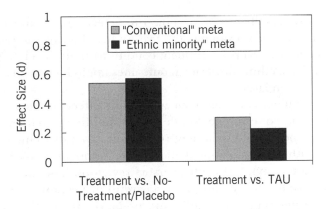

FIGURE 29.2. Mean effect sizes for conventional (Weisz et al., 1995, 2006) versus ethnic minority (Huey & Polo, 2008) youth treatment meta-analyses (TAU, treatment-as-usual).

here are "research therapies" (Weisz, Huey, & Weersing, 1998) that involve (1) recruited versus clinic-referred youth; (2) homogenous samples with one focal problem; (3) highly structured, manualized treatment; and (4) clinicians with extensive training and supervision. Thus, with few exceptions, it is unclear how well these treatments translate to ethnic minority youth in "real-world" mental health settings.

ETHNICITY AS A MODERATOR OF TREATMENT EFFECTS

Another important question concerns whether EBTs are differentially effective for European American versus ethnic minority youth. We addressed this issue by summarizing 13 randomized trials that tested ethnicity as a moderator of treatment effects (Huey & Polo, 2008). A significant moderator effect (i.e., a treatment condition x ethnicity interaction effect) would indicate that treatment was more efficacious for one ethnic group versus another. We found that eight of 13 studies showed no significant moderator effects, two showed stronger treatment effects for European Americans, and three showed stronger effects for minorities.

Beyond individual trials, several investigators have used meta-analyses to test whether treatment outcomes differ as a function of youth ethnicity. These studies found that effect sizes for treatment of ADHD (Fabiano et al., 2009) juvenile offending (Wilson, Lipsey, & Soydan, 2003), phobic/anxiety disorders (Silverman, Pina, & Viswesvaran, 2008), and diverse problems in usual care settings (Weisz et al., 2006) did not differ significantly for European Americans compared with other ethnic groups. Moreover, our meta-analysis (Huey & Polo, 2008) showed no significant effect size differences across ethnic minority groups (i.e., African American vs. Latino vs. mixed/other non-White).

There are several ways to explain these results. Because most studies show no ethnicity effects, one interpretation is that EBTs are equally potent regardless of youth ethnic background; in other words, the data could support the ethnic invariance perspective. However, another possibility is that the results are indeterminate given methodological concerns. First, because true ethnicity effects are likely in the small to medium range,

null findings may have resulted from low power to detect significant treatment moderators (Huey & Polo, 2008). For example, the five studies showing moderator effects had
larger average samples ($n = 84$ per treatment condition) than the eight null studies ($n = 61$ per condition). Thus, ethnic disparity in outcomes might have been apparent in more
studies had samples been larger.

Second, the complexity of treatment moderator effects often makes appropriate
interpretation difficult. For example, Rohde, Seeley, Kaufman, Clarke, and Stice (2006)
found that cognitive-behavioral treatment (CBT) was superior to life skills training for
depressed White youth, but no treatment effects were found for non-White youth (mostly
"mixed" or "other" ethnicity). Although a cursory review of these findings might suggest
that CBT is ineffective for non-White youth, a careful inspection of outcomes by condition and ethnicity argues for an alternative interpretation: that CBT is equally potent for
both groups, whereas life skills training is particularly efficacious for non-White youth.
Similarly, Lochman and Wells (2004) found that Coping Power (a social skills intervention for aggressive youth) reduced substance use for White but not Black youth, although
a review of posttreatment means suggests these results were driven by particularly strong
effects of the comparison condition on Black youth. Thus, for both studies, results that
initially appeared to favor European American youth were actually more ambiguous.

Third, the inclusion of culturally adapted therapies may have masked potential disparities in treatment response. Because many of the 13 treatments included culture-
responsive elements, this may have enhanced the therapeutic experience for minority
participants and thus minimized the possibility of differential outcomes by ethnicity. For
example, Silverman et al. (1999) found that group CBT was efficacious for youth with
anxiety disorders, with no evidence of differential outcomes for Caucasian and Latino
youth (i.e., ethnicity did not moderate treatment effects). However, investigator efforts
to "sensitize therapists to issues specific to working with multicultural populations" (Silverman et al., 1999, p. 996) may have been particularly beneficial to Latino participants
and thus mitigated potential disparities. Given the limited sample size, this possibility
was not evaluated by the investigators.

In summary, evidence for ethnic disparities in youth EBT outcomes is equivocal,
with most studies showing no significant moderator effects. However, it is possible that
null effects result from either low power to detect significant moderator effects or the
failure to account for the potential benefits of incorporating cultural content in standard EBTs. The influence of cultural adaptations on psychotherapy outcomes for ethnic
minority youth is explored more directly in the next section.

EFFECTS OF CULTURE-RESPONSIVE TREATMENTS

A third question addresses whether culture-responsive treatments are more effective
than standard treatments for ethnic minority youth. Although efforts to generate cultural competence guidelines are emerging, there is no consensus concerning what it
means for a treatment to be culturally adapted or tailored (Fuertes & Gretchen, 2001).
Our recent review (Huey & Polo, 2008) revealed a number of culture-responsive elements that were incorporated into the design and implementation of youth EBTs with
ethnically diverse samples. Table 29.2 summarizes these approaches and specifies which

TABLE 29.2. Culture-Responsive Elements in Evidence-Based Treatments for Ethnic Minority Youth

Category	Adaptation	Ethnicity
Counselor training/ education/experience	Sensitizing therapists to issues specific to working with ethnic minorities	Latino/Hispanic
	Family resource specialist to assist clinical team in understanding client cultures	Multiracial Hawaiian
	Experience working with ethnic minority populations	Latino/Hispanic
Counselor–client match	Counselor–youth or peer–youth ethnic match	African American, Latino/Hispanic
	Counselors/peers with common cultural experience or background	African American
	Counselor–youth language match	Latino/Hispanic
Therapy content	Vignettes, examples, materials changed to make more "culturally sensitive"	African American, Latino/Hispanic
	Address intergenerational, cultural conflict	Latino/Hispanic
	Use of cultural themes, symbols, content	Latino/Hispanic
Other/miscellaneous/ vague	Treatment individualized to deal flexibly with sociocultural differences	African American
	Cultural agents involved in treatment development	African American
	Miscellaneous adaptations for culture or diversity	African American, Latino/Hispanic
	Use of clients' cultural/ethnic strengths	African American

Note. Data from Huey and Polo (2008).

ethnic groups were targeted. These include, for example, efforts to use therapists of the same ethnicity as the youth/families receiving treatment. Others have incorporated changes to the protocol during the development of the intervention or during the training of therapists. In some cases, adaptations also consist of modifying the content of treatment manuals to provide examples that are more applicable to ethnic minority participants.

Unfortunately, only a handful of studies over the past 30 years have assessed how culture-responsive modalities affect youth therapy outcomes. Correlational studies generally show that counselor–client ethnic match is associated with positive treatment outcomes for African American, Mexican American, and Asian American youth (e.g., Flicker, Waldron, Turner, Brody, & Hops, 2008). However, correlational methods leave open the possibility that ethnic match is not a true causal factor.

A better approach is to conduct randomized trials comparing standard EBTs with culturally modified versions of the same EBTs. Although this approach is increasingly common in the youth prevention and adult treatment literature (e.g., Botvin, Schinke, Diaz, & Botvin, 1995; Huey & Pan, 2006), our search identified only two experimental studies that have assessed the importance of culture-responsive approaches in evidence-based treatment for youth. Szapocznik, Rio, et al. (1986) compared BSFT with bicultural effectiveness training (a culturally enhanced adaptation of BSFT) in a randomized trial with behaviorally disordered, Cuban American youth. No significant group differences were found at posttreatment, suggesting that cultural enhancement offered no additional benefits. In a recent study, McCabe and Yeh (2009) compared standard parent–child interaction therapy (PCIT) with culturally modified PCIT and TAU in a randomized trial for externalizing Mexican American youth. They found that culturally modified PCIT was superior to TAU for most youth and parenting outcomes, but standard PCIT was superior to TAU for only a few outcomes. However, standard and culturally modified PCIT did not differ significantly for any outcomes. Thus, results from both studies show no clear outcome enhancements from cultural adaptations, although small sample sizes in both studies ($n < 20$ per group) suggest that power may have been inadequate to detect significant differences.

To address this question in our meta-analysis (Huey & Polo, 2008), we directly compared two types of clinical trials: those evaluating culture-responsive EBTs and those evaluating standard EBTs (i.e., treatments with no apparent culture-responsive elements). We used a conservative approach (i.e., the clinical trial suggested treatment was modified for minority youth) and liberal approach (i.e., supplementary sources suggested the treatment was modified for minorities) to classify treatments as culture-responsive. Fifty percent of treatments were culture-responsive using the conservative definition, whereas 70% were culture-responsive based on the liberal definition. Figure 29.3 shows that, regardless of definition, no significant differences were found for standard versus culture-responsive treatments.

Thus, although efforts have been made in a number of studies to consider culture/ethnicity when treating ethnic minority youth, we cannot say whether cultural adaptations result in enhanced treatment outcomes. Although two randomized trials and our meta-analysis show mostly null effects, methodological problems limit what conclusions can be drawn. Existing studies probably lack adequate statistical power, and cultural elements of most treatments are often missing or poorly specified. As a result, null effects

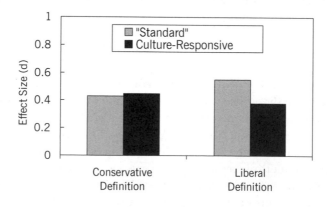

FIGURE 29.3. Mean effect sizes for standard versus culture-responsive treatments, based on conservative versus liberal definition. Differences between standard and culture-responsive treatments not significant. Data from Huey and Polo (2008).

may reflect design limitations or a lack of identification of potent cultural elements that have a more direct impact on treatment effects. Clearly, experimental research is needed to discern the effectiveness of various cultural adaptations with ethnic minority youth.

ENGAGING ETHNIC MINORITY YOUTH IN TREATMENT

As a final issue, we discuss approaches aimed at increasing participation and engagement of ethnic minority youth in mental health treatment. Research indicates that a large proportion of at-risk minority youth do not receive the mental health services they need (Kataoka, Stein, Nadeem, & Wong, 2007), and that utilization rates are lower than those for European American youth (Garland et al., 2005). When they do receive treatment, ethnic minority youth are more likely to terminate prematurely (Miller, Southam-Gerow, & Allin, 2008), attend fewer sessions (Bui & Takeuchi, 1992), and show less clinical improvement (Weersing & Weisz, 2002) than European American youth. Even when receiving EBTs, dropout rates for African American and other ethnic minority youth are often higher than for European American youth (e.g., Kazdin & Whitley, 2003). These data suggest that, in addition to focusing on symptom reduction and functional improvement, research is needed on how interventions can address individual, socioeconomic, cultural, and structural barriers that may determine whether or not ethnic minority families enroll and are retained when offered EBTs.

A number of strategies have been utilized to increase participation in treatment and reduce unilateral termination, including several that have focused on ethnic minority populations. Some of the earliest research in this area focused on single prompts as an engagement method. These studies found that verbal (e.g., telephone) or written (e.g., letter) prompts immediately before a scheduled session significantly increased treatment attendance for poor minority adults and families (e.g., Hochstadt & Trybula, 1980; Planos & Glenwick, 1986).

Subsequent efforts have used more elaborate strategies for recruiting and retaining ethnic minority families. McKay, Stoewe, McCadam, and Gonzales (1998) evaluated the effects of two engagement strategies in an urban mental health agency serving predominately low-income ethnic minority children and adolescents. The authors randomly assigned families to one of three conditions: (1) a 30-minute telephone call before the intake appointment; (2) the same telephone call combined with an in-person engagement interview also conducted before the intake appointment; or (3) usual intake procedures. The engagement interventions included an exploration of both within-family and environmental barriers and problem solving to address these obstacles. Families who received the phone call alone or the combined call and interview were more likely to show up to their scheduled appointments. However, relative to those who received the usual intake procedures, only those in the combined call/interview condition showed improved attendance in subsequent scheduled appointments.

Szapocznik and colleagues' (1988) intervention, strategic structural systems engagement (SSSE), uses family therapy techniques (e.g., joining and restructuring) to reduce resistance and increase the initial engagement of adolescents and their families in treatment. In the first randomized trial of this intervention, Latino families who had an adolescent involved in substance use and received SSSE were significantly more likely to attend the intake and less likely to drop out of treatment than those who received a control condition simulating usual care procedures (Szapocznik et al., 1988). A second trial of SSSE, also involving an exclusively Latino sample (Santisteban et al., 1996), confirmed its efficacy in increasing engagement, as measured by increased rate of attendance of the intake interview and subsequent therapy sessions. Moderator analyses revealed that Cuban Americans were significantly less likely to engage than non-Cuban American Latinos.

More recently, one of us has been involved in the adaptation of a brief intervention inspired by the work of a community nonprofit organization from Lawrence, Massachusetts (see *www.rightquestion.org*). This educational strategy, The Right Question Project-Mental Health (RQP-MH), aims to increase the level of participation in treatment-related decisions of individuals receiving services and reduce their likelihood of dropping out of care. This strategy has been successfully implemented with adult outpatients from ethnic minority backgrounds, particularly immigrant Latinos (see Alegría et al., 2008). Using three 45-minute sessions, the intervention teaches participants to identify important decisions that are relevant to their care and to generate carefully constructed questions directed to their providers. Through this process, participants shift their role from being a passive recipient of information to feeling more empowered to make collaborative decisions and shape their course of treatment in partnership with their therapists and other providers. In a quasi-experimental design, we found that, relative to those receiving usual care, RQP-MH participants reported significantly higher engagement in their interactions with mental health providers. Furthermore, RQP-MH participants were also significantly more likely to attend scheduled sessions and less likely to drop out of care (Alegría et al., 2008). We have further refined the intervention and are testing it in a randomized trial. A version of this program for youth with mental health problems and their parents is also being developed.

In sum, a few strategies exist and others are being developed to increase treatment participation and retention of ethnic minority youth and their families. The vast majority have focused on the initial engagement of clients and devote less effort to reducing dropout postintake. These interventions are not yet available in manual form, which may facilitate dissemination in community settings or integration into existing EBT protocols. Also, engagement strategies for Asian American and Native American youth and families were not found, and the vast majority of the work has been done with African Americans and Latinos. Interestingly, one strength of available engagement strategies is that, in contrast to many EBTs, they have been developed and tested in community settings and compared with usual care procedures. Experimental designs evaluating the impact of EBTs with or without engagement components are much needed, including those conducted in laboratory and naturalistic settings.

DIRECTIONS FOR RESEARCH

Overall, our appraisal of EBT research with ethnic minority youth is fairly optimistic. A number of EBTs exist for African American and Latino youth with diverse problems, and ethnic minorities generally benefit as much as European Americans. Although treatments are often adapted for ethnic minorities, compelling evidence was not found for the need to use separate or specialized procedures to treat ethnic minority youth. Finally, evidence suggests that several successful strategies exist for engaging and retaining minority youth and families in treatment.

Of course, these conclusions must be qualified, given the limited and often inadequate research on treatment issues with minority youth. In an earlier article (Huey & Polo, 2008), we offered six recommendations for improving the quality of psychotherapy research with ethnic minority youth. These included (1) expanding the number of clinical trials with ethnic minority youth, particularly those from immigrant and non-English-speaking backgrounds; (2) focusing greater attention on ethnicity, nativity, and related factors as moderators of treatment effects; (3) consistently describing investigator efforts to make treatments culture-responsive; (4) rigorously assessing whether cultural adaptations enhance treatment effects with minorities; (5) ensuring that sample sizes are appropriate for evaluating key research questions regarding minority youth; and (6) assessing culturally appropriate outcomes. Next, we briefly offer two additional agenda items for future research.

Address Diversity Issues in Treatment Manuals

Although treatment manuals have been critical for the operationalization and dissemination of EBTs, with few exceptions (Rosselló & Bernal, 1996) they do not provide guidelines for how to implement core techniques to serve youth of diverse backgrounds or directly address how to consider culture when working with ethnic minorities. Assuming that culture-responsive adaptations are useful for minorities, it is important to specify how to implement such strategies. One approach is to develop supplementary guides to use in conjunction with therapy manuals that specify how to adapt treatments for particular minority groups (Huey & Pan, 2005, 2006). However, there is also a need for illustrations in mainstream manuals that demonstrate flexible applications of modules with youth and families of different ethnic groups, socioeconomic backgrounds, and settings. For example, a therapist who is teaching a module on activity selection for mood enhancement may benefit from having examples of how this skill can be implemented with youth living in rural or suburban areas as well as youth of poor and urban backgrounds. Fortunately, increased attention has been given to case studies focused on youth of culturally diverse backgrounds participating in CBTs (e.g., Ngo et al., 2008).

Assess Within-Group Differences in Treatment Response

Earlier we discussed whether minorities and European Americans differ in how they respond to treatment; yet it is also critical to test for within-group differences to avoid the assumption of ethnic minority homogeneity of therapy response. For example, limited research suggests that immigration and acculturation status may determine which minorities respond optimally to standard or culturally adapted treatment {Martinez & Eddy, 2005; Pan, Huey, & Hernandez, 2009; Telles et al., 1995). None of these studies included ethnic minorities with preexisting behavioral/emotional problems, however. Thus, future research should assess what culture-related factors determine whether an EBT is efficacious for particular ethnic minority youth.

Assuming that an EBT with demonstrated efficacy for one ethnic group will be equally efficacious across all ethnic minority groups can also be problematic. For example, in a prevention trial, Cardemil, Reivich, Beevers, Seligman, and James (2007) compared ethnic minority youth randomly assigned to either the Penn Resiliency Program (PRP) or a no-treatment control group. PRP focuses on teaching cognitive and social problem-solving skills to youth at risk for depression. A differential effect (fewer depressive symptoms and negative automatic thoughts) in favor of PRP was found for Latino youth, but not for African American youth.

A related question is whether particular modes of treatment, such as family- or group-based interventions, are optimal for ethnic minority youth compared with other approaches. Some initial work in this area leads to very different conclusions. Several randomized trials with Latino youth found no outcome differences between conjoint family therapy versus one-person therapy (Szapocznik, Kurtines, Foote, Perez-Vidal, & Hervis, 1986) or group-based versus individual therapy (Rosselló, Bernal, & Rivera-Medina, 2008). However, a meta-analysis by Waldron and Turner (2008) comparing family, group, and individual interventions for adolescents with substance use problems found significant disparities. Whereas individual and family treatments were efficacious, group CBT effects were much smaller and indistinguishable from control conditions among studies with predominantly Latino youth. Thus, group-focused interventions may be less effective than other interventions for Latino youth with drug use problems. Waldron and Turner (2008) suggest that poor effects for group treatment may be because therapists were less able to attend to cultural factors in group settings compared with individual and family therapy contexts.

As a final note, findings regarding comparisons across cultural groups should be interpreted with caution given the economic, social, and educational disparities that are a reality in the United States. Ethnic comparisons are often fraught with ambiguity because culture and ethnicity are often confounded with risk factors such as lack of insurance, poverty, and a host of other factors which can also directly impact treatment effects. Thus, strong claims about treatment efficacy with ethnic minorities without attention to these other variables should be avoided.

CONCLUSIONS

Despite these concerns, significant progress has been made regarding our understanding of EBTs for ethnic minority youth. The evidence is particularly strong for African American and Latino youth, who represent the two largest ethnic minority groups in the United States. Many gaps remain, however, and much more work is needed to address critical questions concerning what treatments are efficacious for which minority youth, what mechanisms account for clinical change for ethnic minority youth in treatment, and which factors enhance or impede treatment efficacy for these youth. Of special concern is whether these "minority" EBTs can be transported effectively to real-world clinical practice, particularly because ethnic minorities with mental health needs are less likely than European Americans to receive evidence-based care (Wang, Berglund, & Kessler, 2000). We hope that greater attention will be directed toward dissemination efforts, with the ultimate goal of increasing EBT access and use for ethnic minority youth in community settings.

REFERENCES

Alegría, M., Polo, A., Gao, S., Santana, L., Rothstein, D., Jimenez, A., et al. (2008). Evaluation of a patient activation and empowerment intervention in mental health care. *Medical Care, 46*, 247–256.

Botvin, G. J., Schinke, S. P., Diaz, T., & Botvin, E. M. (1995). Effectiveness of culturally focused and generic skills training approaches to alcohol and drug abuse prevention among minority adolescents: Two-year follow-up results. *Psychology of Addictive Behaviors, 9*, 183–194.

Bui, K. V. T., & Takeuchi, D. T. (1992). Ethnic minority adolescents and the use of community mental health care services. *American Journal of Community Psychology, 20*, 403–417.

Cardemil, E. V., Reivich, K. J., Beevers, C. G., Seligman, M. E. P., & James, J. (2007). The prevention of depressive symptoms in low-income, minority children: Two-year follow-up. *Behaviour Research and Therapy, 45*, 313–327.

Chambless, D. L., Baker, M. J., Baucom, D. H., Beutler, L. E., Calhoun, K. S., Crits-Christoph, P., et al. (1998). Update on empirically validated therapies, II. *The Clinical Psychologist, 51*, 3–16.

Fabiano, G. A., Pelham, W. E., Jr., Coles, E. K., Gnagy, E. M., Chronis-Tuscano, A., & O'Connor, B. (2009). Evidence-based treatments for attention-deficit hyperactivity disorder: A meta-analysis of behavioral treatments. *Clinical Psychology Review, 29*, 129–140.

Flicker, S. M., Waldron, H. B., Turner, C. W., Brody, J. L., & Hops, H. (2008). Ethnic matching and treatment outcome with Hispanic and Anglo substance-abusing adolescents in family therapy. *Journal of Family Psychology, 22*, 439–447.

Fuertes, J. N., & Gretchen, D. (2001). Emerging theories of multicultural counseling. In J. G. Ponterotto, J. M. Casas, L. A. Suzuki, & C. M. Alexander (Eds.), *Handbook of multicultural counseling* (pp. 509–541). Thousand Oaks, CA: Sage.

Garland, A. F., Lau, A. S., Yeh, M., McCabe, K. M., Hough, R. L., & Landsverk, J. A. (2005). Racial and ethnic differences in utilization of mental health services among high-risk youth. *American Journal of Psychiatry, 162*, 1336–1343.

Hall, G. C. N. (2001). Psychotherapy research with ethnic minorities: Empirical, ethical, and conceptual issues. *Journal of Consulting and Clinical Psychology, 69*, 502–510.

Hochstadt, N. J., & Trybula, J., Jr. (1980). Reducing missed initial appointments in a community mental health center. *Journal of Community Psychology, 8*, 261–265.

Huey, S. J., Jr., & Pan, D. (2005). *One-session treatment supplemental manual: Cultural adaptations for phobic Asian Americans*. Los Angeles: Department of Psychology, University of Southern California.

Huey, S. J., Jr., & Pan, D. (2006). Culture-responsive one-session therapy for phobic Asian Americans: A pilot study. *Psychotherapy: Theory, Research, Practice, and Training, 43*, 549–554.

Huey, S. J., Jr., & Polo, A. J. (2008). Evidence-based psychosocial treatments for ethnic minority youth. *Journal of Clinical Child and Adolescent Psychology, 37*, 262–301.

Kataoka, S., Stein, B. D., Nadeem, E., & Wong, M. (2007). Who gets care?: Mental health service use following a school-based suicide prevention program. *Journal of the American Academy of Child and Adolescent Psychiatry, 46*, 1341–1348.

Kazdin, A. E., & Whitley, M. K. (2003). Treatment of parental stress to enhance therapeutic change among children referred for aggressive and antisocial behavior. *Journal of Consulting and Clinical Psychology, 71*, 504–515.

Lochman, J. E., & Wells, K. C. (2004). The Coping Power program for preadolescent aggressive boys and their parents: Outcome effects at the 1–year follow-up. *Journal of Consulting and Clinical Psychology, 72*, 571–578.

Martinez, C. R., Jr., & Eddy, J. M. (2005). Effects of culturally adapted parent management training on Latino youth behavioral health outcomes. *Journal of Consulting and Clinical Psychology, 73*, 841–851.

McCabe, K., & Yeh, M. (2009). Parent child interaction therapy for Mexican Americans: A randomized clinical trial. *Journal of Clinical Child and Adolescent Psychology, 38*, 753–759.

McCabe, K., Yeh, M., Hough, R. L., Landsverk, J., Hurlburt, M. S., Culver, S. W., et al. (1999).

Racial/ethnic representation across five public sectors of care for youth. *Journal of Emotional and Behavioral Disorders, 7,* 72–82.

McKay, M. M., Stoewe, J., McCadam, K., & Gonzales, J. (1998). Increasing access to child mental health services for urban children and their caregivers. *Health and Social Work, 23,* 9–15.

Miller, L. M., Southam-Gerow, M. A., & Allin, R. B., Jr. (2008). Who stays in treatment? Child and family predictors of youth client retention in a public mental health agency. *Child and Youth Care Forum, 37,* 153–170.

Ngo, V., Langley, A., Kataoka, S. H., Nadeem, E., Escudero, P., & Stein, B. D. (2008). Providing evidence-based practice to ethnically diverse youth: Examples from the Cognitive Behavioral Intervention for Trauma in Schools (CBITS) program. *Journal of the American Academy of Child and Adolescent Psychiatry, 47,* 858–862.

Pan, D., Huey, S. J., Jr., & Hernandez, D. (2009). *Culturally-adapted versus standard exposure treatment for phobic Asian Americans: Treatment efficacy, mediators, and moderators.* Manuscript submitted for publication.

Planos, R., & Glenwick, D. S. (1986). The effects of prompts on minority children's screening attendance at a community mental health center. *Child and Family Behavior Therapy, 8,* 5–13.

Pollard, K., & Mather, M. (2009). U.S. Hispanic and Asian population growth levels off. Retrieved August 20, 2009, from the Population Reference Bureau Web site, *www.prb.org/Artie les/2009/hispanicasiall.aspx.*

Rohde, P., Seeley, J. R., Kaufman, N. K., Clarke, G. N., & Stice, E. (2006). Predicting time to recovery among depressed adolescents treated in two psychosocial group interventions. *Journal of Consulting and Clinical Psychology, 74,* 80–88.

Rosselló, J., & Bernal, G. (1996). Adapting cognitive-behavioral and interpersonal treatments for depressed Puerto Rican adolescents. In E. D. Hibbs & P. S. Jensen (Eds.), *Psychosocial treatments for child and adolescent disorders: Empirically based strategies for clinical practice* (pp. 157–185). Washington, DC: American Psychological Association.

Rosselló, J., Bernal, G., & Rivera-Medina, C. (2008). Individual and group CBT and IPT for Puerto Rican adolescents with depressive symptoms. *Cultural Diversity and Ethnic Minority Psychology, 14,* 234–245.

Santisteban, D. A., Szapocznik, J., Perez-Vidal, A., Kurtines, W. M., Murray, E. J., & LaPerriere, A. (1996). Efficacy of intervention for engaging youth and families into treatment and some variables that may contribute to differential effectiveness. *Journal of Family Psychology, 10,* 35–44.

Silverman, W. K., Kurtines, W. M., Ginsburg, G. S., Weems, C. F., Lumpkin, P. W., & Carmichael, D. H. (1999). Treating anxiety disorders in children with group cognitive-behavioral therapy: A randomized clinical trial. *Journal of Consulting and Clinical Psychology, 67,* 995–1003.

Silverman, W. K., Pina, A. A., & Viswesvaran, C. (2008). Evidence-based psychosocial treatments for phobic and anxiety disorders in children and adolescents. *Journal of Clinical Child and Adolescent Psychology, 37,* 105–130.

Szapocznik, J., Kurtines, W. M., Foote, F., Perez-Vidal, A., & Hervis, O. (1986). Conjoint versus one-person family therapy: Further evidence for the effectiveness of conducting family therapy through one person with drug-abusing adolescents. *Journal of Consulting and Clinical Psychology, 54,* 395–397.

Szapocznik, J., Perez-Vidal, A., Brickman, A. L., Foote, F. H., Santisteban, D., Hervis, O., et al. (1988). Engaging adolescent drug abusers and their families in treatment: A strategic structural systems approach. *Journal of Consulting and Clinical Psychology, 56,* 552–557.

Szapocznik, J., Rio, A., Perez-Vidal, A., Kurtines, W., Hervis, O., & Santisteban, D. (1986). Bicultural effectiveness training (BET): An experimental test of an intervention modality for families experiencing intergenerational/intercultural conflict. *Hispanic Journal of Behavioral Sciences, 8,* 303–330.

Telles, C. M., Karno, M., Mintz, J., Paz, G., Arias, M., Tucker, D., et al. (1995). Immigrant families coping with schizophrenia: Behavioural family intervention v. case management with a low-income Spanish-speaking population. *British Journal of Psychiatry, 167,* 473–479.

Waldron, H. B., & Turner, C. W. (2008). Evidence-based psychosocial treatments for adolescent substance abuse. *Journal of Clinical Child and Adolescent Psychology, 37*, 238–261.

Wang, P. S., Berglund, P., & Kessler, R. C. (2000). Recent care of common mental disorders in the United States: Prevalence and conformance with evidence-based recommendations. *Journal of General Internal Medicine, 15*, 284–292.

Weersing, V. R., & Weisz, J. R. (2002). Community clinic treatment of depressed youth: Benchmarking usual care against CBT clinical trials. *Journal of Consulting and Clinical Psychology, 2*, 299–310.

Weisz, J. R., Huey, S. J., Jr., & Weersing, V. R. (1998). Psychotherapy outcome research with children and adolescents: The state of the art. In T. H. Ollendick & R. J. Prinz (Eds.), *Advances in clinical child psychology* (Vol. 20, pp. 49–91). New York: Plenum.

Weisz, J. R., Jensen-Doss, A., & Hawley, K. M. (2006). Evidence-based youth psychotherapies versus usual clinical care: A meta-analysis of direct comparisons. *American Psychologist, 61*, 671–689.

Weisz, J. R., Weiss, B., Han, S. S., Granger, D. A., & Morton, T. (1995). Effects of psychotherapy with children and adolescents revisited: A meta-analysis of treatment outcome studies. *Psychological Bulletin, 117*, 450–468.

Wilson, S. J., Lipsey, M. W., & Soydan, H. (2003). Are mainstream programs for juvenile delinquents less effective with minority youth than majority youth? A meta analysis of outcomes research. *Research on Social Work Practice, 13*, 3–26.

30

Adapting Cognitive-Behavioral Therapy for Depression to Fit Diverse Youths and Contexts

Applying the Deployment-Focused Model of Treatment Development and Testing

SARAH KATE BEARMAN, ANA UGUETO, ALISHA ALLEYNE, and JOHN R. WEISZ

OVERVIEW: DEPRESSION AND ITS TREATMENT

The Clinical Problem: Youth Depression

Depression is among the most prevalent and impairing conditions to afflict youths (i.e., children and adolescents). Epidemiological studies show 12-month prevalence rates exceeding 6% for major depressive disorder (MDD) and 10% for dysthymic disorder; point prevalence of adolescent MDD alone has been estimated at 3–8 % (see, e.g., Zalsman, Brent, & Weersing, 2006). By age 18, nearly one-fourth of all youths will have experienced a depressive disorder (Zalsman et al., 2006).

Youth depression predicts low academic achievement and school failure, substance abuse and dependence, and, later in life, unemployment and early parenthood (e.g., Fergusson & Woodward, 2002). It is associated with high rates of psychiatric comorbidity and increased risk of attempted and completed suicide, the third leading cause of death among American adolescents (Zalsman et al., 2006). Few could question the need for effective intervention.

Treatments for Youth Depression to Date: How Successful?

Over the past two decades, a number of youth depression treatment programs have been tested in randomized controlled trials (RCTs; see excellent examples elsewhere in this volume). The most extensively tested treatment approach is cognitive-behavioral therapy

(CBT), but other approaches (e.g., interpersonal therapy) are building an evidence base as well. Although numerous studies of CBT, interpersonal therapy, and other approaches have shown significant effects in RCTs, the nature of the evidence warrants close attention.

In a recent examination of the evidence base, Weisz, McCarty, and Valeri (2006) conducted a meta-analysis of 35 RCTs of youth depression treatment. The mean weighted least squares effect size (ES) across studies was only 0.34, about midway between commonly used benchmarks for small (0.20) and medium (0.50) effects. Compared with the mean ES for a large sample of RCTs for child and adolescent conditions other than depression, the depression mean was significantly lower. Cognitively focused depression treatments (e.g., CBT) showed a mean effect of 0.35. The meta-analysis showed that treatments for youth depression have had beneficial effects but modest effects on average.

The meta-analysis also revealed how few studies have been conducted under conditions that closely resemble actual clinical practice with depressed youths and how few compared the target treatments with active interventions, such as those delivered in actual clinical practice. When steps were taken in study design to better match the conditions of clinical practice, the mean effects were smaller. For example, the mean ES was 0.27 for studies in which practicing clinicians delivered the target treatment, 0.24 for studies in which the treatment took place in clinical practice settings, and 0.24 for studies in which target treatments were tested against active control conditions such as usual clinical care. These findings were echoed by a broader meta-analysis (Weisz, Jensen-Doss, & Hawley, 2006) in which the mean effect size of previously tested evidence-based treatments for a variety of youth problems and disorders dropped to 0.30 when the treatments were compared with usual clinical care, and a number of the evidence-based treatments failed to outperform usual care.

Taken together, these findings have suggested to our research group the need for a body of evidence on the effects of evidence-based treatments—for depression and other conditions—within the contexts in which youth mental health care typically occurs and in comparison to the usual treatment that would otherwise be available in those contexts. The evidence thus far suggests that treatment effects may be reduced as we move from the often optimizing conditions of what is called *efficacy* research, in which researchers exert considerable control over participant and therapist selection, treatment settings, and study conditions, to the broad genre often referred to as *effectiveness* research, in which treatments are tested with representative referred youths, treated by practitioners, and in clinical service settings, and particularly when outcomes of target treatments are compared with outcomes obtained in usual clinical care. This, in turn, suggests that one useful goal in treatment development and testing may be building interventions that can be used effectively within everyday clinical practice contexts and building a body of evidence on treatment effects within those contexts. This perspective has shaped our work on the youth depression treatment front.

PRIMARY AND SECONDARY CONTROL ENHANCEMENT TRAINING AND THE DEPLOYMENT-FOCUSED MODEL OF TREATMENT DEVELOPMENT AND TESTING

In presenting our research program, we describe both the treatment approach and the model of treatment development that has guided the work.

Treatment Overview

Our treatment approach, primary and secondary control enhancement training (PAS-CET; Weisz, Gray, Bearman, & Stark, 2008), is a cognitive-behavioral intervention that has been under study since its initial efficacy trial a decade ago (Weisz, Thurber, Sweeney, Proffitt, & LeGagnoux, 1997). It is focused on helping youngsters cope with depression by developing skills in achieving primary control (changing objective conditions); e.g., using problem-solving skills to resolve an upsetting dilemma) and secondary control (adapting to objective conditions so as to control their subjective emotional impact; e.g., changing cognitions, finding a silver lining in an otherwise distressing situation). PASCET has been used with youngsters ages 8–14, across a spectrum from moderately symptomatic youths to those with depressive disorders, and in both individual and group treatment formats.

Although a number of CBT protocols have shown significant benefit in RCTs, these protocols are not widely used in most everyday practice settings. As we noted earlier, tests of the protocols are not typically carried out within clinically representative conditions or with comparison to usual clinical care, facts that may limit the application of CBT into everyday care. One of our central goals with PASCET has been to pursue treatment development and testing with an eye toward the ingredients needed for ultimate deployment to everyday intervention contexts where youth depression is referred for care and is treated by practitioners. This goal has led us to follow the model described next.

The Deployment-Focused Model of Treatment Development and Testing

Our work has followed the deployment-focused model (DFM) of treatment development and testing (described in Weisz, 2004). The DFM describes a series of procedures designed to promote the development of evidence-based treatments that can be used effectively within everyday practice contexts (i.e., in clinical service settings; e.g., community clinics, schools, hospitals), with youngsters who are normally referred to those settings, and with treatment delivered by the professionals who work in those settings. The model stresses the need to move toward research designs in which the outcomes of a treatment developer's intervention are compared with the outcomes of usual clinical care in the most relevant settings. The model does endorse the value of traditional efficacy trial RCTs that optimize experimental control, particularly in the early stages of treatment development. However, the DFM also assumes that treatments designed for and tested under efficacy conditions may not perform optimally when transported to everyday treatment contexts unless they are adapted to fit those contexts. Figure 30.1 illustrates this concept.

Accordingly, the DFM outlines processes for treatment adaptation and for tests of how successful the adaptation has been. Another goal of the DFM is to generate, over time, a body of evidence on the boundary conditions (e.g., moderators) and change processes (e.g., mediators) associated with treatment impact that will have a high level of external validity, because it is derived from research in the practice context. In short, this model seeks to ensure that tests in clinical practice contexts occur and to produce treatments that are designed and equipped to work well in those contexts. Several procedures are delineated in the model. In our view, the order and exact nature of the procedures may differ across different treatments, but we believe that some form of all these procedures will be needed for optimum fit of treatment to context.

**Deployment-Focused Model for the Transition
from Efficacy Testing to Use in Practice**

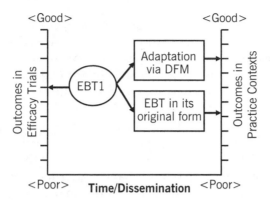

FIGURE 30.1. An assumption of the deployment-focused model (DFM): As interventions are transported from efficacy trials to representative practice contexts, effects will be enhanced to the extent that the interventions have been adapted to fit the contexts (EBT, evidence-based treatment). From Weisz (2004).

• *Theoretically and clinically guided construction, refinement, and manualizing of the treatment protocol.* One key process is the development, refinement, pilot testing, and manualizing of the treatment protocol. Theory and evidence on the nature and treatment of the target condition, plus the clinical literature (e.g., published case studies) and input from clinicians who have treated youngsters with that condition, are used to guide the design of treatment components and to plan clinically sensitive ways of presenting those components in sessions. The goal is production of (1) a treatment protocol that is well grounded in the theoretical, empirical, and clinical literature on the target condition (e.g., depression); (2) a manual that conveys treatment components clearly to the therapist and includes clinically appropriate means of presenting those components to clients; and (3) engaging and clinically appropriate supporting materials (e.g., youth practice book) that convey key ideas, and related exercises, directly to the participants. The treatment protocol should grow out of a clearly articulated model of the condition being treated, the mechanisms by which change in that condition is brought about through the treatment protocol, and characteristics of the context within which the treatment is to be used.

• *Initial efficacy research to establish potential for benefit.* Early in the treatment development process, efficacy research is an appropriate way to assess whether the treatment has the potential to generate beneficial effects. Although in some cases investigators may need to begin their exploration with an open trial, the effectiveness agenda will need to include a randomized trial in which the treatment protocol is compared with a condition that controls, at least, for the passage of time plus any effects of pre- and postassessment. The focus of the efficacy research may be the study of symptomatic individuals, not clinically referred cases, to avoid exposing severely disturbed individuals to an untested intervention. To maximize investigator control, investigators may focus the research on participants who are recruited and not necessarily referred for care, with the intervention provided by research employees and in settings controlled by the investigator. Positive findings of the efficacy research will provide evidence that the intervention has the potential to benefit the target population, justifying efforts to undertake adaptation and testing in the target treatment context.

- *Single-case applications in practice settings, with progressive adaptations to the protocol.* The process of adaptation can be guided by a series of single-case tests with the kinds of individuals and in the kind of setting for which the treatment is ultimately intended. Whether these tests use single-case experimental designs (e.g., ABAB design) or consist of less formal tryouts of the intervention procedures will depend partly on available resources and how much the treatment procedures need to be modified during the treatment episode. Whatever the specific procedures, the single-case aspect of the DFM is expected to be the context for modifying the treatment protocol to ensure goodness of fit with the clients, practitioners, and service setting for which the treatment is intended while maintaining adherence to the model of change that guides the treatment program. Guided by information from treatment of these individual cases, treatment developers may make changes in the nature of the treatment components, the ways the components are presented to clients and family members, and the materials used to guide therapists and clients through the treatment.

- *Effectiveness—tests of implementation and transportability.* Central to the DFM is testing of the candidate treatment within representative practice conditions. Key elements include delivery of the candidate treatment (1) to individuals who meet criteria for the target problems and who are representative of those typically seen in the target setting, (2) by clinicians who typically provide care in the setting, (3) with treatment delivered within the target setting, and (4) with outcomes compared with those of usual care in the setting. In an ideal world, introducing these elements in separate studies would sharpen inferential power in the early stages of research. Early tests that encompass all these elements concurrently may lead to findings that are difficult to interpret; for example, when findings fall short of the outcomes achieved in prior efficacy research, it may be difficult to determine whether the findings reflect inappropriateness of the protocol for referred youths, a mismatch between the protocol and setting constraints, clinician difficulty in using the procedures, or other factors. On the other hand, a series of studies in which only one representativeness dimension is varied at a time, followed by manipulation of strategically selected combinations of dimensions, could be so time consuming and costly as to be impractical. Reality constraints may require investigators to combine multiple elements, even in early stages. Whatever the sequence, the ultimate goal is research in which the primary dimensions are combined within the same trial, with the adapted protocol and procedures tested within the target setting, with youngsters referred to that setting through normal pathways, with treatment provided by clinicians employed in that setting, and with random assignment of clinicians and children to the candidate protocol or usual care. To the extent that these tests show the adapted treatment protocol to be more effective than usual care, an important goal of the DFM will have been attained: development of evidence-based intervention that can improve outcomes for children who are referred to clinical service settings when they are treated in those settings by the clinicians who work there.

- *Tests of sustainability in practice contexts.* Knowing that an effective intervention has been developed is valuable but is not the end of the process. Research is needed to address sustainability of the treatment program within the setting. The agenda may include research on the nature and extent of training and case supervision needed before clinicians can independently deliver the treatment effectively, clinician factors that predict continued use with fidelity, organizational characteristics associated with sustained support for continued use, and even cost and reimbursement factors that influence the likelihood of continued use. A key objective in sustainability research will be to understand what ingredients are needed to ensure that the treatment continues to be used effectively in the setting after the researchers and the research support are gone.

Additional Foci of Effectiveness and Sustainability Research

In addition to the primary objectives described for effectiveness and sustainability research, important questions about the nature and boundary conditions of treatment effects can be addressed via appropriate variations in study design. The variations may include (1) dismantling designs to ascertain the necessary and sufficient components of the treatment protocol, (2) moderator analyses to identify the kinds of youths with whom the treatment works well, and not so well, (3) mediator analyses to assess what change processes are associated with treatment benefit, (4) cost and cost-effectiveness analyses to probe costs in relation to benefits, (5) studies of personnel or organizational factors in the setting that relate to how effective the treatment is, and (6) tests of variations in treatment procedures, packaging, training, and delivery designed to improve outcomes within the setting. The results of such studies should produce a mosaic of information about the target treatment, its most essential ingredients, the factors that enhance or undermine its success, the boundary conditions therapists need to know when deciding whether to use it with children of particular demographic and clinical characteristics, the change processes that account for its effects, and procedural modifications that may magnify effects or extend their duration. Of course, for many treatments, there is already a body of efficacy research that may include dismantling studies, moderator tests, mediation analyses, and the like. However, because the clients, therapists, and conditions of treatment in efficacy trials may differ in significant ways from those of everyday clinical care, it seems quite possible that answers to the questions will differ in important respects from answers found in efficacy trials.

CHARACTERISTICS OF THE TREATMENT PROGRAM

PASCET is both a complete protocol and a work in progress, undergoing continuing adaptation and testing via the DFM. Initial development of the protocol was guided by empirical, theoretical, and clinical literature, particularly that bearing on the connection between youth depression and low levels of perceived control; the two-process model of control (e.g., Weisz, Rothbaum, & Blackburn, 1984), in particular, posits two broad pathways through which individuals attempt to obtain control. *Primary control* involves efforts to influence objective conditions in ways that increase rewards and decrease punishment. *Secondary control* entails efforts to control the psychological impact of objective conditions (without changing the objective conditions). Examples of primary control include resolving a regularly occurring stressor by changing behavioral strategies or doing problem solving with friends; examples of secondary control include altering one's interpretation of an apparent social slight ("My friend was having a bad day and just didn't feel like talking") or finding a silver lining in an otherwise bad event ("I forgot my lunch money, but my friends gave me food—cool!"). The relevance of clinical and research literature was evident from an early stage; these primary and secondary control skills mapped nicely onto skills often emphasized in CBT for youth depression (cf. Lewinsohn, Clarke, Hops, & Andrews, 1990; Stark, 1990).

PASCET is currently composed of 18 individual sessions designed for youths ages 8–15 years. The protocol includes options for parent and school involvement. Therapists use a detailed manual, and youths use a practice book that highlights and illustrates treatment components and skills and guides between-session practice assignments. The first 15 sessions focus on specific coping skills; the last three are individually tailored to help youngsters apply the skills they find most useful.

ACT and THINK Skills

PASCET uses the acronym "ACT and THINK" to present the core coping skills. ACT skills, which emphasize primary control, include (1) **A**ctivities that solve problems (sequential problem solving); (2) **A**ctivities that boost mood (planning pleasant activities); (3) **C**alming (using progressive muscle relaxation, imagery, and focused breathing); and (4) **T**urn on my positive self (practicing and implementing positive self-presentation). After the youth has acquired the ACT skills, the therapist discusses the distinction between conditions children can and cannot readily change. This discussion provides a segue into the second component of PASCET: THINK skills, intended for conditions that are hard to alter: (1) **T**hink positive (generating realistic, helpful thoughts to replace distorted or unhelpful cognitions); (2) **H**elp from a friend (finding social support); (3) **I**dentify the silver lining (finding something positive that is made possible by otherwise negative conditions); (4) **N**o replaying bad thoughts (using distracting activities to minimize unproductive rumination); and (5) **K**eep on using the ACT and THINK skills (persevering despite setbacks and failures; developing and using a Plan A, B, and C).

The remaining sessions entail continued practice of the youngster's best fit ACT and THINK skills to address distressing situations, with favorite skills sequenced as Plan A, B, and C. Additionally, in the final sessions, the youth completes an end-of-treatment project (e.g., a booklet telling "my story," a poster showing his or her favorite skills) designed to represent the skills the youth has learned. The project can serve as a prompt for use in the future, when problems arise and the youngster needs to use PASCET coping skills.

Practice Book and Mood Boosters

Throughout the treatment protocol, in-session activities and between-session practice of skills are supported by written exercises and reminders in the ACT and THINK practice book. To encourage practice of learned coping skills, youths can earn rewards for completing practice assignments and completing the relevant practice book pages. Accumulated stamps and stickers (tracked in early pages of the practice book) may be exchanged for rewards according to a prize schedule developed with parent input.

Throughout treatment, mood boosters are used to provide on-the-spot practice in using the relevant ACT and THINK skills to lift mood. When therapists note changes in youths' presentation that indicate sadness, irritability, or boredom, they use these as opportunities to demonstrate the relevance of the skills. The procedure is as follows: (1) youth rates current mood on a "feelings thermometer," (2) youth carries out an activity with the therapist that is likely to elevate mood (e.g., trash can basketball, a relaxation exercise), (3) youth rerates mood. If the activity is chosen wisely, mood ratings tend to rise, showing the youth the power of the activities. If mood fails to rise, the therapist emphasizes the value of learning, through these simple experiments, which activities are truly mood boosting and which are not.

EVIDENCE ON THE EFFECTS OF TREATMENT

Consistent with the DFM, PASCET was initially tested in an efficacy trial with symptomatic youths to assess its potential for benefit (Weisz et al., 1997). Participants were 48 elementary school students, with a mean age of 9.6 years; 46% (22) were girls, and 38% (18) were a minority (primarily African American). Therapists were research team members. Children were selected for treatment based on elevated scores on a standardized self-report depression inventory and interviewer-administered rating scale. Children were randomly assigned to PASCET or a no-treatment control group, which permitted both posttreatment and 9 month follow-up assessment (i.e., a wait-list control group would have precluded meaningful follow-up). Assessments administered at posttreatment and 9-month follow-up showed significantly greater reductions in depressive symptoms for the PASCET group than the control group. In addition, relative to the control group, children in the PASCET condition were more likely to transition from above the normal range for depressive symptoms to within the normal range on both measures at posttreatment (50% vs. 16%) and 9-month follow-up (62% vs. 31%). The findings suggested that PASCET had the potential to produce beneficial effects.

Consistent with the DFM, a series of single-case applications of PASCET was used to adapt the protocol for use in the practice setting for which it was ultimately intended (i.e., community mental health clinics). In these field tests, advanced clinical trainees, supervised by both senior clinic staff and the PASCET developer (J. Weisz), delivered the protocol and generated adaptations as needed to fit the clientele and clinicians in the setting. Modifications included shifting from group to individual format (groups pose many difficulties in a community clinic setting), lengthening the protocol (e.g., to permit more practice of core skills), adding parent and school contact components (parents and teachers typically initiate youth clinic referrals), strengthening certain skill components (e.g., problem-solving and social presentation skills proved especially important to clinic-referred youths), streamlining organization of the manual for community clinician use, and adding new ways of introducing the core skills to youngsters and boosting homework completion.

With these modifications in place, consistent with the DFM, we undertook an initial test of the transportability of PASCET to community clinics (Weisz et al., 2009). In this trial, we randomized community clinic practitioners to be trained and supervised in the use of PASCET or to continue providing care as usual for depressed youths. The therapists treated 57 clinic-referred youths (56% girls) ages 8–15 (33% Caucasian, 26% African American, 26% Latino). Most were from low-income families, and all had depressive disorders (plus multiple comorbidities). All youths were randomized to PASCET or usual care and treated until normal termination. At posttreatment, depression symptom measures were at subclinical levels for most youths, and 75% of the sample no longer met criteria for a depressive disorder, but the PASCET and usual-care groups did not differ on these outcomes. However, compared with usual care, PASCET was significantly (1) more efficient (24 vs. 39 weeks in treatment); (2) superior in parent-rated therapeutic alliance; (3) less likely to be accompanied by additional mental health services, including all psychotropics combined and depression medication in particular; and (4) less costly. The findings showed advantages for CBT in parent engagement, reduced use of medication and other services, overall cost, and possibly speed of improvement, a hypothesis that we hope to test in future research.

Although the clinical outcomes (depression symptoms and diagnoses) were similar for PASCET and usual care, it is useful to note that these outcomes for both groups were quite similar to those found in successful efficacy trials of other CBT approaches. Apart from the clinical outcomes, PASCET appeared to provide a number of advantages over usual care, including increased efficiency and reduced cost. It is worth noting that therapists implementing PASCET were delivering a treatment that was new to them, one that they had not freely selected and in which they had no prior practice before treating study cases (average number of study cases was one per therapist). By contrast, usual-care therapists delivered their own treatments, in which they both confident and highly experienced. Thus, it is possible that our findings reflect, in part, less expert and complete implementation of PASCET than usual care (see Fixsen, Naoom, Blase, Friedman, & Wallace, 2005). This and a number of other possibilities require attention in future steps.

Testing Alternate Forms of PASCET for Other Clinical Contexts

Other forms of PASCET have been developed, generally following DFM principles, for use with depressed youths in contexts other than individually focused treatment in community mental health clinics; testing is underway for each of these (summarized in Table 30.1).

Video-Guided Version of PASCET for Schools

Because a large proportion of American youths receive their primary or sole mental health services in school, we sought to develop a school-friendly form of PASCET, focusing especially on middle school, the age period when depression risk begins to rise. To make PASCET ecologically valid for schools, we used a group format because most significant intervention in schools takes place in groups and we needed to design procedures that could be used by the staff (counselors and others) who most often provide the services in schools. This led us to create a way of delivering PASCET within groups led by busy professionals. To make this interesting for students and to reduce demands on school staff to remember all the details and keep students engaged, we designed and produced a video-guided program, PASCET = VG, along with an accompanying protocol to illustrate each of the PASCET skills. In the video, youth actors play students using various PASCET coping skills to deal with various stressors. The protocol includes thirteen 90-minute sessions. In a typical session, group leaders introduce a PASCET skill (e.g., problem solving), a video segment shows the actors in a situation in which the

TABLE 30.1. Studies Testing PASCET in Different Forms for Different Populations and Contexts

Study	Version of PASCET	Study design	Setting	Type of sample	Sample size; age/grade	Type of control group	Type of therapist	Findings
Weisz et al. (1997)	PASCET	RCT	Elementary schools	Elevated symptoms	N = 48; grades 3–6	No-treatment control group	Researcher therapists	PASCET significantly superior to control group on depressive symptoms
Weisz et al. (2009)	PASCET	RCT	Community clinics	Depressive disorders	N = 57; 8–15 years	Active UC	Clinic therapists	PASCET similar to UC on depression measures but superior on alliance, treatment efficiency, other services and cost
Weisz et al. (study in progress)	PASCET-VG	RCT	Middle schools	Severe symptoms and/or depressive disorders	N = 185; grades 6–7	Enhanced UC	Researcher therapists and school staff	Study in progress
Eckstain & Gaynor (2008)	PASCET plus C-CRET for parents	Open trial	Elementary and middle schools	Depressive disorders	N = 15; grades 3–8	No control group	Researcher therapist	Significant improvement in depressive symptoms, functioning, coping skills, caregiver–child relationships, and parenting stress
Szigethy et al. (2004, 2006)	PASCET-PI	Open trial	Hospital outpatient and inpatient	Depressive disorders + IBD	N = 11; 12–17 years	No control group	Research psychiatrist	Significant reduction in depressive symptoms; 10 of 11 had no depressive disorder
Szigethy et al. (2007, 2009)	PASCET-PI	RCT	Hospital outpatient and inpatient	Severe symptoms + IBD	N = 41; 11–17 years	UC with depression information sheet	Psychiatrists, social workers, and psychologists	PASCET significantly superior to UC in depression symptom reduction, global functioning, and perceived control
Weisz et al. (2009)	PASCET	RCT	Community clinics and school mental health	Severe symptoms and/or depressive disorders	N = 60; 8–13 years	UC, modular version of PASCET	Clinic therapists	Study completed in May, 2009; data analyses underway
	PASCET within a modular manual	RCT	Community clinics and school mental health	Severe symptoms and/or depressive disorders	N = 60; 8–13 years	UC, PASCET	Clinic therapists	Study completed in May 2009, Data analyses underway

Note. PASCET, primary and secondary control enhancement training; VG, video guided; PI, physical illness; RCT, randomized controlled trial; IBD, inflammatory bowel disease; UC, usual care; C-CRET, caregiver–child relationship enhancement training.

skill is needed, one scene shows (ineffective) coping in the absence of the skill and then (effective) coping via the skill, and the group discusses what the video showed and how students in the group might use that skill in their lives. Additional exercises give the students practice in applying the skills.

We are now testing an initial version of PASCET-VG in a school-based trial. The trial thus far includes 185 sixth and seventh graders with elevated depressive symptoms (identified through a two-step screening and assessment process). Within each of the participating public middle schools, the youths have been randomly assigned to receive either PASCET-VG delivered by psychology graduate students and postdoctoral fellows or enhanced usual care delivered by staff in the schools (i.e., we pay them for their time to plan and deliver their intervention as well as for an expert consultant of their choice to assist and supervise them). The two conditions are matched precisely for treatment dose. So, as discussed in relation to the DFM, the study includes some elements of representative care in schools (i.e., students drawn from the schools, intervention provided in the schools, dose-matched active usual-care treatment provided by school staff), but it is not a complete effectiveness design (i.e., PASCET-VG is being delivered in this initial trial by research team members, not school staff). We are now in the final year of intervention for this trial.

Targeting Parent–Child Interactions with PASCET

The versions of PASCET discussed thus far include only modest levels of parent (or caregiver) involvement and only a limited focus on what parents can do to address depression in their children. To address this limitation, Eckshtain and Gaynor (2008) have adapted PASCET to include an emphasis on parent training to improve the caregiver–child relationship in ways designed to support depression reduction via PASCET. The enhancement included training in five practices: (1) child–caregiver special time, (2) praise, (3) contingent reinforcement of positive mood and behavior, (4) positive communication training, and (5) family problem solving. This approach, PASCET plus caregiver–child relationship enhancement training (PASCET C-CRET), includes 16 child sessions and seven caregiver sessions.

Thus far, PASCET C-CRET has been studied via an open trial, with a sample of 15 children, ages 8–14 years (mean, 10.27), from grades 3–8, and their parents (both parents for four children, one parent for 11), drawn from three elementary schools and one middle school. All the children scored high on self-report and clinical interview measures of depression symptomatology. All treatment was provided by the treatment developer (Dr. Eckshtain). At posttreatment and at 1- and 6-month follow-ups, depressive symptoms showed statistically significant decreases from pretreatment Children's Depression Inventory scores. Statistically significant improvements were also found on measures of psychosocial functioning, coping skills, caregiver–child relationships, and parenting stress. Benchmarking these results against the RCT literature showed that the changes were similar or superior to those found for CBT and for pharmacotherapy in the most relevant prior studies and were markedly superior to changes seen in control conditions, including pill placebo. In addition, age and negative thoughts moderated change in depressive symptoms, with lower age and fewer negative thoughts at pretreatment predicting more depression reduction. The findings suggest that PASCET C-CRET warrants fuller testing, within a randomized trial.

Adapting PASCET for Physically Ill Children

In addition to youngsters in mental health clinic, school, and family contexts, a third group that warrants special attention are youths experiencing chronic physical illness. Such illness has been found to increase the risk of depression, and the combination of depression and chronic illness has been associated with increased functional impairment, decreased quality of life, less optimal medical outcomes, and even increased mortality (see Szigethy et al., 2004). A particularly relevant group are youngsters who suffer from inflammatory bowel disease (IBD), including Crohn's disease and ulcerative colitis. One research team (Szigethy et al., 2004, 2007) has focused on adapting and testing PASCET for adolescents who suffer from IBD plus depression. The resulting protocol, PASCET-PI includes all of the original PASCET elements combined with a physical illness narrative, social skills training (tailored to the special social challenges faced by these children), and family education sessions (Szigethy et al., 2004).

After hospital-based clinical work developing and adapting PASCET-PI in the context of care for these children, Szigethy et al. (2004) conducted an open trial with 11 adolescents suffering from IBD combined with either major ($N = 9$) or minor ($N = 2$) depression. The treatment developer (Dr. Szigethy) was the therapist in each case. The trial found statistically significant reductions in *Diagnostic and Statistical Manual of Mental Disorders* (fourth edition [DSM-IV]; American Psychiatric Association, 1994) depression symptoms and statistically significant improvements in measures of global psychological and social functioning; in addition, after treatment, 10 of the teens no longer met criteria for any depressive disorder and one met criteria for minor depression, as assessed by a standardized diagnostic interview. These gains held up well at 12-month follow-up (Szigethy et al., 2006).

The open trial was followed by an RCT with 41 youths ages 11–17, all suffering from IBD plus elevated depressive symptoms (Szigethy et al., 2007). The youths were randomized to PASCET–PI ($N = 22$) or usual care (UC; or treatment as usual *in this study*; $N = 19$); UC, in this case, consisted of usual IBD treatment plus an information sheet that described the signs, symptoms, and treatment of depression. PASCET-PI was delivered by six therapists (two psychiatrists, two clinical psychologists, two social workers) trained and supervised by the treatment developer. At posttreatment, the PASCET-PI group showed significantly fewer depressive symptoms and significantly better functioning and higher levels of perceived control than the UC group (Szigethy et al., 2007). Follow-up findings at 6 and 12 months (Szigethy et al., 2009) showed that, compared with the UC group, the PASCET-PI group continued to show lower levels of depressive symptoms and higher level global functioning and also showed less use of psychotropic medication and psychotherapy and even less severe disease classification, despite no differences at pretreatment. This study suggests that PASCET, when appropriately adapted, has the potential to reduce depressive symptoms among youngsters with IBD and may be effectively delivered by trained psychologists, psychiatrists, and social workers in a hospital setting.

DIRECTIONS FOR RESEARCH

Findings of the various studies raise a number of issues for further thought and future research. One of these concerns the interpretation of different findings from different treatment contexts. For a treatment program like PASCET, in which much of the work reflects DFM principles, characteristics of a particular treatment context may lead to treatment and study procedures that are quite different from those used in another treatment context, making comparison across contexts quite difficult. As an example, PASCET-PI enjoyed considerably more success in clinical symptom change in relation to UC in Szigethy et al. (2007, 2009) than in Weisz et al. (2009), but UC in Szigethy et al. involved primarily an information sheet on depression whereas UC in Weisz et al. (2009) entailed 39 weeks of therapy (a significantly larger dose than PASCET cases received). Of course, this difference may well reflect clinical reality in the two treatment contexts; UC focused on depression may be quite sparse for youths being treated for physical illness in hospitals but quite intense for youths treated for depression in mental health clinics. Nonetheless, marked differences in the nature and intensity of UC across different settings may make it harder to find beneficial effects of the target intervention in some contexts than others, complicating interpretation of cross-study differences. Because these and so many other variations may be evident across treatment contexts, it may remain difficult to compare progress of treatment development across contexts.

With that noted, it is clear that the treatment development and testing already done within each context (mental health clinics, schools, families, pediatric care settings) suggest useful next steps for research. As an example, the findings of Weisz et al. (2009) suggest that outpatient clinics may be a particularly challenging context for comparison to usual care; about three-fourths of all treated youths in that study moved from DSM-IV depressive disorders at pretreatment to no depressive disorder at posttreatment. We have considered a number of possible interpretations of the high rate of improvement in the UC condition (e.g., that UC clinicians responded to the competitive situation [UC vs. PASCET]) by keeping cases open until their clients' depressive disorders had remitted or that UC improvement was influenced by the significantly higher rate of antidepressant use in UC than PASCET. However, it is also possible that PASCET can outperform even the high rates of UC improvement in mental health clinics if we provide more extensive therapist training and supervision, which might lead, in turn, to more skilled use of the PASCET protocol. In future research, we may test these and related possibilities.

This, in turn, highlights the need for improved assessment. We have found that traditional measures of fidelity do not provide a very sensitive index of therapist skill and competence in the use of protocol procedures; measuring skilled use (rather than mere coverage of manual content) should be on the agenda for our field. We have also learned that we need richer assessment schedules to tease apart various interpretations of findings. As one example, the fact that UC lasted significantly longer than PASCET in Weisz et al. (2009) but achieved very similar outcomes suggests that PASCET may have produced more rapid improvement. That possibility could be tested via periodic assessments following the same schedule in PASCET and UC. We are moving in this direction in all our current research.

Another issue raised by our research on PASCET concerns the most appropriate approach to treatment of depression in the context of high levels of comorbidity. In most of our work thus far, we have kept to an exclusive focus on depression, once that was identified as a youth's primary treatment focus. In the process, we have had to pay relatively little heed to such significant problems as high levels of anxiety and conduct problems, even though these can interfere with depression treatment. In our recent work in conjunction with Bruce Chorpita and other colleagues from the Network on Youth Mental

Health (e.g., Chorpita, Daleiden, & Weisz, 2005), PASCET has been incorporated into a modular treatment protocol for the integrated treatment of depression, anxiety, and conduct problems in youths ages 8–13 seen in mental health clinics and schools. The treatment protocol combines elements of PASCET with elements of CBT for anxiety disorders and behavioral parent training for conduct problems. Data-informed clinical decision flow charts allow therapists to treat children with comorbid conditions, to shift treatment focus as targeted concerns change during treatment, and to combine elements of various treatment approaches as needed (e.g., teaching parents to give clear instructions and to praise appropriate child behavior can sometimes aid in the treatment of depression). Within the modular treatment, each element of PASCET is a single module that may be used as one session or extended to many sessions and may be used in tandem with other treatment elements from PASCET or in concert with elements of CBT for anxiety or behavioral parent training.

A multisite randomized effectiveness trial of Modular Approach to Therapy for Children with Anxiety, Depression or Conduct Problems (MATCH-ADC) with complex cases referred to community clinics and school mental health services is nearing completion, with 175 children ages 8–13 randomly assigned to receive treatment from clinicians trained in (1) the modular protocol, (2) traditional nonmodular versions of PASCET and protocols for anxiety and conduct problems, or (3) UC (Chorpita & Weisz, 2005). Clinicians who work in the project sites (none research employees) were all randomly assigned to one of the three conditions as well. The findings should help us discern whether there are advantages to embedding PASCET components within a larger frame in order to address comorbidity and change in youngsters' treatment needs over the course of treatment episodes.

CONCLUSIONS

Research on youth depression treatment has generated a number of successes, with the most often replicated findings showing beneficial effects of CBT. However, the evidence also suggests that CBT has not generated large effects, particularly when tested in clinically representative contexts and when compared with active forms of usual clinical care. In this chapter, we have described the DFM, a model designed to generate interventions that will fare well in clinically representative practice contexts and when compared with UC; we have also described steps in the development of PASCET, a form of CBT for depression that is being developed according to principles of the DFM.

Efforts to develop and test PASCET thus far have focused on four contexts, each involving different forms of PASCET: mental health clinics, schools, families, and the pediatric care context where children with chronic illness are treated. Beyond the initial protocol development and individual field tests of PASCET, we have described an initial efficacy trial and an effectiveness trial in which clinically referred youths were treated by clinic-employed practitioners in clinic settings and in which clinicians were randomly assigned to learn and use PASCET or continue their UC procedures. We have also described treatment–outcome research on a video-guided form of PASCET designed for use in schools, another form of PASCET developed to engage caregiver support in alleviating youth depression, and a fourth form of PASCET designed to relieve depression in children facing IBD plus depressive symptoms. We have also described recent efforts to integrate PASCET into a modular treatment protocol in the hope of better addressing the comorbidity and flux in problems that are so often seen in depression treatment.

In the decade ahead, the various forms of PASCET are likely to continue evolving as investigators learn more about how to facilitate its effective use in various treatment contexts. The process could be lengthy, but if it leads to increased access to effective care within everyday treatment contexts the investment may well be worthwhile.

REFERENCES

American Psychiatric Association. (1994). *Diagnostic and statistical manual of mental disorders* (4th ed.). Washington, DC: Author.

Chorpita, B. F., Daleiden, E., & Weisz, J. R. (2005). Modularity in the design and application of interventions. *Applied and Preventive Psychology, 11,* 141–156.

Chorpita, B. F., & Weisz, J. R. (2005). *Modular approach to therapy for children with anxiety, depression, or conduct problems (MATCH-ADC).* Unpublished treatment manual.

Eckshtain, D., & Gaynor, S. T. (2008). *Adding child-caregiver sessions to individual CBT for childhood depression: An open trial.* Manuscript submitted for publication.

Fergusson, D. M., & Woodward, L. J. (2002). Mental health, educational, and social role outcomes of adolescents with depression. *Archives of General Psychiatry, 59,* 225–231.

Fixsen, D. L., Naoom, S. F., Blase, K. A., Friedman, R. M., & Wallace, F. (2005). *Implementation research: A synthesis of the literature* (Publication No. 231). Tampa: University of South Florida, Louis de la Parte Florida Mental Health Institute.

Lewinsohn, P. M., Clarke, G. N., Hops, H., & Andrews, J. (1990). Cognitive-behavioral treatment for depressed adolescents. *Behavior Therapy, 21,* 385–401.

Stark, K. D. (1990). *Childhood depression: School-based intervention.* New York: Guilford Press.

Szigethy, E., Carpenter, J., Baum, E., Kenny, E., Baptista-Neto, L., Beardslee, M. R., et al. (2006). Case study: Longitudinal treatment of adolescents with depression and inflammatory bowel disease. *Journal of the American Academy of Child and Adolescent Psychiatry, 45,* 396–400.

Szigethy, E., Kenny, E., Carpenter, J., Hardy, D. M., Fairclough, D., Bousvaros, A., et al. (2007). Cognitive-behavioral therapy for adolescents with inflammatory bowel disease and subsyndromal depression. *Journal of the American Academy of Child and Adolescent Psychiatry, 46,* 1290–1298.

Szigethy, E., Lobst, E., Fairclough, D., Kenney, E., Gonzalez-Heydrich, J., DeMaso, D., & Noll, R. (2008). *Longitudinal results of cognitive-behavioral treatment for youth with inflammatory bowel disease and depression.* Unpublished manuscript.

Szigethy, E., Whitton, S. W., Levy-Warren, A., DeMaso, D. R., Weisz, J. R., & Beardslee, W. R. (2004). Cognitive-behavioral therapy for depression in adolescents with inflammatory bowel disease: A pilot study. *Journal of the American Academy of Child and Adolescent Psychiatry, 43,* 1469–1477.

Weisz, J. R. (2004). *Psychotherapy for children and adolescents: Evidence-based treatments and case examples.* Cambridge, UK: Cambridge University Press.

Weisz, J. R., Gray, J. S., Bearman, S. K., & Stark, K. (2008). *Therapist's manual PASCET: Primary and secondary control enhancement training* (3rd ed.). Cambridge, MA: Harvard University.

Weisz, J. R., Jensen-Doss, A., & Hawley, K. M. (2006). Evidence-based youth psychotherapies versus usual clinical care: A meta-analysis of direct comparisons. *American Psychologist, 61,* 671–689.

Weisz, J. R., McCarty, C. A., & Valeri, S. M. (2006). Effects of psychotherapy for depression in children and adolescents: A meta-analysis. *Psychological Bulletin, 132,* 132–149.

Weisz, J. R., Rothbaum, F. M., & Blackburn, T. F. (1984). Standing out and standing in: The psychology of control in America and Japan. *American Psychologist, 39,* 955–969.

Weisz, J. R., Southam-Gerow, M. A., Gordis, E. B., Connor-Smith, J. K., Chu, B. C., Langer, D. A., et al. (2009). Cognitive-behavioral therapy versus usual clinical care for youth depression: An initial test of transportability to community clinics and clinicians. *Journal of Consulting and Clinical Psychology, 77*(3), 383–396.

Weisz, J. R., Thurber, C., Sweeney, L., Proffitt, V. D., & LeGagnoux, G. L. (1997). Brief treatment of mild-to-moderate child depression using primary and secondary control enhancement training. *Journal of Consulting and Clinical Psychology, 65*, 703–707.

Zalsman, G., Brent, D. A., & Weersing, V. R. (2006). Depressive disorders in childhood and adolescence: An overview of epidemiology, clinical manifestation, and risk factors. *Child and Adolescent Psychiatric Clinics of North America, 15*, 827–841.

31

Building Evidence-Based Systems in Children's Mental Health

BRUCE F. CHORPITA and ERIC L. DALEIDEN

OVERVIEW

The notion of building evidence-based systems is based on a core set of defining principles abstracted from a large summary of existing evidence-based practices. As such, it does not correspond to any specific treatment protocol but rather is a model of a broader set of organizing principles designed to improve quality of care in children's mental health service systems. Arising out of natural experiments involving the early implementation of evidence-based practices in the state of Hawaii (e.g., Chorpita, Taylor, Francis, Moffitt, & Austin, 2004), our program evolved over time into a broad effort to coordinate multiple, specific evidence-based practices to serve complex client populations with diverse clinical needs by multiple providers in multiple settings using a common infrastructure (e.g., Daleiden & Chorpita, 2005). We define an evidence-based system as one that explicitly organizes its clinical and administrative decision making around the use of data and evidence, with the goal of improving child service quality (Daleiden & Chorpita, 2005). Because the specific implementation of these principles has varied in our work across several contexts (e.g., Chorpita, 2007; Chorpita, Bernstein, Daleiden, & Research Network on Youth Mental Health, 2008; Daleiden, Chorpita, Donkervoet, Arensdorf, & Brogan, 2006), the model itself is first reviewed in terms of those core principles, followed by illustrations of specific applications of those principles across different contexts.

Core Principles

Principle 1: Empirical Epistemology

By definition, the design of an evidence-based system rests on the assumption that publicly verifiable observation is a preferred way of knowing. Evidence can come from a

482

variety of sources and can vary in both quality and suitability for a particular purpose (Daleiden & Chorpita, 2005). Thus, in some instances, it is preferable to evaluate a treatment by examining a child's progress on an objective outcome measure; whereas in other cases a treatment can be evaluated according to its prior success in published randomized trials. A related concept is that evidence is dynamic, and thus sources of evidence that are updatable (e.g., a monthly record of treatment practices being used) and self-correcting sources are preferable to those that are static (e.g., a treatment plan developed in a single narrative format). This principle does not advocate rejection of rationally based and value-based decision making, but available evidence is considered foundational, with rational and value criteria applied incrementally. Thus, expert consensus, clinical judgment, and personal values can and do play a role in decision making but most commonly in those areas for which limited evidence is available.

Principle 2: Parsimony and Efficiency

Although not necessary in an evidence-based system, parsimony and efficiency are desirable properties. For this reason, we emphasize modularity in the design of both interventions (e.g., Chorpita, Daleiden, & Weisz, 2005) and reporting structures (Chorpita et al., 2008) to accelerate progress toward goals with a minimum of effort or complexity. This principle typically requires a definition of the context and boundaries of the system, and the broader the context, the greater the need for modularity and compatibility. Thus, in our work with the Hawaii Department of Health, Child and Adolescent Mental Health Division (CAMHD), it was important to design protocols, measurement strategies, and supervision structures that were maximally compatible across the different settings and service populations within the state.

Figure 31.1 shows an example of the application of the parsimony/efficiency principle in the realm of feedback and data review. The figure shows a basic clinical dashboard (cf. Chorpita et al., 2008; Daleiden & Chorpita, 2005), which summarizes progress ratings in the upper half (the progress pane) and the history of practices in the lower half (the practice pane). To serve efficiency, these dashboards are designed to allow for a rapid visual summary of outcome measures, which can reduce the need for prolonged review and discussion about client case history during decision-making contexts such as clinical supervision. For parsimony, these dashboard reports are typically constructed to serve multiple intervention protocols and approaches as well as multiple different measurement instruments on a common platform. Thus, a standardized interface design is widely applicable across all aspects of the system.

Another common application of the parsimony/efficiency principle is the use of modular design in treatment protocols (Chorpita et al., 2005). Modular design emphasizes such properties as information hiding, in which information becomes available only when needed. Thus, rather than reading and reviewing the entire protocol, a therapist works with each practice component one module at a time. The compatibility and connectivity among modules means that aspects of a treatment protocol can be updated without the need for complete revision (e.g., a new relaxation module can easily be introduced to replace or supplement an existing one).

An extension of this notion of parsimony and efficiency emphasizes the universality of tools and concepts across all aspects of an organization. Thus, large systems benefit from a common language and framework across executive and policy functions, quality

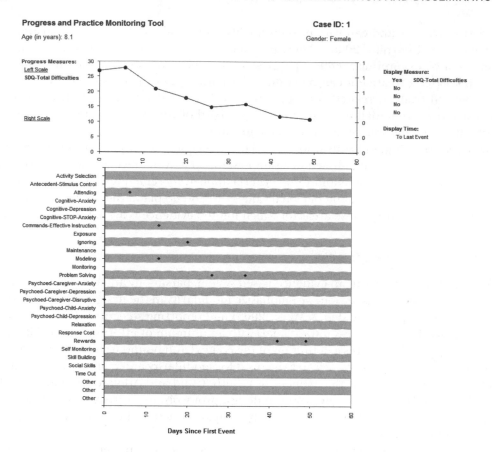

FIGURE 31.1. Example of a clinical dashboard (SDQ, Strengths and Difficulties Questionnaire). From PracticeWise (2008). Copyright 2008 by PracticeWise, LLC. Reprinted by permission.

review functions, practice development functions, billing and administrative functions, and clinical operations. For example, measures used for quality and performance management should be compatible with those inherent in the clinical model proposed by a practice development unit and, likewise, should be compatible with those used by leadership for policy decisions. Different units of the organization should be connected by a common set of measures, concepts, values, and goals.

Principle 3: Visibility

This third principle advocates articulation of explicit models for implicit processes, in other words, to build maps of the decisions and structures that guide the system at all levels. This mapping or modeling can often take the form of diagrams and flow charts and can represent such processes as clinical supervision, treatment authorization, or phone screen. One benefit of modeling these processes is the enhanced reliability afforded by the visibility of the model: thus, a consultation phone call would follow a reliable set of procedures, for example. Such standardization is already common in manualized treatments, but the visibility principle pulls for the documentation of not only the procedures but also the guiding logic that coordinates those procedures and the information sources educating that logic. Thus, even a clinical treatment manual that simply connects step A to step B to step C would preferably be diagrammed to make that flow explicit to its user and to thereby raise awareness of other possible sequences or logic. The idea is to place procedures (such as treatment protocols or clinical management operations) into a coordinating framework representing the larger range of possible values, of which a given procedure is only a single instance.

Many of these models are implicit in most clinical research laboratories that produce and test treatment protocols, and they can include (1) decision models (i.e., those that outline what decisions get made), (2) measurement models (i.e., those that specify informants, instruments, and timing of assessment events such as a pretreatment parent checklist or a posttreatment therapist attitude measure), (3) information/reporting models (i.e., those that specify what information from the measurement model will be made available to people who need it, such as a graph giving a clinician feedback about whether a case is improving), and (4) organizational models (i.e., those that outline roles and permissions of individuals and groups in a system, such as who can inspect medical records, who can provide supervision). Finally, these four types of models can be combined into overall process models, which put everything together to outline what decisions are made by whom using what information gathered in what way and so on.

One example of a clinical process model, adapted from Chorpita et al. (2008), appears in Figure 31.2. This model guides the behavior of clinicians and supervisors and shows how the decisions about a clinical case are handled by referencing various reports or information sources. The diagnostic assessment summary contains a summary of measures outlined in a separate information model and helps to inform the primary diagnosis of the client and hence guide treatment selection. The next four decisions reference different sources of data on a clinical dashboard to guide a supervisor or therapist in how to perform in the face of various clinical events.

Principles in Action: The Four Steps

These three principles govern the basic actions in a system that follows the four steps of the Shewhart or Deming cycle (e.g., Plan-Do-Check-Act or Plan-Do-Study-Act; Shewhart, 1939; Deming, 1982). We tend to use different terms in the mental health context and refer to these as intervention cycles. Intervention cycles are purposeful activities that follow four basic steps of selecting goals, applying procedures, testing results, and refining the intervention. These intervention cycles are essentially the building blocks of all processes in the system, and they link together to form complex and dynamic models that organize behavior within the system to achieve broad system goals.

ILLUSTRATIONS AND APPLICATIONS OF THE MODEL

Details of how these principles and actions are coordinated in an evidence-based system are best understood through illustrations of their application in specific contexts. Our work over the past 12 years has involved several different systems, including uni-

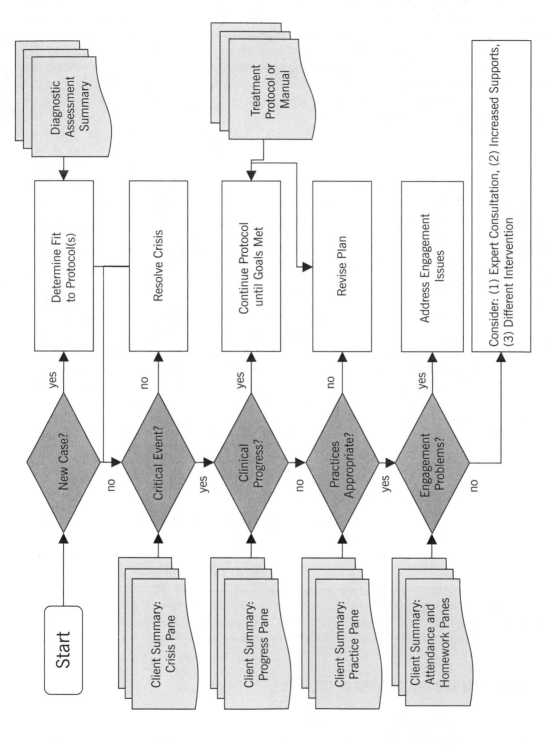

FIGURE 31.2. Example of a clinical process model. Adapted from Chorpita (2007). Copyright 2007 by Guilford Press. Adapted by permission.

versity clinical research laboratories (e.g., University of Hawaii; University of California, Los Angeles), public mental systems (e.g., Hawaii CAMHD, Minnesota Department of Human Services, Western Australia Child and Adolescent Mental Health System), and a multiinvestigator research network (Research Network on Youth Mental Health, John R. Weisz, network director). We review several of these efforts here to illustrate the evidence-based systems model as applied across contexts, and these examples are summarized for comparison in Table 31.1.

Hawaii CAMHD

Goal Setting

The Hawaii CAMHD initiative involved multiple goals related to practice improvement and system functioning. Naturally, there are many goals in a large system involving matters of policy, administration, clinical, and financing processes to name a few. For the sake of comparison, we illustrate a selected number of common goals related to clinical outcomes and service quality. Table 31.1 shows two example intervention cycles in the CAMHD system that are organized to serve those goals.

CAMHD is a statewide system that provides intensive mental health services to youths eligible for such services through Medicaid health insurance, special education program, or juvenile justice involvement through eight regional branches. CAMHD provides crisis stabilization, case management, respite, outpatient, intensive home and community services, and residential services to approximately 2,800 youths per year (Kimhan, Higa-McMillan, & Daleiden, 2008). CAMHD youths represent a diverse group (~60% multiracial) that is predominantly adolescent (mean age, 14.1 years; SD, 2.6; range, 3–20) and roughly two-thirds male (66%). The most common primary diagnoses are disruptive behavior (29%), attention (21%), and mood disorders (20%), although most youths (71%) have multiple diagnoses. Approximately, 40% of youths receive residential services, and this proportion has consistently decreased over the past 5 years.. The first goal in Table 31.1 represents progress on clinical outcomes, which is the central clinical goal of most systems.

Application of Procedures

With that goal in mind, the CAMHD system used several different strategies in the *selection* or design of appropriate treatment procedures. The first among these involved the Blue Menu (e.g., Daleiden & Chorpita, 2005), a one-page tabular summary, printed on blue paper, that represented different child problem areas in the rows (e.g., depression, anxiety) and different levels of strength of evidence in the columns (e.g., best support, no support). Each cell listed practices that corresponded to a level of support and problem combination. Thus, one can find that a treatment with best support for depression is cognitive-behavioral therapy. The CAMHD Blue Menu is updated regularly based on review and coding of the treatment literature.

In addition to the Blue Menu, the CAMHD system publishes a comprehensive evidence review every 2 years—the CAMHD Evidence-Based Services Committee Biennial Report (Chorpita & Daleiden, 2007)—which summarizes characteristics of each intervention in great detail, including, for example, information about service setting,

TABLE 31.1. Examples of Intervention Cycles from Different Applications of the Evidence-Based Systems Model

Domain	Hawaii CAMHD		Minnesota DHS		Child STEPs	
	Outcomes	Practices	Outcomes	Practices	Outcomes	Practices
Goal setting						
Goal	Individual clinical progress	Appropriate practices	Individual clinical progress	Appropriate practices	Individual clinical progress	Appropriate practices
Application of procedures						
Selection	Blue Menu, practice profiles, biennial report, PWEBS database	None	PWEBS database	None	Phase I review	None
Content	Integrated protocols (e.g., MST) supplemented with common elements	Case management	Practitioner guides: content modules	Phone consultation	MATCH content modules	Clinical supervision
Coordination	Program specific for formal treatment programs; statewide training on theory for common elements	None	Practitioner guides: coordination modules	None	MATCH coordination modules	None
Testing effects						
Measurement model	Quarterly CAFAS and MTPS: progress rating	MTPS: practices	SDQ; case-specific measures	MS Excel dashboard data sheet	Weekly phone checklist	Supervisor checklist
Information and reporting model	CAMHMIS clinical reporting module: progress pane	CAMHMIS clinical reporting module: practice pane	MS Excel clinical dashboards: progress pane	MS Excel clinical dashboards: practice pane	Clinical dashboard: progress pane	Clinical dashboard: practice pane
Observed values	CAFAS and MTPS scores	MTPS: practice values	Monthly SDQ and other scores	User entered practice values	Weekly phone checklist scores	Supervisor checklist: reported values

(cont.)

TABLE 31.1. *(cont.)*

Domain	Hawaii CAMHD		Minnesota DHS		Child STEPs	
	Outcomes	Practices	Outcomes	Practices	Outcomes	Practices
Testing effects *(cont.)*						
Expected values	Measure-specific clinical cutoff scores; comparison with caseload; statewide service- and provider-specific progress reports	PWEBS database; statewide service- and provider-specific practice profiles	None	PWEBS database	Comparison with caseload	Supervisor checklist: assigned values
Review and adaptation						
Process	Care-coordination and statewide supervision model	Fidelity and quality review through statewide consultants	Biweekly phone consultation	Biweekly phone consultation	Guided by system consultant	Guided by clinical supervisor

Note. CAMHD, Hawaii Department of Health, Child and Adolescent Mental Health Division; DHS, Department of Health Services; Child STEPS, Child System and Treatment Enhancement Projects; PWEBS, PracticeWise Evidence Based Services; MST, Multisystemic therapy; MATCH, Modular Approach to Therapy for Children; CAFAS, Child and Adolescent Functional Assessment Scale; SDQ, Strength and Difficulties Questionnaire; CAMHMIS, Child and Adolescent Mental Health Management Information System; MTPS, Monthly Treatment and Progress Summary.

background of therapists, ethnicity of study participants, and effect size. The CAMHD biennial report also presents practice profiles that illustrate the common components or practice elements (e.g., relaxation training, cognitive restructuring) of successful treatments for different problem areas (Chorpita & Daleiden, 2009) based on their frequency of use in the evidence-based literature. More recently, Hawaii CAMHD has moved to an online searchable database—PracticeWise Evidence Based Services (PWEBS; Practice-Wise, 2008)—for informing the treatment selection process. Given its similarity with the system being used in the Minnesota Department of Human Services initiative, this database is described in more detail later.

Once a treatment is selected, its content is outlined in treatment manuals and documentation for existing formalized programs, such as multisystemic therapy (MST; Henggeler, Schoenwald, Borduin, Rowland, & Cunningham, 1998) or multidimensional treatment foster care (Chamberlain & Reid, 1998), or more commonly for training materials developed by the CAMHD Clinical Services Office that correspond to the common practice elements across evidence base. The coordination of these procedures is governed by either (1) the program manuals that spell out the logic, sequencing, duration, and related issues relevant to the protocol or (2) guidelines provided by CAMHD Clinical Services Office in statewide trainings regarding how to combine components of evidence-based procedures to build a treatment plan.

Testing Effects

The next step involves establishing a means of gathering data to evaluate the effects of the chosen procedure, in this case the treatment itself. The measurement model for CAMHD requires, among other things, the quarterly administration of the Child and Adolescent Functional Assessment Scale (CAFAS; Hodges, 1998; Hodges & Wong, 1996) by case managers and monthly ratings of treatment progress by service providers (Nakamura, Daleiden, & Mueller, 2007).

This information can be organized to provide feedback in the Child and Adolescent Mental Health Management Information System (CAMHMIS), which contains a clinical reporting module (CRM) that, analogous to the basic clinical dashboard outlined in Figure 31.1, is capable of summarizing outcome scores as well as values from different domains (e.g., practices, diagnoses, interagency involvement) plotted over time. It should be noted that CAMHMIS and the CRM are custom-designed applications that have historically been used to implement these feedback concepts, albeit with varying degrees of implementation success within CAMHD. Under its recent new leadership, CAMHD is currently moving toward replacing CAMHMIS with an electronic health record, which will have the potential to integrate these feedback tools and principles in a more effective manner than in the past. Thus, we provide the following example as an illustration of the implementation of evolving concepts in the CAMHD system rather than of specific tools currently in widespread use in the organization.

Within CAMHMIS, the CRM plots observed values for clinical outcomes and provider practices as well as both literature-based and caseload-based expected values for the clinical dashboards. Literature-based expected values for the outcome measures can be presented as measure-specific benchmarks, such as borderline and clinical range cutoffs and recommended cutoffs for more intensive or residential services. The practice dashboards can display the practice profiles from the ongoing evidence-based services literature review (see biennial report discussed previously) as expected values. In addition, the CRM can issue caseload reports that simultaneously present all active cases for a case manager, which allows for deriving expected values from cross-case comparison. Beyond the CRM, CAMHD regularly produces aggregate reports that summarize the local standard of care in terms of provider-specific and service-specific outcomes and practices.

Reviewing and Adapting

The feedback from the previous step can then be used to determine whether the goal is being met. In all contexts, if the goal is being met, the intervention typically continues or fading and maintenance procedures are introduced. If it is not being met, procedures must be in place to either adapt the intervention (e.g., select a new treatment) or adapt the goal (e.g., modify the treatment or improve the quality of its implementation). In the CAMHD system, this process was designed to be governed at the clinical level through ongoing review by case management staff as well as regional supervisors, supported by statewide practice development consultants as needed. At the regional and system levels, an ever-evolving array of management teams and quality committees are available to guide organizational adaptations. It is possible that the process of examining clinical outcomes initiates a second intervention cycle that targets specific practice-related goals.

Hypothetically, one could imagine that the review process shows that progress toward the goal of positive clinical outcome is not being met, as reflected by outcome measure scores, such that one might then consider whether more appropriate practices could be used toward that goal.

Starting the Next Intervention Cycle

In such cases, a new subgoal would be established: selection of more appropriate practices (represented by column 2 under Hawaii CAMHD in Table 31.1). In Hawaii CAMHD, treatment plan revision is governed primarily by case management and treatment team decision making. The measurement model supporting this goal involves CAMHD's Monthly Treatment and Progress Summary (MTPS; CAMHD, 2008), which is a checklist-type instrument that gathers information on the practices delivered that month by the treating clinician (as well as other data, such as immediate treatment targets and clinician-rated progress). The MTPS is required for all cases in Hawaii's public mental health system and is fully integrated into the routine business operations. By design, the practice element unit of analysis of the MTPS practice checklist corresponds to the same units summarized in the CAMHD biennial report and in the online searchable evidence-based services database. Thus, observed values (what skills were used in the case) and expected values (what skills are used for similar cases in the literature) can be conveniently compared on the same metric on a clinical reporting dashboard delivered through CAMHMIS. This second intervention cycle concludes with a review of practice appropriateness, which could then lead to a number of possible outcomes determined during supervisory review (e.g., continue with plan, dispatch consultant to determine quality/fidelity issues, investigate clinician willingness to use the prescribed practice).

Minnesota Department of Human Services

Goal Setting

Similar work has been done with the Minnesota Department of Human Services (DHS), which provides services statewide to approximately 23,000 children age 0–20 with mental health needs. We can again review the example of a child-outcome related goal to see the parallels between the application of the core principles and steps to a different system.

Application of Procedures

In the Minnesota system, procedures used to achieve outcomes are selected using the department's Evidence Based Services online reporting application, which uses the PWEBS database, an online resource that contains detailed codes on approximately 380 randomized clinical trials and is updated regularly. This online reporting tool summarizes services based on input about specific child characteristics (problem type, age, gender, ethnicity, setting) at different levels of strength of evidence (e.g., best support, good support, minimal support, each operationally defined), and results are provided at multiple levels of analysis, including treatment approaches (e.g., parent management training), specific protocols (e.g., "Coping with Depression for Adolescents"), and practice elements (e.g., time-out, rewards). Users are encouraged to develop a treatment plan based on the common practice elements resulting from the search.

The content or specific steps for how to implement elements of that plan are documented on the Practitioner Guides (PracticeWise, 2009), which is a series of 27 handouts on the most common practice element strategies in the evidence base. Each handout describes a single practice, is no more than one double-sided page, and is modular in nature, such that the procedures can be sequenced together in a variety of different ways to build individualized protocols. Each handout is also independently updatable; such that one technique can be revised without affecting the others. Similar to the Hawaii model, the coordination and sequencing of these treatment procedures are guided by recommendations outlined in state-sponsored training programs.

Testing Effects

The measurement model in the Minnesota DHS initiative uses the Strength and Difficulties Questionnaire (SDQ; Goodman, Ford, Simmons, Gatward, & Meltzer, 2000) and up to four additional client-specific measures chosen by the therapist. The SDQ is administered monthly, whereas other measures may be taken more frequently. The information/reporting model for this initiative uses a progress/practice dashboard similar to the CAMHMIS CRM, but the system is much simpler, yielding a single graphic report that runs on a Microsoft Excel spreadsheet. The Excel dashboard contains data for a single episode of care for a single case and is not interoperable with other medical records or project databases; thus, it requires additional management effort but less technology infrastructure. It is a simple and inexpensive way to provide feedback in the context of this broader model. The Excel dashboard plots observed values only, whereas the expected values are obtained from the online evidence-based systems application.

Review and Adaptation

The feedback on the progress pane of the dashboard informs whether the goal is being met, which is reviewed in a telephone consultation meeting that occurs every 2 weeks. If goals are being met, the current treatment procedures are kept in place. If not, similar to the logic of the CAMHD clinical process model, the supervisor may suggest the use of alternative practices.

Starting the Next Intervention Cycle

In much the same way as in the CAMHD system, a decision to select more appropriate practices is encouraged through a supervisory process, in this case expert consultation. The measurement and information/reporting models in the Minnesota DHS initiative involves the therapist report of the use of specific modules in the Practitioner Guides, and these values are plotted on the practice pane of the dashboard display (e.g., see Figure 31.1). Although the Excel dashboard does not display expected values for the practice components, clinicians are encouraged to use the online evidence-based systems application to determine the evidence for the practices chosen, given the child's particular clinical and demographic characteristics. Thus, expected values for practices can be obtained but are not visually displayed on the dashboard in this instance.

Child System and Treatment Enhancement Projects

These principles have been applied in yet another context as part of a large multisite clinical trial, coordinated by the Research Network on Youth Mental Health, a collaborative network sponsored by the John D. and Catherine T. MacArthur Foundation (Weisz et al., 2003). The clinical trial is one of several large studies in the Child System and Treatment Enhancement Projects (Child STEPs) portfolio. The clinical trial was designed to serve youths ages 8–13 in community clinic and school settings using real-world providers supported through training and consultation. The project involved, among other things, the use of a multiproblem modular treatment protocol (Modular Approach to Therapy for Children [MATCH]; Chorpita & Weisz, 2009) and a clinical dashboard to guide the supervision and consultation procedures (Chorpita et al., 2008).

Goal Setting

As with other applications of the evidence-based system approach, the goal of improving child outcomes provides one of the best illustrations of the underlying logic of the model. In the Child STEPs clinical trial, this goal was a major aim of the investigation.

Application of Procedures

The selection of procedures for meeting the goal of clinical outcomes was based on a review of the child clinical treatment outcome research (Weisz, Jensen-Doss, & Hawley, 2005), which lead to the selection of three existing evidence-based treatment manuals for one experimental condition (standard manualized treatment) and the design of the modular, multiproblem manual (i.e., the MATCH protocol) (Chorpita & Weisz, 2009) for another study condition (i.e., modular manualized treatment). Both conditions were intended to reflect the systems-level approach of preparing community- and school-based therapists to meet multiple types of problems, with the modular approach designed for enhanced parsimony and efficiency relative to the standard manualized condition. In the modular group, specific content was packaged in discrete descriptions of therapy procedures (known as *content* modules), and their selection, arrangement, and sequencing were guided by flow charts specific to various child problem areas (coordination modules; cf. Chorpita et al., 2005).

Testing Effects

The impact of the intervention was tested in a variety of ways, including the use of weekly problem checklists administered to child and caregivers over the telephone. Scores from this weekly phone checklist (Chorpita, Reise, Weisz, Grubbs, Becker, & Krull, 2009) were plotted on a clinical dashboard for supervisory review with expert consultants in a weekly consultation conference call. The dashboard used a progress pane that allowed for the display of these scores (among others in a larger measurement model). Only observed values were plotted; benchmarks for improvement were informally applied based on consultant expectations (i.e., consultant feels the case should be improving more quickly) and formally applied through the use of dashboard summaries that compared all cases in a caseload, which thereby allowed for formal comparisons of degree of improvement among study cases.

Review and Adaptation

Within the modular treatment condition, the Child STEPs model called for a supervisory and consultant review of the outcome measures to guide possible adaptation to the protocol. Adaptations to the protocol content and sequence were structured by the MATCH flow charts. For example, if a youth begins exhibiting problem behaviors that interfere with treatment for depression, the flow chart would suggest departure from depression procedures to work on disruptive behavior until such time as the therapist could return to working on the depression effectively. The role of the supervisors and consultants in the project was to assist in the judgments about whether clinical interference was sufficient to warrant adaptation to the treatment plan as well as other decisions about whether to add or omit therapy modules based on the child's individual presentation.

Starting the Next Intervention Cycle

As with the other examples, the intervention cycles in the Child STEPs context are designed to initiate subgoals when performance expectations are not met. In this example, a lack of clinical improvement might suggest that the current procedures are not appropriate, such as the use of cognitive procedures with a child who seems unresponsive to them. In this case, the supervisor might then intervene with the therapist to suggest omission of a cognitive restructuring module and to proceed to a problem-solving training module. These new practices are plotted on the clinical dashboard practice pane, and in the Child STEPs application observed practice values (e.g., the diamonds in Figure 31.1) are always plotted along with expected practice values. Expected values are visually represented by open circles and reflect the supervisors' suggestions about the next practice module to employ (in this example, problem solving training). Thus, the diamonds that fall within circles indicate that the therapist is following the plan agreed to with the supervisor, diamonds without circles represent errors of commission (e.g., continued use of cognitive procedures, in this example), and circles without diamonds represent errors of omission (e.g., failure to proceed to problem-solving training, in this example).

EVIDENCE OF EFFECTS

The evidence-based system model evolved as a set of strategies to improve care by taking advantage of the existing evidence base for children's mental health and by implementing many of its common procedures and administrative practices, such as monitoring, feedback, supervision, and specific therapeutic techniques into existing clinical structures. The model was not designed as a practice package in and of itself. The fact that it has recently been discussed in programmatic terms is more of a reflection of how the

mental health field is currently operating (i.e., with a penchant for intervention packages, preferably manualized) than a foundational set of design principles. Our initial
goal was more focused on designing the type of system that could support multiple specific evidence-based practices along with providing empirically based guidance for clients, regions, and services, and so on, whether or not gold standard specialized evidence-
based practices were available or feasible.

Currently, if the evidence-based system model is conceptualized as a practice package, then we are still waiting for solid data regarding its efficacy. The closest thing to
a gold standard test of one application of this model currently underway is the Child
STEPs randomized clinical trial, which is comparing modular manualized treatment
with standard manualized treatment and usual care. The findings from this study are
eagerly awaited, but some less stringent evidence of effects is already available.

Because the evidence-based system approach emerged from quality improvement
efforts, the early empirical support emerged from performance improvement projects
and system evaluations conducted by the Hawaii CAMHD. Much of the evaluation information is available on the CAMHD website and as a series of annual evaluations and
quarterly performance reports beginning in 2002 (see *hawaii.gov/health/mental-health/
camhd/index.html*). Further, Daleiden et al. (2006) published a 10-year summary evaluation of youth outcomes from 1996–2005. The first analysis examined a statewide random
sample of cases that were assessed by trained interagency monitoring teams, who conducted record reviews, interviewed family members and service providers, and completed
a service-specific, structured case review protocol (Foster & Groves, 1997). Results indicated that the percentage of cases rated as acceptable in child status increased from 48%
in fiscal years 1996–1997 and stabilized at about 93–94% during fiscal years 2003–2005.
According to the authors' summary "Youth receiving public mental health services today
are more likely to function better than the youth receiving services prior to the reform.
The measured improvement became evident after the period of administrative reorga-
nization and capacity expansion, and during the period of expanded care coordination,
performance management, and information systems development. The evidence-based
services initiative began approximately halfway through the period of improvement. The
specific causes and time course of their effects are not testable in this uncontrolled historical analysis. Nevertheless, because the performance improvements preceded the evidence-based services initiative, this initiative was not responsible for initiating change,
but may have contributed to maintenance of the growth trajectory" (p. 753).

To provide a more in-depth analysis of within-client change during the period when
the system stabilized (2002–2005), the authors also examined the typical monthly rate
of improvement as measured by the quarterly CAFAS administrations. Here the authors
concluded that "over the four-year period, the admission and discharge characteristics
of the population were relatively stable, the average rate of improvement accelerated,
and the average length of service was notably reduced" (p. 754). In retrospect, it appears
as though the rate of youth improvement and length of service reductions peaked during 2004, yet as of late 2008 youths were still improving at roughly twice the rate that
they were in early 2002 and the reduced lengths of service were maintained (Kimhan et
al., 2008). On the bright side, these performance gains were sustained over an extended
period of time despite reduced funding, service array adjustments, progressive conver-
sion to a civil service workforce, and ongoing introduction of a new personnel. Unfortunately, additional performance gains have not materialized, and even gold standard

evidence-based service programs have witnessed periods of relative strength and weakness.

In addition to evaluation of the global outcomes, numerous process improvement studies have been conducted. One specific illustration from CAMHD relates to the improvement of service planning. During the reform, CAMHD committed to coordinated service planning (akin to wraparound planning), provided training and mentorship in planning, and proffered requirements for use with all youths. As is common, anecdotal reports indicated that "a policy is not a practice," and so a performance improvement effort was therefore initiated. The effort progressively targeted the three phases of increasing (1) the quantity of timely service plans, (2) the quality of service plans, and (3) the use of service plans in coordinating care.

The first two indicators evolved into quarterly performance measures that have been publicly reported since 2002, whereas the third became a special study (Young, Daleiden, Chorpita, Schiffman, & Mueller, 2007). The percentage of youths with a current service plan increased from a low of 52% in fiscal year (FY) 2002, peaked at a high of 90% during FY 2005–2006, and was currently reported at 85% in early FY 2009. The quality of service plans, as measured by a rating scale completed quarterly by regional quality assurance specialists for a random sample of plans, has progressively increased from a low of 58% in FY 2002 to 92% in early FY 2009.

The third phase involved the coding of both coordinated service plans and provider-specific treatment plans based on the treatment targets and practice elements that are measured with the MTPS and the biennial report (see earlier discussion). This allowed for evaluation of the degree to which the targets and practices advocated by the youth's treatment team were congruent with the targets and practices pursued by the provider actually treating the youth. Findings from the first 2 years of this study indicated that overall congruence was modest between these plans (i.e., 44% of targets and 40% of practices in the coordinated service plan were also recorded in the provider's treatment plan) and increased nonsignificantly (+5% for both targets and practices) during the first annual remeasurement period of the study.

Such process-based improvement studies do not support the overall efficacy of the evidence-based system model, but they illustrate how the application of the core principles and intervention cycles consistently produced change in targeted phenomenon related to the delivery of evidence-based services. However, our years of experience indicate that active systems often behave like living and breathing organisms. That is, efficacy and effectiveness are not static but dynamic features of the system. Programs that have been found to be effective for several years (e.g., MST in Hawaii) may cycle through phases of ineffectiveness. Therefore, we strongly advocate for ongoing evaluation and performance management throughout the life span of clients, programs, and systems.

DIRECTIONS FOR RESEARCH

Studying the impact of evidence-based designs within systems involves challenges not typically faced by specific evidence-based practices. For example, tests of the full approach could require such methods as random assignment of organizations or systems to different conditions with different design specifications. Studies of this scale are often prohibitively large and logistically complicated. Nevertheless, many of the principles and ideas of the evidence-based system approach are testable in a smaller, controlled manner by selecting a single application of a principle in contrast to a control condition. For example, because it is believed that parsimony is important, one could comparatively test protocols with higher and lower degrees of structure and complexity, but that otherwise involve the same procedures, such as the MATCH protocol (highly structured, albeit flexible) versus the Practitioner Guides (limited structure). These protocols could be tested not only for their comparative efficacy but for the degree to which therapists find them useful and report intention to continue using them outside the research context. A usual-care control group (presumably even less structure) would provide an interest third group for comparison. In a similar manner, one could test the empirical principal by randomizing therapists in a system to conditions with and without decision support tools, such as the PWEBS database or clinical dashboards, to see whether selection or design of a treatment approach is differentially effected or whether treatment outcome differs as a result of instrumental feedback. Of course, crossing these factors to examine interactions can lead to a host of other design possibilities (e.g., modular protocol vs. usual care crossed with feedback vs. no feedback) that allow for the examination of the interaction and possible synergy among these various design principles and their specific applications.

That said, it is difficult to know whether these system principles can, in fact, be implemented true to form in a randomly selected subset of an organization under study. Indeed, it may be that a substantial portion of the impact of evidence-based system design is mediated by that design's effects on creating an evidence-based, data-fluent organizational culture, which could be harder to establish when applied only to a randomly selected subset of that organization's members. Thus, an accompanying line of research that examines the impact of such principles on organization culture, particularly as a mediator of system effectiveness, is likely to be important as well.

CONCLUSIONS

The principles outlined previously are intended to be generalizable to a wide variety of clinical contexts and settings. The model, therefore, affords some advantage in terms of the potential scope of the application of its principles; however, these advantages are also limited by the need to customize and individualize their manifestation in each new context. As the brief illustrations above presented previously application of the principles of an evidence-based system can look quite different across different contexts. This also adds to the empirical burden of evaluating this model as well. Indeed, each application of the model warrants evaluation in its own separate context, such that positive results in the CAMHD system should not necessarily generalize to the community and school-based mental health context of the Child STEPs clinical trial. This also raises issues regarding whether differences across these applications may be associated with differential effectiveness. For example, is the MATCH protocol equally effective as the Practitioner Guides in a given context? Is a static method of protocol selection such as the Blue Menu as effective as a dynamic searchable database such as PWEBS? Each application of this model to date has occasioned adaptations and variations whose differential effects are largely unknown.

A separate issue that we have noted across applications of the model involves the gaps in our use of empirical approaches to all things in the system. For example, the use of supervision to change therapist behavior does not have as formal a selection and application value in Table 31.1. Often this shortcoming can be resolved through reliance on theory and professional consensus in the absence of data; however, in many cases, such data do exist (e.g., literature on management, training, coaching, education) but are simply less conveniently available to members of the organization. Future applications of this model should strive to bring a similar level of discipline in organizing a hierarchy of evidence to inform decisions in the organization other than simply those that are purely clinical in nature.

Finally, this chapter focused on outcome and practice improvement cycles. Nevertheless, improvement cycles focused on intervention targets (e.g., youth strengths and needs, business processes) and other aspects of the implementation contexts (e.g., work design and technology, workforce, communication, leadership, group structure, organizational culture, funding mechanisms) are also important domains to address when building evidence-based systems (cf. Daleiden & Chorpita, 2005; Hamilton & Daleiden, 2009).

ACKNOWLEDGMENTS

This work was supported in part by the Research Network on Youth Mental Health, a collaborative network funded by the John D. and Catherine T. MacArthur Foundation, and the State of Hawaii, Department of Health, Child and Adolescent Mental Health Division.

REFERENCES

Chamberlain, P., & Reid, J. B. (1998). Comparison of two community alternatives to incarceration for chronic juvenile offenders. *Journal of Consulting and Clinical Psychology, 66*, 624–633.

Child and Adolescent Mental Health Division, Hawaii Department of Health. (2008). Instructions and codebook for provider treatment and progress monthly summary. Honolulu: Author. Available at *hawaii.gov/health/mental-health/camhd/library/pdf/paf/paf-001.pdf*.

Chorpita, B. F. (2007). *Modular cognitive-behavioral therapy for childhood anxiety disorders*. New York: Guilford Press.

Chorpita, B. F., Bernstein, A. D., Daleiden, E. L., & Research Network on Youth Mental Health. (2008). Driving with roadmaps and dashboards: Using information resources to structure the decision models in service organizations. *Administration and Policy in Mental Health and Mental Health Services Research, 35*, 114–123.

Chorpita, B. F., & Daleiden, E. L. (2007). *2007 Biennial report: Effective psychosocial interventions for youth with behavioral and emotional needs*. Honolulu: Hawaii Department of Health Child and Adolescent Mental Health Division. Available at *hawaii.gov/health/mental-health/camhd/library/pdf/ebs/ebs012.pdf*.

Chorpita, B. F., & Daleiden, E. L. (2009). Mapping evidence-based treatments for children and adolescents: Application of the distillation and matching model to 615 treatments from 322 randomized trials. *Journal of Consulting and Clinical Psychology, 77*(3), 566–579.

Chorpita, B. F., Daleiden, E. L., & Weisz, J. R. (2005). Modularity in the design and application of therapeutic interventions. *Applied and Preventive Psychology, 11*, 141–156.

Chorpita, B. F., Reise, S., Weisz, J. R.., Grubbs, K., Becker, K. D., & Krull, J. (2009). *Evaluation of the*

Brief Phone Checklist: Child and caregiver phone interviews to measure clinical progress. Manuscript submitted for publication.

Chorpita, B. F., Taylor, A. A., Francis, S. E., Moffitt, C. E., & Austin, A. A. (2004). Efficacy of modular cognitive behavior therapy for childhood anxiety disorders. *Behavior Therapy, 35,* 263–287.

Chorpita, B. F., & Weisz, J. R. (2009). *Modular approach to therapy for children with anxiety, depression, traumatic stress, and conduct problems (MATCH-ADTC).* Satellite Beach, FL: PracticeWise.

Daleiden, E., & Chorpita, B. F. (2005). From data to wisdom: Quality improvement strategies supporting large-scale implementation of evidence based services. *Child and Adolescent Psychiatric Clinics of North America, 14,* 329–349.

Daleiden, E. L., Chorpita, B. F., Donkervoet, C. M., Arensdorf, A. A., & Brogan, M. (2006). Getting better at getting them better: Health outcomes and evidence-based practice within a system of care. *Journal of the American Academy of Child and Adolescent Psychiatry, 45,* 749–756.

Deming, W. E. (1982). *Out of the crisis.* Cambridge, MA: MIT Center for Advanced Engineering Study.

Foster, R., & Groves, I. (1997). *Case-based review protocols.* Tallahassee, FL: Human Systems and Outcomes.

Goodman, R., Ford, T., Simmons, H., Gatward, R., & Meltzer, H. (2000). Using the Strengths and Difficulties Questionnaire (SDQ) to screen for child psychiatric disorders in a community sample. *British Journal of Psychiatry, 177,* 534–539.

Hamilton, J., & Daleiden, E. (2009). Evidence-based practices in child and adolescent psychiatry and psychology. In M. Dulcan (Ed.), *American psychiatric publishing textbook of child and adolescent psychiatry* (pp. 525–540). Arlington, VA: American Psychiatric Publishing.

Henggeler, S. W., Schoenwald, S. K., Borduin, C. M., Rowland, M. D., & Cunningham, P. B. (1998). *Multisystemic treatment of antisocial behavior in children and adolescents.* New York: Guilford Press.

Hodges, K. (1998). *Child and Adolescent Functional Assessment Scale (CAFAS).* Ann Arbor, MI: Functional Assessment Systems.

Hodges, K., & Wong, M. M. (1996). Psychometric characteristics of a multidimensional measure to assess impairment: The Child and Adolescent Functional Assessment Scale (CAFAS). *Journal of Child and Family Studies, 5,* 445–467.

Kimhan, K., Higa-McMillan, C., & Daleiden, E. L. (2008). *Annual evaluation fiscal year 2008.* Honolulu: Hawaii Department of Health, Child and Adolescent Mental Health Division.

Nakamura, B. J., Daleiden, E., & Mueller, C. W. (2007). Validity of treatment target progress ratings as indicators of youth improvement. *Journal of Child and Family Studies, 16,* 729–741.

PracticeWise. (2008). *Evidence-Based Youth Mental Health Services Literature Database.* Available from *www.practicewise.com.*

PracticeWise. (2009). *PracticeWise Practitioner Guides.* Retrieved August 1, 2009, from *www.practicewise.com.*

Shewhart, W. A. (1939). *Statistical method from the viewpoint of quality control.* New York: Dover.

Weisz, J. R., Chorpita, B. F., Duan, N., Glisson, C., Green, E. P., Hoagwood, K. H., et al. (2003). *Research network on youth mental health: Evidence-based practice for children and adolescents.* Los Angeles: University of California.

Weisz, J. R., Jensen-Doss, A., & Hawley, K. M. (2005). Youth psychotherapy outcome research: A review and critique of the literature. *Annual Review of Psychology, 56,* 337–363.

Young, J. T., Daleiden, E., Chorpita, B. F., Schiffman, J., & Mueller, C. W. (2007). Assessing stability between treatment planning documents in a system of care. *Administration and Policy in Mental Health and Mental Health Services Research, 6,* 530–539.

32

Nationwide Dissemination of Effective Parenting Interventions

Building a Parenting Academy for England

STEPHEN SCOTT

OVERVIEW

In countries around the world, there is considerable concern for the well-being of children. Carefully collected survey evidence suggests there is a high prevalence of problems, and in Britain these have become more frequent over the last 30 years (Collishaw, Maughan, Goodman, & Pickles, 2004). The authoritative Office for National Statistics (ONS) surveys of 2004 found that 10% of children and adolescents had mental health disorders with significant impairment (ONS, 2004). On the other hand, there have also been several improvements in their lives, as described later. Many of these time trends are likely to be related to the substantial changes in the day-to-day experiences children have undergone in recent decades and to changes in the structure of society. To improve the lot of children will require high-level political action, for example, to relieve relative poverty and make neighborhoods better places to live. However, recent evidence suggests that a sizable portion of the difficulties—and sizable opportunities for making things better for children—lies in the quality of parenting they receive. This is true for emotional and behavioral well-being, educational achievement, and also health outcomes such as obesity.

This is not to say that parenting has been getting worse; indeed, there is some evidence to suggest it has been getting better. However, as expectations for children are raised, improving the quality of parenting provides one route to make their lives happier and more productive. Up to now, availability of evidence-based parenting programs has been patchy, to say the least, in all countries. The first part of this chapter aims to explain how the case was made to the British government that expanding the quality of parenting support across the nation was a good idea. The notion did indeed catch on with politicians, who accepted the argument with some enthusiasm and have increased parenting support greatly. The remainder of the chapter describes how we are trying to improve the quality of the expanded parenting workforce.

The Problem

A recent major review of conditions in Britain, entitled *A Good Childhood* (Layard & Dunn, 2009), noted that in many ways our children are living better than ever. They are more educated and sick less frequently than ever before; they are more open and honest about themselves and more tolerant of human diversity in all its forms. Yet there is also widespread unease about our children's experience: the commercial pressures they face, the violence they are exposed to, the stresses at school, and the increased emotional distress. The survey evidence supports these fears. More young people are anxious and troubled. As Figure 32.1 shows, the proportion of 15- to 16-year-olds in Britain experiencing significant emotional difficulties rose substantially between 1974 and 1999, remaining roughly stable thereafter. In addition to increased disorders such as depression and anxiety, there has been an increase in everyday worries; those most often listed involved family relationships, weight, and schoolwork. The same increase is true for behavioral problems, including hyperactivity and antisocial behavior, as Figure 32.2 shows (Collishaw et al., 2004).

These problems are connected with the changing world in which children are growing up both outside and inside the family. In the outside world, many influences (e.g., new media, including the Internet) expose children to commercial and lifestyle influences unknown before, and the pressure of school exams is greater than ever. Relative poverty affects more children than in most of the last 50 years. Children's experiences within the family have also changed: More families now break up and more mothers work outside the home.

While these concerns for children are present across the developed world, they seem to be particularly acute in Britain and the United States. A 2007 UNICEF report showed how children are faring in all 21 of the world's richest countries. The report began with

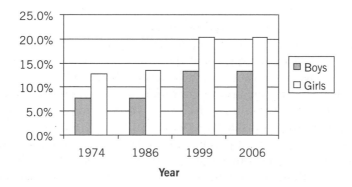

FIGURE 32.1. Percentage of 15- to 16-year-olds suffering from emotional difficulties.

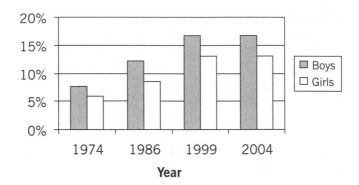

FIGURE 32.2. Percentage of 15- to 16-year-olds suffering from behavioral difficulties.

an overall ranking of the 21 countries, in which Britain was rated lowest and the United States second to last. Britain and America have more broken families than other countries, and our families are less cohesive in the way they live and eat together. The proportion of children living in poverty (defined as less than half the median income) is higher: 10% in most rich countries, 16% in England, and 22% in the United States. Our children are rougher with each other. They are at greater risk of poor health as a result of risky behaviors related to eating, drugs, and teenage sex, and they are less inclined to complete their education. There are marked differences in educational attainment according to income level. In England, about 20% of children are eligible to receive free school meals on account of family poverty. In 2008, 31% of these children attained a good reading level at age 6 compared with 52% of those from higher income families; similar disparities occur in the United States (Waldfogel & Washbrook, 2008). In summary, despite many improvements in society and standards of living, children are not as happy, as well adjusted, or achieving their potential as well as we might wish.

Conceptual Model: The Contribution of Parenting to Child Well-Being

In all countries, many of these concerns need to be addressed by a range of social and political actions at local, national, and international levels. Possible solutions may not be so easy to enact and might encompass, for example, better physical environment and housing, better schools, fairer pay and tax policies, firmer regulations regarding children's access to drugs and unsuitable video material, and so on. Not all disparities will be eliminated by changing the quality of the world children are brought up in; some differences will be due to constitutional factors, including intelligence.

However, when considering how to improve matters, in addition to political action, the quality of children's relationships with their parents is important because it has the potential to moderate these outside experiences and help children cope with them. Of even greater importance, a good parent–child relationship[1] can generate experiences from within the family that provide children with the bedrock of emotional security and social skills to cope with life in a strong, resilient way so they experience fewer problems. Parents are thus a core potential resource because they can buffer children's experiences from the outside world and can nurture them with strength from within the family.

A wealth of observational literature confirms that the quality of the parent–child relationship has a strong association with child outcomes, especially social adjustment and educational attainment (O'Connor & Scott, 2007). Of course, the relationship is not a one-way affair, and in recent years many studies have shown how both the quality of the relationship and child outcomes are influenced by the child's temperament and genetic makeup. However, this does not mean that parenting is irrelevant. Studies that disentangle genetic and rearing effects confirm that parenting effects are especially powerful in the genetically vulnerable. For example, Bohman (1996) found by age 17 children whose birth parents had been alcoholic or criminal and who were adopted into a favorable family environment had a 12% rate of delinquency vs. 40% for those adopted into an unfavorable parenting environment; the difference was much less for children without the genetic liability. Similar considerations apply for intellect: Typical studies find that early-adopted infants raised by parents employed in professional occupations later had an IQ ~12 points higher than those raised by blue-collar workers. Particular genotypes are now being identified that confer increased susceptibility to parenting style (Belsky, Bakermans-Kranenburg, & van IJzendoorn, 2007). For children living under high-risk conditions, the quality of parenting they receive is especially critical. Parents often experience stress from everyday living and this, combined with the increased risks children face in their own neighborhoods makes it harder to raise children optimally.

In a multivariate analysis of the factors that account for the disparities in cognitive attainment seen in 4-year-olds in the United States, Waldfogel and Washbrook (2008) noted that, after controlling for demographic factors, including income and maternal education, parenting style emerged as the single largest domain explaining the poorer cognitive performance of low-income compared with middle-income children, accounting for 33% of the gap in language (4.4 percentile points of the 13-point gap). The particular parenting dimension of maternal sensitivity and responsiveness accounted for more than half of the effect on its own. A second important aspect was the home learning environment. This includes parents' teaching behaviors in the home as well as their provision of learning materials and activities, including books and CDs. Taken together, parenting style and home learning environment accounted for between one-third and one-half of the gaps between low- and middle-income children. These studies, therefore, suggest that if parenting could be improved, major improvements might accrue for children's experiences and life chances.

Government Initiatives to Promote Children's Well-Being

Across the world there has been increasing governmental recognition that what goes on at home is not exclusively a private matter. In 2005 the United Nations called for a worldwide ban on corporal punishment. In the United States, both the Surgeon General and the Substance Abuse and Mental Health Services Administration have called for wider dissemination of evidence-based parenting programs. In Britain the new Labour Party government elected in 1997 made it a priority to give all children a fair chance to achieve their potential and to try to reduce social inequalities. Disrespectful, antisocial, and criminal behavior by youths was a particular concern, as was poor educational attainment. The association of these difficulties with poverty is strong, and a range of initiatives to address child poverty and disadvantage were launched. For example, at a macroeconomic level, strategies were put into place to get more families from less advantaged backgrounds into employment so their incomes would be boosted; new child care programs were offered as an incentive to women to find employment.

Considerable financial resources were deployed in urban regeneration projects in deprived areas and increased income support given to poorer families. Disappointingly, however, this did not appear to have much impact on either youth crime and antisocial behavior or inequalities in educational attainment. While it would be too simplistic to state that diverting money and resources into poor areas did not seem to work, nonetheless it has led to the question, "Poverty of what?" Government-commissioned reviews of crime implicated family factors as major contributors, as did reviews on the source of educational inequalities, which concluded that parental stimulation and interaction style had a great effect.

Many initiatives were implemented to improve outcomes for children. For example, in a manner not unlike Head Start in the United States, the British government introduced Sure Start centers into the most deprived areas to support families with children ages 0–3, at a cost of about $1,500 million (£1,000 million). Major policies were announced aimed at children's achievement and well-being (notably Every Child Matters in 2005 and the Children's Plan in 2007) and youth antisocial behavior (Respect in 2006 and Youth Action Plan in 2007). Continuing this family focus, in 2007 a Minister for Children was appointed as part of the new Department for Children, Schools and Families (DCSF) ministry.

In keeping with increased appreciation of the evidence outlined previously, over the last 2 years, the DCSF has introduced a considerable number of specific parenting initiatives to increase the number of professionals working with parents: for example, Parenting Early Intervention Pathfinder projects to help to parents in disadvantaged areas experiencing difficulties, a parenting expert for each local authority, a parent support adviser in each school, and Family Intervention Projects for the most difficult cases. Thus, there has been a large commitment to investing in parenting services for children.

MAKING THE CASE FOR AN ACADEMY

The fact that the government has been willing to apply insights from family psychology on such a large scale has been exciting. Professionals and academics have had a unique chance to influence policy for the good of children. However, much of the recent research about what makes psychological interventions cost-effective in widespread dissemination needed to be better addressed, it seemed. From 2005–2006 my colleagues and I made a number of presentations to the government and joined the Respect taskforce, a concerted effort led by Prime Minister Tony Blair and Home Office Minister John Reid to reduce antisocial behavior. Three issues in particular were highlighted in our presentations to the government, as discussed next.

High Long-Term Cost of Child Antisocial Behavior and Social Exclusion

The first point to make was the financial effects of ineffective intervention. Our team published a study showing that by age 27 individuals in England who had oppositional and conduct disorders since age 10 cost society 10 times more than controls (Figure 32.3; Scott, Knapp, Henderson, & Maughan, 2001). This was conservatively estimated

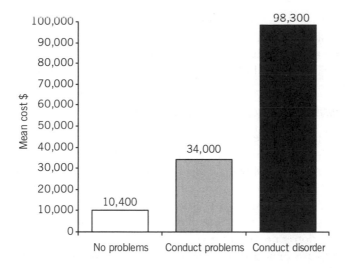

FIGURE 32.3. Long-term cost of child antisocial behavior to age 27 years.

based on actual documented service use. For those with added indirect expenditures such as victim costs, the figures are far higher. For example, Cohen (2005) estimated that the cost of successfully treating high-risk youths in the United States was $1.7–$2.3 million (£1.2–£1.6 million) by the time they reached their mid-20s. Because of the great financial burden, interventions start becoming cost-effective even with relatively modest effect sizes (in Figure 32.3, a modest shift to the left), always provided that the effects are enduring. The Washington State Institute for Public Policy (2004) has reviewed the likely costs and benefits of adopting a portfolio of evidence-based interventions across whole regions and concluded that deploying a range of programs is likely to provide savings.

Some Interventions Are Not Effective

While the drive toward evidence-based practice is becoming increasingly accepted in the mental health context, albeit variably implemented, this way of thinking is less well known among the wide range of those who work with parents. Moreover, when known, it is not necessarily accepted. This is relevant because several evaluations of parenting interventions show they are not always effective; in this regard they resemble other child mental health interventions (Weisz, Doss, & Hawley, 2005). In particular, generic counseling approaches, although very popular with parents, do not necessarily improve child outcomes (Scott, 2008). From the Cambridge–Somerville study onward, studies have shown that one cannot assume that a well-intentioned program will do good, and indeed there is a chance that it may be positively harmful. Yet untested programs that lack many of the ingredients shown to work are widely used in England; for example, one compendium of approaches in current use lists more than 140, of which fewer than 10% have any published evidence base.

In contrast, well-run trials that paid attention to choosing evidence-based programs and that employed skilled therapists and emphasized fidelity to the manual had good results. For example, our team carried out a controlled trial of an evidence-based parenting program (the basic 12-week Incredible Years program), which was delivered in multiple sites to clinically referred cases in ordinary practice treated by local clinicians. This showed that under these real-life conditions a good effect size (1.1 *SD*) was achievable by paying attention to therapist skill (Scott, Spender, Doolan, Jacobs, & Aspland, 2001).

The Role of Therapist Skill in Successful Dissemination

As Weisz and Gray (2008) have emphasized, making interventions work under university efficacy trial conditions is different from going to scale in the real world, where results are often disappointing. In the prior trial, we analyzed the impact of therapist skill rated from videotapes of sessions by observers blind to child outcomes and related it to child antisocial behavior rated by semistructured interview. The results are summarized in Figure 32.4. They show a strong effect of skill, with the workers least skilled in implementing the model doing no good for children.

These findings are in accord with others; for example, the Washington State Institute for Public Policy (2004) found that when therapists delivering functional family therapy were rated by trainers, clients of those rated as more skilled had a later reoffending rate of 18% compared with 28% in controls, but clients of those rated as less skilled had a rate of 32%. Once again, the less skilled therapists had no effect.

SETTING UP THE ACADEMY

Our team made presentations along these lines to many government departments, including the Treasury, the Prime Minister's Strategy Unit, and the DCSF. Of course, many other interested parties from a wide range of backgrounds influenced government, too. Following this, in 2006 Tony Blair launched the Respect agenda to tackle antisocial behavior, which included setting up the National Academy for Parenting Practitioners

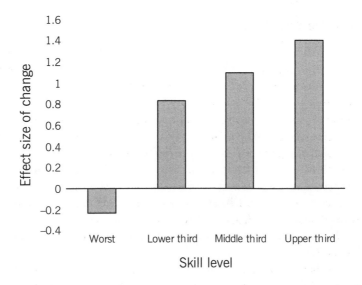

FIGURE 32.4. Reduction in child aggression according to therapist skill.

(NAPP) to improve the quality of the parenting workforce. King's College London (Institute of Psychiatry), in conjunction with two parenting charities, won the competitive bid to set this up, and it was launched in November 2007.

With a budget of $50 million (£30m) for its first 3 years, the academy's mission is "to transform the quality and size of the parenting workforce across England so parents can get the help they need to raise their children well" (see *www.parentingacademy.org*). A potential advantage of such an organization operating in England is the relatively centralized system of government. Whereas in the United States and some European countries, states and local authorities can to a substantial extent determine their own standards and budgets, in England more than 90% of local spending is determined by central government directives. Therefore, in setting up their new parenting services, if local authorities follow academy guidelines, which they are encouraged to do by the government, the academy influence could be substantial.

The Workforce Development and Training Program

As noted, there is a huge expansion of jobs for staff working with parents in England (with currently perhaps 20,000 practitioners, although numbers vary according to definitions). However, many of these personnel are unfamiliar with evidence-based ways of working. There are many levels of skill among practitioners (e.g., from an untrained, unpaid worker in a charity giving support for a few hours a week to a doctoral-level clinical psychologist working full time). We wished to change practice as quickly as possible. We, therefore, decided to put the greater part of our initial workforce development effort into direct training of relatively highly qualified practitioners so they could deliver more substantial evidence-based programs. The plan is that by training the more qualified staff who are higher up in the organization, there is greater chance of their culture changes cascading down, too. A number of plans are being implemented:

- Direct training in evidence-based programs for 3,400 practitioners.
- Ongoing supervision of practitioners to refine their skills.
- Training in basic skills for less qualified parenting practitioners
- Influencing of commissioners to purchase better programs by offering an online rating of their quality and research evidence base.
- Assisting local authorities to organize effective, sustainable services.

We decided that expanding evidence-based training by offering it for free countrywide is an immediate way to promote an evidence-based approach. To begin with, children at serious risk of poor outcomes because of behavioral problems have been prioritized. Programs have been selected that have a reasonable evidence base and sufficient training capacity. Free participation in Triple P, The Incredible Years, Strengthening Families, and Mellow Parenting courses were offered initially (2007–2008); this is being complemented in the next rounds (2009–2010) with a range of additional evidence-based programs (see *www.parentingacademy.org* for details).

From Practitioner to Parent and Child

Some of the factors that we believe mediate the influence of practitioners on child well-being are presented in Figure 32.5. We are trying, where possible, to influence these. For

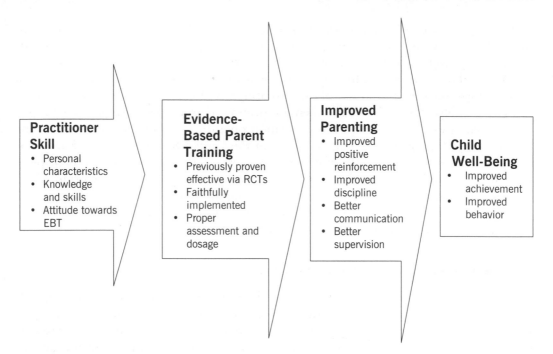

FIGURE 32.5. Steps linking practitioner skill to child well-being (EBT, evidence-based training; RCTs, randomized controlled trials).

example, we do not offer a 3-day training course and then leave trainees to their own devices, we ask providers to build in ongoing supervision and consultation sessions. The aim is to achieve greater fidelity to the model being used and higher levels of practitioner skill.

From Agency to Practitioner

We are also keen to embed recent knowledge regarding what promotes effective dissemination. Even if practitioners have reasonable levels of skill and use proven programs, this does not necessarily guarantee better parent and child outcomes. To gain persistent benefits across a locality requires well-organized services. Some of the factors that link the service organization context with successful delivery by practitioners are set out in Figure 32.6. We are trying to address these factors. For example, we have appointed regional network managers, who are setting up local communities of practitioners and managers.

Our own surveys, in line with research by others, suggest that practitioners believe it is often lack of support at the management level rather than lack of practitioner enthusiasm that hampers effective practice. Therefore, we are also including training days just for commissioners and managers so they have a clear picture of what a model service might look like in terms of planning, skills mix, and facilities. Repeatedly underpinning this is the attempt to persuade them that practitioners should focus on services that measure effectiveness, not just volume of activity.

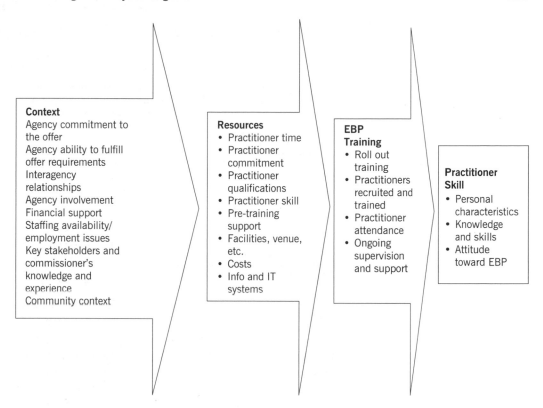

FIGURE 32.6. Steps linking contextual factors to practitioner skill (IT, information technology; EBP, evidence-based program).

The training offer in basic skills for less qualified parenting practitioners covers a range of subjects, such as building and maintaining relationships with parents. Additionally, the academy is delivering 40 one-day good-practice workshops, which cover subjects such as working with fathers, black and ethnic-minority groups, parents of children with disabilities, and parents with substance abuse. The focus is on *what works* in each subject area. Moving forward, there are many activities that we would like to pursue. For example, one major way to improve standards would be to influence the content of curricula taught to trainees. Currently, in our view, there is insufficient teaching of evidence-based approaches in many courses in the country, from those for nannies or people working in nurseries to social work and counseling degrees. We shall try to address this in future years. The academy workforce development plan is closely connected to its research, and this is now addressed.

GENERATING EVIDENCE OF EFFECTIVE WAYS OF WORKING THROUGH RESEARCH

The research and development plan is designed to serve practitioners so they deliver more effective services, not to generate abstract findings. It works at three different levels (Table 32.1): investigation of which parenting styles are associated with good child out-

TABLE 32.1. Ways of Generating the Evidence Base to Improve Practice

	Level		
Activity	Parenting styles	Intervention effectiveness	Service delivery
Evaluate	Determine which aspects are crucial for child outcomes	Assess in variety of ways, from tool kit to randomized controlled trials	Determine effectiveness of on-the-ground delivery and what factors drive it
Refine	Develop better assessment methods; improve treatment targets	Improve interventions (e.g., shorten, add elements)	Alter delivery arrangements (e.g., managerial setup, which families are seen, which staff recruited, what training and supervision they receive)
Disseminate	Include new assessment methods in training	Inform and train practitioners in improved ways of working	Change commissioning criteria, hold regional seminars, etc.

comes; study of which intervention programs are effective; and research on how service delivery should be improved. Across all levels, the aim is not just to collect information, but also to then refine measures, programs, and services and disseminate them. There are three work streams: the measurement of parenting, the development and testing of promising interventions, and the improvement of commissioning and delivery of training. In addition to the appointment of the current author as director of research, a new professor of parenting studies has been appointed. As a check on the research quality and to support it, there is an independent scientific advisory group with clinical scientists from universities in the United Kingdom and the United States.

Measurement of Parenting

Relative Usefulness of Different Methods

Assessing parenting skills and problems is the cornerstone of many child and parent services, yet systems of measurement in England are typically very variable and rarely evidence based. Although several specific measures of parenting can be found in the scientific literature, there is currently no reasonably standard way of assessing parenting. The relative usefulness of questionnaires, interviews, and direct observation in regular practice is uncertain: What should and can be disseminated for effective community use is not clear, and many practitioners use no or unvalidated systems.

A number of methods of assessing parenting are being compared in the trials described next. Some interesting findings have already been generated. First, a short form of the well-known Alabama Parenting Questionnaire is as effective as the long one: using three questions per subscale (thus, with five subscales, 15 questions) were as effective as nine (total of 42 questions) in predicting observed parenting. Second, the responses by teenagers predicted observed parenting better than those by parents. Third, when assessing the parenting of 5- to 6-year-old children, measures using attachment concepts predicted attachment security better than those derived from social learning theory, whereas the reverse was true for conduct problems. This suggests that both conceptual approaches to measurement are important and perhaps should be used in practice. We are now trying to shorten the observation coding scheme so it can be used more easily in everyday practice.

Parenting of Children Who Seem Unresponsive to Discipline

A second line of work that also aims to characterize parenting is investigating the different pattern of parent–child relationships in which the children have emotionally volatile versus emotionally cold (callous–unemotional) traits. The latter children are of particular concern because they seem not to respond to usual types of rewards and sanctions; typically, they show early-onset antisocial behavior. By adolescence, many are on their way to becoming chronic offenders, and many go on to be diagnosed with antisocial personality disorder or labeled as psychopathic. These children are relatively insensitive to punishment, and so attempts to use discipline are ineffective and can be extremely frustrating and distressing to parents. On the other hand, these children are highly reward driven and may be sensitive to reward-based interventions applied carefully within positive parent–child attachments. The plan is to carefully measure the strategies these parents use and observe what, if anything, seems to work.

For this population, new interventions are being tried and refined to make parenting programs more effective. This includes attempts to increase children's emotional awareness by developing emotion language via simple and regular parent–child conversations that cultivate autobiographical memory and language for the children's emotional experiences. Preliminary data from Salmon, Dadds, Allen, and Hawes (2009) showed that parents can achieve significant increases in emotion talk, and this may add to improvement in conduct problems, although the trial was too small to show a significant difference.

Development and Testing of Promising Interventions

The development and evaluation of promising treatments for the United Kingdom is a high priority for NAPP research. Currently, two randomized controlled trials (RCTs) of well-developed interventions are underway: functional family therapy (FFT) for teenage antisocial behavior, and Supporting Parents on Kids Education in Schools (SPOKES) for younger children. Additionally, three trials are using case series to refine new interventions for high-need families, for foster parents, and also for callous–unemotional children, as described previously.

FFT for Teenage Delinquency

A considerable body of evidence has linked child and adolescent delinquency with criminality in adulthood. There is a small population of young people who are harmful to others: They cause damage and upset and make the public feel unsafe; they are expensive in the societal resources they consume, not only in the youth justice system but in extraeducational and training effort, social services, and community and neighborhood safety as well. Teenage pregnancy and drug addiction are common. Cost-effective approaches are sorely needed.

FFT in this population has strong evidence from the United States and is less intensive and expensive than more elaborate interventions such as multisystemic therapy

(MST). However, it has never been used in England, and Program success in the United States does not guarantee success elsewhere: A large trial of MST in Canada did not find FFT effective. This RCT will prove whether FFT works in England.

Improving Behavior and Reading in Elementary School Children

As noted, several research studies have shown that variations in the quality of young children's interactions and learning experiences with their parents are major determinants of social inequalities, which are a particular governmental concern. This RCT aims to determine how best to improve matters.

The intervention is for practitioners working with parents of 5- to 6-year-old children in elementary/primary school. Children are screened by teachers and parents and selected because of moderate disruptive behavior (top 25% of the class). The intervention aims to improve four characteristics key to child success: effective parenting, child social behavior, child ability to concentrate, and child reading ability. Originally, it comprised The Incredible Years program for 12 weeks followed by a new program that taught parents how to read with their children, in the SPOKES project (Sylva, Scott, Totsika, Ereky-Stevens, & Crook, 2008). The first trial of the intervention showed good outcomes, but a subsequent trial with universal admission criteria and less skilled staff led to improved parenting but unchanged child outcomes (Scott, O'Connor, & Futh, 2006). To settle its effectiveness and to demonstrate which elements lead to which changes, this trial included four arms: It compares a parenting program for child behavior (The Incredible Years [to our knowledge no one has studied whether this improves literacy]) versus a literacy program (which, in turn, may also improve behavior) versus both combined (to see whether they act synergistically) versus minimal contact.

Families with High Needs

A small number of families have multiple problems where generally chaotic parenting is especially likely to give rise to unruly, disruptive antisocial behavior among both younger children and teenagers. They are of considerable concern to the government, which has set up Family Intervention Projects to help them. The aim is to develop and evaluate a manualized intervention for these parents, who have a great need for services but are least likely to access and engage in traditional interventions because of the complex array of individual, family, and social factors that impact on their everyday functioning. After the manual has been created, it will be field trialed in a case series of 40 families.

Carers of Fostered Children

Most fostered children are taken into public care because they have been very poorly parented, often with severe abuse or neglect. They do especially poorly on all indexes of life success (e.g., they are greatly overrepresented in prison populations; in England, only 12% pass five or more general certificate exams by age 16 vs. 55% of the general population). There are few good-quality parenting programs specifically designed for foster carers of children beyond infancy. Typically, practitioners seeking an evidence-based approach have to take a program designed for biological families with secure attachments and try to adapt it. None has proper trial evidence of effectiveness in England.

The Fostering Changes program (Pallett, Scott, Blackeby, Yule, & Weissman, 2002) is designed specifically for this client group, and there are two publications showing positive changes for fostered children.

However, the Fostering Changes program is based on social learning theory principles and does not specifically address either attachment issues or educational underachievement. An observational study is underway investigating the links between fostered children's attachment patterns to their birth parents and their foster carers and their educational attainments and interpersonal style. The plan is that insights from this study and the wider literature will inform a revision of the manual. One early finding is that nearly all of the fostered children had insecure attachment patterns toward their birth parents, and the majority (two-thirds) carried forward an insecure pattern toward their foster carers. An implication is that the manual should be revised to enable foster carers to be aware of how the children they look after may signal distress and how they may provide comfort despite it apparently not being sought. Another finding is that the IQ of the fostered children is 20 points lower than for control children attending similar inner-city schools. An implication is that carers may need to be given strategies to gain knowledge and confidence to demand that teachers ensure children are given instruction appropriate to their children's level. The manual will be tested and refined in a series of pre–post case studies.

For both high-need and foster families, the new programs are being refined across the country because of a close relationship between the academy and the DCSF, which is promoting testing of the new manualized approaches across several regions. This seems like a good collaboration because it should lead to refinement of the intervention to work in real-life conditions across diverse contexts, thus making the intervention more acceptable and so, one hopes, more effective. Ideally, in due course, RCTs will be underway.

Improving the Commissioning of Parenting Programs and Delivery of Training

Better Commissioning through a Guide to Program Quality

Currently, there are more than 140 parenting programs available in England. They vary greatly in theoretical orientation, quality of written materials or manuals, sophistication of training available for practitioners, and evidence of effectiveness. Over the last year, most of the 150 local authorities in England (each with about 300,000 inhabitants, 70,000 of whom are children) have appointed a parenting commissioner, whose job it is to develop a parenting strategy and purchase services. The commissioner's background is likely to be in local government administration, often with relatively little exposure to an evidence-based approach regarding interventions for children.

Commissioners need to know which programs are "fit for purpose" for improving parenting and child outcomes, so they have a sound basis to decide which approaches to drop and which to use because they are effective. The academy has a two-stage evaluation process: online self-evaluation by the program developer and then evaluation by academy staff. For the latter, we have begun with the programs that are most widely used in England and that have the strongest evidence base. We have developed detailed criteria to carry out the evaluations, published online (*www.commissioningtoolkit.org*) using the Parenting Programme Evaluation Tool. There are four dimensions, each rated on a 5-point scale:

1. The quality of specification of the interventions (i.e., the level of interventions and for whom they are intended).
2. Whether the content is based on empirically tested theory and is clearly documented in a manual so that it can be replicated.
3. The quality of the procedures for training and supervision of practitioners.
4. The evidence of effectiveness on parenting and child outcomes.

This approach is different from most current evaluation schemes of effective interventions, which usually just have the last dimension, evidence of effectiveness from trials, as seen, for example, in the approaches used by the Blueprints for Violence Prevention (2009) or the American Psychological Association (Chambless & Hollon, 1998). We added the first three dimensions because we wanted to promote interventions that were both effective and replicable because they had well-developed training procedures, and we did not want to penalize programs that had the right ingredients and excellent training procedures but insufficient resources to mount a RCT of their effectiveness.

There is a political dilemma here. On the one hand, the evaluations could be entirely based on outcome evidence and only endorse programs that have excellent RCT evidence. This would certainly stop the use of ineffective programs. However, it might well also shortly lead the majority of parenting practitioners to unemployment, which would likely have large political repercussions. It would also eliminate those programs that have good constituents and training procedures but that lack the financing for proper trial evaluation. It would favor the handful of programs that are commercially backed and well evaluated, risking setting their approach in stone; any new, innovative program trying to take the field forward inevitably would not have good trial evidence.

On the other hand, being totally permissive would be to keep friends but to let down children and parents by allowing them to take part in interventions that are very unlikely to benefit them. We have, therefore, taken an approach that includes all four dimensions noted previously. This allows commissioners to consider using a program of high quality that does not yet have evidence of effectiveness. For program developers that have a potentially strong program, we offer advice on where it might benefit from being stronger: Our aim is to be helpful and raise standards. The limitation here is our own staff time and the fact that we do not need scores of programs addressing the same client group.

As we proceed, we are starting to move from general programs mainly for child antisocial behavior to specialist programs (e.g., for children with attention-deficit/hyperactivity disorder [ADHD] or for ethnic minorities). We use a rigorous evaluation procedure: Three assessors each rate the program material blind to the developer's own ratings. Interrater reliabilities have been high, with intraclass correlations on the dimension ranging from 0.87–0.96 for each of the four rated dimensions. One of the risks of our approach is that it is principally a paper exercise; we do not have the resources to inspect how a program is working or how practitioners are trained. For the time being, we have to take the program developers' word. However, we are in close touch with practitioners and have close links with several commissioners, so we believe we have a reasonably accurate picture of what actually goes on.

The effectiveness of the tool kit can be assessed in the immediate short term by the number of visitors to the website (currently more than 1,000 per week since its launch), in the medium term by the opinions of commissioners as revealed in a survey currently being undertaken, and in the longer term by improved quality of local programs and by the increased commissioning of programs that achieve a good rating.

Ensuring the Quality and Effectiveness of Training

The academy needs to know the effectiveness of the training it commissions directly itself. It, therefore, has a research strand monitoring this. In the pilot phase, we simply measured the numbers trained, their qualifications and whether they went to practice their new skills as taught. We found that two-thirds of trainees had a university education (fewer than on comparable courses run in Europe), but that only 35% of trainees went on to run parenting groups as intended by the developer: Most of the remainder were using their skills in their one-to-one work. To raise numbers in the next round, we are requesting greater details from managers about their plans to implement training as intended before we offer free participation. This seems to be leading to managers thinking through more thoroughly how to set up their parenting services, and we will see whether a higher percentage of the next round of trainees implement programs as intended.

In the next phases of our training, we plan to measure increases in trainee understanding of the principles of the course taken. In later phases, we plan to measure trainees' skill level, initially as assessed by the trainer but subsequently using independent assessment by videotape in a subsample. The ultimate aim is to assess how many cases they see, what the results are (using the free instruments described previously), and what the barriers were to implementing a high-quality service. This will give an accurate picture of the numbers of practitioners using an evidence-based approach in England, their level of skill, and whether they are improving the lives of families and children. Through this activity, we hope to identify ineffective training that needs to be modified or dropped.

DIRECTIONS FOR RESEARCH

The academy's research program operates at several levels: from close observation of the parent–child relationship to discover which elements are fundamental to good child outcomes, through trials to refine and test interventions so they can be implemented well under everyday conditions, to testing the effectiveness of large-scale training ventures. Over the next 3 years, we aim to answer the following questions for each program tested:

1. Does the intervention work? For example, how much does it reduce antisocial behavior and improve child adjustment, increase educational attainment, or improve family relationships?

2. How does it work? Is the main effective ingredient, for example, increased limit setting by parents or more rewards for desirable behavior? This sort of analysis helps determine which ingredients of a program should be kept, modified, or dropped. As well as measuring basic outcomes before and after the intervention, in each of the trials

we are measuring three potential sets of mediators before, during, and after intervention: parenting behavior, parental attributions toward the child, and parental sense of agency/effectiveness.

For example, it could be that for the parenting program with younger children (The Incredible Years), in which from the first session parents are practicing new behaviors, change occurs first in parenting behavior, followed by improvements in child behavior, after which parental attributions and a better sense of agency follow. In contrast, in FFT, the postulated pattern of change is attributions and sense of agency first followed, by parenting behaviors and then youth behavior. When the interventions fail to work, it should be possible to investigate whether it was due to parents' failure to alter their negative attributions of the child, to some or all aspects of parents' behavior, or to the child's insensitivity to parental change. Of course, different mechanisms may operate in different families, but we will begin to address these questions.

3. Are the effects short lived or more enduring: Have the children relapsed a year after the parents took the program, or are their life chances genuinely improving?

4. For whom does it work? Are the interventions more effective with younger or older children, those with more severe or milder problems, or those with two parents or single parents? For ethnic-minority families as much as for white British families? At present, even the best parenting programs only work for about two-thirds of children, leaving one-third unchanged. We need to identify why.

5. What other difficulties are revealed by the assessment (e.g., ADHD, dyslexia, depression, abusive parenting styles) and how do these affect response to the intervention?

6. What is the acceptability of the intervention to (1) parents, (2) youths, (3) frontline practitioners, and (4) senior managers and commissioners?

7. Is the program cost-effective?

8. How difficult was it to implement the intervention to a high-quality level? What is the relationship between practitioner fidelity and skill level and outcome? How good do practitioners need to be?

For the dissemination of training, if we can get practitioners to collect data on their subsequent practice, we should be able to address the impact of qualifications, experience, commitment, and skill to effectiveness. The answers to all these questions should lead to more effective interventions on the ground.

CONCLUSIONS

There are many unanswered questions for the field. At the basic science level, they include discovering the parenting styles that are most effective with particular subgroups of children, from those with ADHD to those with callous–unemotional traits. Currently, these children do not respond especially well to parenting interventions. We need to understand more about the links between different genotypes and differential susceptibility to parenting. At a practical level, we need far more population-level trials to ascertain what proportion of hard-to-reach families can be engaged and the cost-effectiveness of widening access to parenting education. For example, it would be good to see the long-term value of parenting classes for teenagers in schools, even before they become fathers and mothers. Given the shortage of practitioners, it would be beneficial to know the proportion of the population who will do well will self-administered programs (e.g., by using the Internet?) It is hoped that research in the next few years will answer some of these questions.

Being part of the development of an ambitious and unique venture to try to improve parenting interventions on a national scale has been exciting. To ensure the future of this venture in an uncertain financial and political climate, it may in due course be prudent to merge with a larger organization concerned with the development of professionals who work with children. Whatever structure ensues, we will continue to build on the foundations of the academy. We will work with the government to apply psychological knowledge about the parent–child relationship systematically in order to promote to a better, fairer childhood across the country.

NOTE

1. In this chapter, for the sake of brevity, the term "parenting" is used somewhat interchangeably with the term "parent–child relationship."

REFERENCES

Belsky, J., Bakermans-Kranenburg, M. J., & van IJzendoorn, M. H. (2007). For better and for worse: Differential susceptibility to environmental influences. *Current Directions in Psychological Science, 16*, 300–304.

Blueprints for Violence Prevention. (2009). *Selection criteria.* Retrieved April 26 2009, from *www.colorado.edu/cspv/blueprints/criteria.html.*

Bohman, M. (1996). Predisposition to criminality: Swedish adoption studies in retrospect. In G. Bock & J. Goode (Eds.), *Genetics of criminal and antisocial behaviour—CIBA Foundation Symposium 194* (pp. 99–114). Chichester, UK: Wiley.

Chambless, D. L., & Hollon, S. D. (1998). Defining empirically supported therapies. *Journal of Consulting and Clinical Psychology, 66*, 7–18.

Cohen, M. A. (2005). *The costs of crime and justice.* New York: Routledge.

Collishaw, S., Maughan, B., Goodman, R., & Pickles, A. (2004). Time trends in adolescent mental health. *Journal of Child Psychology and Psychiatry, 45*, 1350–1362.

Layard, R., & Dunn, J. (2009). *A good childhood.* New York: Penguin.

O'Connor, T. G., & Scott, S. (2007). *Parenting and outcomes for children.* York, UK: Joseph Rowntree Foundation.

Office for National Statistics. (2004). *Mental health of children and young people in Great Britain.* London: Author.

Pallett, C., Scott, S., Blackeby, K., Yule, W., & Weissman, R. (2002). Fostering changes: A cognitive-behavioural approach to help foster carers manage children. *Adoption and Fostering, 26*, 39–48.

Salmon, K., Dadds, M., Allen, J., & Hawes, D. (2009). Can emotional language skills be taught during parent training for conduct problem children? *Child Psychiatry and Human Development, 40*(4), 485–498.

Scott, S. (2008). Parenting programs. In M. Rutter, D. Bishop, D. Pine, J. Stevenson, S. Scott, E. Taylor, et al. (Eds.), *Rutter's child and adolescent psychiatry* (5th ed.) Oxford, UK: Blackwell Science.

Scott, S., Knapp, M., Henderson, J., & Maughan, B. (2001). Financial cost of social exclusion: Follow up study of antisocial children into adulthood. *British Medical Journal, 323,* 191–194.

Scott, S., O'Connor, T., & Futh, A. (2006). *What makes parenting programmes work in disadvantaged areas?: The PALS trial.* York, UK: Joseph Rowntree Foundation.

Scott, S., Spender, Q., Doolan, M., Jacobs, B., & Aspland, H. (2001). Multicentre controlled trial of parenting groups for childhood antisocial behaviour in clinical practice. *British Medical Journal, 323,* 194–197.

Sylva, K., Scott, S., Totsika, V., Ereky-Stevens, K., & Crook, C. (2008). Teaching parents to help their children read: A randomized controlled trial. *British Journal of Educational Psychology, 78,* 435–455.

Waldfogel, J., & Washbrook, E. (2008, June). *Early years policy.* Paper presented at the Sutton Trust-Carnegie Summit: Social Mobility and Education Policy, New York.

Washington State Institute for Public Policy. (2004). *Outcome evaluation of Washington State's research-based programs for juvenile offenders.* Olympia, WA: Author.

Weisz, J. R., Doss, A. J., & Hawley, K. M. (2005). Youth psychotherapy outcome research: A review and critique of the evidence base. *Annual Review of Psychology, 56,* 337–363.

Weisz, J. R., & Gray, J. S. (2008). Evidence-based psychotherapy for children and adolescents: Data from the present and a model for the future. *Child and Adolescent Mental Health, 13,* 54–65.

33

The International Dissemination of the Triple P—Positive Parenting Program

MATTHEW R. SANDERS and MAJELLA MURPHY-BRENNAN

OVERVIEW

The Importance of Parenting Interventions

There is increasing international recognition of the importance of service providers and agencies delivering evidence-based interventions to promote the well being of children and youths. The main aim of these providers is to prevent serious problems involving young people, including major mental health problems, child maltreatment, antisocial behavior, and drug and alcohol abuse (Graeff-Martins et al., 2008).

Policy initiatives from regions as diverse as Australasia, Europe and the United Kingdom, North and South America, the Middle East, and Asia have led to unprecedented interest on the role of parenting in the promotion of children's well-being and the prevention of maltreatment and mental health problems in children.

As a reflection of this interest, the Council of Europe has called on each of its 47 member states to establish positive parenting programs. The British government has considered the provision of parenting services to be sufficiently important that it has established the National Academy of Parenting Practitioners to promote the use of evidence-based parenting interventions in England. Similar national initiatives to improve the availability of evidence-based parenting programs (EBPPs) have occurred in most Scandinavian countries and in various European countries such as Germany, Belgium, Switzerland, and the Netherlands. The United Nations has recently released a draft report that examines how to make existing EBPPs available to developing countries in a culturally appropriate manner. The Commonwealth Government of Australia and all state governments have policies and funding streams to support parents in the task of raising their children. Interest in promoting parenting programs is not confined to wealthier regions such as North America, the United Kingdom, and Europe but has also occurred in Asia, the Netherlands Antilles, and the Middle East.

Is Interest in Parenting Programs Justified?

Concern about the need for parenting programs stems from the high prevalence rates of social, emotional, and behavioral problems in children. Evidence from behavior genetics research, as well as epidemiological, correlational, and experimental studies, shows that parenting practices have a major influence on children's development (Collins, Maccoby, Steinberg, Hetherington, & Bornstein, 2000). Risk factors such as poor parenting, family conflict, and marriage breakdown strongly influence children's risk of developing various forms of psychopathology. Specifically, a lack of a warm, positive relationship with parents; insecure attachment; harsh, inflexible, or inconsistent discipline practices; inadequate supervision of and involvement with children; marital conflict and breakdown; and parental psychopathology (particularly maternal depression) increase the risk that children will develop major behavioral and emotional problems (Loeber & Farrington, 1998). Parenting interventions, derived from social learning, functional analysis, and cognitive-behavioral principles, are among the most powerful interventions available and are the treatment of choice for a number of developmental problems in toddlers and preschool-age children (Sanders, 1999).

Parental Engagement in Parenting Programs

Despite the strength of the evidence, relatively few parents who might benefit from EBPPs actually participate. Although access to parenting intervention is improving in many countries, EBPPs are not widely available, especially outside of major metropolitan areas or in poorer underserved communities. Poor participation by parents in parenting groups is a formidable barrier to widespread effective implementation of parenting group programs.

In a recent survey of 722 working parents in the United Kingdom, Sanders et al. (2009) found that only 2% of parents had completed a parenting program even though 90% said they would participate in one if it was offered at work. Furthermore, although parenting groups are widely advocated in the parent training field, only a minority of parents (i.e., 27%) wanted to participate in a group program. In fact, no delivery modality (e.g., group, individual, seminar, web based, telephone based) was accounted for by more than 30% of parents. These findings confirm that contemporary parents are looking for alternative flexible ways of accessing parenting advice. The major consequence of low program availability, limited program options, and nonoptimal participation rates is inadequate program reach.

Limited program reach means that most families who could benefit from parenting programs do not complete them. When relatively few families derive the benefits of EBPPs, the potential for these programs to reduce the prevalence of problematic outcomes for children in the entire population is markedly weakened. This has led to the development and trialing of alternate forms of reaching parents with parenting information, including media, primary care, and self-directed approaches (Sanders & Turner, 2002). We have argued previously (e.g., Sanders & Turner, 2002) that a comprehensive evidence-based, multilevel system of parenting support is required to ensure that positive parenting programs are more widely available. In the current chapter, we build on this thesis by making a case for the use of an evidence-based system of training and dissemination to diffuse positive parenting methods in the professional community.

Toward an Evidence-Based Public Health Model of Parenting Support

Effective dissemination of EBPPs is critical for evidence-based research to have any significant community impact. Of the parent training programs that have been disseminated to date, many have been delivered late in the developmental trajectory as interventions for children with diagnosed conduct problems, for high-risk children already showing signs of behavioral disorder, or for families notified for abuse or neglect rather than as prevention programs. It is our contention that to reduce prevalence rates of family dysfunction and emotional and conduct problems in children and adolescents, a population approach that addresses the broader ecological context of parenting (e.g., Biglan, 1995) as well as the knowledge, skills, and confidence of parents is required. The Triple P—Positive Parenting Program is an example of a multilevel parent and family support system.

The empirical basis of Triple P is not the focus of this chapter and has been detailed elsewhere (e.g., Sanders, 1999, 2008). Triple P has been featured prominently in four different meta-analyses, which have concluded that the intervention is effective in reducing behavior problems in children (e.g., Nowak & Heinrichs, 2008).

WHAT IS THE TRIPLE P—POSITIVE PARENTING PROGRAM?

Triple P was developed by Sanders and colleagues at the University of Queensland, Australia, as a multilevel system of parenting intervention to improve the quality of advice available to parents (see Sanders, 1999). The system aims to prevent severe behavioral, emotional, and developmental problems in children and adolescents by enhancing parents' knowledge, skills, and confidence. It incorporates five levels of intervention on a tiered continuum of increasing strength for parents of children from birth to age 16. The suite of multilevel programs in Triple P is designed to create a family-friendly environment that supports parents in the task of raising their children (Table 33.1). It specifically targets the social contexts that influence parents on a day-to-day basis. These contexts include the mass media, primary health care services, child care and school systems, work sites, religious organizations, and the broader political system. The multilevel strategy is designed to maximize efficiency, contain costs, avoid waste and overservicing, and ensuring that the program has wide reach in the community.

Self-Regulation: A Unifying Framework for Supporting Parents, Children, Parenting Service Providers, and Agencies

A central goal of Triple P is the development of an individual's capacity for self-regulation. This principle applies to all program participants, from parents to service providers and researchers. Self-regulation is a process whereby individuals are taught skills to change their own behavior and become independent problem solvers but in a broader social environment that supports parenting and family relationships (Karoly, 1993). In the case

TABLE 33.1. Triple P Model of Parent and Family Support

Level of intervention	Target population	Intervention methods	Practitioners
Level 1 Media-based parent information campaign Universal Triple P	All parents interested in information about parenting and promoting their child's development.	Coordinated media and health promotion campaign raising awareness of parent issues and encouraging participation in parenting programs. May involve electronic and print media (e.g., community service announcements, talk radio, newspaper, magazine editorials).	Typically coordinated by media liaison officers or mental health or welfare staff.
Level 2 Health promotion strategy/brief selective intervention Selected Triple P Selected Teen Triple P	Parents interested in parenting education or with specific concerns about their child's development or behavior.	Health promotion information or specific advice for a discrete developmental issue or minor child behavior problem. May involve a group seminar process or brief (up to 20 minutes) telephone or face-to-face clinician contact.	Parent support during routine well-child health care (e.g., child and community health and welfare staff).
Level 3 Narrow-focus parent training Primary Care Triple P Primary Care Teen Triple P	Parents with specific concerns as above who require consultations or active skills training.	Brief program (about 80 minutes over four sessions) combining advice, rehearsal, and self-evaluation to teach parents to manage a discrete child problem behavior. May involve telephone or face-to-face clinician contact or group sessions.	Same as for Level 2.
Level 4 Broad-focus parent training Standard Triple P Group Triple P Group Teen Triple P Self-directed Triple P Self-directed Teen Triple P	Parents wanting intensive training in positive parenting skills. Typically parents of children with behavior problems such as aggressive or oppositional behavior.	Broad focus program (10 hours over 8–10 sessions) focusing on parent–child interaction and the application of parenting skills to a broad range of target behaviors. Includes generalization enhancement strategies. May be self-directed or involve telephone or face-to-face clinician contact or group sessions.	Intensive parenting interventions (e.g., mental health and welfare staff and other allied health and education professionals who regularly consult with parents about child behavior).

(cont.)

TABLE 33.1. *(cont.)*

Level of intervention	Target population	Intervention methods	Practitioners
Stepping Stones Triple P	Families of preschool children with disabilities who have or are at risk of developing behavioral or emotional disorders	A parallel 10-session individually tailored program with a focus on disabilities. Sessions typically last 60–90 minutes (with the exception of three practice sessions, which generally last 40 minutes).	Same as above.
Level 5 Intensive family intervention modules Enhanced Triple P	Parents of children with behavior problems and concurrent family dysfunction such as parental depression or stress or conflict between partners.	Intensive individually tailored program with modules (60–90 minute sessions), including practice sessions to enhance parenting skills, mood management and stress coping skills, and partner support skills.	Intensive family intervention work (e.g., mental health and welfare staff).
Pathways Triple P	Parents at risk of maltreating their children. Targets anger management problems and other factors associated with abuse.	Modules include attribution retraining and anger management.	Same as above.

of parents learning to change their parenting practices, self-regulation is operationalized to include the following five aspects.

1. *Promotion of self-sufficiency.* Parents must become independent problem solvers so they use their own resources and become less reliant on others in carrying out their parenting responsibilities. Self-sufficient parents are viewed as having the necessary resilience, personal resources, knowledge, and skills they require to parent confidently with minimal or no additional support.

2. *Increasing parental self-efficacy.* This refers to a parent's belief that they can overcome or solve a specific parenting problem. Parents with high self-efficacy have more positive expectations that change is possible. Parents of children with behavior problems tend to have lower task-specific self-efficacy in managing their daily parenting responsibilities (Sanders & Woolley, 2005).

3. *Using self-management tools.* Self-management refers to the tools and skills that parents use to enable them to change their parenting practices and become self-sufficient. These skills include self-monitoring, self-determination of performance goals and standards, self-evaluation against some performance criterion, and self-selection of parenting strategies. Because each parent is responsible for the way they choose to raise their children, parents select which aspects of their own and their child's behavior they wish to work on.

4. *Promoting personal agency.* The parent is encouraged to "own" the change process. This involves encouraging parents to attribute changes or improvements in their family situation to their own or their child's efforts rather than to chance, age, maturational factors, or other uncontrollable events (e.g., spouse's poor parenting or genes).

5. *Promoting problem solving.* It is assumed that parents are active problem solvers and that the intervention needs to equip parents to define problems, formulate options, develop a parenting plan, execute the plan, and evaluate the outcome, revising the plan as required. However, the training process needs to assist parents to generalize their knowledge and skills so they can apply principles and strategies to future problems, at different points in a child's development, and to other relevant siblings in a family.

These same self-regulation skills can be taught to children by parents in developmentally appropriate ways. Attending and responding to child-initiated interactions and prompting, modeling, and reinforcing children's problem-solving behavior promote emotional self-regulation, independence, and problem solving in children. Self-regulation principles can also be applied in the training of service providers to deliver different levels of the intervention and in troubleshooting implementation difficulties or staffing problems within an organization (Sanders & Turner, 2002).

Principles of Positive Parenting

The five core positive parenting principles (Table 33.2) that form the basis of the program were selected to address specific risk and protective factors known to predict positive developmental and mental health outcomes in children. Table 33.3 shows how these principles are operationalized into a range of specific parenting skills (see Sanders, 1999, for a more complete overview).

Program Development, Implementation, and Quality Assurance Issues

Design of Resources

A public health intervention requires a range of high-quality practitioner and parent resources. We have sought to apply the concept of self-regulation to the development of these resources. The type of parent resources used depends on the level of intervention, type of delivery modality, and how the resource was originally designed to be used. Where possible, the information included in parenting materials depicts solutions or strategies that have been subjected to empirical evaluation. In the absence of definitive trials, materials were developed based on evidence-based principles and strategies that have been shown to work for similar problems. Where evidence is available for different strategies, those different options are presented.

The principle of sufficiency means that the minimally sufficient information (i.e., just enough) is used to solve a problem. For example, although there are a large number of tip sheets dealing with specific developmental issues or behavioral problems, workbooks, and DVDs that are all part of the Triple P system, we advocate only using

TABLE 33.2. Principles of Positive Parenting

Principle	Description
A safe and engaging environment	Children of all ages need a safe, supervised, and therefore protective environment that provides opportunities for them to explore, experiment, and play. This principle is essential to promote healthy development and to prevent accidents and injuries in the home (Peterson & Saldana, 1996).
A positive learning environment	Although this involves educating parents in their role as their child's first teacher, the program specifically teaches parents to respond positively and constructively to child-initiated interactions (e.g., requests for help, information, advice, and attention) through incidental teaching and other techniques to assist children to learn how to solve problems for themselves.
Assertive and consistent discipline	Triple P teaches parents specific child management and behavior change strategies that are alternatives to coercive and ineffective discipline practices (such as shouting, threatening, or using physical punishment). These strategies include selecting ground rules for specific situations; discussing rules with children; giving clear, calm, age-appropriate instructions and requests; planned ignoring; logical consequences; quiet time (nonexclusionary time-out); and time-out.
Realistic expectations	This involves exploring with parents their expectations, assumptions, and beliefs about the causes of children's behavior and choosing goals that are developmentally appropriate for the child and realistic for the parents. Parents who are at risk of abusing their children are more likely to have unrealistic expectations of children's capabilities.
Taking care of oneself as a parent	Parenting is affected by a range of factors that impact on a parent's self-esteem and sense of well-being. All levels of Triple P specifically address this issue by encouraging parents to view parenting as part of a larger context of personal self-care, resourcefulness, and well-being and by teaching parents practical parenting skills.

those resources that are actually needed to resolve a problem. Achieving a good outcome depends on providing clear, understandable parenting information with enough detail so that parents can decide whether the depicted strategy is acceptable to them, can follow the suggested solution, and can generalize the strategy to other situations. Giving parents more information than they require can lead to information overload and redundancy and is just as problematic as providing insufficient information.

Engagement of Families

Program design strategies to improve engagement include offering tailored versions of the programs for specific high-need groups (e.g., parents of a child with a disability, maltreating parents) as well as observational documentary and lifestyle television programs that deliver evidence-based parenting messages through the mass media. The workplace has also been used effectively as a context to deliver Triple P seminars and groups because of its convenience for parents (Martin & Sanders, 2003). Implementation of an incentive program can also increase engagement: Heinrichs (2006) found that, among high-risk, low-income German parents offering a small financial incentive increased participation rates.

TABLE 33.3. Core Parenting Skills Introduced in Triple P

Basic skills					Enhanced skills		
Parent–Child relationship enhancement skills	Encouraging desirable behavior	Teaching new skills and behaviors	Managing misbehavior	Anticipating and planning	Self-regulation skills	Mood and coping skills	Partner support skills
• Spending brief quality time • Talking with children • Showing affection	• Giving descriptive praise • Giving nonverbal attention • Providing engaging activities	• Setting a good example • Using incidental teaching • Using "ask, say, do" • Using behavior charts	• Establishing ground rules • Using directed discussion • Using planned ignoring • Giving clear, calm instructions • Using logical consequences • Using quiet time • Using time-out	• Planning and advanced preparation • Discussing ground rules for specific situations • Selecting engaging activities • Providing incentives • Providing consequences • Holding follow-up discussions	• Monitoring children's behavior • Monitoring own behavior • Setting developmentally appropriate goals • Setting practice tasks • Self-evaluation of strengths and weaknesses • Setting personal goals for change	• Catching unhelpful thoughts • Relaxation and stress management • Developing personal coping statements • Challenging unhelpful thoughts • Developing coping plans for high-risk situations	• Improving personal communication habits • Giving and receiving constructive feedback • Having casual conversations • Supporting each other when problem behavior occurs • Problem solving • Improving relationship happiness

Promoting and Maintaining Program Fidelity

The maintenance of program fidelity can be extremely difficult if professionals work in isolation, and there is no workplace culture to support evidence-based interventions. Program drift can occur unless program adherence is supported by an organization's leadership so that a workplace culture around evidence-based practice is given more than lip service. Other threats to effective implementation include difficulty in accessing necessary program resources, defunding of a program, and change in policy that gives lower priority to prevention and early intervention services for children. Strategies to minimize the extent of this drift include surveying practitioners to identify aids and barriers to program implementation, the development of a survey for program managers to assess organizational readiness to support an evidence-based program, and the provision of ongoing technical advice and support to agencies implementing the program.

Commitment to Research

The Triple P model as a form of behavioral family intervention evolved within a scientific tradition that valued rigorous evaluation of outcomes and pursuit of greater understanding about what intervention works for whom and under what circumstances. Ensuring that the program has an adequate evidence base that demonstrates efficacy and effectiveness has meant that all aspects of the intervention system, including different levels of intervention, modes of delivery, and programs targeting specific problems and age groups, must be subjected to empirical scrutiny. This scientific agenda is necessary to ensure the program continues to evolve in the light of new evidence. To assist with this task, an international network of researchers in Australia, North America, Asia, and Europe has been formed to promote scientific inquiry into all aspects of the program and its dissemination. This networking has led to a series of international collaborations (e.g., Prinz, Sanders, Shapiro, Whitaker, & Lutzker, 2009) and also independent replications that contribute to the growing body of evidence concerning the intervention.

The Sociopolitical Environment

Broader Sociopolitical Context

The implementation of a public health model takes time to become properly embedded within a community. This implementation occurs in a broader sociopolitical environment, which includes:

1. Availability of political support and advocacy that transcends political party allegiance, government entities, and other policy-related institutions. A public health intervention is always vulnerable to changes of government or leadership within funding agencies. Consequently, program advocates who are prepared to publicly support a program need to be nurtured.
2. Availability of recurrent funding to ensure that a program can become embedded within an institution and can be sustained over time.
3. Having social marketing and community advocacy strategies that link parents to appropriate support services without overwhelming those services.

4. Having strong consumer advocates.
5. Having a public relations strategy designed to communicate to government, service providers, and the public about the progression of an initiative.

Challenges Arising from the Differing Perspectives of Stakeholders

Although many different stakeholders need to come together for the benefit of children, occasional misunderstandings are inevitable because of the differing perspectives and priorities of funders, disseminators, researchers, service providers, and parents (consumers). Understanding the broader motivational contexts within which each stakeholder operates can help to promote mutuality of respect and teamwork and a willingness to meet agreed-on obligations, particularly those relating to participation in evaluation.

A Multidisciplinary Workforce and "Turf Wars"

In a public health intervention, programmers usually seek to make parenting interventions as broadly accessible as possible. One way to do this is to involve service providers from many disciplines. The Triple P System Population Trial in South Carolina, for example, has been training psychologists, social workers, parent educators, preschool directors, nurses, physicians, counselors, and others in the delivery of Triple P (Prinz et al., 2009). This strategy ensures that many families have access to programming and that no discipline can monopolize the program. It assumes that agencies and organizations promote, or at least do not interfere with, broad participation across disciplines.

Service providers, agency administrators, and program disseminators have the collective professional responsibility to overcome barriers that interfere with client access to needed assistance. Turf wars take at least two forms. The more common definition of territoriality is when one agency maintains that certain services or families are that agency's sole province. The more troubling form is when an agency denies services to specific families by claiming that the service or family is not their responsibility. This type of turf war is probably driven by an agency's financial exigencies, but the consequence is that families might not receive the services they need. Strategies that promote better understanding of the respective and complementary roles of different disciplines and organizations can improve access to services by families needing support (e.g., across agencies and multidiscipline-based training).

Program Utilization

The public health approach to parenting services is relatively new but very promising. However, its success can be compromised if insufficient numbers of trained service providers become regular program users or, as a consequence of this, insufficient numbers of parents participate. Provider utilization of Triple P has been dependent on three factors: whether providers complete the full training process, including accreditation (Seng, Prinz, & Sanders, 2006); practitioners' self-efficacy after training; and the level of organizational support providers receive (Turner, Nicholson, & Sanders, 2009).

We have used a number of strategies to promote continued program use following initial training. These include establishing a web-based support network for service providers and their managers or supervisors (*www.triplep.net* and *www.triplep.org*), the assignment of dissemination staff to provide technical support, the promotion of peer supervision groups, briefing days for line managers to enable them to better support staff in their organization, and the development of web tools for easier, more convenient program use.

SELF-REGULATION APPROACH TO INTERNATIONAL DISSEMINATION

We have taken an ecological or systems–contextual approach to dissemination, which views professionals' consulting practices as being a complex interaction between the quality of the intervention, the skills training, and the posttraining environment. Dissemination does not commence until a program has undergone rigorous scientific evaluation with significant positive outcomes for parents and children. With the empirical validation of an intervention satisfied, two complementary perspectives underpin our dissemination efforts.

First, our dissemination efforts are based on the same self-regulatory approach used in our parent education programs. The focus here is on promoting professional behavior change through self-directed learning and personal responsibility for skill development (e.g., Karoly, 1993). We propose that practitioners are more likely to implement a new program if they are given appropriate training and support to feel confident in their ability to implement the program and are taught skills to monitor, set personal goals, self-evaluate, and improve their consulting practices. Practitioners are encouraged to actively problem solve so they become more confident and trust their own judgment and become less reliant on others in making clinical decisions. As with the parenting sessions, an active skills training process is incorporated into Triple P training for practitioners to enable skills to be modeled and practiced.

Second, our systems-contextual approach aims to support practitioners' program use in their workplace. Professional change is thought more likely to occur when managers, administrators, and professional colleagues support the adoption of the innovation (Backer, Liberman, & Kuehnel, 1986) and when supervision, feedback, and support are available.

Consequently, an effective dissemination process must not only adequately train practitioners in the content and processes of an intervention, but it must also strategically form alliances with participating organizations to ensure that program adoption is supported by administrators and staff (Backer et al., 1986). Central to this is the identification of at least one internal advocate, or champion, from an organization who can foster internal support for the program and the development of strategies for informing administrators about the distinguishing features of the intervention, its potential benefits, and the procedures and cost of adoption. Triple P has introduced a training and accreditation program and a range of workplace support strategies in line with its ecological perspective, as outlined next.

THE TRIPLE P SYSTEM OF PROFESSIONAL TRAINING

The effective dissemination of Triple P required a cost-effective method of training the professional workforce. Over a 3-year period (1996–1998), a standardized professional training program was developed for all levels of Triple P intervention. In designing the training program, several principles were adhered to, discussed next.

Active Skills-Based Training

To be effective, the program adopted a skills training approach that involved a combination of didactic input, video and live demonstration of core consultation skills, small-group exercises to practice skills, problem-solving exercises, course readings, and competency-based assessment. This assessment included a written quiz and live or video-taped demonstration by participants to show that they had mastered core competencies specific to the level of training undertaken.

Brevity and Cost-Effectiveness

If the evidence-based programs were designed as a university-based course, employers would be reluctant to release staff for training. Consequently, Triple P training was designed to be relatively brief to minimize disruption to staff schedules and to reduce the need for relief workers while staff undertook training. The training experience was structured to include background reading, attendance at a 1- to 5-day training workshop (based on the level of intervention), and attendance at a 1-day accreditation workshop 8–12 weeks after initial training.

Data Responsiveness

An evidence-based program must continue to evolve on the basis of evidence. Hence, every course is carefully evaluated and feedback elicited on the training course content, quality of presentation, opportunities for active participation, and practitioners' overall consumer satisfaction. Practitioner feedback is incorporated into revisions of the training program.

Viability of the Training Program

Because we have had no specific grants to disseminate the program, a training cost structure was required that was affordable for agencies and individuals and financially viable. The training program was originally conducted by training staff from the Parenting and Family Support Centre at the University of Queensland. However, as demand for training increased, a new entity was established to manage all aspects of program dissemination. This entity, Triple P International was licensed by the University of Queensland to conduct training on its behalf on a self-sustaining basis. Hence, the research and development functions were consolidated within the university, and the training and dissemination functions became part of Triple P International, a one-stop shop that handles Triple P publications, video production, and dissemination.

Eligibility to Participate

The Triple P system of intervention uses a wide range of professions in the health, education, and social service sectors to deliver the program. The only requirement is that participants have professional training in psychology, medicine, nursing, social work, counseling, or another related field that has provided prior exposure to principles of child development. Most training courses involve an interdisciplinary mix and bring together participants with quite diverse backgrounds, theoretical orientations to working with families, and varied clinical experience. Although the training is cognitive-behavioral in theoretical orientation, we have found that prior exposure to this orientation is not essential for participants to successfully implement the program.

Course Requirements

Successful completion of a Triple P training course and accreditation involves the following: completion of set readings; attendance at a training course; and completion of accreditation requirements, including a quiz to demonstrate knowledge of theory, program content, and process issues involved in consulting with families. Initially, we conducted Triple P training with accreditation being optional. Since 1998, accreditation has been incorporated into the training process, and only practitioners who complete accreditation requirements can be considered properly trained to deliver the interventions.

Selection, Training, and Accreditation of Trainers

Courses are typically conducted by clinical or educational psychologists with training and experience in the field of behavioral family intervention. Professionals invited to become trainers undergo an intensive 2-week training program. After initial induction, trainers are provisionally accredited and can begin conducting training, under supervision, from Triple P International. To be considered fully trained, trainers have to complete a skills-based accreditation process. Trainers do not work independently and use standardized materials, which serves to ensure program integrity.

Maintaining the Quality of Training

To maintain intervention integrity, it is essential that the training process itself is carefully controlled to minimize program drift at source. To prevent program drift, all trainers use standardized materials (including participant notes, training exercises, and training videotapes demonstrating core skills) and adhere to a quality assurance process. Trainers become part of a trainer network and have to adhere to a quality assurance process to maintain their accreditation.

CHALLENGES IN DISSEMINATION

Disseminating a program developed in the Southern Hemisphere is not an easy or straightforward process. Apart from the fact that Australia is seen by most Europeans, North Americans, and Asians as a considerable distance away, there are special communication challenges because of time zone differences. Despite these challenges, the Triple P system has been disseminated, to varying degrees, across 17 countries, testifying to the robustness of the training program and adaptability to different cultural groups.

Creating an Evidence-Based System of Professional Training

Engaging a motivated workforce to deliver Triple P requires strategic planning by organizations, key stakeholders, and funding bodies. Engaging a workforce that is committed to professional development, accepting of change, and willing to embark on evidence-based practices with line management support will ensure better program usage and uptake. To achieve these outcomes, standardized professional training programs have been developed for all levels of Triple P intervention. In addition to the core training courses, combined and extension courses are available to suit the service delivery modalities of the organization, ensuring wherever possible a goodness of fit that also takes into account the professional development needs of staff. Courses vary from 1–5 days in duration for part 1 (i.e., initial training) with an additional day scheduled 2–3 months posttraining for part 2 (i.e., accreditation).

Promoting and Maintaining Program Quality

The establishment of a quality assurance system has been imperative not only to increase consumer confidence and Triple P's credibility at a broader community level but also to improve work processes and efficiency and enable the organization to improve provision of services to families.

The Triple P disseminating team provides consultative support to organizations to ensure smooth program transition and implementation for new providers (e.g., troubleshooting obstacles). However, their optimal goal is to impart knowledge and skills to managers and organizational representatives so that organizations are empowered to work independently and learn to celebrate their successes and problem solve issues internally.

Creating an environment for the successful rollout of Triple P also requires adequate provision of funding for program implementation, including professional training for staff and implementation resources for families, which will allow organizations to build solid foundations to enhance future sustainability. Of particular importance is that organizations have the infrastructure in place to adequately manage training, especially when large-scale rollouts of Triple P occur with short timelines, typically reliant on funding releases and subsequent early-onset dates for the start-up phase of the operation. Organizations can work toward this process by lowering perception of barriers to implementation of Triple P by providing the necessary workplace supports to increase practitioner self-efficacy (e.g., line management support, setting realistic targets for program uptake, opportunities for ongoing professional development).

The Triple-P Approach to Workplace Support

Our approach has focused on the goals of internal advocacy, supervision, and administrative support. It has been further informed by a survey of more than 1,000 professionals following training in Primary Care Triple P (Turner et al., 2009), which identified a number of barriers for primary care staff in delivering the program following training. Many of the common barriers were related to the posttraining work environment, such as integration of the program with their usual caseload or responsibilities, access to supervision, and ability to schedule after-hours appointments. To circumvent such issues and maximize agency support for the introduction of Triple P, the following strategies have been used. These strategies have been developed through the statewide dissemination of Triple P within the Queensland Health Department.

Information and Administrative Support

The Triple P team endeavors to provide information and support specific to the needs of each agency adopting the program. Support is provided at a number of levels. We provide an orientation for administrators, supervisors, or managers with clear information about the program being introduced (e.g., its evidence base, format, target populations), training and accreditation procedures, and expectations of the agency and staff members to be involved in implementing the program (e.g., flexible work hours to allow for late appointments and evening groups). This has been achieved through orientation briefings, development of procedural guidelines and performance targets, regular updates and reviews of performance targets, and assistance in identifying and overcoming any barriers to implementation. We also aim to support practitioners implementing the program by ensuring that staff have access to adequate training, supervision (see following discussion), and resources and providing strategies and materials for program promotion (e.g., brochures and posters, sign-up sheets displayed at schools and community centers, press releases). We also provide regular updates on Triple P research and dissemination to agencies and practitioners via a biannual newsletter and web pages (e.g., *www.triplep.net*).

Promotion of Supervision Networks

Research has identified the importance of ongoing supervision in psychological practice for promoting greater utilization of the training and for maintaining program fidelity in a dissemination strategy (e.g., Henggeler, Schoenwald, Liao, Letourneau, & Edwards, 2002). In the dissemination of Triple P, we encourage the establishment of peer support networks and adopt a self-regulatory approach to supervision. These self-regulatory skills enable practitioners to direct their own learning, skill acquisition, and problem solving subsequent to participating in skills-training workshops.

Consultation Backup

Ongoing contact with program inventors has also been proposed to support program implementation in dissemination efforts (Backer et al., 1986). The Triple P team has encouraged practitioners to access backup consultative support posttraining and provides constant support via e-mail contact, teleconferences, staff meetings, and update seminars to address administrative issues (e.g., data management, performance indicators), logistical issues (e.g., avoidance of accreditation workshops because of anxiety, referral strategies), and clinical issues (e.g., dealing with specific populations, clinical process problems) identified by practitioners. These contacts actively engage agency staff in troubleshooting.

Strategies for Defusing Misinformation and Resistance

Our efforts to inform staff and management of the program, respond to their concerns about its introduction, and engage them in the process of dissemination go a long way to defusing potential organizational resistance. We have also developed strategies to address misinformation or myths about Triple P that have come to our attention. Often these myths (e.g., "It only works with middle-class families," "It's inflexible," "It's too behavioral") are based on hearsay rather than experience or evidence or are contrary to evidence. The approach we take, and encourage others to take, is to be open and nondefensive and, wherever possible, to let the data do the talking.

CHALLENGES AND OPPORTUNITIES FOR INTERNATIONAL DISSEMINATION

Working with Different Nationalities

Triple P has been implemented with many diverse cultures since its large-scale international dissemination approximately 10 years ago. Our experience since then tells us that there are more similarities than differences across nations as parents worldwide have similar concerns about raising their children. Parent support practitioners (PSPs) working with these diverse families voice issues that have a consistent theme (e.g., engagement of hard-to-reach families, low-literacy families) and pose challenges to program usage globally. To date, Triple P training programs have followed the same standardized format across all countries supported by translated resources. To fully appreciate the different and unique aspects of a culture, training is tailored to account for contextual factors with both minority groups and culturally diverse populations. As Triple P continues to gain international acceptance in different countries (e.g., Middle East) and among different minority groups (e.g., indigenous populations), consideration may need to be given to the delivery of training, translation of professional resources, and modification of processes required for accreditation (e.g., video demonstration of skills by trained professionals vs. live delivery) when dealing with developing nations with limited professional resources (e.g., Southeast Asia).

Provision of Ongoing Support

Triple P recognizes the need to provide ongoing professional support to newly trained practitioners and organizations to ensure quality practice, especially during the initial year of training and impementation. Given the expanse of Triple P dissemination worldwide, the following model was used extensively within the United Kingdom as part of Triple P's involvement with the British government's Respect projects. This ongoing support model is made up of two components: (1) technical assistance, defined as the provision of information using a self-regulatory process that guides best practice in program delivery (e.g., addresses clinically relevant issues such as application of strategies and generalization of parenting strategies); and (2) Consultative support, which encapsulates the sharing of knowledge in a self-regulatory context to enhance the dissemination process (e.g., discussing issues related to engagement of families, sustainability, training of practitioners). A central goal of this self-regulatory model is the development of an organization's capacity for self-regulation and, ultimately, independence.

Tailoring EBPPs

Tailoring strategies has enabled Triple P to be used in a diverse range of cultural and delivery contexts. Triple P's flexible tailoring philosophy encourages PSPs to preserve the key or essential elements of the program but gives them freedom to change or adapt examples to make them more relevant to specific client populations. Through this type of tailoring, core concepts and procedures are preserved but the idiosyncratic needs of particular parent groups are also attended to (e.g., parents of multiples, parents of gifted children or those with special needs, intellectual disability, autism spectrum disorder, chronic illness such as asthma). We have also used consumer preference surveys to solicit parents' and practitioners' views on the cultural appropriateness and relevance of parenting procedures, materials (written and DVD), program features, and delivery methods (Sanders et al., 2008). Interestingly, Sanders et al. showed that the most important program design feature, endorsed by 94% of parents as being "very important," was that it had been proven to work. This finding confirms the importance consumers attach to programs having an evidence base.

Tailoring of Training Methods

As Triple P training is disseminated to a broad range of service providers, the delivery of training courses has to be customized to a certain extent to cater to the special characteristics and needs of the trainee. This can be accomplished by ensuring that trainers are familiar with the local context, including where different providers work, their role in providing parenting support, their professional backgrounds, and level of experience. A good trainer must be flexible enough to attend to the experience and learning styles of the group while ensuring that essential content is properly covered. This tailoring can involve selection of audience-relevant case examples and illustrations, drawing on the knowledge, experience, and expertise of the group, and pointing out the variant and invariant features of the program.

Fidelity Monitoring and Concerns about External Intrusion

Some EBPPs have extensive systems of external fidelity monitoring to promote competent use of a program. The Triple P quality assurance monitoring system adopts a self-regulatory framework, where the responsibility for fidelity resides with the agency rather than the disseminator.

DIRECTIONS FOR FUTURE RESEARCH

The task we have undertaken in creating the Triple P system is to develop and properly test the efficacy and effectiveness of a full suite of parenting programs tailored to the needs of individual parents. Such an ambitious undertaking requires the sustained commitment of a number of prevention scientists and a dissemination organization that can translate findings from research into accessible programs for the community.

Parenting in Developing Nations

The next stage in the evolution of parent support programs is to develop and evaluate culturally appropriate and relevant adaptations of existing programs for use in developing nations. Countries where human life is characterized by poverty, war, famine, disease, and natural disasters have very different needs. Parents and children living in these traumatic conditions may benefit from parental support by well-trained local providers, typically well-respected professionals and community members.

Education of Key Stakeholders and Policy Advisers

Barriers exist as budget cycles, short-term vision for the political agenda and allocation of funding, and changes with elected parliaments make it difficult to secure longer term funding despite the societal advantages of adopting Triple P. One of the benefits of the Triple P system is that it not only has a strong evidence base but can be easily implemented as part of core business, with a proven track record in dissemination within government and nongovernment bodies worldwide. To ensure long-term funding and program survival, key stakeholders and policy advisers must be engaged and their support secured.

Optimizing the Benefits of New Technologies

Despite the proliferation of parenting websites, there is little evidence to refute or support the efficacy of this method of knowledge dissemination. Specifically, randomized trials are needed to determine whether web-based delivery of parent information advice changes parenting practices or children's behavior.

CONCLUSIONS

This chapter has documented the evolution of the Triple P—Positive Parenting Program as a multilevel-system EBPP designed to reduce the prevalence rates of social, emotional, and behavioral problems in children. The program continues to evolve in the light of new evidence showing that it can be successfully implemented in diverse cultural contexts. The challenge remains to implement procedures that promote fidelity and program use by service providers in a way that advances professional development and delivers the program in a manner that is effective.

REFERENCES

Backer, T. E., Liberman, R. P., & Kuehnel, T. G. (1986). Dissemination and adoption of innovative psychosocial interventions. *Journal of Consulting and Clinical Psychology, 54,* 111–118.

Biglan, A. (1995). Translating what we know about the context of antisocial behaviour into a lower prevalence of such behaviour. *Journal of Applied Behaviour Analysis, 28,* 479–492.

Collins, W. A., Maccoby, E. E., Steinberg, L., Hetherington, E. M., & Bornstein, M. H. (2000). Contemporary research on parenting: The case for nature and nurture. *American Psychologist, 55,* 218–232.

Graeff-Martins, A., Flament, M., Fayyad, J., Tyano, S., Jensen, P., & Rohde, L. (2008). Diffusion of efficacious interventions for children and adolescents with mental health problems. *Journal of Child Psychology and Psychiatry, 49,* 335–352.

Heinrichs, N. (2006). The effects of two different incentives on recruitment rates of families into a prevention program. *Journal of Primary Prevention, 27,* 345–366.

Henggeler, S. W., Schoenwald, S. K., Liao, J. G., Letourneau, E. J., & Edwards, D. L. (2002). Transporting efficacious treatments to field settings: The link between supervisory practices and therapist fidelity in MST programs. *Journal of Clinical Child and Adolescent Psychology, 31,* 155–167.

Karoly, P. (1993). Mechanisms of self-regulation: A systems view. *Annual Review of Psychology, 44,* 23–52.

Loeber, R., & Farrington, D. P. (1998). Never too early, never too late: Risk factors and successful interventions for serious and violent juvenile offenders. *Studies on Crime and Crime Prevention, 7,* 7–30.

Martin, A. J., & Sanders, M. R. (2003). Balancing work and family: A controlled evaluation of the Triple P—Positive Parenting Program as a work-site intervention. *Child and Adolescent Mental Health, 8,* 161–169.

Nowak, C., & Heinrichs, N. (2008). A comprehensive meta-analysis of Triple P—Positive Parenting Program using hierarchical linear modeling: Effectiveness and moderating variables. *Clinical Child and Family Psychology Review, 11,* 114–144.

Peterson, L., & Saldana, L. (1996). Accelerating children's risk for injury: Mothers' decisions regarding common safety rules. *Journal of Behavioural Medicine, 19,* 317–331.

Prinz, R. J., Sanders, M. R., Shapiro, C. J., Whitaker, D. J., & Lutzker, J. R. (2009). Population-based prevention of child maltreatment: The U.S. Triple P system population trial. *Prevention Science, 10*(1), 1–12.

Sanders, M. R. (1999). The Triple P—Positive Parenting Program: Towards an empirically validated multilevel parenting and family support strategy for the prevention of behavior and emotional problems in children. *Clinical Child and Family Psychology Review, 2,* 71–90.

Sanders, M. R. (2008). The Triple P—Positive Parenting Program as a public health approach to strengthening parenting. *Journal of Family Psychology, 22,* 506–517.

Sanders, M. R., Haslam, D. M., Stallman, H. M., Calam, R., & Southwell, C. (2009). *Designing effective interventions for working parents: A survey of parents in the U.K. workforce.* Manuscript in preparation.

Sanders, M. R., Ralph, A., Sofronoff, K., Gardiner, P., Thompson, R., Dwyer, S., et al. (2008). Every family: A population approach to reducing behavioral and emotional problems in children making the transition to school. *Journal of Primary Prevention, 29,* 197–222.

Sanders, M. R., & Turner, K. M. T. (2002). The role of the media and primary care in the dissemination of evidence-based parenting and family support interventions. *The Behavior Therapist, 25,* 156–166.

Sanders, M. R., & Woolley, M. L. (2005). The relationship between maternal self-efficacy and parenting practices: Implications for parent training. *Child: Care, Health and Development, 31,* 65–73.

Seng, A. C., Prinz, R. J., & Sanders, M. R. (2006). The role of training variables in effective dissemination of evidence-based parenting interventions. *International Journal of Mental Health Promotion, 8,* 19–27.

Turner, K. M. T., Nicholson, J. M., & Sanders, M. R. (2009). *The role of practitioner self-efficacy, training, program and workplace factors on the implementation of an evidence-based parenting intervention in primary care.* Manuscript submitted for preparation.

34

From Policy Pinball to Purposeful Partnership[1]

The Policy Contexts of Multisystemic Therapy Transport and Dissemination

SONJA K. SCHOENWALD

OVERVIEW

The promise of multisystemic therapy (MST; Henggeler, Schoenwald, Borduin, Rowland, & Cunningham, 2009) for juvenile offenders—reducing criminal activity and substance use, preventing out-of-home placement, improving youth and family functioning, and cost savings—has led service systems, payers, practitioners, and families in 32 states and 10 nations to establish MST programs. Delivering on that promise, no matter how new or how seasoned the MST therapist or program, is the function of the quality assurance and improvement system used by MST Services, LLC and its 21 Network Partner organizations—collectively, the purveyors of MST (Fixsen, Naoom, Blase, Friedman, & Wallace, 2005)—to support the transport and implementation of MST in diverse communities and cultures. Prior publications review the theory, research, and experience informing the journey toward evidence-based transport and implementation of MST; the MST quality assurance/quality improvement system; and empirical evidence supporting linkages among components of that system and youth outcomes in usual-care settings (Schoenwald, 2008). To recap, therapist adherence to MST has been found to predict short- and long-term youth behavioral and criminal outcomes and consultant and supervisor adherence to predict therapist adherence and youth outcomes.

The purpose of this chapter is to consider the interplay of policy initiatives with MST transport, implementation, and dissemination. Two disclaimers are warranted. First, although published research has identified factors at multiple levels of the practice context affecting the implementation and outcomes of MST in usual-care settings, we lack such evidence with respect to factors affecting the diffusion (naturally occurring adoption) and dissemination (proactive efforts to promote adoption) of MST. This chapter is thus based largely on our experiences and their consistency with theory and research in other fields (e.g., technology transfer, diffusion of innovation, organizational implementation of innovation, and health services).

Second, the circumstances that have facilitated the transport of MST may not characterize prospects for the transport of other empirically tested psychosocial treatments for youths. To wit:

1. The initial transport and subsequent diffusion of MST was demand driven: Service provider organizations and government agencies asked for MST even before we had developed any transport capacity.
2. The government agencies were legally mandated to serve the target population for which MST was originally designed: juvenile offenders.
3. Serving that target population was very costly for the government because "service" consisted primarily of incarceration, residential treatment, and other out-of-home placements.
4. Evidence from randomized trials supported the long-term clinical and cost-effectiveness MST for this target population and preceded its transport.

These circumstances created a public health context for the transport of MST, albeit primarily in the juvenile justice sector and via implementation by private provider organizations.

A PUBLIC HEALTH PERSPECTIVE ON THE TRANSPORT OF MST

As explicated elsewhere (Schoenwald & Henggeler, 2004), a public health perspective assumes that both a specific target population and the general population benefit from a treatment for the target population. The providers and recipients of the treatment are dispersed across diverse communities in which local norms govern perceptions of illness, access to care, and health care practices (Institute of Medicine, 2001). Yet the risk to the target population and general public is sufficient that a specific intervention must be effectively delivered in the context of these local variations. Regulations and legal mandates can be used to provide at least a "floor" and "ceiling" for local and individual variations in a practice (Ferlie & Shortell, 2001) and are among mechanisms used in public health strategies (Thornicroft & Tansella, 1999).

In the case of MST, chronic and violent juvenile offenders constitute the target population of interest to public systems and their contracted service provider organizations. The demonstrated benefits of MST for this population (decreased recidivism, out-of-home placement, and behavior problems, among others) translate into greater community safety and cost savings for public service systems. The transport of MST thus occurs in the context of legal mandates governing the custody of juvenile offenders (i.e., incarceration, residential treatment facility, group home) and services provided to them. Note, however, these mandates do not necessarily require effective or evidence-based services to be provided.

Legal Mandates and Evidence-Based Treatment Implementation

Legal mandates (laws) do not guarantee that effective treatments will be implemented. Mandates can build a floor and ceiling for practice, for example, terminating funding for demonstrably ineffective programs like boot camps for juvenile offenders. Conversely, with or without changes in law, regulations and budgetary actions often affect clinical practices. In our experience, legal mandates can affect MST implementation and outcomes through their impact on service parameters, service funding, definition of the target population eligible for service, and the time and scale on which they are enacted.

Service Parameters

Some examples of service parameters affecting implementation are as follows: personnel allowed to deliver the service (e.g., physicians, licensed social workers); medical necessity criteria governing client eligibility for the service; and requirements regarding treatment session duration, frequency, participants, and length of treatment episode. Sources of such requirements include referral, funding, and collateral agencies. For example, even when a referring juvenile justice agency and Medicaid payer endorse the short duration (4–5 months) of MST, a judge or probation chief may require a youth to stay in treatment for a yearlong term of probation, a major aberration of MST protocols.

Funding

Legal mandates activated in the absence of sufficient resources to implement a treatment can corrupt its implementation and sustainability. Four funding issues seem critical to mandates designed to support the import and implementation of evidence-based treatments like MST.

1. If it is more profitable to a local provider organization to deliver a treatment of unknown effectiveness (e.g., residential treatment) to a specific target population than to deliver an evidence-based treatment for that population (e.g., MST), odds are low that the evidence-based treatment will substantially penetrate that market of service providers. So long as one or more service systems that contracts with provider organizations for youth services is willing to support the relatively more lucrative residential rate, then penetration of an effective and less costly alternative will be limited.

2. Where evidence exists that model-specific training and implementation support are needed to sustain treatment fidelity and associated client outcomes, then funding must be provided for the training and ongoing implementation support.

3. Funding must be adequate to subsume the start-up costs associated with staffing and initial training incurred before services can be delivered and billed.

4. Adequate "fit" is needed between the payment mechanism and demand characteristics of the treatment. For example, fee-for-service billing mechanisms requiring therapists to document 15-minute increments of service fit poorly with several hallmark features of MST: variable and functionally driven duration of sessions; therapist travel to the homes, schools, and neighborhoods and attendance at court hearings and probation meetings; and frequent telephone contact with the family and others participating in treatment. In contrast, case rates and daily rates better accommodate these features

of MST. Accordingly, during the MST program development process, the MST purveyor, payers, and provider organizations work together to craft a financial plan for the proposed MST program, align reimbursement mechanisms as much as possible with the contours of MST, and assess sufficiency of funding to sustain the program from start-up to full operation. Although decisions about funding levels and program reimbursement mechanisms ultimately lie with the service systems funding the MST program, stakeholders often attempt such alignment in the interest of increasing the likelihood that the new program will be successful. When alignment cannot be optimized, the semiannual program implementation review enables all parties to monitor the extent to which misalignment may contribute to problems with program implementation and outcomes.

Target Population

The implementation and outcomes of an evidence-based treatment can degrade when a mismatch exists between the population mandated to receive services and that for which evidence of treatment effectiveness exists. When mismatch in target population is apparent from the inception of a new initiative or mandate, the development of an MST program is not pursued. A state child welfare system seeking to import standard MST as an antidote for child abuse and neglect is one such example. Often, however, the potential fit between a target population of interest and MST is not clear, because criteria stakeholders use to define the population do not map directly onto the clinical and functional criteria characterizing youths effectively treated with MST. For example, when a class action suit is successfully brought against a state, those mandated to receive services might be identified on legal grounds. Examples include youths court ordered to residential placement without prior access to community-based alternatives, youths in detention whose mental health services are suspended as a result of the detention, and youths with individualized education plans denied mental health services. In such cases, the conjoint task of the model developers, purveyors, and stakeholders is to consider the overlap in the class action and MST treatment populations and to develop strategies that support treatment with MST of appropriate youths.

An alternative strategy is to test scientifically treatment modifications specified for the target population in question. In collaboration with the Department of Health in Hawaii, for example, a continuum of MST-based services for Felix Class youths was developed and tested (Rowland et al., 2005). The Felix Class encompassed juvenile offenders and youths with psychiatric histories resembling participants in a randomized controlled trial testing an MST adaptation for youths experiencing psychiatric crises (Henggeler et al., 2003). The experimental MST continuum services were funded by the state, with the research conjointly funded by the state and the Annie E. Casey Foundation. Collaborating with the state in response to this suit catalyzed the launch of standard MST programs for juvenile offenders in Hawaii. Although the continuum was dismantled after the research and Felix settlement ended, the standard MST programs continue to operate.

Finally, even when an MST program is established for the appropriate target population, net widening to other populations can occur over time for a variety of reasons. An organization contracted by a juvenile justice system to provide MST to offenders may be asked by another service system, such as mental health, to serve ostensibly similar populations. Because youths with serious antisocial behavior and in trouble with the law may also be involved with mental health or child welfare systems, some youths referred by other systems do indeed reflect the population MST was designed to serve. Others, however, do not.

Time and Scale

Mandates often embody two sources of potential mismatch with MST implementation: time and scale. Mandates typically call for the broad use, within a fairly short time period, of a new type of service. Sometimes state juvenile justice or mental health agencies inform contracted service provider organizations that a new mandate requires bringing new services on line within 3 to 6 months. The steps of MST program development cannot be accomplished so quickly, however, without risking a mismatch between the program and needs of the community, fidelity of implementation, and sustainability. For simpler technologies, such as new medications or brief diagnostic screens, establishing an aggressive timeline for broad penetration within the provider community may suffice to facilitate adequate, large-scale implementation. For interventions requiring multiple changes in practitioner behavior, multiple strategies are likely required to ensure adequate implementation, and wide, rapid deployment may corrupt implementation (Grimshaw et al., 2001). Requiring numerous provider organizations to implement a complex treatment on a short timeline outstrips the capacity of the organizations and purveyors of evidence-based treatments to ensure the treatment can be delivered as intended to the effect desired by the mandating agency.

THE DIFFUSION OF MST: THE *S*-SHAPED CURVE

As noted in this chapter's disclaimer, we have not conducted prospective studies of the rate of MST diffusion or of factors affecting that rate. However, some information is available about the number of programs established in the 12 years since MSTS was founded. This information suggests that the trajectory of MST transport and diffusion to date resembles the *S*-shaped rate of adoption of innovation first observed in research on the uptake of agricultural technologies (Rogers, 1995). The *S*-curve describes a rate of adoption that begins with a small number of early adopters, accelerates fairly quickly when mainstream adopters begin to sign on, slows as mainstream adoption continues, and then accelerates again until the innovative practice becomes the new status quo, when adoption plateaus or even declines slightly. Within the first 5 years of transport, 100 MST teams were established, and in the subsequent 7 years a growth rate of approximately 25% annually resulted in expansion to 425 teams in 2008. However, with only 10% of juvenile offenders in the United States receiving any evidence-based treatment, including MST, it is premature to assert that MST has significantly penetrated the mainstream of practice for this population.

Starting the S-Curve: MST Transport Begins

Key events in the chronology of MST transport are depicted in Figure 34.1, and the research, practice, and policy contexts that intertwined to influence these events are described in the remaining sections of this chapter. Between 1986 and 1990, results were published in academic journals of a quasi-experimental study of MST with delinquent

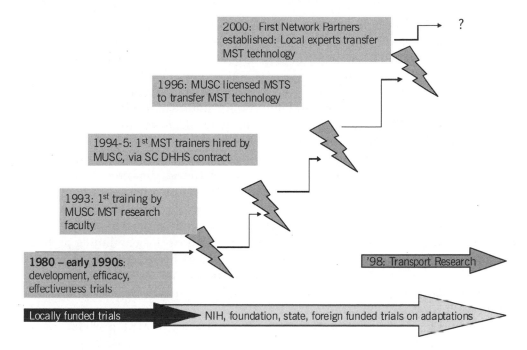

FIGURE 34.1. Seminal events in Multisystemic therapy (MST) transport capacity building and research (MUSC, Medical University of South Carolina; MSFTS, MST Services, LLC; SC DHHS, South Carolina Department of Health and Human Services; NIH, National Institutes of Health).

youths and of small-scale university-based efficacy trials of MST for other populations (see Chapter 17 by Henggeler and Schaeffer, this volume). Results supporting the clinical and cost-effectiveness of MST in a community-based randomized trial in South Carolina of MST with chronic, violent offenders were first published in 1992, with long-term results published in 1993. Long-term results from a university-based trial in Missouri were published in 1995, and additional community-based trials underway in South Carolina were providing promising findings. The community-based trials were launched in collaboration with the South Carolina Departments of Juvenile Justice and Mental Health, which helped fund the MST and control condition services. These state agencies thus knew the study results before they were published and expressed interest in replicating MST throughout the state. Presentations of the clinical and cost-effectiveness findings at national juvenile justice and mental health conferences prompted queries from officials and service provider organizations from other states. Hence, the demand to transport MST to usual-care settings began, and, as described subsequently, two federal initiatives catalyzed that demand.

In 1993 and 1994, several private and three public service provider organizations treating juvenile offenders sought the model developers' assistance in establishing MST programs. Initially, faculty at the Family Services Research Center (FSRC), Medical University of South Carolina (MUSC), provided training and ongoing consultation in MST teams in these organizations on a "moonlighting" basis. The faculty could not, however, retain their research productivity and at the same time adequately meet the needs of the therapists and provider organizations attempting MST implementation. Hence, funding was sought to hire experienced professionals to provide such training and supervision. Because the training focused on clinicians in community-based provider organizations rather than university faculty or students, the university's ability to offer support for such training positions was constrained.

In 1994, the South Carolina Department of Health and Human Services, having received a federal block grant to support family preservation services, asked the FSRC to provide training in MST to such programs and invited faculty to collaborate in establishing standards for Medicaid reimbursement for MST. This created the first opportunity to cultivate expertise in MST and MST training among individuals other than model developers and faculty. Because state dollars paid the trainer salaries, however, trainers could not assist clinicians and organizations outside of the state. Once again, a moonlighting arrangement was established to support off-hours training for out-of-state provider organizations. Again, the arrangement did not meet the needs of organizations attempting to develop and implement MST programs. In 1996, to address this continuing problem, MUSC and the treatment developers established a university-licensed, for-profit technology transfer company, MST Services, LLC (MSTS), that could charge training fees to support the salaries of trainers on a full-time basis. Under this agreement with MUSC, MSTS licenses provider organizations to use MST to treat appropriate youth populations. The MSTS website, *www.mstservices.com*, includes a list of MST provider organizations and the status of their license (full, provisional, or terminated). Policymakers, public systems administrators, clinicians, and consumers can use this site to determine whether a particular provider organization operates a licensed MST program.

Upward Movement on the S-Curve: Key Federal Policy Initiatives

Two federal initiatives incubating in the early 1990s came to fruition shortly after MSTS was founded and stimulated additional demand for MST. The Office of Juvenile Justice and Delinquency Prevention (OJJDP) and the Center for Mental Health Services (CMHS), Substance Abuse and Mental Health Services Administration (SAMHSA), funded initiatives for target populations experiencing high rates of out-of-home placement and poor clinical, functional, and service system outcomes. The agencies took very different approaches to this task, and both catalyzed community interest in MST.

OJJDP Focus on Effective Treatments for Juvenile Offenders

Under the leadership of then-Director Shay Bilchick, OJJDP undertook to reduce juvenile delinquency and attendant incarceration and long-term deleterious effects on youths, families, communities, and taxpayers. Four strategies, identified next, focused on identifying and supporting the broader use of *effective* juvenile justice prevention and intervention strategies. These strategies stimulated demand for MST among state and county juvenile justice agencies and the organizations with which they contracted to treat juvenile offenders.

1. With the Juvenile Justice and Delinquency Prevention Council, Colorado Division of Criminal Justice, OJJDP cofunded a comprehensive review of research on effective youth violence prevention and intervention programs. This review was undertaken by leading delinquency researcher Delbert Elliott, Center for

the Study and Prevention of Violence (CSPV) at the University of Colorado at Boulder, and his colleagues. This review produced the Blueprints for Violence Prevention (Elliott, 1998).

2. Through the federal Juvenile Accountability Block Grants (JABG) program (*www.ojjdp.ncjrs.org/jabg/overview.html*), OJJDP provided grants to states for activities to reduce juvenile offending and criteria for measuring the effects of funded activities.

3. OJJDP awarded a grant to CSPV to help disseminate and evaluate the dissemination of the evidence-based Blueprints programs.

4. OJJDP provided seed funding (1) to develop manuals and measures for key aspects of MST implementation (supervision, expert consultation, program administration) and a rudimentary computerized fidelity and outcomes tracking system and (2) to conduct a pilot study of the viability of their use in nine states already implementing MST.

Because the initial Blueprints dissemination grant program did not include resources to support or monitor model-specific implementation or monitor youth outcomes, MSTS worked together with states asking Blueprints for MST to identify funding sources to provide such support. Purveyors of several other Blueprints models followed suit. The ensuing dialogue among the Blueprints model developers and purveyors, the leadership of the Blueprints initiative, and communities attempting to import the models resulted in a revision of the Blueprints dissemination strategy to include implementation support and measurement of fidelity and outcomes.

SAMHSA/CMHS Focus on Systems Change

In 1992, following several years of modest funding to improve children's mental health services via the National Institute of Mental Health Child and Adolescent Service System Program (Stroul & Friedman, 1986), the federal Comprehensive Community Mental Health Services for Children and Their Families Program began. This program provided grants to states and communities to develop systems of care to improve the access, array, and child- and family-centered nature of community-based mental health services for youths with severe emotional disturbances (SED). This system of care (SOC) initiative expanded to the majority of states within a decade of its inception.

Under the auspices of the SOC initiative, some state departments of mental health sought to import MST to treat SED youth. At the time, the aforementioned randomized trial of an MST adaptation for youths in psychiatric crises was underway and yielding promising short-term results. Thus, the MST model developers and MSTS agreed to help service provider organizations contracted by departments of mental health to implement MST with the case mix of youths falling under the SOC umbrella. This experience unfolded over 2–3 years, during which it became clear that effective treatment for some youths would require the clinical, administrative, and service adaptations being tested in the randomized trial. Evidence of the longer term outcomes of that trial were not yet known, however, and only the project director, psychiatrist, and clinical staff participating in the trial had the expertise to train and support therapists. By mutual agreement, the model developers, MSTS, and several SOC sites chose to discontinue the use of MST or to shift the target population served to juvenile offenders.

The SOC experience, among others, contributed to the creation by the MST developers and purveyors of a rubric identifying specific adaptations of MST for different populations. This rubric conveys the status of the evidence base with respect to (1) the effectiveness of those adaptations and (2) the transfer of training and clinical support expertise from the adaptation developers to purveyors needed to support community-based implementation (the adaptations rubric is available online at *www.mstservices. com*). By virtue of this discernment process, and as reflected in the SAMHSA-sponsored National Registry of Evidence-based Programs and Practices (*www.nrepp.samhsa.gov*), adaptations of MST for specific populations tested in randomized trials are now identified for stakeholders. In sum, it is incumbent on the developers and purveyors of an evidence-based treatment to engage interested stakeholders in discussion of the risks and benefits of applying that treatment to populations for which it has not been tested and, as occurred in the Hawaii example among others, to consider undertaking together research to test adaptations and alternatives before taking them to scale.

State Initiatives

State initiatives contributing to the diffusion of MST have taken several different forms and illustrate how mandates and policies can catalyze, but not guarantee, the uptake, implementation, and diffusion of evidence-based treatments. In some states, like Washington and Florida, the legislature identified juvenile crime and the associated community safety risks and costs as sufficiently onerous problems to warrant new legislation. In 1997, Washington was the first state to legislate, through the Community Juvenile Accountability Act (CJAA), the use of research-based programs to reduce juvenile crime cost-effectively. In a process that paralleled the Blueprints review, the Washington State Institute on Public Policy (WSIPP; *www.wsipp.wa.gov*) selected programs on the basis of a national research literature review; WSIPP was also contracted to evaluate the performance of the programs as implemented in Washington. Counties chose the programs they wished to implement, and service funding was partially provided by the CJAA, with federal (JABG) and Blueprints dollars contributing to the cause. Some of the chosen programs were not launched because the mechanisms for training and technical assistance had not been developed; others were implemented but yielded poorer outcomes than anticipated and were thus discontinued. Three counties established MST teams as a result of this initiative.

In 2003, the Florida legislature undertook a statewide initiative to import evidence-based treatments for juvenile offenders and evaluate the effects of those treatments in Florida. The legislation was discharged through the state Department of Juvenile Justice in a new program called Redirection. Redirection imported only models whose implementation and outcomes were favorable in Washington and other states, and MST and Functional Family Therapy were imported. At the time, research linking the MST quality assurance system components and youth outcomes, and specification of infrastructure and program practices, had advanced considerably. Accordingly, the legislature and Department of Juvenile Justice collaborated with purveyors of MST to create the infrastructure, funding, and regulations to support implementation. The regulations were thus more closely aligned than was the case when Washington pioneered the import of MST.

In the intervening years, a number of states sought to import one or more evidence-based treatments and then to expand the reach of those treatments throughout the state. States differed, however, in their approach to the task. The states' strategies can be conceptualized on a continuum from centralized to laissez-faire. Connecticut, for example, pursued a centralized approach to the import and expansion of MST. There the Department of Children and Families (DCF), responsible for serving youths in state custody, initiated the import of MST as aftercare for juvenile offenders released from out-of-home placements. State-funded evaluations of MST were favorable, and these, along with political pressures to improve services for juvenile offenders not in state custody, prompted the Court Support Services Division (CSSD) of the judicial branch to support statewide expansion of MST. Today, DCF and CSSD jointly fund a private provider organization as the Network Partner to provide training and quality assurance to all MST programs in the state. The state agencies directly reimburse contracted provider organizations for delivering MST to youths and families.

Ohio provides an example in the middle of the continuum between centralized and laissez-faire strategies to take evidence-based treatments to scale. Although the import of MST was initiated in 1996 as a result of a governor's office initiative to improve and evaluate services for juvenile offenders, the growth of MST accelerated via the state's establishment in 1999 of Coordinating Centers of Excellence (CCOEs) across all state departments (health, education, welfare, juvenile justice, mental health). The state provided infrastructure funds to support each CCOE; and the CCOE then established its own strategies for identifying practices it wished to import or develop. Within the Department of Mental Health, the Center for Innovative Practices (CIP) was established in 2003. The CIP collaborates with the local mental health boards (which control services and funds), consumer advocacy groups, universities, and sister agencies to identify and support a variety of clinical practices. As an MST Network Partner, the CIP provides the quality assurance/quality improvement system to MST programs in Ohio; the state, however, does not fund that endeavor. Thus, CIP, like MSTS and many Network Partners, pays the salaries of the training experts via contracts with provider organizations. Those organizations are paid (via services contracts) by local mental health boards to deliver MST to youths and families.

Finally, Colorado presents an example of highly decentralized, nonpublicly funded diffusion of MST. The first MST teams in Colorado were established with funding from the aforementioned federal JABG and Blueprints dissemination programs. The subsequent expansion of programs, however, was spearheaded by private provider organizations. Today, the MST Network Partner in Colorado, the Center for Effective Interventions, supports the majority of MST programs in Colorado, New Mexico, and neighboring states but receives no state or county support or sponsorship for these activities. As occurs in Ohio and Connecticut, state and county agencies contract directly with provider organizations to serve youths and families with MST.

International Parallels

The continuum of centralized to laissez-faire dissemination of MST is also apparent among international sites. Space constraints prevent elaboration on this point, but interested readers can find details in recent publications (Ogden, Christensen, Sheidow, & Holth, 2008; Schoenwald, Heiblum, Saldana, & Henggeler, 2008). Norway provides an example of a highly centralized strategy, akin to that taken in Connecticut. A Norwegian government initiative launched in 1997 to provide evidence-based treatments to the nation's youths enabled counties and collaborating municipalities to select the treatments they wished to implement. In 1999, four counties launched MST teams; today MST Norway, a Network Partner funded by the Norwegian government, supports MST programs in 17 of the 19 counties in Norway. Denmark is more similar to Ohio, in that the government provides infrastructure support to an umbrella agency, but the decision to start an MST program is locally made and funded. Finally, the Netherlands is more similar to Colorado, as private provider agencies are spearheading the import of MST and its dissemination.

Nudging Up the S-Curve: The Role of Financing Policies

In 1994, South Carolina's state Medicaid, juvenile justice, and mental health agencies provided the FSRC a first opportunity to collaborate in crafting a financing strategy to support the deployment of MST. This yearlong process included developing medical necessity criteria, clinical standards, management standards, outcomes standards, and reimbursement levels and mechanisms that would neither reward "creaming" of youths and families to serve only those less complex problems nor truncate services to collect payment prior to treatment completion. That Medicaid standard, with some revisions, continues to fund MST programs in South Carolina today, 9 years after the Medicaid agency and university agreed to suspend the university-based training of all family preservation programs in the state, most of which served child welfare populations. Currently, the state Medicaid, mental health, and juvenile justice agencies support, in collaboration with MSTS, MST programs for juvenile offenders and other youths with serious antisocial behavior at imminent risk of placement.

Nebraska and New Mexico are examples of states that also undertook the import of MST using Medicaid funding. In Nebraska, Mid Plains Rehabilitation Health Center, in collaboration with the regional Medicaid authority (Nebraska Department of Health and Human Services, Region III), began this process in 1997. Mid Plains leveraged CMHS/ SAMHSA funding for systems of care for the initial import of MST and then quickly developed a Medicaid-based revenue stream to sustain and expand MST in the state. In New Mexico, the process took longer. Before importing MST, the state's DCF had developed a Medicaid managed care program for all publicly funded behavioral health services. The sustainability and expansion of MST in New Mexico now occurs under the auspices of Medicaid managed care, but the leadership of pertinent state agencies and provider organizations worked for almost 3 years to achieve their goal of funding MST in this way. Because the sources of funding for MST programs vary within and across states, and because Medicaid coverage terms and reimbursement rates vary across states, the extent to which financing strategies for MST developed in one locale or state can generalize to another, or to other evidence-based treatments, is unclear. Examples of funding mechanisms and strategies government agencies and private service provider organizations use to develop and sustain evidence-based treatment programs, including MST, are, however, described in a recent document authored by members of the National Implementation Research Network and MST Network Partners (George, Blase, Kanary, Wotring, Bernstein, & Carter, 2008).

Moving Further Up the S-Curve: The Role of MST Network Partners

By 2000, provider organizations that had expanded their MST programs became eager to cultivate the expertise needed to train their own staff in MST, as did the state and local government agencies supporting these programs. To meet the demand for expansion, MST Network Partners were established in organizations and sites with strong track records developing and sustaining MST programs. Network Partners have the capacity to carry out the entire MST transport and implementation process from preimplementation site assessment through training, ongoing consultation, and quality assurance and improvement. The growth in the number of MST programs from 100 to 425 teams over the last 7 years has occurred primarily through the Network Partners. This expansion seems a function of two phenomena: (1) Network Partners seeking to expand their reach and capacity in the private sector and (2) government agencies seeking to bring MST to their cities, counties, states, or nations. In the latter case, government agencies continue to ask MSTS to develop and incubate new programs and to transfer oversight for the programs to a Network Partner in a nearby geographical region, or develop a new Network Partner absent a regional option, when adequate implementation and sustainability are evident.

Going to Scale: From Policy Pinball to Purposeful Partnership

Observers of public policy development have long noted that the process of coming to a decision to create a mandate is often unruly and unpredictable. An observation made more than 20 years ago remains applicable today: "In contrast to a problem-solving model in which people become aware of a problem and consider alternative solutions, it is more accurate to postulate in the case of public policy that solutions float around, in and near government, search for problems to which to become attached or political events that increase their likelihood of adoption" (Kingdon, 1984, p. 191, as cited in Morris, 2000).

In discussing the role of policy in the improvement of mental health services, John A. Morris, professor at the University of South Carolina and former state mental health director and American College of Mental Health Administration president, has proposed the metaphor of "policy pinball" for the process by which scientific evidence makes its way into practice. Morris suggests conceptualizing an intervention (e.g., medication, evidence-based treatment) as a pinball launched by the flippers of science, which, via repeated collision with three bumpers—politics, economics, and current practice—either accrues points for the player to yield a high-scoring win (evidence changes practice) or returns to the gutter. Applying this metaphor to the prospects for the transport and dissemination of evidence-based treatments, one might conceive the passive dissemination of information about treatments as a gutter ball, destined to roll back down the board once it hits the bumpers of policy, economics, and practice and perhaps before it even reaches one or more of these bumpers. An evidence-based treatment (ball) launched with training and implementation support shown to affect outcomes may fare better among the bumpers and generate a score, but the number of clinicians using the treatment and, therefore, the number of consumers benefiting from it may be low. To achieve a high-scoring game in which science changes practice in a sustainable way (the evidence-based practice is built in to the service infrastructure), persistent and coordinated maneuvering among the interplay of economic, political, and practice forces is likely needed. This metaphor suggests at least three things that ring true from our experience with the transport and diffusion of MST and that are consistent with pertinent theory and research on technology transfer and dissemination discussed next.

Collaboration Is Essential and Perpetual

As illustrated in this chapter and evidenced in social marketing research (Andreason, 1995), mandates can stimulate demand for an intervention and help sustain its implementation if sufficient resources and alignment of regulations are present. Thus, individuals and organizations seeking to transport an evidence-based treatment for a particular population would do well to cultivate and align the interests and resources of agencies with legal and financial mandates to care for that population. Achieving this starting place for transport is seldom a linear process, even for a target population such as juvenile offenders in the United States, whose custody and service are the responsibility of government agencies. This is in part because mental health services are provided predominantly by privately held organizations operating multiple programs, each of which may be funded by several different public agencies. The decision to adopt and implement an innovation—in this case MST—is thus fundamentally not made by an individual but by a system, and thus the decision process is more complicated (Rogers, 1995).

Moreover, "system" is a misnomer, because even within a single public entity with mandated authority for a target population, such as a county juvenile justice system, other units within that system (e.g., the state-level department of juvenile justice) and other systems with legal authority over the youths (probation, juvenile court) and with responsibility for the provision of service funding (e.g., a Medicaid funding agency) are in play. Each of these may be on its own trajectory with respect to the awareness, consideration, adoption, and implementation of one or more innovations for one or more target populations. The degree of communication and collaboration among them varies considerably across locales and time. Thus, to shift pinball movement from repeated ricocheting between bumpers requires nurturing collaboration among established economic, political, and practice forces and the purveyors of the new treatment.

Effective Treatments Do Not Guarantee Effective Programs

In each locale, the intervention program built between the floor and ceiling of laws and regulations can vary in ways that can attenuate implementation and outcomes, even when the program is designed to deploy an evidence-based treatment. Research on the implementation of innovations in organizations in general, and of evidence-based interventions specifically, indicates that specification and monitoring of organizational policies and practices are needed to support the implementation of a particular treatment technology (Dane & Schneider, 1998; Klein & Knight, 2005; Mihalic, 2004). Early experiences with MST transport illustrated the need to adapt existing organizational policies and practices to better fit the demand characteristics of MST. For example, personnel policies based on the contours of office-based outpatient service fit poorly with the irregular hours, round-the-clock availability, and home and community deployment of service that characterize MST. Thus, an organizational manual with guidelines, strategies, and resources for developing and sustaining MST programs was developed early in the transport process (Strother, Swenson, & Schoenwald, 1998). In addition, although government and private entities establish their own strategies for taking MST to scale in their locales, the responsibility for ensuring the adequate implementation of MST during this process lies conjointly with the organization operating the program and purveyors of MST. When a state or local dissemination strategy or regulation, or the internal policy or practice of a service organization, threatens the integrity of MST implementation and outcomes, then the organization and MST purveyor work together, and with pertinent stakeholders, to generate solutions that preserve integrity.

Purveyor Organizations Are Critical

Taking a complex evidence-based treatment like MST to usual-care settings has to be someone's job. Getting the pinball to stay on the boards is hard work, and the ball can roll into the gutter after an errant bounce on any bumper even before a program is established. The game can also end absent sufficient training and ongoing clinical support to ensure adequate implementation and achieve the promised outcomes. Accordingly, purveyor organizations dedicated to treatment transport have been developed for MST and several other evidence-based treatments for youths (see Schoenwald & Henggeler, 2003).

DIRECTIONS FOR RESEARCH

This chapter was developed to illustrate the interplay of laws and policy initiatives with the transport, diffusion, and dissemination of MST. Its goal was to facilitate the work of stakeholders in children's mental health seeking to expand the use of effective treatments and to develop and test such treatments in practice contexts. Still needed, however, is a sound evidence base regarding the nature and interplay of the most salient predictors of the effective transport, implementation, and dissemination of evidence-based treatments. Such evidence is needed to develop and test programmatic strategies to extend the reach of evidence-based treatments in usual care. The strategies may vary as a function of the treatment itself, the client population it is designed to serve, and the organizations and service systems in which most of that population is served. Thus, research is needed to identify common and distinct processes characterizing the effective transport and implementation of different treatments and classes of treatments. Finally, to disseminate treatments for conditions not yet identified as public safety or health concerns, demand must be stimulated. Social marketing theory and research may be instructive in this regard. To cultivate demand for a product or service, social marketing approaches evaluate the particular contexts, motivations, resources, and behaviors of distinctive consumer groups and tailor marketing efforts accordingly. Insofar as the distinct stakeholders in mental health can be likened to distinctive consumer groups, such strategies may be effective, and research is needed to test this proposition.

CONCLUSIONS

Anecdotal evidence suggests policymakers increasingly, but not indiscriminately, support the use of evidence-based treatments to enhance the public health. Two indicators of change are particularly apparent. First, whereas a decade ago federal mental health service funding agency policies did not recognize implementation support and measurement as necessary for the uptake of evidence-based treatments, several now advise against attempting to import prevention or intervention models for which model-specific technical assistance is not available. Second, government agencies are now asking MST purveyors to assume their own oversight and management functions in three areas: (1) quality of MST implementation, (2) efficient utilization of service capacity, and (3) client outcomes. This interest echoes developments in the history of managed care, during which third-party payers for health care—private insurers and government agencies—initially contracted with managed care organizations to treat patients and then contracted with administrative service organizations to take on the oversight functions for the managed care organizations previously held by the insurance company or state agency.

Requests from state governments that MST purveyors take this role present both opportunities and challenges. The challenges of greatest concern are a potential mismatch of the mission and culture of the organization doing the asking and the organization asked to help. The state agencies doing the asking, clearly dedicated to the public good, are charged with ensuring compliance with regulations and policies. The mission of MST purveyors is to facilitate the learning and performance of therapists, supervisors, and expert consultants and to support their capacity to implement MST with the fidelity needed to achieve desired youth outcomes. The mismatch lies in the compliance focus of the state and the learning and performance focus of MSTS and its Network Partners. The goal shared by the state and MST purveyors—achieving positive and measurable outcomes for youths—provides common ground for initial dialogue on this topic. Whether government oversight functions should or can be efficiently and effectively contracted to MST purveyors is, however, a new and as yet unanswered question.

ACKNOWLEDGMENTS

Preparation of this chapter was supported by the National Institute on Drug Abuse (Grant No. DA018107), the Annie E. Casey Foundation, and the John D. and Catherine T. MacArthur Foundation. The views presented in this chapter are those of the author alone and do not necessarily reflect the opinions of the Anne E. Casey or John D. and Catherine T. MacArthur Foundations. Sonja K. Schoenwald is a board member and stockholder in MST Services, LLC, which has the exclusive licensing agreement through MUSC for the dissemination of MST technology. I am grateful to John A. Morris for so graciously allowing the reprisal of key constructs from the title and body of his previously published article for this chapter and for his review and feedback on an earlier draft of this chapter. Special thanks to Keller B. Strother for providing helpful feedback on several chapter drafts and checking the accuracy of information about MSTS and its Network Partners.

NOTE

1. This title takes its inspiration, with permission, from John A. Morris's (2000) article, "Playing Policy Pinball: Making Policy Analysis Palatable," *Administration and Policy in Mental Health, 28,* 131–137.

REFERENCES

Andreason, A. R. (1995). *Marketing social change.* San Francisco: Jossey-Basss.
Dane, A. V., & Schneider, B. H. (1998). Program integrity in primary and early secondary prevention: Are implementation effects out of control? *Clinical Psychology Review, 18,* 23–45.

Elliot, D. S. (Series Ed.). (1998). *Blueprints for violence prevention.* Boulder: Regents of the University of Colorado.

Ferlie, E. B., & Shortell, S. M. (2001). Improving the quality of health care in the United Kingdom and the United States: A framework for change. *The Milbank Quarterly, 79,* 281–315.

Fixsen, D. L., Naoom, S. F., Blase, K. A., Friedman, R. M., & Wallace, F. (2005). *Implementation research: A synthesis of the literature* (FMHI Publication No. 231). Tampa: University of South Florida, Louis de la Parte Florida Mental Health Institute, National Implementation Research Network.

George, P., Blase, K. A., Kanary, P. J., Wotring, J., Bernstein, D., & Carter, W. M. (2008). *Financing evidence-based programs and practices: Changing systems to support effective service.* Denver, CO: Child and Family Evidence-Based Practices Consortium.

Grimshaw, J. M., Shirran, L., Thomas, R., Mowatt, G., Fraser, C., Bero, L., et al. (2001). Changing provider behavior: An overview of systematic reviews of interventions. *Medical Care, 39,*(8, Suppl. 2), II-2–II-45.

Henggeler, S. W., Rowland, M. D., Halliday-Boykins, C., Sheidow, A. J., Ward, D. M., Randall, J., et al. (2003). One-year follow-up of multisystemic therapy as an alternative to the hospitalization of youths in psychiatric crisis. *Journal of the American Academy of Child and Adolescent Psychiatry, 42,* 543–551.

Henggeler, S. W., Schoenwald, S. K., Borduin, C. M., Rowland, M. D., & Cunningham, P. B. (2009). *Multisystemic treatment of antisocial behavior in children and adolescents* (2nd ed.). New York: Guilford Press.

Institute of Medicine. (2001). *Crossing the quality chasm: A new health system for the 21st century.* Washington, DC: Author.

Klein, K. J., & Knight, A. P. (2005). Innovation implementation: Overcoming the challenge. *Current Directions in Psychological Science, 14*(5), 243–246.

Mihalic, S. (2004). The importance of implementation fidelity. *Emotional and Behavioral Disorders in Youth, 4,* 83–86, 99–105.

Ogden, T., Christensen, B., Sheidow, A. J., & Holth, P. (2008). Bridging the gap between science and practice: The effective nationwide transport of MST programs in Norway. *Journal of Child and Adolescent Substance Abuse, 17*(3), 93–109.

Rogers, E. M. (1995). *Diffusion of innovations* (4th ed.). New York: Free Press.

Rowland, M. D., Halliday-Boykins, C. A., Henggeler, S. W., Cunningham, P. B., Lee, T. G., Kruesi, M. J. P., et al. (2005). A randomized trial of multisystemic therapy with Hawaii's Felix Class youths. *Journal of Emotional and Behavioral Disorders, 13*(1), 13–23.

Schoenwald, S. K. (2008). Toward evidence-based transport of evidence-based treatments: MST as an example. *Journal of Child and Adolescent Substance Abuse, 17,* 69–91.

Schoenwald, S. K., Heiblum, N., Saldana, L., & Henggeler, S. W. (2008). The international implementation of multisystemic therapy: Evaluation and The Health Professions [Special issue]. *International Translation of Health Behavior Research Innovations, I,* 211–225.

Schoenwald, S. K., & Henggeler, S. W. (2003). Current strategies for moving evidence-based interventions into clinical practice: Introductory comments. *Cognitive and Behavioral Practice, 10,* 275–277.

Schoenwald, S. K., & Henggeler, S. W. (2004). A public health perspective on the transport of evidence based practices. *Clinical Science and Practice, 11,* 360–363.

Strother, K. B., Swenson, M. E., & Schoenwald, S. K. (1998). *The MST organizational manual.* Charleston, SC: MST Institute.

Stroul, B., & Friedman, R. (1986). *A system of care for children and youth with severe emotional disturbances.* Washington, DC: Georgetown University Child Development Center, National Technical Assistance Center for Children's Mental Health.

Thornicroft, G., & Tansella, M. (1999). *The mental health matrix: A manual to improve services.* Cambridge, UK: Cambridge University Press.

IV

CONCLUSIONS AND FUTURE DIRECTIONS

35

The Present and Future of Evidence-Based Psychotherapies for Children and Adolescents

JOHN R. WEISZ and ALAN E. KAZDIN

Efforts to help children are as old as parenthood, but over time some of these efforts morphed into a set of formal professional strategies known collectively as psychotherapy. We traced some of this historical evolution in Chapter 1, noting the many decades required for psychotherapy with young people to become a subject of scientific study. The study of evidence-based psychotherapies for children and adolescents is now a fast-moving target, and the pace of research, indexed by the development of new treatments and the acceleration of published evidence, is ballistic. This is reflected in diverse ways, including the expansion in the number of treatments encompassed within this volume relative to the first edition (Kazdin & Weisz, 2003) and the addition of a new section devoted entirely to research on implementation of treatments in new populations and new settings. The chapters reflect an impressive blend of intelligence, creativity, and perseverance—sheer hard work by talented clinical scientists pursuing treatments that work for children and adolescents. In this volume, these scientists have summarized valuable work on a variety of specific intervention programs, highlighted critical ethical and legal issues, spelled out the need for a solid developmental foundation, probed what is known about ethnic and cultural variations in relation to outcome research, and offered historically informed and insightful perspectives on the implementation and dissemination issues that are now moving to front and center in the field.

Taken together, the chapters paint a vivid picture of the state of the field. The chapters nicely complement what we know about general trends from broad-based reviews and meta-analyses of published trials (e.g., Kazdin, Bass, Ayers, & Rodgers, 1990; Weisz, 2004; Weisz & Weiss, 1993; Weisz, Weiss, Alicke, & Klotz, 1987; Weisz, Weiss, Han, Granger, & Morton, 1995). The meta-analyses have shown fairly consistently that treated youngsters in randomized controlled trials (RCTs) show better outcomes after treatment than at least 70% of comparable youngsters in control groups, on average; the effects are relatively specific to the problems and disorders targeted in treatment, not just general improvements in overall adjustment or "feeling better" (Weisz, 2004), and they hold up well, at least across the 5- to 6-month periods characteristic of most follow-up assessments (Weisz, 2004). The chapters in this book take us beyond these generalizations, describing specific treatments that produce the effects, summarizing the evidence on those treatments, and characterizing the contexts within which the treatments have been used and tested as well as the new frontiers into which the research is now pushing.

CHALLENGES FOR THE FUTURE

The chapters also convey some of the challenges that need to be confronted in the next era of research. We discuss these challenges in the following sections and summarize them in Table 35.1.

Coverage of Conditions and Types of Dysfunction

The accounts presented in these chapters tell us a good deal about the breadth of coverage of youth problems and dysfunction in current treatment research. Tested treatments have now been developed to address multiple internalizing conditions within the anxiety cluster (see Franklin, Freeman, & March, Chapter 6; Kendall, Furr, & Podell, Chapter 4; and Pahl & Barrett, Chapter 5, this volume) including posttraumatic stress disorder following maltreatment and other forms of trauma (Cohen, Mannarino, & Deblinger, Chapter 19, this volume); depressive disorders (see Bearman, Ugueto, Alleyne, & Weisz, Chapter 30; Clarke & DeBar, Chapter 8; Jacobson & Mufson, Chapter 10; Stark, Streusand, Krumholz, & Patel, Chapter 7; and Weersing & Brent, Chapter 9, this volume); mul-

---

TABLE 35.1. Challenges for the Future in Evidence-Based Psychotherapy

1. Expand coverage to forms of dysfunction that lack evidence-based psychotherapies, and address boundary conditions (e.g., age constraints) that limit the range of therapies
2. Build evidence-based psychotherapies that are more fully informed by developmental science
3. Broaden the array of theoretical models tested, encompassing more of the treatment models widely used in practice
4. Test an enriched array of treatment packaging and delivery models to address well-known complexities (e.g., comorbidity, episodic conditions, heterogeneity within conditions)
5. Extend scope, duration, and density of outcome assessment to increase the information value of findings across constituencies and to permit fair comparisons to usual care
6. Build and strengthen research on how therapist behavior and the therapeutic relationship relate to treatment engagement, completion, and outcome
7. Delineate the effective range of evidence-based psychotherapies in regard to youth and family clinical and demographic characteristics
8. Use dismantling and related designs to identify necessary and sufficient conditions for treatment benefit
9. Use multiple strategies (mediation analysis and much more) to identify mechanisms of change that explain why evidence-based psychotherapies work
10. Develop and test evidence-based psychotherapies under clinical practice conditions to foster robust treatment design and garner evidence on effectiveness in clinical care
11. Build models and evidence on treatment implementation and transportability to guide the application of evidence-based psychotherapies to new populations and contexts

tiple externalizing conditions ranging from chronic disobedience and aggression to the disruptive behavior disorders and criminal behavior (see Forgatch & Patterson, Chapter 11; Henggeler & Schaeffer, Chapter 17; Kazdin, Chapter 14; Lochman, Boxmeyer, Powell, Barry, & Pardini, Chapter 15; Smith & Chamberlain, Chapter 16; Webster-Stratton & Reid, Chapter 13; and Zisser & Eyberg,, Chapter 12, this volume) and attention-deficit/hyperactivity disorder(ADHD; Pelham, Gnagy, Greiner, Waschbusch, Fabiano, & Burrows-MacLean,, Chapter 18, this volume); autism and related disorders along the spectrum (see Koegel, Koegel, Vernon, & Brookman-Frazee, Chapter 21; and Smith, Chapter 20, this volume); habit problems such as enuresis (Houts, Chapter 23, this volume); eating disorders (Robin & Le Grange, Chapter 22, this volume); and substance abuse (see Liddle, Chapter 27; and Waldron & Brody, Chapter 26, this volume). Indeed, the problems and disorders for which evidence-based psychotherapies now exist encompass the concerns that bring the great majority of children and adolescents into clinical care.

That said, many *Diagnostic and Statistical Manual of Mental Disorders* (fourth edition; American Psychiatric Association, 1994) diagnoses that can be applied to children and adolescents lack evidence-based psychotherapies for this age range, and some of our field's success stories carry caveats and boundary conditions. As an example, psychosocial treatment success with ADHD has been largely limited to preadolescents, and some of the most beneficial parent training programs for conduct problems and disorder also may not travel so well up the developmental ramp into adolescence (see Dishion & Patterson, 1992). So, although evidence-based psychotherapies exist for many conditions that propel youths into treatment, there are treatment orphans, and some successful treatments carry caveats that represent empirical challenges for the future.

Attention to Developmental Science

One strategy for broadening the array of treatments and the developmental range within which treatments have impact might be to draw more heavily from developmental science. As Holmbeck, Devine, and Bruno (Chapter 3, this volume) emphasize, the principles and findings of developmental psychology, and developmental science more broadly, are rich in their implications for treatment development and design. Research on cognitive, social, personality, and neuropsychological development, and child–caregiver interactions from infancy through adolescence, might well undergird and inform the creation of treatments for a broad range of dysfunction. Despite this clear potential for developmentally informed intervention, developmental science and clinical science have not been closely linked, and few treatments appear to have been prompted or much informed by developmental theory or findings.

Instead, treatments for juvenile internalizing conditions appear to be primarily downward extensions of interventions originally developed for adults. Most treatments for juvenile externalizing conditions, habit-related problems (e.g., enuresis, substance abuse), and disorders on the autism spectrum appear to have drawn most heavily from behavioral theory and research and to some extent cognitive and family systems theory, not developmental science. Perhaps this is not a problem. After all, evidence indicates that the treatments described in this volume generate real benefit, on average. However, the evidence also shows that a substantial percentage of youngsters receiving these treatments apparently do not benefit.

A key question for our field is whether youth treatment fit and breadth of benefit might be enhanced if interventions were built on a more substantial understanding of the characteristics and capacities of children at different developmental periods and the developmental trajectories that create opportunities for change. As one of many examples, it is possible that the cognitive-behavioral technique of having children identify and critique their own cognitions (e.g., cognitions associated with depression, with anxiety, or with interpersonal aggression) might work well for youngsters who have achieved the developmental capacity to observe and reflect on their own thinking (see, e.g., Flavell, 2000) but not so well in youngsters who have not. In this and other respects, there appear to be multiple logically appealing connections between developmental and clinical science. To date, unfortunately, those seemingly logical connections have not been investigated and exploited very fully in ways that dramatically alter the nature or use of interventions; potentially relevant work on the developmental psychopathology front (see Cicchetti & Hinshaw, 2002; and Holmbeck et al., Chapter 23, this volume) may eventually have this effect.

Coverage of Theoretical Perspectives on Youth Treatment

The evidence-based psychotherapies encompass several of the influential theoretical perspectives that have guided youth treatment historically but certainly not all the relevant theories. Behavioral (operant, classical, and modeling) approaches are common among the tested treatments, as are cognitive-behavioral applications; and family systems perspectives are evident in some treatments (e.g., Robin & Le Grange, Chapter 22, this volume). However, numerous other schools of therapy (e.g., psychodynamic, client centered, humanistic) are largely missing from the roster. A similar pattern is evident in meta-analyses of published treatment–outcome research (Kazdin, Bass, et al., 1990; Weisz et al., 1987, 1995), with the great majority of the studies in those meta-analyses testing behavioral and cognitive-behavioral therapies (CBT).

A problem with this state of affairs is that many of the nonbehavioral treatment models that are common in clinical practice are rarely found in the research literature (see, e.g., Kazdin, Siegel, & Bass, 1990; Weersing, Weisz, & Donenberg, 2002). We have a strong and rapidly growing evidence base on treatments that are not so widely used in practice, and we have a weak and barely growing evidence base on the approaches that are widely used. The treatment models service providers use and trust clearly warrant more attention in clinical trials than they have received to date. The disparity between the scope of evidence and the scope of practice is illustrated by a recent count identifying more than 550 named therapies used with children and adolescents (see Kazdin, 2000b) only a tiny percentage of which have been subjected to empirical test. The field could profit from research that broadens the array of empirically tested treatment models. Researchers who take on this challenge will find no shortage of candidate models.

Intervention Delivery Strategies and Models

The intervention programs described in this volume convey a broad and broadening array of models for providing treatment content to the child and family. To be sure, the most common model follows the tradition of weekly office visits with a therapist. However, investigators have pushed the boundaries with diverse strategies and models:

- Embedding core principles and skill illustrations within videotaped vignettes for parents (Sanders & Murphy-Brennan, Chapter 33; and Webster-Stratton & Reid, Chapter 13, this volume)
- Embedding critical concepts and lessons in stories or videos for youths (Malgady, Chapter 25; Bearman et al., Chapter 30; and Webster-Stratton & Reid, Chapter 13, this volume)
- Using therapists as coaches, guiding parents as they interact with their children in real time (Zisser & Eyberg, Chapter 12, this volume)
- Treating enuresis using home-based behavioral training with a urine alarm (Houts, Chapter 23, this volume)
- Building intervention into summer day camp programming (e.g., Pelham et al., Chapter 18, this volume)
- Supplementing a core depression protocol with posttherapy booster sessions (Clarke & DeBar, Chapter 8, this volume)
- Therapy in motion, using a peripatetic-therapist-in-the-youth's-environment model (Henggeler & Schaeffer, Chapter 17; and Schoenwald, Chapter 34, this volume)
- Guiding child welfare program youths by teaching behavioral skills to foster care providers (Smith & Chamberlain, Chapter 16, this volume)
- Teaching parents and others in the children's environment to use early intensive behavioral intervention (Smith, Chapter 20, this volume) or pivotal response training (Koegel et al., Chapter 21, this volume) with children on the autism spectrum
- Teaching behavioral skills to parents via highly readable books with DVD guidance included (e.g., Kazdin & Rotella, 2008)

Although the current array of treatment packaging and delivery strategies is impressive, it seems likely that continued creativity will be needed in the future to address the variety of ways youth dysfunction presents in relation to treatment (see Kazdin, 2000a, 2000b; Kazdin & Weisz, 1998; Weisz, 2004). The episodic, recurrent nature of many youth conditions may call for models that encompass regular periodic monitoring of the child's status, or checkups, with treatment resumed as needed (see Clarke & DeBar, Chapter 8, this volume). The likelihood that not all youths diagnosed with the same disorder will manifest all symptoms of that disorder or need all the same treatment elements suggests the potential value of modular treatment strategies (see Chorpita, Daleiden, & Weisz, 2005; Chorpita & Daleiden, Chapter 31, this volume). As an example, some youths treated for depression do not manifest marked cognitive distortion, and others seem to have strong social skills; for such youths, a treatment program in which cognitive and social skills training are optional modules could make for enhanced efficiency.

As a third illustration of how our treatment delivery models may need to be stretched, we note that most evidence-based psychotherapies are focused on a single condition or homogeneous cluster of them. By contrast, most treated children do not present with only one problem or diagnosis, or even one at a time (Angold, Costello, & Erkanli, 1999; Jensen & Weisz, 2002), and even conditions that may seem quite different superficially, such as depression and conduct disorder, often co-occur. The fact that different problems and diagnoses coincide so regularly suggests that we need models for blending and combining elements of some rather distinct treatments, a task that could engage some of our best minds for many years.

Scope, Duration, and Density of Outcome Assessment in Treatment Research

The body of evidence surveyed in this book illustrates how outcome assessment has expanded in scope, intensity, and rigor over the years. In the best research, child dysfunction is now assessed from multiple perspectives, often including youth, parent, and teacher report, and ideally including direct observation of the treated youths' behavior. Formal diagnostic assessment is often included now, in part to assess the clinical significance of treatment-related change. Increasingly, such measures of problems, symptoms, and diagnoses are complemented by assessments of real-world functioning: grades and school behavior reports, for example, and arrests, where relevant. Beyond the treated youths, assessments focus increasingly on dispersion of treatment benefit: for example, increases in parents' child management skills, parenting confidence, parental stress and mental health, and even changes in marital satisfaction associated with changes in child behavior. Consumer satisfaction with treatment is making its way into the outcome literature as well.

Although the increasing breadth and intensity of outcome assessment is a positive feature, some leaders in the field have encouraged further broadening. For example, Hoagwood, Jensen, Petti, and Burns (1996) have argued for tapping such system-related outcomes as the extent to which treatment reduces the use of other mental health services. We would add that there is room for expansion in the duration of outcome assessment as well. In meta-analyses (Weisz et al., 1987, 1995), only about one-third of the published studies have included any assessment other than immediate posttreatment, and for that one-third the mean follow-up lag time was 5–6 months after the end of treatment. As a consequence, we know relatively little about the long-term holding power of the effects generated by most treatments and thus little about whether or when there may be a need for treatment supplements, booster sessions, and the like to maintain gains.

Measurement density also needs attention in future work. In some areas of treatment research (e.g., depression), there is increasing interest in the impact of treatment on pace of recovery. Regardless of whether outcomes at the end of treatment show a target treatment to be superior to a control or comparison condition, it may be important to know whether the target treatment accelerated relief and symptom reduction. Reducing the duration of suffering is valuable in its own right, but in addition efficiency is a concern of many who pay the costs of mental health care, and frequent assessment is required to gauge efficiency. Another reason to move toward denser schedules of assessment is the increasing emphasis on comparisons between structured, protocol-guided treatments and usual clinical care (see Weisz, Jensen-Doss, & Hawley, 2006). In such comparisons, the duration of usual care cannot be controlled (otherwise, the care is not "usual"), and thus it is not possible to match the protocol-guided treatment and usual care on treatment length or dose. With frequent (e.g., weekly or monthly), routine assessment on outcome measures of interest, trajectories of change can be monitored and compared across treatment conditions in ways that do not require artificially limiting the duration of usual care.

Treatment Benefit as a Function of Therapist Behavior and the Therapeutic Relationship

The treatment–outcome research literature is particularly strong in describing intervention procedures but weak in helping therapists build a warm, empathic relationship and a strong working alliance with the children and families who receive the interventions. This gap is striking, even stunning, in light of the widespread belief that quality of the therapeutic relationship or alliance is critical to success in most treatment encounters. Indeed, many child therapists rate the therapeutic relationship as more important than the specific techniques used in treatment (Motta & Lynch, 1990; Shirk & Saiz, 1992), and some treated children may agree, including those receiving evidence-based treatments. Kendall and Southam-Gerow (1996), for example, found that children treated for anxiety disorders using the Coping Cat program rated their relationship with the therapist as the most important aspect of treatment.

Clinical scientists are now building a body of evidence aimed at (1) defining what a positive therapeutic relationship is, (2) establishing how best to measure it, (3) identifying therapist characteristics and behaviors that foster it, and (4) testing the extent to which such a relationship actually predicts outcome when evidence-based psychotherapies are used. In the treatment of children, both child–therapist and parent–therapist alliance may need to be understood; in fact, the two may show different patterns of association with treatment attendance, engagement, and outcome (see, e.g., Hawley & Weisz, 2005). Progress is now being made in assessing and understanding the roles of child and parent alliance, using youth-report and parent-report assessment of therapeutic alliance (e.g., Kazdin, Whitley, & Marciano, 2006; Shirk & Saiz, 1992) as well as an observational approach based on coding of actual therapy sessions for child and parent alliance with the therapist (McLeod & Weisz, 2005). Kazdin et al. (2006), for example, found that both child–therapist and parent–therapist alliance predicted therapeutic gains in children treated with evidence-based interventions for externalizing problems (and parent–therapist alliance predicted improved parenting practices); McLeod and Weisz (2005), focusing on treatment as usual for internalizing problems, found that child–therapist alliance predicted therapeutic gains in child anxiety, whereas parent–therapist alliance predicted therapeutic gains in child anxiety and depression. As these findings illustrate, both questionnaire and observational approaches have identified significant associations between alliance and treatment outcome that bear further study (see also Shirk & Karver, 2003).

It seems inherently useful, at any time, to learn all we can about therapist behavior and therapist–youth interactions that predict good treatment outcomes; this can be valuable in usual clinical care (e.g., Hawley & Weisz, 2005; McLeod & Weisz, 2005), and it seems especially timely in relation to structured, protocol-guided treatments (e.g., Kazdin et al., 2006), which may call for a special set of skills. As an example, effective use of such treatments may require agile, multitasking therapists who can maintain attention to a structured treatment plan, remain responsive to what youths and parents bring to the session, find ways to connect the treatment agenda to the youngsters' real-life concerns, nurture a warm relationship, and make sessions lively and engaging. Tests of these and other speculations on therapist–process–outcome connections within evidence-based practice are likely to be a valuable component of the research agenda for many years.

Identifying the Effective Range of Treatments

The youth treatment–outcome literature is much stronger in demonstrating benefit than in identifying the boundary conditions that constrain benefit. For each treatment, we need to know as much as possible about the range of youth and family clinical and demographic characteristics within which the treatments are helpful and outside of which effects diminish. Even the best supported treatments are beneficial for some conditions and some youths but not others, with benefit potentially limited by comorbid conditions, age, socioeconomic status, ethnicity, family configuration, or other clinical and demographic factors; however, until recently, research had left us relatively uninformed about such constraints. Fortunately, the chapters in this volume show a marked increase in attention to these issues since the time of our first edition (Kazdin & Weisz, 2003).

Given the relative youth of our field, it is not surprising that most tested treatments lack provisions for dealing with variations in language, values, customs, child-rearing traditions, beliefs and expectancies about child and parent behavior, and distinctive stressors, resources, values, and preferred learning styles associated with different cultural traditions. Exceptions to this pattern can be seen in the chapters by Malgady (Chapter 25, this volume) and Robbins, Horigian, Szapocznik, and Ucha (Chapter 24, this volume), describing extended efforts to shape interventions specifically for Hispanic youths. It certainly does seem possible that the interplay between cultural factors and treatment characteristics may influence the relationship between child/family and therapist, the likelihood of treatment completion versus dropout, and the outcome of the treatment process (Weisz, Huey, & Weersing, 1998). The chapter by Huey and Polo (Chapter 29, this volume) suggests that, to the extent that evidence is now available, evidence-based psychotherapies may be rather robust across certain ethnic and racial boundaries, but research on this topic is just beginning. We need more research building on the work described by Huey and Polo, Malgady, and Robbins et al. assessing the extent to which treatment persistence, process, and outcome are moderated by race, ethnicity, culture, and a variety of other child and family characteristics and their interaction and testing the extent to which culturally sensitive design and adaptation of therapies improves treatment process and outcome.

Understanding the Necessary and Sufficient Conditions for Treatment Benefit

Among the diverse treatments that are considered evidence based, a substantial subset are omnibus or multicomponent in form, with various concepts and skills brought together in one protocol and with termination considered appropriate only when all the concepts and skills have been covered. For some of these treatments, all the elements may well be needed, but often the evidence base is too poorly developed to clarify just which elements are truly necessary or whether a subset of them, used alone, might be sufficient to produce most of the benefit possible from the treatment. Indeed, it is the absence of such a clear picture that often stimulates development of multicomponent interventions; new concepts and skills are added when in doubt, because it seems that they may help, and *it probably can't hurt.*

One result of this process may be treatments with adipose tissue, components that do not contribute much to the outcomes achieved. For a variety of reasons, including the time and expense of treatment, we need interventions that are as efficient as possible. Treatments that fall short of this goal are apt to clash with the current emphasis on managing costs and professional time. Increasing treatment efficiency will enhance the attractiveness of the interventions to practitioners and payers, improve the teachability of the procedures and time to mastery, and increase the likelihood that children and families will stay the course to the end of treatment. That said, some treatment elements may not enhance outcome directly but may still be useful to retain. For example, elements that enhance the acceptability of treatment, minimize dropout rates, or increase patient and therapist compliance with the treatment regimen may serve as the spoonful of sugar that makes the medicine go down and may be valuable to keep for that reason.

In our field, a traditional pathway to understanding which treatment elements are necessary and sufficient is *dismantling* research, in which various treatment components are broken apart and tested separately and in various combinations. In principle, such research should provide the key to understanding necessity and sufficiency within the evidence-based treatments; but the task is complex when the same protocol includes many elements, because the number of combinations multiplies quickly. A further complication is that different subgroups of youths may respond differently to different subsets of treatment components. All of this means that the dismantling process may be particularly challenging for some of the more complex multicomponent treatments, particularly those targeting complex conditions, but it is these treatments and these conditions for which streamlining may be most needed.

Identifying Mechanisms of Change That Explain Why Treatments Work

The job of streamlining treatments would, of course, be greatly simplified if we knew the specific change processes that make the treatments work. However, at this point, we know much more about what outcomes are produced by evidence-based therapies than about what happens in treatment that actually causes those outcomes (Kazdin, 2000a, 2000b; Shirk & Russell, 1996; Weersing & Weisz, 2002). This is understandable for at least two reasons. First, simple logic dictates that we first find out whether a treatment works so that we can know whether there is a benefit that needs an explanation. Second, figuring out why (i.e., what the causal mechanisms are) is not a simple task or a quick one. These difficulties notwithstanding, the task is critical for the field. Failure to identify core causal processes could mean a proliferation of treatments administered rather superstitiously "because they work" but without an understanding of the change processes that must be set in motion to produce results. This, in turn, would raise the risk of including therapy components that add to treatment burden without actually contributing to change.

To understand *how* treatments actually work, we need a new generation of research on mechanisms underlying change. One element of this process (but *only* one) is testing hypothesized mediators of outcome. Data analytic procedures have been developed for mediation testing (Baron & Kenny, 1986; Holmbeck, 1997; Kraemer, Stice, Kazdin, & Kupfer, 2001; Kraemer, Wilson, Fairburn, & Agras, 2002), and the raw material needed for such procedures exists in many treatment investigators' data sets. A review by Weersing and Weisz (2002) noted that 63% of clinical trials in the areas of anxiety, depression, and disruptive behavior included measures of potential mediators in their designs, but only six of the 67 studies surveyed had included any formal mediation test.

As the chapters in this volume show, mediation testing has surged since the Weersing–Weisz review, at least in problem domains for which substantial samples can be obtained for trials. Investigation of proposed mediators is now a part of the youth treatment–outcome research agenda in areas as diverse as depression, anxiety, posttraumatic stress, conduct problems, delinquency, substance use and abuse, and sex offending. Many of the findings support mediational processes that are integral to the treatment models. Some open up areas of debate regarding prominent models. For example, Kolko, Brent, Baugher, Bridge, and Birmaher (2000) failed to find that changes in negative cognitions mediated the effect of CBT on depression, but Kaufman, Rohde, Seeley, Clarke, and Stice (2005) did find the proposed mediational process in a different CBT study. Such conflicting findings can be good for the field, sparking debate and further analysis and ultimately leading to a sharper image of how mediation does and does not operate in relation to prominent treatment models.

Although mediation tests have real value, a case has been made that such tests alone cannot tell us what the mechanisms of change are for any treatment. Kazdin (2007) has noted that mediation tests can be used to explain statistically an association between independent and dependent variables in an outcome study, but the mediators thus identified cannot alone tell us the processes or events that are responsible for change, the reasons why change occurred, or how change came about. Identifying mechanisms of change, Kazdin (2007) notes, requires that investigators (1) demonstrate a strong and specific association among the intervention used, the proposed mediator, and therapeutic change (ideally ruling out alternative plausible processes that are not associated with change); (2) show consistency in the pattern across replications; (3) conduct experimental tests in which the proposed mediator or mechanism is manipulated, demonstrating its impact; (4) establish a timeline in which proposed mechanisms precede their proposed effects; (5) provide evidence of a gradient in which increasing degrees or doses of the proposed mechanism are associated with larger changes in the outcomes of interest; and (6) establish the plausibility of the hypothesized operation of the mechanism vis-à-vis findings in the broader evidence base: Does the proposed mechanism of action make sense in light of what we know based on relevant studies and even common sense?

This rich agenda for establishing mechanisms of change goes far beyond the simple statistics of standard mediation testing and clearly will require extended effort by serious clinical scientists conducting and synthesizing multiple studies within each treatment domain. The work will be challenging, but the payoff could be enormous. With increased understanding of the mechanisms of therapeutic change within the different domains of dysfunction, the prospects will increase for us to (1) identify cross-cutting principles for use in designing, refining, and streamlining interventions; (2) train therapists by teaching them what processes they need to set in motion rather than simply what techniques to use; and (3) understand and reverse treatment failures by focusing on the change processes that need to be activated.

Studying Evidence-Based Psychotherapies in Relation to Clinical Practice

It is instructive to note that not all who share our interest in quality mental health care share our enthusiasm for the evidence-based, manual-guided treatments tested in RCTs (see, e.g., Garfield, 1996; Havik & VandenBos, 1996; Westen, Novotny, & Thompson-Brenner, 2004). Many mental health care professionals have genuine concerns that this new generation of manual-guided treatments is either not relevant to the work they do or not appropriate for the clients they treat. The specific concerns are diverse, but among those frequently mentioned are (1) that the use of prescriptive, manual-guided treatments will limit creativity and innovation and may risk turning therapists into mere technicians who follow cookie-cutter procedures; (2) that manual adherence will interfere with development of a productive therapeutic relationship and constrain the therapist's ability to individualize treatment; (3) that the treatments have only been tested with simple cases with low levels of psychopathology and may not work with more severe and complex cases; (4) that the treatments tend to focus on single problems or disorders and thus may not work with comorbid cases; and (5) that the complexity and volatility of clinically referred individuals and their families make each session unpredictable and a predetermined series of session plans unworkable (for details on some of these arguments, focused especially on evidence-based psychotherapies for adults, see Addis & Krasnow, 2000; Garfield, 1996; Havik & VandenBos, 1996).

Some of these points may not be valid, and others may not apply equally to all evidence-based psychotherapies, but it would be a mistake to simply dismiss the arguments out of hand. At a minimum, we need to understand the concerns that make many practitioners reluctant to use these structured treatments, so that we can grasp and address impediments to EBT implementation in practice settings. A second good reason to attend to the concerns is that some may be quite valid, at least for a number of EBTs; addressing points that are valid could improve the robustness and viability of the treatments (see Weisz & Gray, 2008; Weisz, Jensen-Doss, & Hawley, 2005). One point on which proponents and opponents may agree is that most of the concerns can be construed as empirical questions warranting research attention. In this respect, the different perspectives on evidence-based practice can be valuable heuristically.

Differences between the perspectives of treatment researchers and treatment providers may be understood partly in relation to the distinction between efficacy and effectiveness research. Most research findings on evidence-based psychotherapies are clustered at the *efficacy* end of the continuum (i.e., derived from studies involving carefully arranged and somewhat idealized conditions designed to maximize the opportunity to show treatment effects). For practitioners, the apparent gap between the conditions prevailing in most treatment research and the conditions of actual youth mental health practice raises questions about whether the resultant treatments can work well in a practice context (Weisz & Gray, 2008; Weisz et al., 2006). The efficacy research versus clinical practice gap may include characteristics of the treated individuals (e.g., youths in the clinic may be more severely disturbed, more likely to meet criteria for a diagnosis, more likely to have numerous comorbidities, and less motivated for treatment), their families (e.g., more parental psychopathology, family life event stressors, and perhaps even maltreatment), reasons for seeking treatment (e.g., not recruited from schools or through ads but referred by caregivers because of unusually serious problems or family crisis or even court ordered), the settings in which treatment is done (e.g., more financial forms to complete, more bureaucracy, and sometimes a less welcoming approach in the clinic), the therapists who provide the treatment (e.g., not graduate students or research assistants hired by and loyal to the advisor and committed to her or his treatment research program, but rather staff therapists who barely know the treatment developer or the tested treatment and who may prefer different treatment methods), the incentive system (e.g., not paid by the treatment developer to deliver her or his EBT with close adherence to the manual but rather paid by the clinic to see many cases and with no method prescribed), and the conditions under which therapists deliver the treatment (not graduate students' flexible time, but strict productivity requirements, paperwork to complete, and little time to learn a manual or adhere closely to it).

Such differences between psychotherapy in many RCTs and psychotherapy in clinical practice can lead practitioners to question the relevance of the evidence to their own clinical practice. On the plus side, the same differences may also be viewed as a nascent agenda for treatment researchers. Indeed, the very real-world factors that experimentalists might view as a nuisance (e.g., child comorbidity, parent pathology, life stresses that produce no-shows and dropouts, therapists with heavy caseloads) and thus attempt to avoid (e.g., by recruiting and screening cases, applying exclusion criteria, hiring their own therapists) or control may, in fact, be precisely what we need to include, to understand, and to address if we are to develop psychosocial treatment protocols that work well in practice (Weisz, 2004; Weisz & Gray, 2008). Treatments that cannot cope with these real-world factors may not fare so well in practice, no matter how efficacious they are in well-controlled laboratory trials.

Thus, another critical direction for research on evidence-based psychotherapies is toward clinical practice. Testing treatments under conditions more and more like those of actual practice in mental health service settings may be a way to build especially robust treatments and an evidence base that supports their use in everyday clinical care.

Implementing and Transporting Treatments to New Populations and Context

Even as researchers work to refine treatments for young people and boost their impact and clinical practice relevance, there is exciting work underway addressing the challenges of treatment implementation in new settings. A new section of the book encompasses broad principles of implementation applied to child and adolescent treatment (Fixsen, Blase, Duda, Naoom, & Van Dyke, Chapter 28, this volume) plus examples of research on implementation of treatments in outpatient clinical practice settings (Bearman et al., Chapter 30, this volume), statewide service systems (Chorpita & Daleiden, Chapter 31, this volume), a nation (Scott, Chapter 32, this volume), and across multiple national boundaries (Sanders & Murphy-Brennan, Chapter 33, this volume) and policy contexts (Schoenwald, Chapter 34, this volume).

As the work of implementation and transporting builds and extends, we are apt to see increasingly sophisticated models of how to plan, design, revise, and refine treatments to achieve good fit with particular populations and contexts. The implementation review and analysis by Fixsen et al. (Chapter 28, this volume) provide potential basic elements of one such model, as do reports on the hands-on experiences of other authors in Hawaii and Minnesota (Chorpita & Daleiden, Chapter 31, this volume), England (Scott, Chapter 32, this volume), multiple other nations (Sanders & Murphy-Brennan, Chapter 33, this volume), and multiple policy contexts (Schoenwald, Chapter 34, this volume). An explicit deployment-focused model is described by Bearman et al. in Chapter 30 of this volume (see also Weisz, 2004), proposing steps of treatment development and testing to build interventions that will fit the specific contexts for which they are ultimately intended.

The model-building process will almost certainly need to include attention to the broad array of policy and practical considerations that can work for or against implementation. As one example, a significant impediment to the spread of evidence-based psychotherapies in the United States is that effective use of the treatments requires considerable training and supervision, both of which are more costly for financially strapped clinicians and provider organizations than simply continuing current practice patterns. Because reimbursement is based on units of service rather than which particular treatment is being done, there is little incentive for bringing in new practices. In fact, increased cost paired with no increased income is a clear *dis*incentive working *against* the implementation of new evidence-based practices. As this example illustrates, our models of implementation will likely need to encompass theoretical, clinical, and very practical considerations, including money and the way it must figure into decision making by those who run organizations and provide clinical care.

CONCLUSION

We have come a long way, as a field, from the early precursors described in Chapter 1. After slow ferment between the time of Aristotle and psychoanalytic theory, child and adolescent psychotherapy and related research accelerated quickly through the 20th century, with an output of more than 1,500 youth treatment outcome studies by the year 2000 (see Kazdin, 2000a). As one index of that output, the *Journal of Clinical Child Psychology* devoted an entire issue, in 1998, to articles reporting on 27 youth treatments meeting multiple criteria for the status of "empirically supported psychosocial interventions" (see Lonigan, Elbert, & Johnson, 1998). A recent 10-year update issue of the same journal (Silverman & Hinshaw, 2008) reported on 46 "evidence-based psychosocial treatments." As research intensity and output have surged, so has attention to the responsible conduct of research in relation to ethical and legal issues, as described by Hoagwood and Cavaleri (Chapter 2, this volume). This book brings together descriptions of evidence-based psychotherapies for young people and the evidence on those therapies written by the treatment developers who know them best. These accounts are complemented by a focus on developmental and ethical issues in the field and research on implementation of evidence-based psychotherapies across a range of populations and contexts.

In this final chapter, we have noted several characteristics of the treatments and the evidence that are particularly admirable, including breadth of coverage of significant youth problems and disorders, a creative array of treatment delivery models, an increasingly rich mix of informants and measures in outcome assessment, and recently expanded attention to moderators and mediators of treatment outcome. However, we also find areas in which change is needed and topics that need attention in future research, as outlined in Table 35.1. Among these, we note a need to extend outcome research to treatment models that are widely used in clinical practice but poorly represented in the research literature thus far. We note how little is currently known about the ways therapist behavior and the therapeutic relationship relate to treatment persistence and outcome, particularly in the world of manual-guided treatments. We stress the need to identify mechanisms of action that explain why treatments work. We emphasize the need to understand evidence-based psychotherapies and how they perform in the arena of clinical practice, with more of the research carried out under conditions like those practitioners confront. And we stress the need to build a science and a viable model of treatment implementation and transportability to guide ever-increasing efforts to apply tested interventions in new contexts and with new populations.

Viewed in historical perspective, the trajectory of research on child and adolescent psychotherapy is quite remarkable, particularly in recent decades. The clinical scientists whose work fills this book have built that recent trajectory. We laud the work of these leaders, who have brought us to such a pivotal point in psychotherapy research.

REFERENCES

Addis, M. E., & Krasnow, A. D. (2000). A national survey of practicing psychologists' attitudes toward psychotherapy treatment manuals. *Journal of Consulting and Clinical Psychology, 68*, 331–339.

American Psychiatric Association. (1994). *Diagnostic and statistical manual of mental disorders* (4th ed.). Washington, DC: Author.

Angold, A., Costello, E. J., & Erkanli, A. (1999). Comorbidity. *Journal of Child Psychology and Psychiatry, 40*, 57–87.

Baron, R. M., & Kenny, D. A. (1986). The moderator-mediator variable distinction in social psychological research: Conceptual, strategic, and statistical considerations. *Journal of Personality and Social Psychology, 51*, 1173–1182.

Chorpita, B. F., Daleiden, E., & Weisz, J. R. (2005). Modularity in the design and application of therapeutic interventions. *Applied and Preventive Psychology, 11*, 141–156.

Cicchetti, D., & Hinshaw, S. P. (Eds.). (2002). Prevention and intervention science: Contributions to developmental theory [Special issue]. *Development and Psychopathology, 14*, 667–981.

Dishion, T. J., & Patterson, G. R. (1992). Age effects in parent training outcomes. *Behavior Therapy, 23*, 719–729.

Flavell, J. H. (2000). Development of children's knowledge about the mental world. *International Journal of Behavioral Development, 24*, 15–23.

Garfield, S. L. (1996). Some problems associated with "validated" forms of psychotherapy. *Clinical Psychology: Science and Practice, 3*, 218–229.

Havik, O. E., & VandenBos, G. R. (1996). Limitations of manualized psychotherapy for everyday clinical practice. *Clinical Psychology: Science and Practice, 3*, 264–267.

Hawley, K. M., & Weisz, J. R. (2005). Child versus parent therapeutic alliance in usual clinical care: Distinctive associations with engagement, satisfaction and treatment outcome. *Journal of Clinical Child and Adolescent Psychology, 34*, 117–128.

Hoagwood, K., Jensen, P. S., Petti, T., & Burns, B. J. (1996). Outcomes of mental health care for children and adolescents: I. A comprehensive conceptual model. *Journal of the American Academy of Child and Adolescent Psychiatry, 35*, 1055–1063.

Holmbeck, G. N. (1997). Toward terminological, conceptual, and statistical clarity in the study of mediators and moderators: Examples from the child-clinical and pediatric psychology literatures. *Journal of Consulting and Clinical Psychology, 65*, 599–610.

Jensen, A. L., & Weisz, J. R. (2002). Assessing match and mismatch between practitioner-generated and standardized interview-generated diagnoses for clinic-referred children and adolescents. *Journal of Consulting and Clinical Psychology, 70*, 158–168.

Kaufman, N. K., Rohde, P., Seeley, J. R., Clarke, G. N., & Stice, E. (2005). Potential mediators of cognitive behavioral treatment for adolescents with comorbid major depression and conduct disorder. *Journal of Consulting and Clinical Psychology, 73*, 38–46.

Kazdin, A. E. (2000a). Developing a research agenda for child and adolescent psychotherapy. *Archives of General Psychiatry, 57*, 829–835.

Kazdin, A. E. (2000b). *Psychotherapy for children and adolescents: Directions for research and practice.* New York: Oxford University Press.

Kazdin, A. E. (2007). Mediators and mechanisms of change in psychotherapy research. *Annual Review of Clinical Psychology, 3*, 1–27.

Kazdin, A. E., Bass, D., Ayers, W. A., & Rodgers, A. (1990). Empirical and clinical focus of child and adolescent psychotherapy research. *Journal of Consulting and Clinical Psychology, 58*, 729–740.

Kazdin, A. E., & Rotella, C. (2008). *The Kazdin method for parenting the defiant child.* Boston: Houghton Mifflin.

Kazdin, A. E., Siegel, T. C., & Bass, D. (1990). Drawing on clinical practice to inform research on child and adolescent psychotherapy: Survey of practitioners. *Professional Psychology: Research and Practice, 21,* 189–198.

Kazdin, A. E., & Weisz, J. R. (1998). Identifying and developing empirically supported child and adolescent treatments. *Journal of Consulting and Clinical Psychology, 66,* 19–36.

Kazdin, A. E., & Weisz, J. R. (Eds.). (2003). *Evidence-based psychotherapies for children and adolescents.* New York: Guilford Press.

Kazdin, A. E., Whitley, M., & Marciano, P. L. (2006). Child–therapist and parent–therapist alliance and therapeutic change in the treatment of children referred for oppositional, aggressive, and antisocial behavior. *Journal of Child Psychology and Psychiatry, 47,* 436–445.

Kendall, P. C., & Southam-Gerow, M. A. (1996). Long-term follow-up of a cognitive-behavioral therapy for anxiety-disordered youth. *Journal of Consulting and Clinical Psychology, 64,* 724–730.

Kolko, D. J., Brent, D. A., Baugher, M., Bridge, J., & Birmaher, B. (2000). Cognitive and family therapies for adolescent depression: Treatment specificity, mediation and moderation. *Journal of Consulting and Clinical Psychology, 68,* 603–614.

Kraemer, H. C., Stice, E., Kazdin, A., & Kupfer, D. (2001). How do risk factors work?: Mediators, moderators, independent, overlapping, and proxy risk factors. *American Journal of Psychiatry, 158,* 848–856.

Kraemer, H. C., Wilson, G. T., Fairburn, C. G., & Agras, W. S. (2002). Mediators and moderators of treatment effects in randomized clinical trials. *Archives of General Psychiatry, 59,* 877–883.

Lonigan, C. J., Elbert, J. C., & Johnson, S. B. (1998). Empirically supported psychosocial interventions for children: An overview. *Journal of Clinical Child Psychology, 27,* 138–145.

McLeod, B. D., & Weisz, J. R. (2005). The Therapy Process Observational Coding System–Alliance Scale: Measure characteristics and prediction of outcome in usual clinical practice. *Journal of Consulting and Clinical Psychology, 73,* 323–333.

Motta, R. W., & Lynch, C. (1990). Therapeutic techniques vs. therapeutic relationships in child behavior therapy. *Psychological Reports, 67,* 315–322.

Shirk, S. R., & Karver, M. (2003). Prediction of treatment outcome from relationship variables in child and adolescent therapy: A meta-analytic review. *Journal of Consulting and Clinical Psychology, 71,* 452–464.

Shirk, S. R., & Russell, R. L. (1996). *Change processes in child psychotherapy: Revitalizing treatment and research.* New York: Guilford Press.

Shirk, S. R., & Saiz, C. C. (1992). Clinical, empirical, and developmental perspectives on the therapeutic relationship in child psychotherapy. *Development and Psychopathology, 4,* 713–728.

Silverman, W. K., & Hinshaw, S. P. (Eds.). (2008). Evidence-based psychosocial treatments for children and adolescents: A ten year update [Special issue]. *Journal of Clinical Child and Adolescent Psychology, 37,* 1–301.

Weersing, V. R., & Weisz, J. R. (2002). Mechanisms of action in youth psychotherapy. *Journal of Child Psychology and Psychiatry, 43,* 3–29.

Weersing, V. R., Weisz, J. R., & Donenberg, G. R. (2002). Development of the Therapy Procedures Checklist: A therapist-report measure of technique use in child and adolescent treatment. *Journal of Clinical Child and Adolescent Psychology, 31,* 168–180.

Weisz, J. R. (2004). *Psychotherapy for children and adolescents: Evidence-based treatments and case examples.* Cambridge, UK: Cambridge University Press.

Weisz, J. R., & Gray, J. S. (2008). Evidence-based psychotherapies for children and adolescents: Data from the present and a model for the future. *Child and Adolescent Mental Health, 13,* 54–65.

Weisz, J. R., Huey, S. J., & Weersing, V. R. (1998). Psychotherapy outcome research with children and adolescents: The state of the art. In T. H. Ollendick & R. J. Prinz (Eds.), *Advances in clinical child psychology, Vol. 20* (pp. 49–91). New York: Plenum.

Weisz, J. R., Jensen-Doss, A. J., & Hawley, K. M. (2005). Youth psychotherapy outcome research: A review and critique of the evidence base. *Annual Review of Psychology, 56,* 337–363.

Weisz, J. R., Jensen-Doss, A. J., & Hawley, K. M. (2006). Evidence-based youth psychotherapies versus usual clinical care: A meta-analysis of direct comparisons. *American Psychologist, 61,* 671–689.

Weisz, J. R., & Weiss, B. (1993). *Effects of psychotherapy with children and adolescents.* Newbury Park, CA: Sage.

Weisz, J. R., Weiss, B., Alicke, M. D., & Klotz, M. L. (1987). Effectiveness of psychotherapy with children and adolescents: A meta-analysis for clinicians. *Journal of Consulting and Clinical Psychology, 55,* 542–549.

Weisz, J. R., Weiss, B., Han, S. S., Granger, D. A., & Morton, T. (1995). Effects of psychotherapy with children and adolescents revisited: A meta-analysis of treatment outcome studies. *Psychological Bulletin, 117,* 450–468.

Westen, D., Novotny, C. M., & Thompson-Brenner, H. (2004). The empirical status of empirically supported psychotherapies: Assumptions, findings, and reporting in controlled clinical trials. *Psychological Bulletin, 130,* 631–663.

Author Index

Subject Index